Health Care Management

ORGANIZATION DESIGN AND BEHAVIOR

Fifth Edition

To Walter J. McNerney, M.H.A.,
(1925–2005)
our teacher, friend, and colleague,
for his enormous contributions to health policy and practice.

To our students—past, present, and future—
for their contributions to a better health system.

To Heather, Crosby, Nicolas, and Caden—
for whom all things are possible.

Health Care Management

ORGANIZATION DESIGN AND BEHAVIOR

Fifth Edition

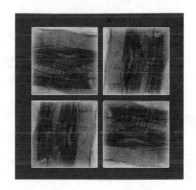

Stephen M. Shortell, PhD

Blue Cross of California
Distinguished Professor of Health Policy and
Management, Professor of Organization Behavior,
Haas School of Business
and Dean, School of Public Health
University of California, Berkeley
Berkeley, California

Arnold D. Kaluzny, PhD

Professor Emeritus of Health Policy and
Administration
and Director Emeritus of the
Public Health Leadership Program,
School of Public Health,
and Senior Research Fellow, Cecil G. Sheps
Center for Health Services Research
University of North Carolina at Chapel Hill
Chapel Hill, North Carolina

and Associates

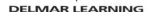

THOMSON

DELMAR LEARNING™   Australia Canada Mexico Singapore Spain United Kingdom United States

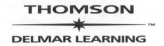

Health Care Management: Organization Design and Behavior, 5th Edition

by Stephen M. Shortell and Arnold D. Kaluzny

Vice President, Health Care Business Unit:
William Brottmiller

Editorial Director:
Matt Kane

Acquisitions Editor:
Maureen Rosener

Developmental Editor:
Laurie Traver

Editorial Assistant:
Elizabeth Howe

Marketing Director:
Jennifer McAvey

Channel Manager:
Tamara Caruso

Marketing Coordinator:
Michele Gleason

Technology Director:
Laurie Davis

Technology Project Manager:
Mary Colleen Liburdi

Production Director:
Carolyn Miller

Production Manager:
Barbara A. Bullock

Art and Design Coordinator:
Drea Porteus

Production Coordinator:
Kenneth McGrath

Project Editor:
Jennifer Luck

Library of Congress-in-Publication Data
Health care management : organization, design, and behavior / [edited
    by] Stephen M. Shortell, Arnold D. Kaluzny.—5th ed.
        p. ; cm.—(Thomson Delmar Learning series in health services
    administration)
        Includes bibliographical references and index.
    ISBN 1-4180-0189-9
    1. Health services administration.
I. Shortell, Stephen M. (Stephen
    Michael), 1944- . II. Kaluzny, Arnold D. III. Series.
    [DNLM: 1. Health Services Administration. W 84.1 H4364 2006]
    RA393.H38 2006
    362.1'068—dc22
2005024671

NOTICE TO THE READER

Publisher does not warrant or guarantee any of the products described herein or perform any independent analysis in connection with any of the product information contained herein. Publisher does not assume, and expressly disclaims, any obligation to obtain and include information other than that provided to it by the manufacturer.

The reader is expressly warned to consider and adopt all safety precautions that might be indicated by the activities herein and to avoid all potential hazards. By following the instructions contained herein, the reader willingly assumes all risks in connection with such instructions.

The publisher makes no representations or warranties of any kind, including but not limited to, the warranties of fitness for particular purpose or merchantability, nor are any such representations implied with respect to the material set forth herein, and the publisher takes no responsibility with respect to such material. The publisher shall not be liable for any special, consequential, or exemplary damages resulting, in whole or part, from the readers' use of, or reliance upon, this material.

INTRODUCTION TO THE SERIES

This Series in Health Services is now in its third decade of providing top-quality teaching materials to the health administration/public health field. Each year has witnessed further strengthening of the market position of each of the principal books in the Series, also reflecting the continued excellence of the products. Each author, book editor, and contributor to the Series has helped build what is widely recognized as the top textbook and issues collection of books available in this field today.

But we have achieved only a beginning. Everyone involved in the Series is committed to further expansion of the scope, technical excellence, and usability of the Series. Our goal is to do more for you, the reader. We will add new books in important areas, seek out more excellent authors, and increase the physical attributes of the book to make them easier for you to use.

We thank everyone, the authors and users in particular, who have made this Series so successful and so widely used. And we promise that this third decade will be dedicated to further expansion of the Series and to enhancement of the books it contains to provide still greater value to you, our constituency.

Stephen J. Williams
Series Editor

v

THOMSON DELMAR LEARNING'S SERIES IN HEALTH SERVICES ADMINISTRATION

Stephen J. Williams, Sc.D., Series Editor

Ambulatory Care Management, third edition
Austin Ross, Stephen J. Williams, and Ernest J. Pavlock, Editors
The Continuum of Long-Term Care, third edition
Connie J. Evashwick, Editor
Essentials of Health Care Management
Stephen M. Shortell and Arnold D. Kaluzny, Editors
Essentials of Health Services, third edition
Stephen J. Williams
Essentials of Human Resources Management in Health Services Organizations
Myron D. Fottler, S. Robert Hernandez, and Charles L. Joiner, Editors
Financial Management in Health Care Organizations, second edition
Robert McLean
Health Care Economics, sixth edition
Paul J. Feldstein
Health Care Management: Organization Design and Behavior, fifth edition
Stephen M. Shortell and Arnold D. Kaluzny, Editors
Health Politics and Policy, third edition
Theodor J. Litman and Leonard S. Robins, Editors
The Hospital Medical Staff
Charles H. White
Introduction to Health Services, sixth edition
Stephen J. Williams and Paul R. Torrens, Editors
Motivating Health Behavior
John P. Elder, E. Scott Geller, Melbourne F. Hovell, and Joni A. Mayer, Editors
Really Governing: How Health System and Hospital Boards Can Make More of a Difference
Dennis D. Pointer and Charles M. Ewell
Strategic Management of Human Resources in Health Services Organizations, second edition
Myron D. Fottler, S. Robert Hernandez, and Charles L. Joiner, Editors
Health Services Research Methods
Leiyu Shi

CONTRIBUTORS

Jeff Alexander, PhD
Richard C. Jelinek Professor of Health
Management and Policy
School of Public Health
University of Michigan
Ann Arbor, Michigan

G. Ross Baker, PhD
Professor
Department of Health Policy, Management
and Evaluation
Faculty of Medicine
University of Toronto

Lawton R. Burns, PhD, MBA
The James Joo-Jin Kim Professor:
Professor of Health Care Systems
and Management
Director, Wharton Center for
Health Management & Economics
The Wharton School,
University of Pennsylvania
Philadelphia, Pennsylvania

Martin P. Charns, DBA
Director
Center for Organization, Leadership &
Management Research
Health Services Research & Development
Service
Department of Veterans Affairs and
Professor and Director

Program on Health Policy & Management
School of Public Health, Boston University
Boston, Massachusetts

Thomas A. D'Aunno, PhD
Novartis Professor of Healthcare Management
Professor of Organizational Behavior
Director, Healthcare Management Initiative
INSEAD, Fontainebleu, France

Amy C. Edmondson, PhD
Professor of Business Administration
Harvard Business School
Harvard University
Boston, Massachusetts

Ann Barry Flood, PhD
Professor of Health Policy and Sociology
Co-Editor-in-Chief, HSR Journal
Chair of PhD Program & of NRSA Pre- and
Postdoctoral Programs
Center for the Evaluative Clinical Sciences at
Dartmouth
Dartmouth Medical School
Hanover, New Hampshire

Myron D. Fottler, PhD
Professor/Director HSA Programs
Department of Health Professions
College of Health and Public Affairs
University of Central Florida
Orlando, Florida

Bruce Fried, PhD
Associate Professor
Director, Residential Masters Program
Department of Health Policy and
  Administration
School of Public Health
University of North Carolina at Chapel Hill
Chapel Hill, North Carolina

Jody Hoffer Gittel, PhD
Assistant Professor
The Heller School for Social Policy and
  Management
Brandeis University
Waltham, Massachusetts

Maria J. Gilmartin, RN, PhD
Senior Research Fellow
Healthcare Management Initiative
INSEAD, Fontainebleau, France

Christian D. Helfrich, PhD
Postdoctoral Fellow
Health Services Research and Development
VA Puget Sound Health System, and
  Research Associate,
Department of Health Services
School of Public Health and Community
  Medicine
University of Washington
Seattle, Washington

Robert S. Hernandez, Dr PH
Professor & Director
Doctoral Program in Administration/Health
  Services
School of Community and Allied Health
  Professions
University of Alabama
Birmingham, Alabama

Timothy J. Hoff, PhD
Associate Professor
School of Public Health,
SUNY at Albany

Albany, New York

Jennifer Illes, PhD
Research Associate
Harvard Business School
Harvard University
Boston, Massachusetts

Arnold D. Kaluzny, PhD
Professor Emeritus of Health Policy and
  Administration and Director Emeritus of the
  Public Health Leadership Program
School of Public Health, and
  Senior Research Fellow,
Cecil G. Sheps Center for Health Services
  Research
University of North Carolina at Chapel Hill
Chapel Hill, North Carolina

John R. Kimberly, PhD
Henry Bower Professor
  of Entrepreneurial Studies;
Professor of Management,
  Healthcare Systems, and Sociology
The Wharton School
University of Pennsylvania
Philadelphia, Pennsylvania, and Novartis
  Professor Healthcare Management at
  INSEAD
Executive Director of the INSEAD-Wharton
  Alliance
Fontainebleau, France

Peggy Leatt, PhD
Professor and Chair
Department of Health Policy and
  Administration
School of Public Health,
University of North Carolina at Chapel Hill
Chapel Hill, North Carolina

Beaufort B. Longest, Jr., PhD
M. Allen Pond Professor and Director
Health Policy Institute of Health Policy
  Management

Graduate School of Public Health
University of Pittsburgh
Pittsburgh, Pennsylvania

Roice D. Luke, PhD
Professor
Graduate Program in Health Administration
School of Allied Health Professions
Medical College of Virginia
Richmond, Virginia

Laura L. Morlock, PhD
Professor and Associate Chair for Health
    Management Program
Department of Health Policy and Management
Johns Hopkins University
Baltimore, Maryland

Margaret A. Neale, PhD
John G. McCoy-Banc One
Corporation Professor
Graduate School of Business
Stanford University
Stanford, California

Stephen J. O'Connor, PhD
Professor and Director,
    Residential MSHA Program
Department of Health Services
    Administration
School of Health Related Professions
University of Alabama at Birmingham
Birmingham, Alabama

Dennis D. Pointer, PhD
Austin Ross Professor
Department of Health Services
School of Public Health and Community
    Medicine,
University of Washington
Seattle, Washington

Jeffrey T. Polzer, PhD
Associate Professor
Harvard Business School

Harvard University
Boston, Massachusetts

Thomas G. Rundall, PhD
Henry J. Kaiser Professor of Organized Health
    Services
Division of Health Policy and Management
School of Public Health
University of California
Berkeley, California

W. Richard Scott, PhD
Professor of Sociology Emeritus
Department of Sociology
Stanford University
Stanford, California

Stephen M. Shortell, PhD
Blue Cross of California Distinguished
    Professor of Health Policy and Management
Division of Health Policy and Management
Dean of the School of Public Health
Professor of Organization Behavior
Haas School of Business
University of California, Berkeley
Berkeley, California

Sharon Topping, PhD
Professor of Management
College of Business & Economic Development
University of Southern Mississippi
Hattiesburg, Mississippi

Stephen L. Walston, PhD
Professor
Graduate Program in Health Administration
School of Public and Environmental Affairs
Indiana University
Indianapolis, Indiana

Bryan J. Weiner, PhD
Associate Professor
Department of Health Policy and
    Administration
School of Public Health

University of North Carolina at Chapel Hill
Chapel Hill, North Carolina

William E. Welton, DrPH, MHA
Senior Lecturer, and Director, Graduate
   Program in Health Services Administration
Department of Health Services
School of Public Health and Community
   Medicine
University of Washington
Seattle, Washington

Gary J. Young, J.D., PhD
Associate Director
Center for Organization
Leadership Management Research
Department of Veterans Affairs
Boston, Massachusetts, and
   Professor and Co-Director Program in
   Health Policy and Management
Boston University School of Public Health
Boston, Massachusetts

Edward J. Zajac, PhD
James F. Beré Professor of Organization
   Behavior
J.L. Kellogg Graduate School of Management
Northwestern University
Evanston, Illinois

Jacqueline Zinn, PhD
Professor
Department of Risk, Insurance and Health
   Care Management
Fox School of Business and Management
Temple University
Philadelphia, Pennsylvania

CONTENTS

P A R T

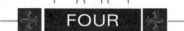

THREE

Operating the Technical System / 171

P A R T

FOUR

Positioning the Organization for Success / 311

P A R T

FIVE

Charting the Future / 455

FOREWORD

There are no thought leaders who have studied the organization design and behavior of health care management in more depth or breadth than Stephen Shortell, PhD, and Arnold D. Kaluzny, PhD. Their work spans over twenty years of a very dynamic transition in the profession of health care management, the structure of health care organizations, and the strategies that have been used to respond to an increasingly complex and challenging environment.

This fifth edition of their work takes this analysis to the next level and reinforces it by giving the reader both the current thinking about health care management skills and competencies and "how management gets done" in organizations. The case histories of health care's leading organizations do a superb job of exemplifying what works and sometimes what doesn't in the twenty-first-century hospital and health system. Interestingly enough they have once again highlighted and updated the several different perspectives regarding how organizations function and have evolved over the years.

One of the important contributions to "system thinking" has been their analysis of managing partnerships, strategic alliances, networking, and other arrangements between and among physicians, hospitals, health systems, and other provider organizations. The reader learns quickly that perhaps the motivating factor for these arrangements may be as important as or more important than the arrangements themselves. It's also clear that the CEO's per-

spective or the need for these "deals" may not be shared by those managers who have to execute them.

The authors' perspective on the management role move very quickly to transformational leadership as the manager is forced to foster the nurturing and creation of a shared vision for the organization. As this evolves an emphasis on values, accountability, commitment, and the characteristics of a learning organization take on increased meaning for managers at every level. Motivation of people, the leadership framework, conflict management, and negotiation are identified as essential factors for success in the twenty-first-century organizations.

Day-to-day management in an organization that has adopted a transformational leadership model requires the effective use and management of groups and teams in these organizations. Two of the text's strongest chapters are the discussion of groups and teams in health services organizations and the design of work for individuals and teams. The descriptions of the challenges in the professions of medicine and nursing in relationship to work design are particularly helpful. These professions seek organizations that function in a predictable way and will support them in times where they are feeling hassled and undervalued.

The lessons in coordination and communication as well as power and politics in health services organizations are a perfect way to reinforce the reasons behind the need for transformational leadership.

"Perceptions are often reality" even though senior-level managers attempt to be sensitive to the needs of the entire organization when allocating resources, managing change, making difficult decisions, conveying bad news, considering management succession, and creating alliances.

In these chapters one of the important concepts that emerge is the increasing importance of human resources management of human capital. Every organization is now expected to have elevated the human resources functions to a level equivalent to the chief financial officer and the chief information officer. Mission, vision, values, culture, organizational norms and behavior, team development, and leadership training have now become an essential factor in organizational success "with a twenty-first-century workforce" in a learning organization.

In the era of "pay for performance" the health care organization will be challenged to demonstrate its ability to assess and demonstrate performance. Quality, efficiency, effectiveness, appropriateness, and productivity are no longer something to aspire to; they are now being measured and are expected. The success of these organizations will depend upon their ability to "Cross the Quality Chasm," adhere to Sarbannes-Oxley, have a prudent cost structure, and be an important community resource, while maintaining and growing market share.

The last two chapters reinforce the importance of lessons learned from our authors through essays on strategy making, creating, and managing the future. The twenty-first-century health care manager will be required to manage their organizations strategically and operationally as well as influence the environment and create and actively manage their future. With Shortell and Kaluzny's guidance, this should be greatly enhanced.

Gail L. Warden
President Emeritus
Henry Ford Health System
Detroit, Michigan

PREFACE

This book is intended for those interested in a systematic understanding of organizational principles, practices, and insights pertinent to the management of health services organizations. While based on state-of-the-art organizational theory and research, the emphasis is on application. While the primary audience is graduate students in health services administration, management and policy programs, the book will also be of interest to undergraduate programs, extended degree programs, executive education programs, and practicing health services executives interested in ready access to the latest developments in organizational and managerial thinking. It is also intended for students of medicine, nursing, pharmacy, social work, and other health professions who will assume managerial responsibilities or who want to learn more about the organizations in which they will spend the major portion of their professional lives. Previous editions have been translated into Polish, Korean, Ukranian and Hungarian and we look forward to the books continued use by our international colleagues.

This fifth edition of the text continues a number of popular features from the fourth edition. These include:

- An explicit list of topics provided at the beginning of each chapter.
- Specific behaviorally oriented learning objectives highlighted at the beginning of each chapter.

- Each chapter includes a list of key terms that readers should be able to define and apply as a result of reading each chapter.
- Each chapter opens with an "In Practice" column describing a practical situation facing a health services organization. Many chapters contain several "In Practice" columns to illustrate the major principles and lessons of the chapter.
- Most chapters incorporate a section called "Debate Time," which poses a controversial issue or presents divergent perspectives to stimulate the reader's thinking.
- A set of comprehensive managerial guidelines concludes each chapter.

All chapters have been updated and revised and where appropriate "In Practice" scenarios are provided with Web site locations for additional background information. The book is organized in five sections or parts. Part 1 provides an overall perspective on the study of health services organizations and the associated managerial role. Part 2 deals with fundamental building blocks of managerial activity involving motivation, leadership, conflict management, and negotiation. Part 3 deals with largely internal organizational issues including work design, coordination and communication, and managing power and political processes. Part 4 focuses on performance issues related to organization design, strategic alliances, innovation and change, and managing for efficiency and effectiveness. The final section focuses on strategic issues and attempts to anticipate future issues that will challenge health services leaders. With the exception of Part 1, which should be read first by all readers because it provides the groundwork for chapters that follow, the remaining parts and chapters can be read in any order depending on instructor and course objectives.

We believe that the major strength of the text is the diversity of the talented authors involved. They have brought multiple perspectives, experiences, skills, and expertise to bear on each chapter. As a result, each chapter is at the frontiers of knowledge with clear applications that illuminate the practice of health services management. We hope that readers enjoy this richness as much as we and our colleagues continue to have in creating it.

Stephen M. Shortell
Berkeley, California

Arnold D. Kaluzny
Chapel Hill, North Carolina

ACKNOWLEDGMENTS

This fifth edition has benefited greatly from feedback from students and faculty over the past five years. They have provided insight and perspective that we have tried to incorporate into the current edition. The authors would like to acknowledge the following reviewers for their feedback on this new edition:

Sharon B. Buchbinder, RN, Ph.D.
Professor and Coordinator
Health Care Management Program
Department of Health Science
Towson University
Towson, Maryland

Rohn Butterfield, MBA
Instructor
Health Services/Health Administration
    Program
University of Southern Indiana
Evansville, Indiana

Donna L. Gellatly, MBA, FHFMA, CPA
University Professor
Health Administration Program
Governors State University
University Park, Illinois

Christopher E. Johnson, Ph.D.
Associate Professor
Department of Health Policy and Management
School of Rural Public Health
Texas A&M University System Health Science
    Center
College Station, Texas

Justin C. Matus, Ph.D., MBA, FACHE
Assistant Professor of Business Administration
Lycoming College
Williamsport, Pennsylvania

Valerie L. Myers, M.A., M.S.W., Ph.D.
University of Michigan School of Public Health
Department of Health Management & Policy
Ann Arbor, Michigan

James T. Ziegenfuss, Jr., Ph.D.
Professor of Management & Health Care Systems
Graduate Programs in Health & Public
    Administration
Penn State University
Middletown, Pennsylvania

Appreciation is also expressed to various friends and colleagues who have contributed to the production of the book. The coordination and integration of the contributing authors was a significant undertaking and we had the privilege to work with excellent colleagues. On the Berkeley side, special thanks are given to Jackie Henderson, Julian Wimbush and Candi Dorali-Martinez.

On the Chapel Hill side, a number of people have given of their time, energy, and patience including Adriane Terrell, who managed the book project and provided research, and Damian Gallina, who assured that all chapters maintained the proper format and that the authors stayed on schedule, and Paul Frellick, who provided editing and general counsel as the book entered the production stage. Special thanks are given to Bill Carpenter and Young Do and their work on the development of the Instructor's Manual. Thanks are also given to Bill Sollecito, the director of the school's Public Health Leadership Program and Tim Carey the director of the university's Cecil G. Sheps Center for Health Services Research who made resources available to complete what seemed an endless task. Finally, we are most grateful to colleagues around the country who provided input to various sections including Rob Haley and Jo Ann Nolin and their contributions to Chapter 15 and the discussion of the allied health professions, Brenda Nevidjon and her reading of Chapter 15 and the discussion of nursing, and Glen Mays for his assistance in updating selected material in Chapter 1.

We also acknowledge the assistance and wise counsel of Maureen Rosener, Elizabeth Howe, and Laurie Traver at Delmar and Terry Routley at Carlisle Publishers for their overall guidance and suggestions in the production of the fifth edition.

Stephen M. Shortell
Berkeley, California

Arnold D. Kaluzny
Chapel Hill, North Carolina

ABOUT THE AUTHORS

Stephen M. Shortell, is the Blue Cross of California Distinguished Professor of Health Policy and Management, Professor of Organization Behavior, and Dean of the School of Public Health, University of California, Berkeley. He also holds appointments at the Haas School of Business, the Department of Sociology, and is an affiliated member at the Institute for Health Policy Studies at the University of California, San Francisco.

He has been the recipient of the Baxter Allegiance Prize for Health Services research, the Gold Medal Award from the American College of Healthcare Executives, the Distinguished Investigator Award from the Association of Health Services Research, and the American Hospital Association Honorary Life Member Award. He is a Distinguished Fellow of Academy Health.

He is an elected member of the Institute of Medicine of the National Academy of Sciences; has served as President of the Association for Health Services Research; and has served as Chairman of the Accrediting Commission for Graduate Education in Health Services Administration. He serves on a number of boards including the National Center for Healthcare Leadership (NCHL), and other Health Research and Educational Trust (HRET) and is a consultant and an advisor to a number of private and public organizations.

Dr. Shortell received his undergraduate degree from the University of Notre Dame, his master's degree in public health and hospital administration from UCLA, and his Ph.D. in the behavioral sciences from the University of Chicago. He is currently conducting research on efforts to improve the quality and outcomes of care particularly in regard to the management of chronic illness.

Arnold D. Kaluzny is Professor Emeritus of Health Policy and Administration, and Director Emeritus of the Public Health Leadership Program, School of Public Health, as well as a Senior Research Fellow in the Cecil G. Sheps Center for Health Services Research and a member of the Lineberger Comprehensive Cancer Center at the University of North Carolina at Chapel Hill.

He has served as a consultant to a number of private research and health service organizations and various international, federal, and state agencies, including Project HOPE, the World Health Organization, various programs and institutes within the National Institutes of Health, the Joint Commission on the Accreditation of Healthcare Organizations, the Department of Veterans Affairs, the Agency for Health Care Policy and Research and the Institute for Medicine of the National Academy of Sciences. From 1991 through 1995, he was a member of the Board of Scientific Counselors for the Division of Prevention and Control at the National Cancer Institute and served as Chairman from 1993 to 1995.

Dr. Kaluzny was a member of the Advisory Panel for Public Health, Pew Health Professions Commission, and chaired the Commission's Advisory Panel for Health Care Management. He also served as Chairman of the Accrediting Commission for Graduate Education in Health Services Administration.

His research has focused on the organizational factors affecting implementation and change of a variety of health care organizations, with specific emphasis given to cancer treatment prevention and control, continuous quality improvement initiatives in both organizational and primary care settings, and most recently, the study of alliances within health care. In all these endeavors, a major focus has been to strengthen the science base of policy and practice.

Teaching responsibilities have included doctoral, masters and executive students. He has served as invited faculty to executive training programs in various countries including China, Poland, Czech Republic, Hungary, and the Baltic countries of Estonia, Latvia and Lithuania.

Dr. Kaluzny received his undergraduate degree from the University of Wisconsin at River Falls, his master's degree in hospital administration from the University of Michigan School of Business, and his Ph.D. in Medical Care Organization-Social Psychology from the University of Michigan.

ONE

Organizations
and
Managers

THE NATURE OF ORGANIZATIONS: FRAMEWORK FOR THE TEXT

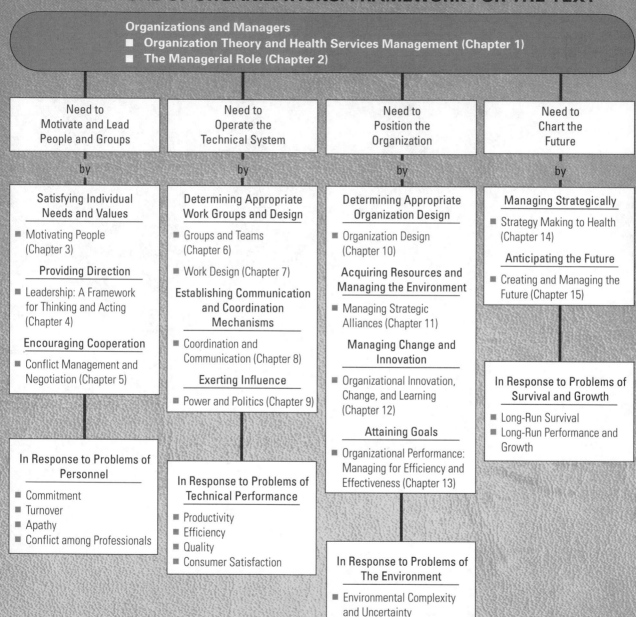

Organizations and Managers
- Organization Theory and Health Services Management (Chapter 1)
- The Managerial Role (Chapter 2)

Need to Motivate and Lead People and Groups	Need to Operate the Technical System	Need to Position the Organization	Need to Chart the Future
by	by	by	by

Satisfying Individual Needs and Values
- Motivating People (Chapter 3)

Providing Direction
- Leadership: A Framework for Thinking and Acting (Chapter 4)

Encouraging Cooperation
- Conflict Management and Negotiation (Chapter 5)

In Response to Problems of Personnel
- Commitment
- Turnover
- Apathy
- Conflict among Professionals

Determining Appropriate Work Groups and Design
- Groups and Teams (Chapter 6)
- Work Design (Chapter 7)

Establishing Communication and Coordination Mechanisms
- Coordination and Communication (Chapter 8)

Exerting Influence
- Power and Politics (Chapter 9)

In Response to Problems of Technical Performance
- Productivity
- Efficiency
- Quality
- Consumer Satisfaction

Determining Appropriate Organization Design
- Organization Design (Chapter 10)

Acquiring Resources and Managing the Environment
- Managing Strategic Alliances (Chapter 11)

Managing Change and Innovation
- Organizational Innovation, Change, and Learning (Chapter 12)

Attaining Goals
- Organizational Performance: Managing for Efficiency and Effectiveness (Chapter 13)

In Response to Problems of The Environment
- Environmental Complexity and Uncertainty
- Technological and Social Change
- Competitive Forces
- Multiple Performance Demands

Managing Strategically
- Strategy Making to Health (Chapter 14)

Anticipating the Future
- Creating and Managing the Future (Chapter 15)

In Response to Problems of Survival and Growth
- Long-Run Survival
- Long-Run Performance and Growth

The unrelenting changes in the health care environment are increasing the demand for organizational and managerial expertise. There is an increased need to manage across organizational boundaries in responding to new treatment technologies, payment mechanisms, consumer preferences, and accountability. The two chapters in this first section take up this challenge by laying the groundwork for the remainder of the book.

Chapter 1, "Organization Theory and Health Services Management," addresses the following kinds of questions:

- What are the main forces influencing the organization and delivery of health services?
- What are the major conceptual frameworks and perspectives for thinking about health services organizations?
- What are the major units of analysis that require managerial attention?

The first chapter suggests the importance of viewing health services organizations from different perspectives drawing on a number of different metaphors to stimulate thinking.

Chapter 2, "The Managerial Role," focuses on the following kinds of questions:

- What are the major ways of viewing the manager's role in the health sector?
- What are the distinctive challenges faced by health care managers and leaders?
- What new skills and knowledge are needed by health services managers and leaders to be successful?

This chapter emphasizes the need for managers and leaders who can successfully integrate multiple roles in promoting and implementing changes to meet the new challenges.

Upon completing the first two chapters, readers should have a clearer understanding of the complexity of the health services manager's role and the need for comprehensive frameworks and approaches that recognize the complexity of the role.

CHAPTER 1

Organization Theory and Health Services Management

Stephen M. Shortell, Ph.D. and Arnold D.Kaluzny, Ph.D.

CHAPTER OUTLINE

- The Changing Health Care System
- Ecology of Health Services Organizations
- Key Dimensions of Health Services Organizations
- Health Services Organizations as Systems
- Areas of Managerial Activity
- Major Perspectives on Health Services Organizations
- Metaphors of Health Services Organizations
- Organization Theory and Behavior: A Framework for the Text

LEARNING OBJECTIVES

After completing this chapter, the reader should be able to:

1. Identify the major forces affecting the delivery of health services.

2. Understand how these major forces affect the role of the health services manager.

3. Identify some of the commonalities and differences among major types of health services organizations.

4. Identify and understand the basic processes that must be accomplished by any organization.

5. Identify and understand the different areas of managerial activity.

6. Identify, understand, and apply the major perspectives and theories on organizations to real problems facing health services organizations.

7. Identify, understand, and apply major metaphors of organizations to the challenges facing health services organizations.

KEY TERMS

Adaptation Function
Biological Organisms
Boundary Spanning Function
Brains
Bureaucratic Theory
Change
Closed System
Complex Adaptive System
Contingency Theory
Differentiation
Evidence-Based Management
External Environment
Governance Function
Health Networks
Health Systems

Holograms
Human Relations School
Innovation
Institutional Theory
Interorganizational
   Relationships
Machines
Macro Approach
Maintenance Function
Management Function
Managerial Competencies
Managing Across Boundaries
Micro Approach
Open System
Organizational Behavior

Playing Fields
Political Systems
Population Ecology Theory
Production Function
Psychic Prisons
Resource Dependence Theory
Scientific Management School
Six Essential Aims
Social Network Perspective
Strategic Management
   Perspective
Tyrants
Vision/Mission/Goals

IN PRACTICE   Henry Ford Health System Positions Itself for the Future

Henry Ford Health System (HFHS) is one of the nation's leading comprehensive, integrated health systems providing acute, specialty, primary, and preventive care services along with a commitment to teaching and research. Founded in 1915 by auto pioneer Henry Ford, it is committed to improving the health and well-being of a diverse community in Detroit and the surrounding southeastern Michigan region. The system is anchored by a 903-bed tertiary care hospital and by the Henry Ford Medical Group, one of the nation's largest group practices with 800 physicians in forty specialties. In addition, the system owns an insurance company, the Health Alliance Plan, which serves more than 3,000 employer groups and 540,000 members. The system has approximately 12,700 full-time equivalent employees; has more than 2.5 million annual patient visits to physicians; admits 65,000 patients to its hospitals; and generates revenue of

$2.4 billion. Overall, more than one million residents in southeast Michigan receive care from HFHS.

As it looks ahead to the end of the first decade of the twenty-first century, HFHS faces a number of challenges including: (1) changing demographics, (2) continuing advances in medical technology and the biomedical sciences, (3) the growth of information technology, (4) workforce shortages and disruptions, and (5) dealing with the implications of globalization. On the demographic front, HFHS will need to find cost-effective ways of managing the increased incidence and prevalence of chronic illness, a more culturally and ethnically diverse population, and an increasingly informed and demanding public. In regard to the continued growth in medical technology and the biomedical sciences, HFHS's investment in clinical research should be of assistance in incorporating the latest advances in basic science and biotechnology into patient diagnosis and treatment. A large part of the HSHS's ability to do this will depend on its continuing efforts to extend its information technology capabilities to manage the growing body of information and knowledge generated and to provide effective interface with patients and the community. The system will also need to contend with shortages in various categories of health professionals, particularly nurses. Further, globalization will have an effect through the outsourcing of functions from the big three auto manufacturers headquartered in the Detroit area. In addition, the systems geographic proximity to Canada will hold implications for both patient flow and supply of health professionals. Cutting across all of these issues will be intensified demands for improved cost and quality performance and greater public accountability.

To meet these challenges, HFHS has developed strategic priorities related to growth; financial stability; development of a county hospital; recruitment and retention of professional staff and employees; system positioning emphasizing integrated and strategic, operating, and financial planning; and continuous attention to quality and cost performance. In the latter regard, HFHS plans to implement half of the National Quality Forum endorsed thirty best practices for the safest hospitals in America and develop an ongoing mechanism to identify and spread quality improvements rapidly throughout the system. Overall they are committed to serving as an ideal model for health care delivery in the United States, including "preparing for and winning the Malcolm Baldrige National Quality Award" (*http://www.henryfordhealth.org*).

CHAPTER PURPOSE

As seen in the example of the Henry Ford Health System, the health services management challenge of the new millenium is to create value for an increasingly diverse and demanding citizenry. *Value* is created when for a given cost or price to the purchaser additional quality features desired by the purchaser are provided or, conversely, when a given level of quality services can be provided at a lower cost or price relative to others from whom purchasers can obtain the services. Providing greater value is a challenge for all health services organizations and to the professionals—both clinical and managerial—associated with them. As noted in a Pew Commission Report on Education for the Health Professions:

> Health services management will become even more challenging, because it is the point where increasing service demands, cost containment strategies, interprofessional tensions, technological change pressures, guidelines implementation, and quality improvement mandates all converge. The managerial function in health services is unique because of the relative autonomy of providers and the complexity of assessing the quality of the services rendered. (Pew Commission, 1993)

The challenges facing Henry Ford Health System (HFHS) in the accompanying "In Practice" are representative of those facing any health care organization. This chapter sets the stage for addressing some of these challenges. We discuss the major forces that influence the health care system; describe the great variety of organizations involved; highlight key approaches, dimensions, perspectives, theories, and metaphors; and indicate how each of the succeeding chapters will address the complex issues that are raised.

THE CHANGING HEALTH CARE SYSTEM

Ultimately the goal of health services managers is to help maintain and enhance the health of the public. While individual citizens hold primary responsibility for their health status, there is much that health services managers working in concert with physicians, nurses, other health professionals, and community leaders can do to assist in the process. This goal may seem strange to some and unrealistic to others. After all, isn't it sufficient simply to care for those who come to you for help and make sure that one's organization retains its financial health in order to provide the requested care? The answer is no. Economic, political, and social forces have moved the health services system beyond the largely reactive acute care paradigm to a more holistic paradigm emphasizing population-based wellness. Some of the major economic, political, and social forces that will influence health care delivery in the next five to ten years are highlighted in Table 1.1. These forces are causing a fundamental shift in the way in which health care is viewed. The major elements of this *shift* are outlined in Table 1.2.

At the core of this shift is the movement away from episodic treatment of acute illness events to the provision of a coordinated continuum of services that will support those with chronic illness and enhance the health status of defined populations. In the evolving health care system of financial incentives for performance, organizations win by helping health care professionals provide services at that point in the continuum of care where the greatest value (i.e., cost-benefit) is provided. They do not win by filling hospital beds or continuing to have key professionals working at cross purposes with each other. These kinds of changes require new and different ways of organizing and managing health care services.

In its seminal work on *Crossing the Quality Chasm,* the Institute of Medicine (2001) identified **six essential aims** for any health care system shown in Table 1.3. Achieving these six aims will require considerable leadership in addition to alignment of incentives among individuals, health care teams, health organizations, and the purchasers, payers, and regulators of health care services. Figure 1.1 provides a framework for thinking about the key changes that must be realized. As shown, the desired outcomes of safety, effectiveness, efficiency, personalization of care, timeliness of care, and equitable care are most immediately a function of high-performing patient-centered teams operating within an organization designed to facilitate the work of those teams. This is referred to as the "care system." It is suggested that developing such care systems will require six major redesign imperatives including: (1) redesigning care processes themselves; (2) making effective use of information technologies; (3) developing the organization's knowledge and skills management capabilities including the ability to transfer knowledge quickly; (4) developing effective teams; (5) developing the ability to coordinate care across patient conditions, services, and settings over time; and (6) using performance and outcome measurements for continuous quality improvement and accountability purposes. All of this takes place within a payment and regulatory environment that will require greater incentives for organizations and the health care teams working within them to make the desired changes to improve care.

Various chapters in this text address each of the redesign imperatives. For example, issues involving the redesign of care processes are covered in Chapters 7, 8, 10, 12, and 13 addressing work design, communication and coordination, organization design, organizational change, and organizational performance, respectively. Issues involving the effective use of information technology are highlighted in Chapter 12 on organizational change and learning and Chapter 13 on organizational

Table 1.1. Nine Forces Influencing Health Care Delivery and Their Implications for Management

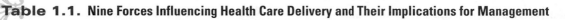

External Force	Management Implication
1. Financial incentives that reward superior performance	▪ Need for increased efficiency, productivity, and quality ▪ Redesign of patient care delivery ▪ Development of strategic alliances that add value ▪ Increased growth of networks, systems, and physician groups
2. Increased accountability for performance	▪ Information systems that facilitate patient-centered care across episodes of illness and "pathways of wellness" ▪ Effective implementation of clinical practice guidelines and related care management processes ▪ Ability to demonstrate continuous improvements of all functions and processes
3. Technological advances in the biological and clinical sciences	▪ Expansion of the continuum of care, need for new treatment sites to accommodate new treatment modalities ▪ Increased capacity to manage care across organizational boundaries ▪ Need to confront new ethical dilemmas
4. Aging of the population and associated increase in chronic illness	▪ Increased demand for primary care, wellness, and health promotion services and chronic care management ▪ Challenge of managing ethical issues associated with prolongation of life
5. Increased ethnic and cultural diversity of the population	▪ Greater difficulty in understanding and meeting patient expectations ▪ Meeting the challenge of eliminating disparities in care provision and outcomes ▪ Challenge of managing an increasingly diverse health services workforce
6. Changes in the supply and education of health professionals	▪ Need for creative approaches in meeting the population's need for disease prevention, health promotion, and chronic care management services ▪ Need to compensate for shortages in some categories of health professionals (i.e., physical therapy, pharmacy, and some areas of nursing) ▪ Need to develop effective teams of caregivers across multiple treatment sites ▪ Need to develop work settings conducive to recruitment and retention
7. Social morbidity (AIDS, drugs, violence, bioterrorism "new surprises")	▪ Ability to deal with unpredictable increases in demand ▪ Need for increased social support systems and chronic care management ▪ Need to work effectively with public health community agencies to address "preparedness" issues
8. Information technology	▪ Training the health care workforce in new information technologies ▪ Increased ability to coordinate care across sites ▪ Challenge of managing an increased pace of change due to more rapid information transfer ▪ Challenge of dealing with confidentiality issues associated with new information technologies
9. Globalization and expansion of the world economy	▪ Need to manage cross-national and cross-cultural patient care referrals ▪ Increasing the competitiveness and productivity of the American labor force ▪ Managing global strategic alliances, particularly in the areas of biotechnology and new technology development ▪ Meeting the challenge of new and reemerging infectious diseases

Table 1.2. Transformation of Health Care

Old View	New View
Emphasis on acute inpatient care	Emphasis on the continuum of care
Emphasis on treating illness	Emphasis on maintaining and promoting wellness
Responsible for individual patients	Accountable for the health of defined populations
Emphasis on tangible physical assets	Emphasis on intangible knowledge/relationship-based assets
All providers are essentially similar	Differentiation based on ability to add value
Success achieved by increasing market share of inpatient admissions	Success achieved by keeping people well
Goal is to fill beds	Goal is to provide care at the most appropriate level
Hospitals, physicians, and health plans are separate	Virtual and/or vertically integrated delivery systems
Care provided by autonomous health professionals	Care provided by health care teams working together in collaboration
Information is a record for health professionals use	Information is a dynamic means for sharing knowledge with patients for their use
Managers run an organization	Managers provide leadership for improving the value of services delivered
Managers coordinate services	Managers actively pursue continuous improvement of quality and individual and community health

Table 1.3. Health System Essential Aims

- *Safe*—patients should receive care and be cared for in an environment that protects them from harm.
- *Effective*—care should be provided based on the best scientific information availabe and services not likely to benefit patients should be avoided.
- *Patient-centered*—care should take into account for individual patient preferences, needs, and values.
- *Timely*—care should be delivered expeditously to meet patient needs with the elimination of waiting time and harmful delays.
- *Efficient*—care should be provided in a manner that avoids all waste—of equipment, supplies, ideas, and energy.
- *Equitable*—care should not vary because of personal characteristics such as gender, ethnicity, geographic location, or socioeconomic status.

performance. Knowledge and skills management are addressed in Chapter 3 on motivation, Chapter 7 on work design, Chapter 8 on communication and coordination, Chapter 10 on organization design, and Chapter 12 on organizational change and learning. Content relevant to developing effective teams are covered in many chapters throughout the text including Chapter 6, which directly addresses the topic of groups and teams, but in addition, Chapter 3 on motivation, Chapter 5 on conflict management and negotiation, Chapter 7 on work design, and Chapter 8 on communication and coordination among others. The issue of developing the ability to coordinate care across settings is addressed in Chapter 7 on work design, Chapter 8 on communication and coordination, Chapter 12 on change, and Chapter 13 on performance. Finally, issues of performance and outcome measurement for quality improvement and accountability purposes are highlighted in Chapter 12 on change, Chapter 13 on performance, and Chapter 14 on managing strategically. In addition, Chapter 2 on

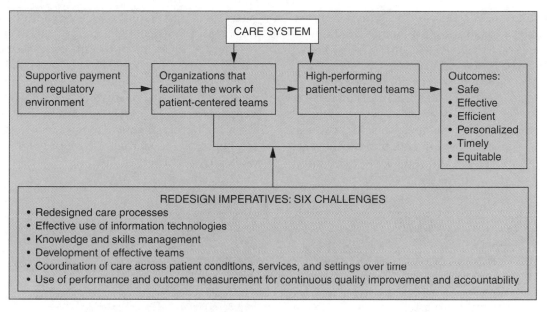

Figure 1.1. Framework for Thinking about Redesign

SOURCE: Reprinted with permission from *Crossing the Quality Chasm: A New Health System for the 21st Century* © 2001 by the National Academy of Sciences, courtesy of the National Academies Press, Washington, D.C.

the managerial role, Chapter 4 on leadership, and Chapter 9 on power and politics present crosscutting ideas and approaches relevant to all of the redesign imperatives.

Meeting the six aims and the associated redesign imperatives requires practicing **evidence-based management** (Walshe & Rundall, 2001; Baker & Wakefield, 2001). Evidence-based management involves the systematic application of the best available evidence for assessing options and making managerial decisions within the context of the organization's mission and values. Each of the chapters that follow presents some of the most recent evidence available for enhancing managerial effectiveness and organizational performance. They are consistent with the three domains of the National Center for Health Care Leadership (NCHL, 2004) competency model involving *transformation* competencies (see Chapters 11, 12, 14, and 15), *execu-*

tion competencies (see Chapters 2, 6 through 10, and Chapter 13), and *people* competencies (see Chapters 3 through 6).

Achieving the six aims also requires a shift in thinking about how to create value in health care delivery taking into account the demographic, technological, and related trends highlighted in Chapter 15. In the past, value was largely created through investment in physical assets involving bricks and mortar (e.g., hospitals, research labs, clinics). But with the information technology and knowledge explosion and the increased emphasis on customer satisfaction, value is now primarily created through the development and application of intellectual capital. Thus, health care executives must provide greater investment in the human capital represented by the health professional workforce and give greater attention to meeting customer preferences. Further, to meet the new demands for accountability and continuous quality improvement greater investment must be made in information technology that can effectively link patients, providers, and payers over time.

It is also important to think about the six aims of safety, effectiveness, efficiency, patient-centeredness, timeliness, and equity on a *population basis* in addition to being desired characteristics of care for individuals. An example of the population-based approach is provided by Group Health Cooperative (GHC) of Puget Sound as discussed in the accompanying "In Practice" vignette.

The key elements involved are: assessing the health needs of the population to be served; understanding how the community uses health and social services; organizing relationships among providers, health plans, and payers to ensure continuity of care; and developing an outcomes reporting system for purposes of internal continuous improvement and external accountability.

IN PRACTICE Group Health Cooperative and Population-Based Health Management

Group Health Cooperative (GHC) is a nonprofit health care system with a 57-year history of serving residents in the Pacific Northwest. It operates as both a health plan and an integrated health care delivery system, and serves more than 500,000 members enrolled in its health maintenance organization (HMO) and point-of-service (POS) product lines. The structure of a capitated, staff-model HMO has long provided the organization with the ability and incentive to monitor patient health status and manage health care utilization prospectively across its member population. However, growing consumer dissatisfaction with tightly managed care and increasing competition from more loosely managed preferred provider organization (PPO) products recently led the organization to retool its approaches to care management. The challenge it faced was to offer consumers more choice and flexibility in health care without losing its ability to improve clinical quality and manage costs and outcomes on a population-wide basis.

Since 1992, GHC has used a collection of clinical guidelines and disease management protocols called Clinical Roadmaps to help physicians provide evidence-based care to defined populations of members with health conditions such as diabetes, asthma, heart disease, and depression. It routinely measures physician performance in adhering to these guidelines and generates comparative feedback reports for physicians to encourage improvements. The Roadmaps, used in combination with electronic registries of patients diagnosed with these conditions, have proven effective in improving quality of care and reducing rates of hospitalization. However, these tools have been much more successful in GHC's staff-model HMO product—where salaried physicians exclusively serve GHC patients—than in its network-model HMO or its point-of-service products that allow members to access care from larger networks of community physicians that serve GHC members along with members of other health care plans. As larger numbers of GHC members have shifted to these other products, the overall impact of GHC's care management processes have diminished.

In response, GHC has adopted several new approaches for enhancing its ability to manage health care utilization and costs. First, it has begun a pay-for-performance initiative within its network HMO that rewards physicians who adhere to established performance standards for the management of patients with chronic diseases. These financial incentives are expected to raise awareness about the Clinical Roadmaps among network physicians and provide a more powerful motivation for adopting and adhering to these guidelines. Second, GHC has implemented several chronic disease self-management programs led by lay health advisors who educate patients about their diseases, the types of health services they should receive, and the steps they can take to prevent disease progression. These programs, which are not dependent on physician participation and adherence, are designed to enable patients to play greater roles in managing their own diseases and demanding appropriate, evidence-based care from their physicians.

GHC also revised several of the care management features of its staff-model HMO in order to make this product more appealing to consumers and competitive with loosely managed products. It eliminated a long-standing policy that required patients to receive a referral from their primary care physician (PCP) before receiving care from a specialist, and simultaneously instituted a policy of guaranteed same-day appointments for PCP visits. These changes offer patients more choices in seeking care—much like a PPO

product—while still encouraging patients to visit their PCP for routine care. Additionally, GHC implemented a secure messaging service that allows patients to e-mail questions to their physicians and other members of their care team with guaranteed response within 24 hours, along with an online medical record that allows patients to access detailed clinical information including diagnostic test results, physician notes and recommendations, and prescription information. Over time, these innovations are expected to encourage greater patient involvement in and adherence to care management process. For additional information, visit http://www.ghc-hmo.com.

References

Mays, G. P.; Trude, S.; Casalino, L. P.; Felland, L. E.; Claxton, G.; Pham, H. H.; Regopoulos, L. E.; Katz, A.; Kinner, K. (Winter 2003). Economic downturn and state budget woes overshadow Seattle health care market. *Community Tracking Study Community Report,* No. 3. Washington, DC: Center for Studying Health System Change.

Mays, G. P.; Claxton, G., & White, J. (2004, August 11). Managed care rebound? Recent changes in health plans' cost containment strategies. *Health Affairs,* Web Exclusive, 427–436.

Drawing on examples such as these, this book focuses on the new attitudes, the new ideas, the new skills, the new behaviors, and the new mind-sets required to manage a continually changing health care system.

The book is divided into three parts. Part 1 lays the foundation with chapters that discuss the manager's role, motivational forces, and leadership issues. Part 2 emphasizes the knowledge, skills, and understanding required to manage interdependent professional work teams in the provision of services across the

continuum of care. Areas covered include negotiation and conflict management, work groups, work design, coordination and communication, and power and influence. Parts 3 and 4 deal with the challenges posed by issues of organization design, the development of interorganizational networks and strategic alliances, the demands for change and innovation, the emphasis on performance accountability, and the importance of positioning the organization strategically. The book concludes with a discussion of the future issues that will challenge health services executives.

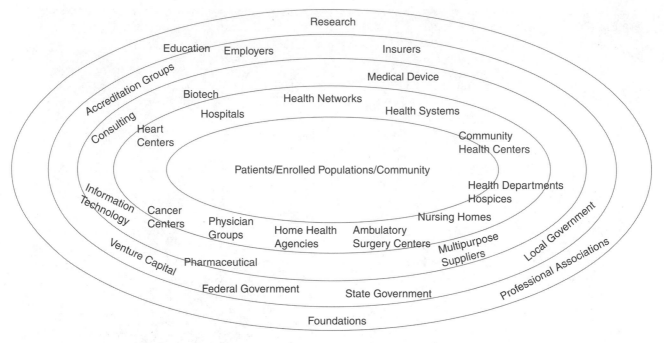

Figure 1.2. **The Concentric Ecology of Organizations in the Health Care Sector**

ECOLOGY OF HEALTH SERVICES ORGANIZATIONS

An organization is formally defined as a group of people who come together to pursue a specific purpose. Most organizations will embody both formal properties reflected in rules, policies, procedures, reporting relationships, and informal properties as expressed by customs, norms, beliefs, values, rituals, and celebrations. Figure 1.2 depicts the great number and variety of organizations engaged in the process by which services are ultimately delivered to patients. Those organizations most directly involved in services to patients, enrolled populations, or the communities at large are shown in the innermost concentric circle. These include not only traditional providers such as physicians and hospitals, but also health networks, health systems, and spe-

cialty "carve-out" organizations, such as cancer centers and heart clinics/hospitals, that focus on single diseases. **Health networks** are defined as strategic alliances or contractual arrangements among hospitals, physicians, and other health services organizations that provide an array of health services to the community. **Health systems** are defined as arrangements among hospitals, physicians, and other provider organizations that involve direct ownership of assets on the part of the parent system (Bazzoli, Shortell, Dubbs, Chan, & Kralovec, 1999). Thus, the key distinction is between the looser financial arrangements present in networks versus the unified ownership of health systems. In reality, many systems will have both owned and nonowned components representing "hybrid" organizations. **Integrated or organized delivery systems** have been defined as a network of organizations that provides or arranges to provide a coordinated continuum of services to a defined population and is willing to be held clinically and fiscally accountable for the outcomes and health status of the population served (Shortell, Gillies, Anderson, Mitchell, & Morgan, 1993).

The next concentric circle reflects the major suppliers to those organizations that directly provide services. These include multipurpose suppliers such as Baxter, General Electric, and 3M; biotech companies such as Amgen, Genetech, and Chiron; medical device companies such as Medtronic and information technology companies such as Cerner and SMS; pharmaceutical companies such as Abbott, GlaxoSmithKline (GSK), Lilly, Pfizer, Hoecht-Marion-Roussel, Bristol-Myers Squibb, and Merck; and consulting firms such as Ernst and Young, Deloitte and Touche, Peat Marwick, and Lewin and Associates.

The third concentric circle reflects the major payers and sources of capital. In addition to private sector employers, business coalitions, and insurers, this group includes federal, state, and local governments and private-sector venture capital firms that supply funding to the biotech, medical device, and pharmaceutical companies for research and development. It is also important to note the federal government's important role in funding biomedical, clinical, and health services research as represented in particular by the National Institutes of Health (NIH), the Agency for Health Care Research and Quality (AHRQ), and Centers for Disease Control (CDC). The federal government also plays an important regulatory role as reflected by the Food and Drug Administration (FDA). Also included in this circle are private-sector accreditation groups such as the Joint Commission on Accreditation of Healthcare Organizations (JCAHCO) that primarily accredits hospitals, the National Committee for Quality Assurance (NCQA) that primarily accredits health plans, and the Foundation for Accountability (FAACT). Examples of private foundations that provide support for innovations in health care delivery are The Commonwealth Fund, The Hartford Foundation, The Henry J. Kaiser Family Foundation, The Milbank Memorial Fund, The Pew Charitable Trusts, The Robert Wood Johnson Foundation, the W. K. Kellogg Foundation, and a number of state foundations. Note should also be made of the Institute of Medicine (IOM) of the National Academy of Sciences (NAS), which is charged by Congress to of-

fer independent objective analysis of a wide range of biomedical, health policy, and health care delivery issues facing the nation and the world.

What is most significant about Figure 1.2 is the growing permeability between the concentric circles. Not only are provider organizations merging and consolidating with each other, but they are also forming linkages with suppliers and payers. Biotech, medical device, and pharmaceutical companies, in turn, are forming alliances with universities. Federal government and private foundation funding is also encouraging the emergence of new partnerships. The clear message for future health care executives is the need for skills, knowledge, and understanding of how to effectively manage such **interorganizational relationships.** Nearly all chapters in this text address this challenge, with Chapters 11 and 14 being particularly relevant.

Figure 1.2 also suggests the immense size, diversity, and complexity of the health care system. On the provider side alone, there are approximately 820,000 physicians, 20,000 medical groups, 1.9 million nurses, 154,000 dentists, 5,800 hospitals, 300 health networks, 300 health systems, 550 health maintenance organizations (HMOs), 17,000 nursing homes, 17,000 home health centers, 4,900 community health centers, 2,000 adult day care centers, and 51 state public health departments. On the education side, there are 126 medical schools, 56 dental schools, 2,364 nursing education programs, 37 schools of public health, and 67 accredited graduate programs in health services management.

While direct health care expenditures comprise about 15% of the gross national product involving more than $1.6 trillion, the actual impact of health care on the American economy through its linkages with other organizations as shown in Figure 1.2 is even more pervasive.

Are Health Services Organizations Unique?

Health services organizations are often described as unique or at least different from other types of organizations, particularly different from industrial organizations. Further, these differences are believed to be significant in the area of management. Among the most frequently mentioned differences are the following:

- Defining and measuring output are more difficult.
- The work involved is more variable and complex.
- More of the work is of an emergency and non-deferrable nature.
- The work permits little tolerance for ambiguity or error.
- The work activities are highly interdependent, requiring a high degree of coordination among diverse professional groups.
- The work involves an extremely high degree of specialization.
- Organizational participants are highly professionalized, and their primary loyalty belongs to the profession rather than to the organization.
- Little effective organizational or managerial control exists over the group most responsible for generating work and expenditures: physicians.
- Dual lines of authority exist in many health care organizations, particularly hospitals, that create problems of coordination and accountability and confusion of roles.

Upon careful examination, it is possible to refute or at least question each of these allegedly distinctive attributes. For example, universities also have difficulty in defining and measuring their product. Is it the number of students graduated or the number of credit hours produced? Is quality measured by grade point average? If so, how much of that is the contribution of the student or of the faculty? A number of other organizations such as police and fire departments are concerned with highly variable, complex, emergency work. Other organizations also have limited ability to tolerate errors or ambiguities (for example, air traffic controllers). Are work activities any more interdependent in health care than in a symphony orchestra? What about the high degree of specialization of activities in a large legal firm? As for control over professional members, do universities or research institutes have any more control over their faculty or investigators than health services organizations have over physicians? Finally, many business and industrial organizations have dual lines of authority. In fact, as discussed in Chapter 10, many firms have institutionalized dual-authority structures through matrix organization designs. Further, the concept of uniqueness can be harmful if it leads health services managers to believe that their job is so much more difficult or different from others that relatively little can be done to improve performance or to learn from the experience of others.

On the other hand, health services organizations may be unusual, if not unique, in that many of them possess all of the characteristics stated above in combination. It is one thing to have little control over professionals when they do not need to interact frequently with others in the organization, such as with a number of research and development units in industry. But it is different when physicians, nurses, and other health professionals are highly dependent on each other in providing and coordinating patient care. The independence of professionals from managerial control is also less of a problem in situations where output is readily defined and measured than where clear performance criteria are still under development and yet external bodies hold the organization responsible for the activities of the relatively independent group of professionals. Thus, it is the confluence of professional, technological, and task attributes that make the management of health services organizations particularly challenging. Further, health services organizations are highly involved with values on a daily basis. For example, cost containment, which is valued by society at large, may frequently conflict with individual client values, such as the desire to recover one's health at almost any cost. In other cases such as abortion, outcomes valued by different parties may be in conflict.

KEY DIMENSIONS OF HEALTH SERVICES ORGANIZATIONS

Seven key dimensions of health care organizations are its (1) external environment, (2) vision/mission/goals, (3) strategies, (4) level of differentiation, (5) level of integration, (6) level of centralization, and (7) ability to adapt and change. Each of these is discussed in turn.

External Environment

One key to an organization's success is having a good understanding of its **external environment**, defined as all of the political, economic, social, and regulatory forces that exert influence on the organization. Environments differ in their complexity, susceptibility to change, and competitiveness. Depending on these attributes, organizations might choose different strategies, structures, and processes to compete successfully (see Chapters 7, 10, 13, and 14, in particular). For example, in markets characterized by a lower degree of managed care activity, health systems are less likely to own health plans and less likely to have salaried relationships with a large number of physicians. In more heavily penetrated managed care markets, one would expect to see greater ownership of health plans and a greater number of salaried relationships with physicians. The challenge is to appropriately match the organizations' strategies and structures to the demands of the environment. In order to deal with these environmental demands, health services organizations are increasingly forming strategic alliances with each other, resulting in a dense web of interorganizational networks (see Chapter 11).

Vision/Mission/Goals

The organization's **vision**, **mission**, and associated **goals** largely dictate the major tasks to be carried out and the kinds of technologies and human resources to be employed. Vision is what the organization aspires to become. Mission is what the organization does. Goals are statements of what the organization needs to achieve to fulfill its potential. Organizations, of course, differ widely in their mission and goals. Three examples of mission statements and statements of values are shown in Table 1.4. An organization's mission and goals have both an external and internal purpose. Externally they communicate what the organization is about to those who may want to use its services (e.g., patients) or in some other way have contact with the organization (e.g., regulators and third-party payers). They help to provide legitimacy, which, in turn, assists in helping the organization acquire needed resources (see Chapter 13). Internally goals serve as a source of motivation and direction (see Chapters 2, 3 and 4).

Strategies

Strategies are plans for achieving the organization's mission and goals and primarily involve positioning the organization to succeed in its environment relative to its competitors. Chapters 11, 13, and 14 emphasize the importance of the manager's role in the development and implementation of strategy. It is believed that in fast-paced turbulent environments characterized by considerable change, flexible, "emergent" strategies are needed, drawing on the best thinking of those closest to the customers. In more stable environments, a more top-down formal planning process may be effective. In reality, most organizations engage in and require both approaches to strategy development and implementation.

The generic content of strategies that health care organizations may adopt include being (1) low-cost providers or (2) differentiating on high quality.

Table 1.4. Three Examples of Mission and Value Statements

Tallahassee Memorial Health Care Mission

With caring hands and hearts, we honorably serve our community and maintain positive, collaborative relationships, by providing compassionate, leading-edge, patient-centered health care for all. We pursue perfection in a trusting and learning environment, thus enhancing the quality of life of those we serve.

Tallahassee Memorial Values
- **I**ntegrity
- **C**ompassion
- **A**ccountability
- **R**espect
- **E**xcellence

Cerner Corporation Mission

Cerner's mission is to connect to the appropriate person, knowledge, and resource at the appropriate time and location to achieve the optimal outcome.

Cerner Values
- Excellence in technology
- Investment in people
- Client service

Chiron Mission

Chiron is a global health care company focused on vaccines, diagnostics, therapeutics, and technology development. Its broad expertise enables an integrated approach to preventing, diagnosing, and treating cancer, as well as infectious and cardiovascular diseases. Chiron's approach is supported by scientific strengths in recombinant proteins, gene therapy, small molecule discovery, and diagnostic instrumentation.

Either of these can be done across-the-board or targeted to specific market niches or customer segments (Porter, 1985). Others have characterized an organization's strategies as being those of a prospector (i.e., almost always first to do anything), analyzer (approaches new developments cautiously with an emphasis on well-thought-out plans), defender (is seldom an innovator; emphasizes cost-effectiveness), and reactor (doesn't have a coherent strategy) (Miles & Snow, 1978). Existing research suggests that in the fast-paced health care environment, organizations using prospector and analyzer strategies appear to do better than those using de-

fender and reactor strategies (Shortell, Gillies, Anderson, Morgan-Erickson, & Mitchell, 1996).

Differentiation

The major way in which organizations compete is through the array of products and services that they offer. This is referred to as **differentiation** and involves the development of specialized knowledge, functions, departments, and viewpoints (Lawrence & Lorsch, 1967). Some pharmaceutical/biotech companies, such as Merck, offer a broad array of drugs across a wide spectrum of diseases, while others, such as Amgen, have a more narrow "pipeline," focusing on only a few. Some consulting firms offer tax, audit, information technology, and strategic services to their health care clients, while others focus only on strategic services. Some community care networks focus on a wide range of health problems in the community, while others focus on a single problem such as teenage pregnancy or domestic violence (Bazzoli et al., 1997). In general, the greater the degree of differentiation, the greater the managerial challenges to appropriately integrate and coordinate the organization's various products and services offerings. Effective approaches for accomplishing this are discussed in Chapters 5 through 8, 10, and 13.

Integration

All organizations require some degree of coordination across specialized functions and processes in order to achieve unity of effort. This is referred to as integration. Organizations that are more differentiated also require a greater degree of integration. The overall managerial challenge is to appropriately match the levels of differentiation and integration to the demands of the external environment (Lawrence & Lorsch, 1967). While integration has been most studied within individual organizations, health services organizations are increasingly required to integrate their activities across organizational boundaries. This has been particularly true with the growth of health networks and systems, many of which develop complex relationships involving hospitals, physician groups, long-term care facilities, and health plans. The integration challenge within the organization involves issues of work group design (see Chapters 6 and 7), communication and coordination (see Chapter 8), and the overall design of the organization (see Chapter 10). The integration challenge of effectively linking the organization to other organizations involves issues of forging strategic alliances (see Chapter 11) and change and innovation (see Chapter 12). It is important to note that these forms of interorganizational arrangements can be either of a vertical

ownership nature or a virtual contractual nature, depending on the costs and benefits associated with each approach (Conrad & Shortell, 1993; Robinson, 1997).

Centralization

Another important dimension of organizations is the extent to which decision making and selected functions are centralized or decentralized. In a centralized health system, for example, more decisions are made by the top management team of the system than by individual hospitals or physician groups. Also, functions such as strategic planning and marketing would be primarily done centrally rather than within each of the hospitals or physician groups. In a decentralized health system, more decisions, strategic planning, and marketing functions would be primarily done within individual hospitals and physician groups and then "coordinated" at the system-wide level. The degree of centralization has important implications for how quickly decisions get made, how effectively decisions are implemented, the ability of the organization to adapt to change, and how well the organization meets the accountability demands of external groups (Bazzoli; Chan, Shortell, & D'Aunno, 2000). The centralization/decentralization issue is further explored in Chapters 9, 10, 12, and 13.

Change/Innovation

As never before, health services organizations are being called on to develop their capacity for **change** and **innovation**. Three points are particularly relevant. First is to recognize that most health care organizations are extremely complex. Hospitals, for example, typically employ up to 260 different professional/occupational groups, each with their own specialized training, norms, beliefs, and views of the world. Second, most health care organizations, particularly on the provider side, are "loosely coupled" (Weick, 1969) in that hospitals, physicians, and health plans often exist through a loose set of contractual

IN PRACTICE Restructuring Chronic Illness Management

An estimated 125 million Americans have at least one chronic illness with half of these having more than one. People with chronic illness account for the majority of health care spending and result in reduced worker productivity and school absenteeism (National Academy on an Aging Society, 2000).

A number of important questions relevant to assessing an organization's readiness to manage chronic illness must be addressed. Some of these include:

- Is the effective management of care for chronically ill patients an important part of the organization's overall mission?
- Do the goals of functional areas within the organization, and the strategies being used to achieve those goals, support the restructuring of chronic illness treatment processes?
- Are purchasers willing to pay for restructured care processes for chronic illness? Is reimbursement for restructured care processes possible under existing payment procedures?
- Is the organizational culture supportive of coordinated team approaches to patient care?
- Can the existing process of caring for the chronically ill be clearly described? Can its shortcomings be identified? Is the need for restructuring clear in light of these shortcomings?
- Can agreement on reasonable performance targets for the restructured care process be reached in light of the perceived shortcomings of the existing process?
- Can key individuals within the organization who will be affected by a restructured chronic illness treatment process be recruited to participate in that restructuring?
- Is there a "process owner" who will assume leadership responsibility in the restructuring process?
- Is there commitment to having patients meaningfully involved in their own treatment?
- Will the organization commit the resources to training and education that the restructured care process needs to function effectively?
- Do existing compensation systems discourage clinicians from participating in chronic illness treatment teams? Can systems be designed and implemented to reward clinicians and patients for team participation?

Adapted from Christianson, J. B., Taylor, R. A., Knutson, D. J. *Restructuring Chronic Illness Management: Best Practices and Innovations in Team-Based Treatment.* San Francisco: Jossey-Bass, 1998: 163–173.

relationships rather than ownership of each other's assets. Thus, new ideas, plans, and strategies require negotiation and persuasion involving a rather extensive decision-making process. Third, as the number of interorganizational relationships has grown, the ripple effects of any single organization's change become magnified. For example, problems can be created when a hospital belonging to a given system decides to enter into an arrangement with an HMO that is not the system's own HMO. The accompanying "In Practice" highlights relevant change management questions for dealing with these kinds of issues within the context of caring for people with chronic illness. These and related issues of managing change in health care organizations are further discussed in Chapter 12 and 15.

HEALTH SERVICES ORGANIZATIONS AS SYSTEMS

Health services organizations are complex social systems. In managing these organizations, there is a constant tension between the need for predictability, order, and efficiency on the one hand and openness, adaptability, and innovation on the other. The need for predictability, order, and efficiency is consistent with a **closed system** view of an organization. The closed system view assumes that at least parts of an organization can be sealed off from the external environment. As such, the management challenge is how to use internal design, productivity improvement tools, and incentives to maximize internal efficiency.

The need for openness, adaptability, and innovation is consistent with an **open system** view (Scott, 1981). This view emphasizes that organizations are parts of the external environment and, as such, must continually change and adapt to meet the challenges posed by the environment. The emphasis is on meeting the needs of external customers and stakeholders with relatively less emphasis given to issues of internal efficiency.

Both approaches are needed to understand and manage health services organizations. While each activity, function, or department of a health services organization can be considered by itself with its unique requirements and expectations, the real payoff lies in recognizing the interdependence of most activities and functions. One set of functions and activities is usually the building blocks for another set, which, in turn, serves as inputs for still others. These sets of functions, activities, and departments serve as internal environments for each other in addition to being influenced by forces in the external environment. The processes that occur in health services organizations can be described in terms of six primary functions: production, boundary spanning, maintenance, adaptation, management, and governance (Katz & Kahn, 1978).

Production

The **production function** provides the product or service and is at the center of most organizational activity. It is represented by the manufacturing of a new drug in a pharmaceutical company, the diagnosis and treatment of patients in a multispecialty group practice, and the alleviation of pain and suffering in a hospice organization. These core production processes can vary on a number of dimensions including complexity, time, use of labor versus capital, and ease with which results can be measured among others.

Boundary Spanning

The **boundary spanning function** focuses on the interface between the organization and its external environment. It is concerned with new developments in technology, reimbursement, regulation, licensure, changing demographics, customer expectations, competitive threats, and related issues. Depending on the size of the organization and its local market environment, these activities will often vary in their complexity and susceptibility to change. Some organizations will establish certain departments that designate specific individuals or functional areas to carry out boundary spanning activities. In other cases, all employees with managerial responsibilities are required to undertake at least some boundary spanning activities.

Maintenance

The **maintenance function** is concerned with both the physical and human infrastructure of the organization. It includes capital acquisition and maintenance as well as employee growth and development. As the rate of change accelerates and as the external environment becomes more threatening, greater demands are placed on the maintenance functions of health services organizations.

Adaptation

The **adaptation function** focuses on change. Using information obtained from the boundary spanning activities of the organization and with knowledge of the organization's production capability and maintenance support systems, the adaptation function helps the organization to anticipate and adjust to needed changes. This may include the need for new programs and services, deletion or modification of existing programs and services, changes in the organization's structure and design, or major changes in the organization's basic strategy. The adaptation function also emphasizes the health services organization's ability to innovate by actively creating changes in its environment. Given the turbulence of the health services environment, the ability of health services organizations to adapt is of growing importance.

Management

Management is a distinct function that cuts across all the other functions and subsystems. In a sense, it is the "head" that organizes, directs, and oversees all of the other functions. It is represented in most health services organizations by the senior management team and key middle managers.

Governance

Although not usually mentioned in traditional texts, **governance** is added as a sixth distinct function because of the important public trust and social accountability responsibilities of health services organizations. It is the function that holds management and the organization accountable for its actions and that helps provide management with overall strategic

direction in guiding the organization's activities. The pressure for greater accountability in regard to patient outcomes, treatment effectiveness, patient satisfaction, cost containment, and ethical use of resources is posing significant challenges to the governance function of health services organizations.

AREAS OF MANAGERIAL ACTIVITY

Figure 1.3 shows the major areas of activity requiring managerial attention. They include the individual, the group/department, the organization as a whole, the network of interorganizational relationships, and the larger environment that interacts with all of the other spheres. The figure also suggests the complexity of the manager's job in attempting to integrate the various levels of activities in positioning the organization to meet its goals and objectives in the face of environmental challenges.

Traditionally, the individual area has been the primary focus of **organizational behavior** or what is sometimes referred to as the **micro approach** to understanding organizations. The emphasis is on examining individuals within organizations. Chapters 2 through 5 deal with clear examples of organizational behavior issues: managers' role relationships, motivation, leadership, and conflict management. The next area shown is the group/department. These activities typically combine both individual issues and organization-wide issues as they influence group behavior. Chapters 6 through 9, dealing with work groups, work design, coordination and communication, and power and politics, address these issues. The organizational and interorganizational areas shown comprise what is often called the **macro approach** to organizational analysis, particularly as they influence and are influenced by the environment. The organizational area issues are the subject of Chapters

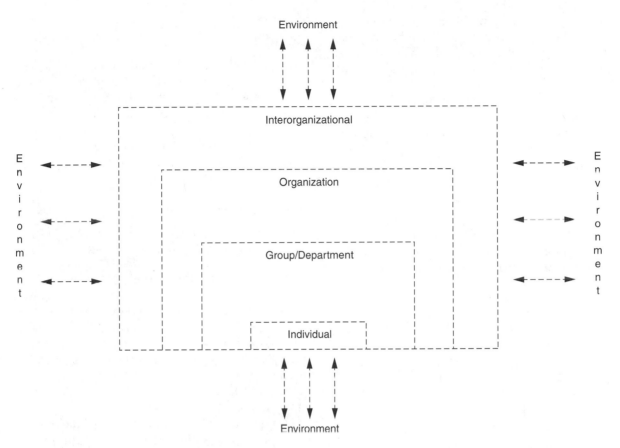

Figure 1.3. Major Areas of Activity

9, 10, 12, 13, and 14. Interorganizational issues are explicitly treated in Chapter 11 on managing strategic alliances. It is important to recognize that these different areas of managerial activity are in reality highly permeable as indicated by the dashed lines. A large part of the executive's job is to manage the complex, dynamic, interactive relationships among the multiple levels. This is what will be required by the leadership of the Henry Ford Health System to deal with the multiple challenges described in the opening scenario of this chapter.

MAJOR PERSPECTIVES ON HEALTH SERVICES ORGANIZATIONS

Everyone has a theory or a perspective on how organizations function. Based on personal experience, we create "mental maps" of what is connected to what and how things happen. In many respects, organization theory consists of the systematic examination of these mental maps of how things work. Over the years, a number of major perspectives of how organizations work have evolved: classical bureaucratic theory, the scientific management school, the human relations school, contingency theory, resource dependence theory, the strategic management perspective, population ecology theory, institutional theory, the social network perspective, and complex adaptive systems. These perspectives can be used to gain insight into the structure and functioning of health services organizations.

Bureaucratic Theory

Classical **bureaucratic theory** is consistent with the closed system approach to organizations and is based on five characteristics.

1. The organization is guided by explicit specific procedures for governing activities.

2. Activities are distributed among office holders.

3. Offices are arranged in a hierarchical fashion.

4. Candidates are selected on the basis of their technical competence.

5. Officials carry out their functions in an impersonal fashion (Weber, 1964).

The bureaucratic organizational form can achieve technical superiority over other forms under certain stable conditions. However, a number of investigators have pointed out dysfunctional consequences of bureaucracy, including its lack of individual freedom, rigidity of behavior, and difficulty in dealing with clients (Gouldner, 1954; Merton, 1957; Selznick, 1966). While most health services organizations are organized along bureaucratic lines to some degree, other forms of organization are better at dealing with rapidly changing environments. The manager's challenge is to decide the extent to which some organizational components might best be organized along bureaucratic lines versus other approaches. Chapters 6, 7, and 10 deal explicitly with this issue.

The Scientific Management School

Closely related to the bureaucratic approach is the **scientific management school** (Gulick & Urwick, 1937; Mooney, 1947; Taylor, 1947). This perspective emphasizes span of control, unity of command, appropriate delegation of authority, departmentalization, and the use of work methods to improve efficiency. The scientific management approach consists of

1. programming the job

2. choosing the right person to match the job

3. training the person to do the job

Much of the early work on job design (see Chapter 7) is based on the scientific management school, as are some current work methods' improvement and operations research approaches. Recent interest in "focused factories"—organizations that specialize in the treatment of selected diseases (e.g., cancer, heart disease, and diabetes)—are largely based on the scientific management school (Herzlinger, 1997).

Using quality of care as an example, the bureaucratic and scientific management approaches would suggest that the quality improvement goals be explicitly defined and that the requirements for achieving these goals be spelled out in detail and expressed in terms of specific job positions and necessary skills. People should then be screened and selected on the basis of defined criteria. The quality improvement function would be hierarchically organized with one department reporting to an overall head who in turn would report to an organization-wide coordinating body. Various rules, policies, and practices would exist for what problems to study, how to study them, and what kinds of information should be generated. The bureaucratic and scientific management schools would help to contribute needed structure to an organization's quality improvement efforts.

The Human Relations School

The focus of the **human relations school** is on the individual. Satisfying individual needs is seen as a worthy goal in itself, not merely a means of achieving other organizational goals (Argyris, 1964; Barnard, 1938; Likert, 1967; McGregor, 1960; Roethlisberger & Dickson, 1939). The approach emphasizes the usefulness of participatory decision making that involves the individual in the organization and the role of intrinsic self-actualizing aspects of work. The approach represents the foundation for many applied organization development efforts and for the reemphasis on empowering individuals associated with total quality management and continuous quality improvement efforts. A number of issues associated with the human relations school are discussed in Chapter 3 on motivation and Chapter 4 on leadership.

The human relations school would emphasize the importance of empowering individuals in the organization to take greater responsibility for improving all aspects of their work. Employees would be given greater autonomy to identify and solve problems. They would be provided with the training and tools to function in this role. A major challenge for organizations in implementing this philosophy of management is to get senior and middle managers to let go of the tendency to want to do things themselves to make sure that they get done right. This requires a culture that is consistently supportive of employee empowerment focused on organizational goals (Rundall, Starkweather, & Norrish, 1998).

Contingency Theory

Proponents of the **contingency theory** (Burns & Stalker, 1961; Lawrence & Lorsch, 1967; Perrow, 1967; Rundall et al., 1998; Thompson, 1967) suggest that a more bureaucratic or "mechanistic" form of organization is more effective when the environment is relatively simple and stable, tasks and tech-

nology are relatively routine, and a relatively high percentage of nonprofessional workers are employed. In contrast, a less bureaucratic or more "organic" form of organization is likely to be more effective when the environment is complex and dynamic, tasks and technologies are nonroutine, and a relatively high percentage of professionals are involved. The more organic organizational form involves decentralized decision making, more participative decision making, and a greater reliance on lateral communication and coordination mechanisms to link people and work units. These mechanisms are appropriate when the environment is complex and nonroutine technologies are involved, because the organization has a greater need for information, expertise, and flexibility. Organic forms of design are better able to respond to these needs. In contrast, where no such demands are made, there is less need for flexibility, and the more traditional bureaucratic approach is likely to be more efficient and effective.

Contingency theorists do not advocate an either/or approach but rather view the process as a continuum from more or less bureaucratic (i.e., mechanistic) to more or less organic. Furthermore, they recognize that different subunits of the organization may be organized differently depending on the specific environments and technologies with which they are involved. Empirical support for contingency theory ideas is mixed depending on whether one is studying the organization as a whole, particular subgroups, or specific individuals (Schoonhoven, 1981). Nonetheless, given the wide variety of health services organizations and different environments in which they operate, the contingency perspective has wide application to health services organizations (Mohr, 1982). The contingency perspective is drawn on throughout this book, including Chapters 7, 8, 10, and 13.

In the case of quality, the contingency perspective would suggest that the quality improvement function might be organized differently depending on the environment faced by each organization, the nature of the clinical problems and other issues being addressed, and the types of employee skills available. For example, in smaller hospitals operating in more stable markets, it may be possible to develop structured approaches to quality improvement and to do so in an orderly fashion by training most employees in quality improvement tools in advance, conducting pilot projects, learning from them, and gradually diffusing them throughout the organization. In more complex hospitals and clinics operating in more dynamic environments, a more flexible approach may be needed. Some of the training may need to occur in a "just in time" fashion, problems may need to be addressed as they arise, and a more flexible structure may need to be used to make rapid changes as required.

Resource Dependence Theory

The **resource dependence theory** emphasizes the importance of the organization's abilities to secure needed resources from its environment in order to survive (Hickson, Hinings, Lee, Schneck, & Pennings, 1971; March & Olsen, 1976; Pfeffer & Salancik, 1978; Strasser, 1983; Williamson, 1981). Those subunits within the organization that have access to key external resources will hold greater power and influence. While organizations desire to maintain their autonomy and remain relatively independent of their environment, they also recognize the need to form certain coalitions or networks to pool resources and reduce transaction costs. The resource dependence perspective, like the strategic management perspective but unlike the population ecology perspective discussed below, assumes that managers can actively influence their environment to reduce unwanted dependencies and enhance survivability. The resource dependence perspective is drawn on in Chapters 2, 9, 11, 13, and 14.

In regard to quality, the resource dependence perspective would emphasize the importance of continuous improvement and total quality management for demonstrating value to purchasers of care. To accomplish this, the organization needs resources from the environment in the form of measurement tools, information systems, and technical expertise to produce valid data on the processes and outcomes of patient care. An organization's ability to exert influence over its environment will depend on how successful it is in demonstrating continuous improvement relative to that of other organizations that patients and purchasers can choose.

Strategic Management Perspective

The **strategic management perspective** emphasizes the importance of positioning the organization relative to its environment and competitors in order to achieve its objectives and ensure its survival (Andrews, 1971; Ansoff, 1965; Ouchi, 1980; Porter, 1980, 1985; Schendel & Hofer, 1979; Shortell & Zajac, 1990; Luke, 2004). The perspective attempts to link environmental forces, internal organizational design and processes, and the strategy of the firm. It suggests that the firm's strategy needs to be consistent with both the external environmental demands and the organization's internal core capabilities and competencies. It is explicitly concerned with issues of organizational performance, arguing that managers and organizational members have discretion in choosing strategies and structures to match the environment in a way that will enhance the organization's performance. Major sub-issues of interest include the different processes by which organizations develop strategies, the formation of strategic alliances, the extent to which organizations are able to successfully change their strategies, and the extent to which organizations vary in their ability to implement strategies. Chapters 11, 13, and 14 of the text highlight many of these issues.

The strategic management and resource dependence perspectives are illustrated by the "In Practice" creation of the Somerbridge Community Health Partnership. The likely success of the partnership will depend on its ability to secure needed resources by aligning its strategies and services with the needs of the population, the partnership's own capabilities, and the larger environmental forces affecting the partnership.

IN PRACTICE

The Somerbridge Community Health Partnership

MICHAEL E. CAPUANO, Mayor, City of Somerville
ROBERT W. HEALY, City Manager, City of Cambridge
In the aftermath of the failed national health care reform debate, the attention of those committed to health care access has again focused closer to home. For many years, using slightly different methods, health and human service providers and community activists in Somerville and Cambridge have worked on local solutions to the health problems confronted by our communities.

Somerville (Massachusetts) and Cambridge (Massachusetts) have a combined population of 170,000. This population is extremely diverse from a socioeconomic, demographic, and cultural perspective. Both cities have experienced significant growth in immigrant populations, with dozens of languages spoken in the homes of these newly arrived residents. Both communities also have extensive health and human service networks and a high level of community activism.

Both Cambridge Hospital and Somerville Hospital have worked for years in collaboration with their respective communities. Separately, both cities conducted community needs assessments in partnership with their community hospitals. This work served to strengthen the connection between the hospitals and residents of each city. It also influenced programs and services provided by the hospitals. However, this work was not coordinated between the two cities until the opportunity for closer collaboration was presented through the community care network (CCN) program.

Through the CCN vision, the Somerbridge Community Health Partnership will facilitate this ongoing community health effort across both cities. The three issue initiatives of Somerbridge—substance abuse, geriatric health and immigrant health—were identified as top priorities through the community needs assessment. It is our dream, as chief executives, that this new collaboration will result in greater opportunities for the residents of our cities as cooperation and improvement guide this project. We truly believe that the Somerbridge partnership will serve as a model of collaboration for other communities to replicate.

Population Ecology Theory

Advocates of the **population ecology theory** (Aldrich, 1979; Delacroix & Carroll, 1983; Hannan & Freeman, 1985, 1989; Kimberly & Zajac, 1985) argue that the environment "selects out" certain organizations for survival. Based on theories of natural selection in biology, the focus is on a given population of organizations rather than on an individual organization. Whether a given organization will succeed depends on where it stands in relation to the population of its competitors and the overall environmental forces influencing that population. As environmental pressures increase, only the stronger, more dominant organizational forms will survive; the weaker forms will cease to exist or will survive only as markedly different forms of organization. In the population ecology approach, unlike the resource dependence and strategic management approaches, there are severe limits on the ability of organizations to adapt. This is expressed in terms of "structural inertia." In this approach, the ability of managers to successfully influence their environments is subsumed to be relatively minor.

The population ecology approach is based on the principles of variation, selection, and retention. Variation involves the continuous development of new organizational forms that add to the variety and complexity in the environment. In health care, examples include freestanding surgery centers, urgent care centers, birthing care centers, hospices, diagnostic imaging centers, fitness centers, and specialty hospitals.

The selection principle states that some of the new organizational forms will fit the external environment better than others. They will be better able to exploit the environment for resources and will move in the same direction that the environmental trends are moving. In health care, ambulatory surgery centers serve as an example as more surgical procedures are being reimbursed on an outpatient basis, and there appears to be a growing trend for consumers to prefer quicker, more accessible, and convenient services.

Retention involves the preservation and ongoing institutionalization of the new organizational form. Those that are valued by the environment in the long run will be retained, while others will fall by the wayside. For example, ambulatory surgery centers may experience relatively long survival (at least until it becomes possible to do most surgery in the patient's home), whereas urgent care centers, faced with stiff competition from physician providers, hospital emergency rooms, and growing regulatory requirements, face a less certain future. The winners may be those organizations that manage to carve out specialized market niches viewed as complementary to other organizations and in which they can act as non-competing sources of patient referrals to other providers.

As health services organizations are faced with increasing cost-containment and competitive pressures, the issues raised by the population ecology perspective become particularly important. In recent years a growing number of general acute care hospitals and HMOs have gone out of business and, as previously noted, a variety of new organi-

zational forms have arisen, including specialty providers in cancer, heart disease, and diabetes. In addition, the hospital industry has been transformed from a largely cottage industry composed of individual hospitals to approximately 600 networks and systems (Bazzoli et al., 1999). These entities, both investor-owned and not-for-profit, are working to find specific niches in the marketplace, focusing in particular on the development of regionally and locally integrated networks of care. While the population ecology perspective tends to minimize the manager's role, it adds an important dimension and challenge to the effective management of health services organizations by emphasizing the importance of networking and coalition building and of developing products and services for specific population segments in which the competitive market forces and related pressures are less threatening (Alexander, Kaluzny, & Middleton, 1986; Carroll, 1984). These issues are further discussed in Chapters 2, 9, 12, 13, and 14.

In the case of quality management, the population ecology approach would suggest that efforts at continuous quality improvement are only germane to the extent that they make the organization form more viable in a changing health care environment. It would emphasize the extent to which quality improvement principles are congruent with the current organization's structure and capabilities. It would suggest that the organization has very little flexibility or ability to modify these approaches if they prove to be inconsistent with its culture and capabilities. If the organization experiences difficulty in incorporating the newer continuous quality improvement approaches, the population ecology school would argue that the organization becomes more susceptible to being "selected against" by other organizations with which the new approach is more compatible.

Institutional Theory

Institutional theory emphasizes that organizations face environments characterized by external norms, rules, and requirements that the organizations must conform to in order to receive legitimacy and support (Alexander & Amburgey, 1987; Meyer & Scott, 1983; Scott, 1987). While technical environments reward organizations for effective and efficient performance, institutional environments emphasize rewarding organizations for having structures and processes that are in conformance with the environment. The rules, beliefs, and norms of the external environment are often expressed in the form of "rational myths" (Alexander & D'Aunno, 1990). Such myths are rational in the sense of being reflected in professional standards, laws, and licensure and accreditation requirements but are myths in the sense that they cannot necessarily be verified empirically. They are, nonetheless, widely held to be true. Conformity with these myths helps the organization to gain legitimacy and support. This conformance is often referred to as "isomorphism" and causes organizations faced with a similar set of environmental circumstances to resemble each other (Fennell & Alexander, 1987). Traditional institutional theorists have emphasized the regulative and normative aspects of rules and conformance (Selznik, 1966), while the "new" institutional theorists have underscored the importance of cultural and cognitive beliefs (Scott, 1995). Institutional theorists have also addressed issues of organizational change highlighting the role played by institutional processes, social processes, and culture (Fligstein, 1990; Powell & DiMaggio, 1991; Scott, Ruef, et al., 2000).

Health services organizations are experiencing a rapid transformation of both their technical and institutional environments. The increased technical pressure for greater efficiency and quality expressed in terms of value is causing health services organizations to change long-established structures (Alexander & D'Aunno, 2003). This is reflected in the reorganization of acute care hospitals as they forge new relationships with physician groups and health plans and the development of new norms and beliefs about what constitutes the effective delivery of health care. This transition results in a great deal of internal conflict that must be managed. Chapter 5 addresses the conflict issues. The implications of the institutional theory perspective on

health services organization are also discussed in Chapters 9, 11, 13, and 14.

From an institutional theory perspective, efforts at continuous quality improvement might be viewed as a response to newly emerging norms and practices within the health services sector. These are being fostered by the Joint Commission on Accreditation of Healthcare Organizations (JCAHO), which has adopted continuous quality improvement as the basis for new accreditation requirements, and by the National Committee for Quality Assurance (NCQA), which has developed quality criteria for health plans. In addition, continuous improvement has been increasingly accepted as a distinguishing feature of an innovative organization with several national awards created to recognize institutions that exert such leadership. Thus, it could be argued that an organization's quality effort is not motivated so much by substantive concerns over its quality or efficiency of care in a competitive marketplace but rather by negative perceptions of external groups if it did not pursue continuous quality improvement (DiMaggio & Powell, 1983; Westphal, Gulati, & Shortell, 1997).

Social Network Perspective

The **social network perspective** emphasizes the importance of social relationships among individuals and groups. The key idea is that all behavior, including economic behavior, is embedded in social relationships. This fundamental precept can be used to understand the behavior of individuals in organizations as well as the diffusion of innovations throughout an organization and interorganizational relationships.

Some key dimensions of the social network perspective include: embeddedness, centrality, strength of ties, direct versus indirect ties, structural equivalence, and structural holes. Embeddedness or density refers to the number of different ways in which two or more units or organizations are linked to each other particularly in regard to their social relationships (Uzzi, 1999). The greater the number of relationships that exist, the more embedded the network. There is some evidence suggesting that more embedded networks offer greater potential to transfer knowledge and facilitate learning (Gulati, 1995; Uzzi, 1997).

Centrality refers to a given unit or an organization's position within the network. It may be thought of being in the middle of relationships or having ready access to others who are connected (Nohria & Berkley, 1992).

Strength of ties refers to the degree or magnitude of ties among individuals, units, or organizations in a given network. It is often measured through frequency of interaction. Ties may also be *direct* or *indirect*. A direct tie occurs when two or more individuals, units, or organizations are not mediated by a third party. Indirect ties involve relationships between two or more individuals, units, or organizations that are mediated by other organizations. Ahuja (2000) has shown that both direct and indirect ties can have a positive impact on an organization's rate of innovation.

Structural equivalence refers to situations in which two individuals, units, or organizations have a tie with a third entity or provide a third entity with the same indirect contacts but the two original units have no direct relationship with each other. They are considered "structurally equivalent" (Burt, 1992) because the third entity gets nothing unique from either of the other ones.

Finally, a structural hole exists in which individuals, units, or organizations "A" and "B" have a tie to "C" but not to each other even though they provide "C" with different indirect contacts. This presents an opportunity for third parties "to fill" the hole or mediate the transactions between the two parties to its own advantage. There is some evidence suggesting that the existence of such holes has a negative impact on organizational innovation (Ahuja, 2000).

The social network perspective is particularly useful to managers and leaders of health services organizations in considering adoption, implementation, and diffusion of clinical and managerial process innovations. The social network perspective complements many of the other perspectives including human relations, resource dependence, institutional theory, strategic adaptation, and complex adaptive

system applications. In the case of implementing total quality management, the social network perspective would underscore the importance of selecting units, divisions, or departments that are centrally located within given networks and that are highly embedded, with a combination of strong and weak ties of a direct and indirect nature.

Complex Adaptive Systems

Complex adaptive systems involve the interaction of people and activities that are highly interdependent but in ways and with outcomes that are not always predictable (Plsek, 2001). Examples include our immune system (Varela & Coutinho, 1991), a colony of ants (Wilson, 1971), the stock market (Mandelbrot, 1999), and most groups of people (Stacey, 1996). Such systems have a number of properties including elements that can change themselves; complex outcomes that can emerge from a few simple rules; nonlinearity of effects in which small changes can result in large effects; emergent creative behavior as an inherent property of the system; orderly properties without a system of central control reflective in the principle of self-organization (Kaufmann, 1995); embeddedness of one system within other systems; and coevolution in which various elements of the system move forward together as they interact over time.

All organizations have features of complex adaptive systems but the perspective is particularly relevant for understanding the complexity of health care organizations operating in a highly uncertain environment (Anderson & McDaniel, 2000; Begun, Zimmerman, & Dooley, 2003). A complex adaptive system perspective views health care organizations as a series of continual experiments to identify the "good" ideas and spread them throughout the organization. Chaos is avoided by the application of simple rules that guide people's behavior and through the development of self-managed groups and teams. Organizations "construct" and shape their environment in addition to being influenced by them.

Organizations and environments "co-evolve" in the case of quality improvement; the complex adaptive system approach would support the use of rapid-cycle plan-do-study-act (PDSA) improvement methods that have been widely used in health care (Berwick, 1998). Such an approach emphasizes the acceleration of experience by planning small changes, studying and learning from those changes, taking corrective action, and identifying those activities and interventions that produce desired results. The emphasis is on developing "good enough" plans to try out and then observing what happens. The focus is also on examining the implications of changes made at one level of the organization on the other levels and anticipating unintended consequences.

Table 1.5 provides a brief summary of how each major theory or perspective would view an organization's quality efforts. It is important to note that none of the perspectives are inherently right or wrong. They are different from each other and incomplete. As such, each represents a partial view of organizational dynamics and can provide input for constructive disagreement and debate, an example of which is highlighted in Debate Time 1.1. It is important to understand the basic assumptions and premises of each perspective, as they can be drawn on in various combinations to provide a greater understanding of how health services organizations operate.

METAPHORS OF HEALTH SERVICES ORGANIZATIONS

The above perspectives are enriched by recasting them as metaphors of health services organizations as shown in Table 1.6 (Morgan, 1986). The eight metaphors are machines, tyrants, brains, playing fields, psychic prisons, biological organisms, political systems, and holograms.

Machines

Classical bureaucratic theory is reflected in the image of the organization as a **machine**. In fact, workers may speak of the organization as a "well-oiled machine." This metaphor reflects the image of an organization as interlocking parts with clearly defined roles that are appropriately meshed together to accomplish the organization's work. Being a well-oiled machine is important for many of the tasks undertaken by health services organizations including the admission of patients into hospitals, the paperwork associated with billing for patient services, the production of a laboratory test, and the processing of a Food and Drug Administration (FDA) application for approval. The downside is that the machines can rapidly become outmoded and inflexible in the face of changing demands and circumstances. An organization whose dominant paradigm is that of a machine that sees order and stability where none exists and rapidly becomes technologically and organizationally obsolete.

Tyrants

Organizations can also behave as **tyrants** or as instruments of domination. In pursuit of their missions, they can lose sight of basic human values and exploit their employees and others either unconsciously or by intent. This may be the basis for many physicians' fears of large complex health services organizations such as the growing health services systems and networks. The mental map that many physicians have is that of the organization as tyrant or potential tyrant restricting their freedom and autonomy and making unilateral decisions without soliciting their input. The tyrant metaphor represents the shadow or dark side of organizational functioning that must be carefully guarded against by the organization's leaders.

Brains

The metaphor of organizations as **brains** places emphasis on the importance of learning, intelligence, and information processing. It is based in part on cybernetic theory, which stresses four key principles.

1. Systems have the capacity to sense, monitor, and scan significant aspects of their environment.

Table 1.5. How Major Perspectives Would View an Organization's Quality Improvement Efforts

Perspective	Point of Emphasis	Contribution
Bureaucratic and scientific management	Explicit goals; hierarchical organization; detailed specifications	Provide needed structure
Human relations	Employee empowerment	Need for a culture supportive of empowerment
Contingency theory	Structure depends on environment, task, technology, and the contingencies facing each unit	Flexible approach needed; adapt efforts to meet the requirements of the situation
Resource dependence	Ability to secure needed resources	Need to demonstrate value through providing reliable and valid data on patient care processes and outcomes
Strategic management	Achieve fit or alignment between the organization's strategy, external enviornment, and internal structure and capabilities	Need to link quality improvement to core strategies and capabilities of the organization
Population ecology	External environmental pressures are primary determinant of success; little managers can do	Highlights powerful role played by external environment; quality improvement efforts alone may not be sufficient if organization is not well positioned within the environment
Institutional theory	External norms, rules, requirements, and relationships cause organizations to conform in order to receive legitimacy; organizations in a similar institutional environment come to resemble each other (i.e., become isomorphic with the environment)	Quality improvement efforts must take into account regulatory and accreditation pressures and public expectations
Social network perspective	All behavior is social in nature, and successful organizations will develop and use social networks to advantage	Adoption, implementation, and transfer of best-quality improvement practices will occur through effective use of social networks
Complex adaptive systems	Organizational elements are highly interdependent, embedded, and unpredictable. Progress is made through experimentation, application of simple rules, and coevolution of the organization and its environment.	Emphasizes importance of experimentation, innovation, and rapid information sharing to facilitate improved performance

DEBATE TIME 1.1   What Do You Think?

In recent years a number of health services organizations and health supplier organizations have either merged, consolidated, or gone out of business. How might this be explained? Population ecology theory, of course, would assert that the environmental variables involving reimbursement rates, competitive factors, technological growth, and societal forces are the primary causes of this organizational restructuring. They would further argue that these organizations and their managers could do relatively little to prevent the eventual outcomes. Basically, the organization was no longer "fit" given the changing environmental forces.

In contrast, the resource dependence and strategic management perspectives argue that organizations have considerable control over their destiny. Through actions taken by organization leaders and members, new strategies, policies and procedures, alliances, changes in structure, and hiring of new or different kinds of people can be initiated in order to improve the organization's "fit" with changing environmental forces and to ensure its viability. They point to examples of organizational "turnarounds" that suggest the reasons why some organizations are restructured or closed, while others survive has more to do with the vision

and talent of the organization and its members than with externally generated environmental forces. Which view is more correct?

Does the Literature Help?

". . . [T]he corporatization of health care in the United States has been precipitated by a transformation of institutional systems rather than by rational or strategic adaptation by individual organizations to changes in their operating environments." (Morgan, 1986)

"Our view is simply that most relevant environmental forces are, in fact, organizationally created and sustained, and thus are subject to organizational influence." (Alexander & D'Aunno, 1990, p. 79)

"The basic feature of the natural selection perspective is that the environment selects the most fit or optimal organizations. The organization is thus seen as relatively powerless to affect the selection process. But our review of some of the research on health care organizations suggests otherwise. Furthermore, from a managerial perspective it is difficult to accept so much organizational fatalism and inevitability." (Shortell & Zajac, 1990, p. 169)

2. Systems can relate this information to the norms that guide system behavior.

3. Systems can detect significant deviations from these norms.

4. Systems are able to initiate corrective actions when discrepancies are detected. (Starkweather & Cook, 1988)

When these conditions hold, a continuous process of information exchange is created between an or-

ganization and its environment allowing the system to operate in a spontaneous self-correcting manner. This operation is characterized by double-loop learning, which involves an ability to take a second look at a situation by questioning the relevance of underlying assumptions (Morgan, 1986, p. 87). The brain metaphor is particularly useful for health services organizations in terms of maximizing the ability of individuals and groups to learn from their environment and make use of the information to create innovative programs and services. It is consistent

Table 1.6. Organizational Perspectives and Metaphors

Organizational Perspectives	Relevant Metaphors
Classical bureaucratic theory →	Machines Tyrants
Human relations school →	Brains Playing fields Psychic prisons
Contingency theory →	Biological organisms Brains
Resource dependency theory →	Political systems Playing fields
Strategic management perspective →	Biological organisms Holograms
Population ecology theory →	Biological organisms
Institutional theory →	Biological organisms
Social network perspective →	Playing fields Political systems
Complex adaptive systems →	Biological organisms Holograms

with the human relations school's emphasis on personal growth and development.

Playing Fields

Organizations can also be viewed as **playing fields** or stages upon which individuals perform their "art." For health services organizations, this frequently involves a complex performance by many different talented individuals. These professionals—physicians, nurses, therapists, technologists, researchers, executives, and many others—have a highly developed sense of professionalism and professional identity. As such, they frequently clash as one culture emphasizes its beliefs and values relative to others in competing for resources. The result is often "tribal warfare," which must be managed (Ar-

gyris, 1982). The challenge is to create a larger overall sense of organizational identity and culture that can embrace the individual cultures of the different health professionals. Social networks can be viewed as playing fields for promoting desired behavior. When this is done, the goals articulated by the human relations school are met, and people are able to work effectively in performing interdependent tasks.

Psychic Prisons

Organizations can also be viewed as places where people are trapped by their own perceptions, ideas, and beliefs whether consciously or unconsciously. Often this is reflected in the tendency to avoid conflict, to avoid anxiety-provoking situations, or to strive to maintain one's sense of identity and self-esteem. These issues can be particularly important in health services organizations because, as noted above, individuals identify strongly with their professional disciplines. When these needs are concretized in a way that allows no room for other perspectives or viewpoints, the result is indeed a **psychic prison** stifling organizational learning, innovation, and the ability to adapt. It is the negative side of the human relations school's emphasis on personal growth and development.

Biological Organisms

In recent years it has become popular to think of organizations as **biological organisms**; that is, as different species that must adapt to their environments in the process of birth, growth, decline, and eventual death. It is concerned with the issue of how the organization becomes fit to survive in its environment. As shown in Table 1.6, contingency theory, strategic management perspective, population ecology theory, institutional theory, and complex adaptive systems each contain major aspects of the biological organism metaphor. Contingency theory primarily emphasizes internal organization design and fit, while the strategic management perspective emphasizes the fit of the organization's strategy with its environment. The population ecology approach emphasizes the strength of the external forces that essentially select out various organizational species for survival. Institutional theory suggests that one way in which organizations can succeed is to mimic or match the values and norms contained in the environment in order to maintain necessary legitimacy and credibility with environmental sources of sanctions and power. Complex adaptive systems remind us that organizations co-evolve with their environment and in ways that may be unpredictable in advance due to emergent properties of the coevolution process itself. The biological organism metaphor highlighting the interplay of the organization with the environment over time can provide many useful insights for health services managers. Organizations of different sizes and at different stages in their existence require different resources and different strategies to ensure success.

Political Systems

Organizations, of course, can also be viewed as **political systems** in which various groups and actors vie for control of important resources. Organizations are ruled by whomever controls these resources and decides how they are used to accomplish the interests of various groups. Given the many different kinds of professionals working in or affiliated with health services organizations, the political system metaphor is particularly salient. Physicians, executives, nurses, researchers, and others often vie for control over important resources to push their own view of what is good for the organization. The political system metaphor is closely aligned with the playing field metaphor in which the organization essentially serves as the playing field or battleground for control. When things get out of control, health services organizations can turn into psychic prisons or tyrants. Resource dependence theory and the social network perspective are consistent with the political system metaphor as they focus on the ways in which organizations acquire and control needed resources.

Holograms

A **hologram** is an object in which each of the parts contains the entire essence of the overall object or image. As a result, the overall object or system can continue to function even when specific parts malfunction or are removed. While this metaphor is often used in conjunction with the brain metaphor and can be considered an important aspect of the brain metaphor, we believe that treating it separately provides some special insights. In a holographic structure the intent is to design the whole into the parts and to create a redundancy of parts so that a range of functions can be performed rather than just a single specialized activity. Designing health services organizations as holograms emphasizes the need for flexibility, creativity, change, and innovation. An organization's culture, its design, and its information-processing capabilities are facilitators of holographic properties. These are properties of complex adaptive systems. The metaphor is also consistent with the strategic management perspective's emphasis on viewing the organization as a whole in positioning its various elements to deal with outside forces while at the same time recognizing the interplay between those forces and internal organizational components. The idea is to see the organization's strategy as being expressed in the task and function of an individual worker as well as in the accumulation of worker activities across multiple tasks; that is, the "part–whole relationship." Viewing health services organizations as holograms can provide powerful insights contributing to the need for integrating multiple components of health services delivery into a more coherent whole. A micro example is provided by the cross-training of workers such that more functions and activities are contained in a single individual. A macro example is provided by the efforts of some health services organizations to develop regionally based vertically integrated delivery systems to provide more coordinated care across the range of patient needs.

These metaphors are intended to challenge the reader's thinking about health services organizations and to provide a lens for interpreting the chapters that follow. While they are presented in a sequential and categorical fashion, it is important to note that they represent a continuum of perspectives that may overlap each other. Having learned about them, revisit the issues posed in Debate Time 1.1. Have your views of these issues changed?

ORGANIZATION THEORY AND BEHAVIOR: A FRAMEWORK FOR THE TEXT

As discussed in the various perspectives and metaphors above, the essence of management is to motivate people and groups to carry out technical tasks for the attainment of organizational goals and at the same time to position the organization for long-run survival and growth as it charts the future. These dimensions of the managerial challenge are outlined in Figure 1.4, which provides a basic framework for the book and a focus for the development of specific **managerial competencies**.

The book is divided into five parts. The first is an introductory part that provides an overview of perspectives on the management of health services organizations (Chapter 1) and an analysis of the evolving role of management in these organizations (Chapter 2). This is followed by four parts corresponding to the managerial activities of motivating and leading people and groups, operating the technical system, positioning the organization for success, and charting the future.

Managers must motivate and lead people to ensure high levels of commitment, stability, and cooperative behavior. This is accomplished by satisfying individual needs and values (Chapter 3), by providing direction (Chapter 4), and by managing conflict and negotiation processes (Chapter 5). These needs are primarily met by drawing on the manager's execution and people competencies.

Managers must also operate the technical system in response to challenges of technical performance involving productivity, efficiency, quality, and customer satisfaction. This is accomplished by determining the appropriate work groups and work design (Chapters 6 and 7), establishing communication and coordination mechanisms (Chapter 8), and using appropriate influence processes (Chapter 9). These challenges are primarily met by drawing on the manager's execution and people competencies.

Organizations operate within a constantly changing environment, and managers must position the organization for success by determining effective organizational design (Chapter 10), acquiring resources and managing interorganizational relationships (Chapter 11), managing change, innovation, and learning (Chapter 12), and attaining organizational goals (Chapter 13). These demands draw heavily on the manager's transformational competencies.

Finally, organizations function through time, and managers must be responsive to the challenges of long-term survival and growth of the organization. This is accomplished by managing strategically (Chapter 14) and anticipating the future (Chapter 15). The framework presented in Figure 1.4 is intended as a departure point, not a point of closure, for the reader's own synthesis of the material that follows.

DISCUSSION QUESTIONS

1. As you think about the challenges facing Henry Ford Health System in the opening scenario, which of the major perspectives on organizations (bureaucratic, scientific management, human relations, contingency, resource dependence, strategic management, population ecology, institutional social network perspective, and complex adaptive system) would offer you the most assistance? Defend your choice.

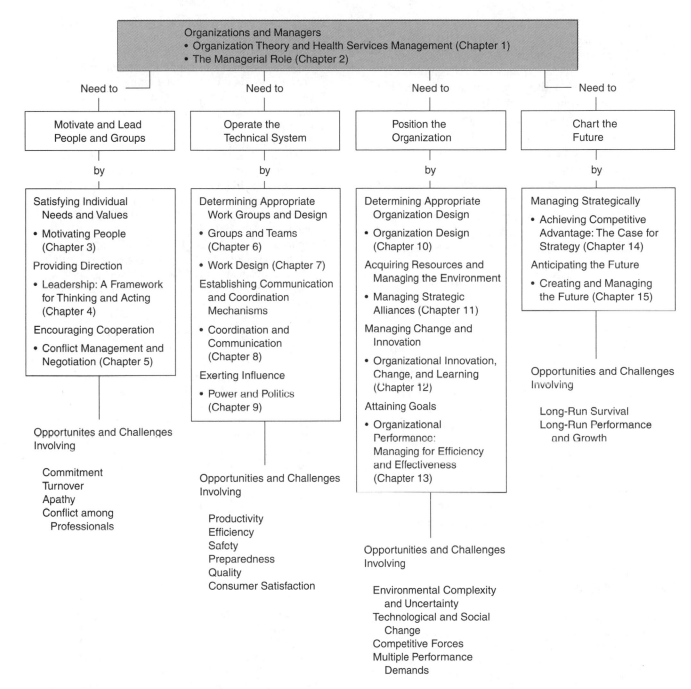

Figure 1.4. The Nature of Organizations: Framework for the Text

2. During the past decade, hundreds of hospitals have closed, merged, or entered into various strategic alliances. How would you attempt to explain this reorganization? In addressing this question, refer to Debate Time 1.1 and consider the resource dependence, strategic management, population ecology, institutional and complex adaptive system perspectives on organizations.

3. Several community health centers have hired you as a consultant to help them form an umbrella organization that in turn would be merged with the local county health department. Which of the metaphors of organizations (machine, tyrant, brain, playing field, psychic prison, biological organism, political system, hologram) would provide you with the greatest insight as you take on this assignment? Defend your choice.

4. State whether you agree or disagree with the following statement: For the most part, health services organizations are no different from most other organizations. Indicate the specific reasons for your agreement or disagreement and develop at least two reasons in addition to those presented in the chapter.

5. Networks and alliances are marriages of money and convenience. Systems are marriages of commitment and values. Develop arguments and counterarguments for each statement.

REFERENCES

Ahuja, G. (2000). Collaboration networks, structural holes, and innovation: A longitudinal study. *Administrative Science Quarterly, 45*(3), 425–455.

Aldrich, H. (1979). *Organizations and environments.* Englewood Cliffs, NJ: Princeton Hills.

Alexander, J. A., & Amburgey, T. L. (1987). The dynamics of change in the American hospital industry: Transformation or selection? *Medical Care Review, 44,* 279–321.

Alexander, J. A., & D'Aunno, T. A. (1990). Transformation of institutional environments: Perspectives on the corporatization of U. S. health care. In S. S. Mick and Associates, *Innovations in health care delivery: Insights for organizational theory* (pp. 53–85). Ann Arbor, MI: Health Administration Press.

Alexander, J. A., & D'Aunno, T. A. (2003). Alternative perspectives on institutional and market relationships in the U.S. health care sector. In S. Mick W. Wyttenbach (Eds.), *Advances in Health Care Organization Theory,* (pp. 45–77). San Francisco: Jossey-Bass.

Alexander, J. A., Kaluzny, A. D., & Middleton, S. C. (1986). Organizational growth, survival and death in the U. S. hospital industry: A population ecology perspective. *Social Science and Medicine, 22,* 303–308.

Anderson, R. & R. McDaniel. (2000). Managing health care organizations: Where professionalism meets complexity science. *Health Care Management Review, 25*(1), 83–92.

Andrews, K. R. (1971). *The concept of corporate strategy.* Homewood, IL: Dow Jones-Irwin.

Ansoff, H. I. (1965). *Corporate strategy: An analytic approach to business policy for growth and expansion.* New York: McGraw-Hill.

Argyris, C. (1964). *Integrating the individual and the organization.* New York: John Wiley & Sons.

Argyris, C. (1982). *Reasoning, learning, and action.* San Francisco: Jossey-Bass.

Baker, G. R., & Wakefield, D. (2001). Domains and core competencies for effective evidence-based practice—Quality improvement. *Journal of Health Administration, Special Issue,* 177–186.

Barnard, C. I. (1938). *The functions of the executive.* Cambridge, MA: Harvard University Press.

Bazzoli, G. J., Chan, B., Shortell, S. M., & D'Aunno, T. (2000). The financial performance of hospitals belonging to health networks and systems. *Inquiry,* Fall, 234–252.

Bazzoli, G. J., Shortell, S. M., Dubbs, N., Chan, C., & Kralovec, P. (1999, February). A taxonomy of health networks and systems: Bringing order out of chaos. *Health Services Research, 34.*

Bazzoli, G. J., Stein, R., Alexander, J. A., Conrad, D. A., Sofaer, S., & Shortell, S. M. (1997). Public-private collaboration in health and human service delivery: Evidence from community partnerships. *The Milbank Quarterly, 75*(4), 533–561.

Begun, J. W., Zimmerman, B., & Dooley, K. J. (2003). Health care organizations as complex adaptive systems. In S. Mick & M. Wyttenbach (Eds.), *Advances in Health Care Organization Theory,* (pp. 253–288). San Francisco Jossey-Bass.

Berwick, D. M. (1998). Developing and testing changes in delivery of care. *Annals Internal Medicine, 128*(8), 651–656.

Bogue, R., & Hall, C. H. (Eds.). (1995). *Health network innovation their systems through collaboration.* American Hospital Publishing.

Burns, T., & Stalker, G. M. (1961). *The management of innovation.* London: Tavistock.

Burt, R. S. (1992). *Structural holes: The social structure of competition.* Cambridge, MA: Harvard University Press.

Carroll, G. R. (1984). Organizational ecology. *Annual Review of Sociology, 10,* 71–93.

Christianson, J. B., Taylor, R. A., & Knutson, D. J. (1998). *Restructing chronic illness management: Best practices and innovations in team-based treatment.* San Francisco, CA: Jossey-Bass.

Conrad, D. A., & Shortell, S. M. (1993, Fall). Integrated health systems: Promise and performance. *Frontiers of Health Services Management, 13*(1), 3–42.

Delacroix, J., & Carroll, G. R. (1983). Organizational foundings: An ecological study of newspaper industries of Argentina and Ireland. *Administrative Sciences Quarterly, 28,* 274–291.

DiMaggio, P. J., & Powell, W. W. (1983). The iron cage revisited: Institutional isomorphism and collective rationality in organizational fields. *American Sociological Review, 48,* 147–160.

Fennell, M., & Alexander, J. A. (1987). Organizational boundary spanning and institutionalized environments. *Academy of Management Journal, 30,* 456–476.

Fligstein, N. (1990). *The transformation of corporate control.* Cambridge, MA: Harvard University Press.

Gouldner, A. (1954). *Patterns of industrial bureaucracy.* New York: Free Press.

Gulati, R. (1995). Does familiarity breed trust? The implications of repeated ties for contractual choice in alliances. *Academy of Management Journal, 38,* 85–112.

Gulick, L., & Urwick, L. (1937). *Papers on science of administration.* New York: Columbia University Press.

Halverson, P. K., Kaluzny, A. D., McLaughlin, C. P., & Mays, G. P. (1998). *Managed care and public health.* Gaithersburg, MD: Aspen Publishers, Inc.

Hannan, M. T., & Freeman, J. H. (1985, April). Structural inertia and organizational change. *American Sociological Review,* 149–164.

Hannan, M. T., & Freeman, J. H. (1989). *Organizational ecology.* Cambridge, MA: Harvard University Press.

Herzlinger, R. (1997). *Market driven health care.* Reading, MA: Addison-Wesley.

Hickson, D. J., Hinings, C. R., Lee, C. A., Schneck, R. E., & Pennings, J. M. (1971). A strategic contingencies theory of intraorganizational power. *Administrative Science Quarterly, 16,* 216–229.

Institute of Medicine. (2001). *Crossing the quality chasm: A new health system for the 21st century.* Washington, DC: National Academy Press, 6.

Katz, E., & Kahn, R. (1978). *The social psychology of organizations* (2nd ed.). New York: John Wiley & Sons.

Kauffman, S. A. (1995). *At home in the universe.* Oxford, England: Oxford University Press.

Kimberly, J. R., & Zajac, E. J. (1985). Strategic adaptation in health care organizations: Implications for theory and research. *Medical Care Review, 42,* 267–302.

Lawrence, P., & Lorsch, J. (1967). *Organization and environment.* Cambridge, MA: Harvard University Press.

Likert, E. (1967). *The human organization.* New York: McGraw-Hill.

Luke, R. (2004). *Health care strategy.* Chicago, IL: HAP/AUPHA.

March, J. G., & Olsen, J. P. (1976). *Ambiguity and choice in organizations.* Bergen, Norway: Univeristetsforlaget.

McGregor, D. (1960). *The human side of enterprise.* New York: McGraw-Hill.

Merton, R. K. (1957). Bureaucratic structure and personality. In *Social theory and social structure.* New York: Free Press.

Meyer, J. W., & Scott, W. R. (1983). *Organizational environments: Ritual and rationality.* Beverly Hills, CA: Sage.

Miles, R. E., & Snow, C. C. (1978). *Organizational strategy, structure, and process.* New York: McGraw-Hill.

Mohr, L. B. (1982). *Explaining organizational behavior.* San Francisco: Jossey-Bass.

Mooney, J. E. (1947). *Principles of organization.* New York: Harper & Row.

Morgan, G. (1986). *Images of organization.* Beverly Hills, CA: Sage Library of Social Research.

National Academy on an Aging Society. (2000). Workers and chronic conditions: Opportunities to improve productivity. Retrieved from http://www.partnershipforsolutions.org/pdf_files/workers.pdf

National Center for Health Care Leadership (2004) Competency Model 2.0, Chicago IL.

Nohria, N., & Berkley, J. D. (1992). The virtual organization: Bureaucracy, technology and the imposition of control. In C. Heckscher & A. Donnellon (Eds.), *The post bureaucratic organization: New perspectives on organizational change,* (pp. 32–47). Thousand Oaks, CA: Sage Publications.

Ouchi, W. G. (1980). Markets, bureaucracies, and clans. *Administrative Science Quarterly, 24,* 129–141.

Perrow, C. (1967). A framework for the comparative analysis of organizations. *American Sociological Review, 32,* 194–208.

Pew Commission on Education for the Health Professions, Health Care Administration. (1993). Philadelphia: Pew Charitable Trusts.

Pfeffer, J., & Salancik, G. R. (1978). *The external control of organizations.* New York: Harper & Row.

Plsek, P. (2001). Redesigning health care with insights from the science of complex adaptive systems. In *Crossing the quality chasm: A new health system for the 21st century* (pp. 309–322), Washington DC: National Academy Press.

Porter, M. E. (1980). *Competitive strategy: Techniques for analyzing industries and competitors.* New York: Free Press.

Porter, M. E. (1985). *Competitive advantage: Creating and sustaining superior performance.* New York: Free Press.

Powell, W. W., & DiMaggio, P. J. (Eds.). (1991). *The new institutionalism in organizational analysis.* Chicago: University of Chicago Press.

Robinson, J. (1997, March). Physician-hospital integration and the economic theory of the firm. *Medical Care Research and Review, 54*(1), 3–24.

Roethlisberger, F. J., & Dickson, W. J. (1939). *Management and the worker.* Cambridge, MA: Harvard University Press.

Rundall, T., Starkweather, D., & Norrish, B. (1998). *After restructuring: Empowerment strategies at work in America's hospitals.* San Francisco: Jossey-Bass, Inc.

Schendel, D. E., & Hofer, C. W. (1979). *Strategic management: A new view of business policy and planning.* Boston: Little, Brown.

Schoonhoven, C. B. (1981, September). Problems with contingency theory: Testing assumptions hidden within the language of contingency "theory." *Administrative Science Quarterly, 26,* 349–377.

Scott, W. R. (1981). Developments in organization theory, 1960–1980. *American Behavioral Scientist, 24,* 407–422.

Scott, W. R. (1987). The adolescence of institutional theory: Problems and potential for organizational analysis. *Administrative Science Quarterly, 32,* 493–512.

Scott, W. R. (1995). *Institutions and organizations.* Thousand Oaks, CA: Sage Publications.

Scott, W. R., Ruef, M., et al. (2000). *Institutional change and healthcare organizations: From professional dominance to managed care.* Chicago, IL: Chicago University Press.

Selznick, P. (1966). *TVA and the grass roots.* New York: Harper & Row.

Shortell, S. M., Gillies, R. R., Anderson, D. A., Mitchell, J. B., & Morgan, K. L. (1993, Winter). Creating organized delivery systems: The barriers and facilitators. *Hospital and Health Services Administration, 38*(4), 447–466.

Shortell, S. M., Gillies, R. R., Anderson, D. A., Morgan-Erickson, K., & Mitchell, J. B. (1996). *Remaking health care in America: Building organized delivery systems.* San Francisco: Jossey-Bass Publishers.

Shortell, S. M., & Zajac, E. J. (1990). Health care organizations and the development of the strategic management perspective. In S. S. Mick and

Associates, *Innovations in health care delivery: Insights for organization theory* (pp. 144–180). Ann Arbor, MI: Health Administration Press.

Stacey, R. D. (1996a). *Complexity and creativity in organizations.* San Francisco: Berrett-Koehler.

Stacey, R. D. (1996b). *Strategic management and organizational dynamics.* London: Pittman Publishing.

Starkweather, D., & Cook, K. S. (1988). Organization-environment relations. In S. M. Shortell & A. D. Kaluzny (Eds.), *Health care management: A text in organization theory and behavior* (2nd ed.) (p. 352).

Strasser, S. (1983, Winter). The effective application of contingency theory in health settings: Problems and recommended solutions. *Health Care Management Review,* 15–23.

Taylor, F. (1947). *Scientific management.* New York: Harper & Row.

Thompson, J. D. (1967). *Organization in action.* New York: McGraw-Hill.

Uzzi, B. (1997). Social structure and competition in interfirm networks: The paradox of embeddedness. *Administrative Science Quarterly, 42*(1), 35–67.

Uzzi, B. (1999). Embeddedness in the making of financial capital: How social relations and networks benefit firms seeking financing. *American Sociological Review, 64,* 481–505.

Varela, F., & Coutinho, A. (1991). Second generation immune networks. *Immunology Today, 12*(5), 159–166.

Walshe, K., & Rundall, T. (2001). Evidence-based management: From theory to practice in healthcare delivery. *The Milbank Quarterly, 29*(3), 438.

Weber, M. (1964). *The theory of social and economic organization.* Glencoe, IL: Free Press.

Weick, K. E. (1969). *The social psychology of organizations.* Reading, MA: Addison-Wesley Publishing Co.

Westphal, J. D., Gulati, R., & Shortell, S. M. (1997). Customization or conformity? An institutional and network perspective on the content and consequences of TQM adoption. *Administrative Science Quarterly, 42,* 366–394.

Williamson, O. E. (1981). The economies of organization: The transaction cost approach. *The American Journal of Sociology, 87,* 548–577.

Wilson, E. O. (1971). *The Insect Societies.* Cambridge, MA: Harvard University Press.

CHAPTER 2

The Managerial Role

William E. Welton, Dr. P.H., M.H.A.

CHAPTER OUTLINE

❧ Framing the Managerial Role from a Behavioral Perspective

❧ The Practice of Management in Health Care Organizations: Integrating Organizational Process Management and Professional Leadership Roles and Skills

❧ Placing the Health Care Management Role in a Strategic Perspective

❧ Exploring Health Care's Distinctive Context and Executive Leadership Requirements

❧ Crossing the Quality Chasm: Distinctive Challenges for Health Service Managers

❧ Developing a Standardized Knowledge Base for Professional Leadership and for Health Care Managers within the Health Care Industry

LEARNING OBJECTIVES

After completing this chapter, the reader should be able to:

1. Understand the managerial role and how it is derived from organization and management theory.

2. Recognize the executive leadership challenges posed by the need to integrate and align internal organization structure and culture with the external environment.

3. Understand the strategic context of organizational effectiveness and its implications for managerial action.

4. Understand the relationship between enterprise management and clinical systems management roles in health care delivery organizations, including the challenges in integrating these important roles within complex health care delivery systems and communities.

5. Understand the requirements of and interactions among systemic organizational structure, managerial process management, and executive leadership roles in assuring high-quality organizational management.

6. Recognize the importance and special challenges associated with managing and leading within the "distinctive" health care context.

7. Recognize the special challenges to executive leaders and organizational managers of health care delivery systems that are associated with addressing the aims and challenges posed by the Institute of Medicine in its watershed report, *Crossing the Quality Chasm: A New Health System for the 21st Century* (2001).

8. Recognize the importance of viewing management as an integrated and integrating activity, requiring strong conceptual, transformational, execution, and people skills applied within an emerging context of professional leadership competencies.

KEY TERMS

Organizational Adaptation
Clinical Care System(s)
Conceptual Skills
Conceptual/Mental/System Models
Enterprise System(s)/Management Role(s)

Executive Leadership Role
Execution Skills
External Environment
Human Relations
Integrating Skills
Managerial Accountability
Mental Models

Organizational Framework
Organizational Transformation
Strategic Management
Transformational Leadership Role
Value-Oriented Leadership

❦ IN PRACTICE   A Medical Center in Transition (1) . . . The CEO Perspective

September 1985. James Varnum, president and CEO of the Mary Hitchcock Memorial Hospital (MHMH) in Hanover, NH, reflected on the viable strategic options confronting the hospital and on the seven-year path he had taken to reach this point.

The hospital, preparing to enter its ninth decade of operation, had a rich history of service to the northern New England region (predominantly the Upper Connecticut River Valley). Since its founding in 1893, the hospital had been the primary teaching hospital for the Dartmouth Medical School (DMS), the nation's fourth oldest medical school, founded in 1797. This role was disrupted from 1914 through 1970 by Dartmouth College's decision to suspend its granting of the MD degree. In 1966, Dartmouth College decided to reestablish its role as an MD degree-granting institution, graduating its first

modern MD class in 1973. The decision required the support of three key partners to provide clinical training experiences for its medical students. These three partner organizations were: the MHMH; the Hitchcock Clinic (HC), a more than 120-member multi-specialty medical group practice founded in 1927 and serving as the MHMH medical staff for half a century; and the Veteran's Hospital in nearby White River Junction, Vermont.

The MHMH/HC clinical partnership (1927 through 1977) developed a strong regional and national reputation. During this period, MHMH and HC operated as organizational partners, developing an extremely strong and collaborative culture based on clinical and service excellence. Neither organization controlled the other. By 1970, however, the college, hospital, and clinic all agreed on the

(continues)

need to create a new organizational vehicle through which they could cooperate in the critical joint functions of program planning, investment, and development required to build a modern academic medical center. Those involved recognized the need to invest in new facilities, new programs, and additional faculty and clinical leadership to support a three-part mission of providing medical education, medical research, and clinical services. They decided to form a "shared service organization," the Dartmouth-Hitchcock Medical Center (DHMC) (http://www.dhmc.org) through which they could accomplish the goal of developing the medical center.

It was into this mix that Varnum, a Dartmouth College graduate and an experienced academic medical center hospital CEO, arrived in 1978. He succeeded William L. Wilson, a highly respected CEO who retired following a distinguished 30-year career. Varnum's principal job was to move MHMH into its new role as the principal teaching hospital for DMS, while maintaining the MHMH board's long-standing commitment to community-accountable governance and to the provision of efficient and effective clinical services. As he arrived, it was clear that the newly enhanced mission would require significant investments in new facilities and equipment, new tertiary clinical programs, and enhanced educational programs. It was also clear that the hospital's partners were looking to MHMH to provide the majority of resources to make these investments. From the hospital's perspective, its trustees were supportive of assuming these responsibilities—but only under a strong shared program planning organization, operated under a strong and publicly accountable shared governance structure. This would require a significant transformation of the complicated series of bilateral and trilateral business and organizational relationships among the medical center partner organizations. It would be a daunting task, requiring several years to complete.

CHAPTER PURPOSE

As described in the unfolding events involving James Varnum and his colleagues at the Mary Hitchcock Memorial Hospital, effective management requires an understanding of the context of health care and of the interpersonal and/or interinstitutional dynamics as they evolve over time. Health care organizations are distinctively complex and strategically managed social structures that operate within a dynamically changing "open system"—the health system. Health care managers must play a combination of executive leadership, organizational management, and strategic management roles on behalf of both

their business enterprises and the clinical and business service components within them. In this context, the health care manager is principally concerned with assuring appropriate and timely organizational adaptation and transformation. We will explore this overarching theme throughout this chapter.

The health care system provides a unique product—personal health services. Core managerial roles within any given "health system" organization must assure continuous access to the types and quantities of resources required to ensure the organization's long-term survival. At the same time, managers must assure the safety, efficacy, efficiency, and quality of services provided. Health care managers and executive leaders must complete this task by influencing and/or controlling:

1. Interactions between the organization and its systemic environment(s), and the

2. Rate and extent of organizational transformation and adaptation, and by assuring the

3. Appropriateness and mix of services offered, while assuring the quality, safety, efficacy, efficiency, and profitability of the organization's core products and services relative to market and community needs.

FRAMING THE MANAGERIAL ROLE FROM A BEHAVIORAL PERSPECTIVE

While significant time can be spent discussing details of traditional formulations of the managerial role, it is important to note that these traditional descriptions of the managerial role tend to emphasize tasks, activities, and processes. Such descriptions must be integrated with a broader discussion of executive leadership and managerial behavior. At its core, management is an integrated and dynamically applied activity. This work takes place within a context of dynamic system change and evolution. Thus, the following discussion will focus on these concepts rather than on a more traditional description of tasks, activities, and processes. This is a particularly important consideration given our focus on the strategically oriented **transformational leadership role** of management in assuring timely and appropriate organizational adaptation to environmental challenges and opportunities.

Core Management Roles

Mintzberg and his colleagues have made some of the most insightful observations about managerial roles, the nature of managerial work, and basis of man-

agement behavior (Mintzberg, 1990; Mintzberg, 1994; Mintzberg & Gosling, 2003). In a key early article Mintzberg (1990) defined ten roles of managers and organized them into three domains—interpersonal, informational, and decisional.

1) Interpersonal roles
   a) Figurehead
   b) Leader
   c) Liaison
2) Informational roles
   a) Monitor
   b) Disseminator
   c) Spokesperson
3) Decisional roles
   a) Entrepreneur
   b) Disturbance handler
   c) Resource allocator
   d) Negotiator

Although each of these roles is self-descriptive, it is important to view them together as an integrated system of roles. As described by Mintzberg (1990), these "ten roles are not easily separable   and, in all cases the interpersonal, informational, and decisional roles remain inseparable."

Mintzberg (1994) subsequently extended his thinking, noting that: "The integrated job of managing has been lost in the conventional ways of describing it—as individual behaviors, such as leading, controlling, communicating, and so on." Instead, he presents a model of the management job, beginning with the manager at the center of the model and working out, layer by layer, to include: (a) the person in the job, (b) the frame of the job, and (c) the agenda of the work (Mintzberg, 1994).

The Person in the Job

Managers bring a unique combination of personal values, personal experience, and personal stylistic preferences to their job assignments. One of the most important issues in this context is the element of personal experience, the combination of personal skills and competencies developed over time, and a set of personal knowledge elements gained through formal and informal means. Managers integrate the knowledge gained into **mental models** they use to guide their interpretation of environmental conditions and actions and their assumptions about whether and when to take action.

Each combination of elements is unique to each individual manager, meaning that any given individual with managerial responsibilities is likely to interpret or react somewhat differently when confronted with the same environmental or organizational stimuli. Thus, the fundamental importance of the person in the job is apparent.

The Frame of the Job

Mintzberg (1994) defines the "frame" of the job as the mental set the incumbent uses to carry out the job. The frame is a combination of four elements: organizational purpose, organizational perspective, organizational positions, and organizational conceptualization. All these elements are integrated into a single context—the frame—for each management job.

The organizational purpose involves decisions to create a given organizational unit, assign responsibility to maintain effective functioning of that unit, and adapt the unit to new conditions. Organizational perspective involves defining an overall approach to managing the organizational unit, including defining or managing vision, mission, and culture. Peter Drucker (1994) noted the importance of these decisions in his seminal article, "The Theory of the Business." The definition of organizational position involves decisions about organizational and unit location within and relating to its systemic environment. This also includes decisions about what markets will be served, what products will be produced, what structures and systems will be designed, and what facilities will be built (Mintzberg, 1994). Organizational conceptualization involves the process of "thinking through the purpose, perspective, and positions of a particular unit to be managed over a period of time" (Mintzberg, 1994).

The Agenda of the Work

Beyond defining the frame of the job and assigning managers to work within that frame, no actions are more important than setting the agenda of the work to be done.

Agenda setting, priority setting, and work scheduling are fundamental to management work. Managers define the set of organizational issues they will consider and the scheduling of these issues for consideration and action. They make these agenda-setting and work-scheduling decisions, of course, within the context of the individual characteristics and framing elements described above.

Managers execute their managerial roles by acting simultaneously on three levels: (a) the information level, where emphasis is given to communicating and controlling activities; (b) the people level, where emphasis is given to leadership and linking activities; and (c) the action level, where emphasis is given to "doing," whether inside or outside the organizational unit. Mintzberg (1994) notes the difference between "doing inside" where managers manage projects and solve problems, and "doing outside" where managers negotiate deals and relationships and manage them over time.

Finally, Mintzberg (1994) argues that managerial style affects the quality of managerial work in three important ways:
1) The roles a manager favors
   a) Conceptual style
   b) Administrative style
   c) Interpersonal style
   d) Action style
2) The way the manager elects to perform those roles
   a) Approaches to linking
   b) Approaches to conceiving
   c) Approaches to leading
3) The approaches the manager takes to initiate action
   a) Deductive approaches
      i) Cerebral or deliberate style
   b) Inductive approaches
      i) Insightful style

Through this analysis, the management role clearly emerges as complex and integrated. In many ways, we can describe it as art, informed by science and uniquely applied in the context of organizational and personal experience.

Integrating Management Roles and Mind-Sets

Having described managerial roles and managerial application and practice characteristics in the general terms above, there is yet one more set of considerations to complete the picture—the mind-set of the managers as they fulfill their responsibilities. Gosling and Mintzberg (2003) recently observed that managers tend to operate from one or more of five mind-sets that they use to relate to the world within which they function. The authors identify the importance of: (a) a "reflective" mind-set in managing "self," (b) an "analytic" mind-set in managing organizations or organizational units, (c) a "worldly" mind-set to aid in managing organizational context, (d) a "collaborative" mind-set to aid in managing relationships, and (e) an "action" mind-set to assist in managing organizational change and transformation.

In considering requirements to integrate managerial roles within structure, context, and behavior, selection of mind-set may often be the determining factor in how the manager performs his or her assigned responsibilities (see Debate Time 2.1). Gosling and Mintzberg (2003) conclude their analysis by observing:

> We need distinct labels for them, but they obviously overlap, and they are more than mere words. They are more than metaphors too. . . . Imagine the mind-sets as threads and the manager as weaver. Effective performance means weaving to create a fine, sturdy cloth. You analyze, and then you act. However, that does not work as expected, so you reflect. You act some more, then find yourself blocked, realizing you cannot do it alone. You have to collaborate. But to do that you have to get into the world of others.

Then more analysis follows, to articulate the new insights. Now you act again—and so it goes, as the cloth of your effort forms.

Applying these important concepts within complex health service organizations, public health departments, regulatory agencies, etc., requires leaders and managers to begin with a clear understanding of the context, nature, and work of the organization. We can gain such an understanding by developing a clear organizational model to guide management and leadership action. Such a model is proposed and discussed in the following section.

THE PRACTICE OF MANAGEMENT IN HEALTH CARE ORGANIZATIONS: INTEGRATING ORGANIZATIONAL PROCESS MANAGEMENT AND PROFESSIONAL LEADERSHIP ROLES AND SKILLS

Organizational entities or enterprises within the health care system consist of a broad range of health care enterprises (i.e., hospitals and/or other institutional care organizations, such as long-term care, home care, and rehabilitative care facilities), as well as physician practice organizations, supply chain organizations, professional groups, insuring organizations, educational institutions, policy organizations and programs, and technology-based organizations. All of these organizational entities operate within one or more market environments, whether within an individual delivery system context or within this broader health system context. Each organizational entity within this complex system is, in turn, operating strategically to accomplish its own strategic objectives and to assure long-term access to the organizational, human, and capital resources necessary to meet these objectives.

DEBATE TIME 2.1   What Do You Think?

As noted in the foregoing discussion, management is a highly integrated job and it is often practiced in highly complex organizational environments. Yet, managers are often faced with the reality that they cannot do everything and that they must select priorities for their own direct involvement and depend on others to support the top management agenda. It is here that managers are faced with an often-difficult class of decisions of delegation, direction, and control. It sounds good to talk about empowering others, sharing power, and teaching people to lead them, in part because these ideas appeal to basic values that emphasize the inherent importance of each individual. However, in the final analysis, the buck has to stop somewhere in organizations, and that is with top management. This is not to say that developing others in the organization and delegating or sharing decisions with them does not work. These can be extremely effective management tools in the right circumstances. However, in reality, some subordinates just are not comfortable with more responsibility or do not have the skills to solve

problems as well as the manager can. In addition, empowering multidisciplinary, cross-organizational teams to grapple with problems, rather than referring them up the management hierarchy for solution, can be time consuming, can create confusion across departments, and can obfuscate who is responsible for results. Perhaps most important, it must be remembered that in the real world, not all the actors in an organization share the organization's goals. Or even if they do, the natural inclination to try to further one's own interests through the organization may be more motivating. As a result, managers could delegate decision-making opportunities only to find the participants "running away with the store." Selective empowerment and carefully proscribed delegation can be effective tools, however. Organizations work best when top management retains final decision-making authority and everyone knows it, and when the most critical or difficult decisions are not left in the hands of others all over the organization. What do you think?

Moreover, all these components operate within a dynamic and rapidly evolving scientific and technical environment. The continuously changing nature of the systemic interactions places a premium on any given organization's ability to initiate and manage processes of learning, adaptation, and transformation.

Figure 2.1 presents a systemic model of the health care system, allowing the reader to enter the system through the eyes of patients. The central focus of the model is a typical delivery organization, which can be any of a number of institutional types (i.e., hospital, medical practice, long-term care facility, home care program, hospice program, etc.).

The critical point is that patients enter the enterprise through a relationship with their "clinician." This "clinician" specifies the profile of clinical services required to best serve the patient's needs, directs and evaluates the clinical care of the patients within the enterprise, and serves as the patient's advocate to assure optimal outcomes. The health care enterprise (system) provides required clinical services to the patient within one or more of a number of **clinical care systems** (e.g., cardiac, trauma, obstetric, orthopedic, neurological, etc.). Clinical care system managers are responsible to enterprise-level (i.e., organization-wide) executive leaders for the appropriateness, effectiveness, safety, quality,

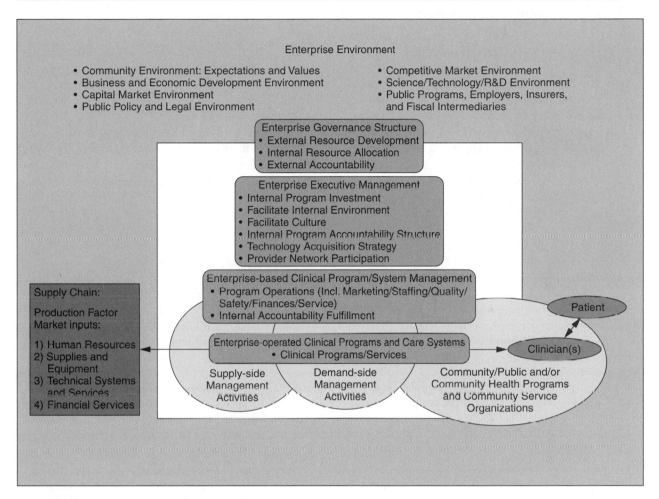

Figure 2.1. Health Care Clinical Enterprise Model

SOURCE: Reprinted with permission from William E. Welton, Dr. P.H., M.H.A., University of Washington, 2004.

and efficiency of the clinical services rendered to the patient within each clinical care system.

Each health care enterprise usually contains and supports several such clinical care systems. In this regard, each of these several clinical care systems operates within the internal environment of the broader health care enterprise (i.e., culture, human resource policies, technology infrastructure, information processes, business processes, and clinical processes). Each clinical care system depends on enterprise-level managers for acquisition and in-

vestment of capital in technology, facilities, and clinical resources required to achieve clinical effectiveness and sustainable strategic advantage. Each clinical care system also depends on its enterprise management and governance structure to assure access to critical elements of the enterprise environment. Elements include such things as institutional licensure, Medicare certification, JCAHO for example, or other accreditation, obtained from the public policy and legal environment and funds from the capital market environment, etc.

In the final analysis there are two fundamental management roles within each health care enterprise—enterprise-level management and clinical system management. Both of these are critical to strategic success and managers must integrate both effectively. While the clinical system management role must focus on the provision and safety of direct services to patients, the enterprise-level managers must manage the enterprise's relationship and interaction with the external environment, and they must manage the rate of organizational adaptation to changes and opportunities within the external environment.

Chapter 1 noted the inherent tension between an organization's needs for predictability, order, and efficiency with those of openness, adaptability, and innovation when operating within an open-systems context. It also noted the importance of six primary processes required to achieve organizational objectives and accountabilities: production, boundary spanning, maintenance, adaptation, management, and governance. Enterprise executives and clinical process managers are responsible for developing and overseeing these functions and for assuring organizational adaptation and economic transformation within the systems they manage. They do this through appropriate integration and application of these six organizational processes.

The organizational and management literature strongly supports the notion of management practice as a process. Authors address a range of important concepts and processes, including competitive strategy (Porter, 1985), competitive strategy and health care (Porter & Teisberg, 2004; Luke, Watson, & Plummer, 2004), strategic management processes (Hill & Jones, 2002), systems management processes (Anderson & Johnson, 1997), technology and organizations (Perrow, 1984), organizational evolution processes (Nelson & Winter, 1982), and metamorphic organizational change processes (Tushman & Romanelli, 1985). Others have made significant contributions to the literature in the areas of leadership (Kotter, 2001), organizational learning (Argyris, 1999; Sterman, 2000), change management (Kotter, 1996), organizational trans-formation (Bridges, 1991), organizational change (Hayes, 2002; Burke, 2002), and executive leadership (Zaccaro, 2001). Taken together, the contributions of these and others all argue strongly for development of an integrated process-based view of the managerial role.

Garvin (1998) for example has presented such a "process-based view" of management, defining the management role in terms of both management processes and organizational processes for which enterprise executives and clinical process managers are broadly accountable. Within this process-oriented context, one must view organizational management as a highly integrated, intuitive, dynamic, and evolving function.

Metaphorically, managers sit at the "strategic apex" (Mintzberg, 1989) of a systemic triangle where—through their exercise of personal and professional leadership—they act to assure that organizational structure is managed and the process-oriented management roles discussed above are properly organized and executed. In order to understand the management role more completely, one can view the core organization in a triangular, systemic context (Figure 2.2). The base of this triangular system appears as systemic organizational structure, and the two sides of the triangle are organizational and management processes and organizational management. At the center of the triangle is the organization's technology and production core. The three sides of the triangle enclose the organization's internal environment, in which the technology and production core are immersed as the organization embarks on a quest for resources and legitimacy from the external environment.

The components of each side of the triangle are presented below:

System Organization Structure

1. Mission

2. Strategies, goals, and accountabilities

3. Production function, including support of organizational "core competences" (Prahalad &

Hamel, 1990), production technology, and information technology

4. Strategic affiliations

5. Organizational culture

Management and Organizational Processes

Building on Garvin's (1998) "process-based view" of management, below are the components of management and organizational processes.

1) Management processes, including:
    a) Direction-setting processes
        i) Learning about the organization and its problems through a broad range of interactions and assessments and continued probing
        ii) Framing an agenda to be pursued through conscious reflection and intuitive experience
        iii) Aligning individuals through communication, motivation, rewards, and punishments, often using new or established communication processes
        iv) Framing, testing, and revising initiatives
    b) Negotiating and selling processes
        i) Framing and presentation of issues and proposals
        ii) Deciding how to solicit help and present proposals in ways that appeal to others yet meet one's basic objectives
        iii) Building and maintaining network contacts and communication processes
        iv) Building and managing coalitions
        v) Applying the above in horizontal and vertical organizational contexts
    c) Monitoring and controlling processes
        i) Ensuring organizational operation as planned
            (1) Detect (systemic) perturbations relating to unexpected shocks and disturbances

(2) Initiation of corrective action
(3) Restoration of the organization to its previous equilibrium

2) Organizational processes, including:
    a) Work processes (i.e., operational and administrative production or support processes)
        i) Customer, transformation, and supply-chain systems serving external or internal customers requiring alignment to achieve mutual support
        ii) Redesign processes to improve quality, cut costs, reduce cycle times, or otherwise enhance operating performance
        iii) Activities to decrease fragmentation and improve cross-functional integration
    b) Behavioral processes
        i) Decision-making processes (lengthy, complex, slow to change, subject to managerial control)
        ii) Communication processes (interpersonal, within-group, and intergroup interaction)
            (1) Nature, direction, and quality of information flows
            (2) Interrelationships among group members and stances toward one another
            (3) Tenor and tone of group work
        iii) Organizational learning
            (1) Knowledge acquisition
            (2) Knowledge interpretation
            (3) Knowledge dissemination
            (4) Knowledge retention
    c) Change processes (i.e., longitudinal and dynamic processes with four stages over organizational or individual life cycles)
        i) Creation
        ii) Growth
        iii) Transformation
        iv) Decline

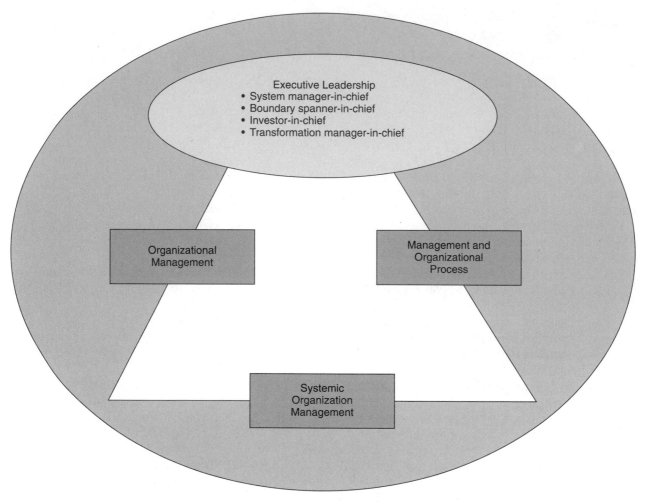

Figure 2.2. Framing the Managerial Role

SOURCE: Reprinted with permission from William E. Welton, Dr. P.H., M.H.A., University of Washington, 2004.

Organizational Management

Kotter (2001) makes the distinction between organizational management and executive leadership when he says ". . . leadership and management are two distinctive and complementary systems of action. Each has its own function and characteristic activities. Both are necessary for success in an increasingly complex and volatile business environ-

ment. . . . Leadership is about coping with change." Following this distinction, the notion of organizational management forms the third side of the management triangle in Figure 2.2. Kotter (2001) notes that organizational management "is about coping with complexity . . . without good management complex enterprises tend to become chaotic in ways that threaten their very existence. Good management brings a degree of order and consistency to key dimensions like the quality and profitability of products (and services)." He goes on to note that:

> Companies manage complexity first by planning and budgeting—setting targets or goals for the future, establishing detailed steps for achieving those targets, and then allocating resources to accomplish those plans . . . Management develops the capacity to achieve its plan by organizing and staffing—creating an organizational structure and set of jobs for accomplishing plan requirements, staffing the jobs for accomplishing plan requirements . . . with qualified individuals, communicating the plan to those people, delegating responsibility for carrying out the plan, and devising systems to monitor implementation . . . Management ensures plan accomplishment by controlling and problem solving—monitoring results vs. the plan in some detail, both formally and informally, by means of reports, meetings and other tools, identifying deviations, and then planning and organizing to solve the problems. (Kotter, 2001)

Executive Leadership Work at the Organization's Strategic Apex

At the top of Figure 2.2 is the executive leadership role (as distinguished from his concept of the organizational management role) and is defined as "coping with (organizational) change (and adaptation) . . . in a more competitive and volatile business environment . . . (that is characterized by) faster technological change, increased competition and increased deregulation . . ." (Kotter, 2001). This critical role applies at the model's strategic apex. It is here that fundamental leadership decisions are made as to whether or not, when, and

how to embark on significant organizational adaptations to perceived threats and opportunities within the organization's operating environment (see "In Practice," p. 54). In describing his concept of the relationship between the executive leadership and organizational management roles, Kotter (2001) notes that ". . . the real challenge (to organizations) is to combine strong (executive) leadership and strong management and use each to balance the other."

In Figure 2.2, the executive leader performs a combination of four fundamental and interrelated leadership roles, critical to executive management's overall responsibility to guide organizational adaptation and transformation:

1. Organizational system manager-in-chief

2. Boundary spanner-in-chief

3. Resource developer/investor-in-chief

4. Transformation manager-in-chief

In this context, the executive leader is accountable to organizational and environmental governance structures for the effective and efficient use of resources, for defining and achieving strategic goals, and for assuring access to resources essential to fulfilling expectations of customers and stakeholders. Ultimately, one can broadly define each of these executive leadership roles:

1. As organizational system manager-in-chief, the manager bears primary responsibility for structuring and maintaining the organizational system to achieve strategic goals efficiently and effectively. The executive leader must assure the development and maintenance of internal environments and systems required to assure safe, efficient, and effective operation and to assure commitment of valuable human resources.

2. As boundary spanner-in-chief, the executive leader links interests, programs, and operating elements within the organization to those within the larger health system. The executive

must use a combination of personal skills (i.e., knowledge, technical and political skills, discretion, and influence) to exert control both inside and outside the organization.

3. As resource developer/investor-in-chief, the executive leader assures access to essential human, technological, organizational, and capital resources, while assuring conformance with cus-

tomer, community, regulatory, legal, licensure, and accreditation expectations and requirements.

4. As transformation manager-in-chief, the executive leader acts to influence and/or control the initiation of and the rate and extent of organizational transformation and adaptation to a broad range of organizational or systemic stimuli and reactions.

IN PRACTICE   A Medical Center in Transition (2) . . . The Leadership Challenge

It was clear to Varnum that his major role as CEO would be to provide the high-level executive leadership required to transform the structure of the hospital's historical relationships with the clinic and the medical school. These relationships were a complex mix of "enterprise-level" relationships and "clinical system organization and managerial" relationships. Redefining them would require high-level negotiations to address significant changes in organizational responsibilities and resource commitments.

At the same time, Varnum recognized the importance of operating the hospital in its new and evolving role as a teaching hospital within the academic medical center. Thus, shortly after his arrival, he hired as his new chief operating officer William Welton, who was experienced in the operational management of complex academic medical centers. Welton's role would be to support Varnum's work in transforming the hospital organization, in contributing to the transformation of the medical center, and in helping to execute hospital programs and responsibilities within the medical center and the community. This would also require skills in managing changes in the organization's clinical service culture and in developing more productive approaches to managing the clinical portion of the larger

enterprise. Varnum would also look to Welton to suggest the physical form that a new integrated medical center facility should take to become a more integrated academic medical center (while conserving on capital costs).

During the next seven years, Varnum and Welton worked closely together to transform MHMH into a fully functioning and efficient academic teaching hospital operation, emphasizing excellence in execution, and to create a new set of clinical facilities that would support long-term growth and regional and national leadership. Throughout this period, characterized by significant change at the enterprise and clinical operations level of the hospital, both Varnum and Welton recognized the importance of maintaining the organization's strong commitment to its valuable human resources. Because of the long-term clinical partnership between MHMH and the Hitchcock Clinic and the highly integrated nature of the facilities and communications support and human resources support functions, this commitment applied equally to hospital and clinic employees, including the physicians who also served as the MHMH medical staff and as the DMS clinical faculty.

At this time, the hospital's clinical care systems were adapting to major changes in the nation's health care system, including introduction of

Medicare's diagnostic related groups (DRG) reimbursement system and an increasing movement of clinical care and technology from inpatient to ambulatory venues. Both had significant implications for allocation of revenue generation opportunities between the hospital and clinic, for higher levels of competition between the two organizations, and for the redefinition of managerial roles and responsibilities.

By September 1985, the operational transformation was largely complete. Most of the enterprise-level relationships required to operate the medical center had been renegotiated or newly established. For seven years, however, the partner organizations had struggled with the question of what new facilities should be built, who should pay for them and in what proportion, and how important governance-level decisions would be to allow the hospital trustees to agree to undertake the $225 million construction project, while incurring the $150 million in debt. It was clearly a "fork in the road," and the immediate answers to these questions were neither clear nor agreed-upon.

With collaborative leadership at the governance and CEO levels, a group of board, medical leadership, and executive management personnel from the three collaborating organizations and the DHMC worked to create an even more effective decision-making structure.

It was at this point that all three of the principal partners (i.e., hospital, clinical, and college) agreed on a common assessment of environmental forces affecting the hospital's potential to finance the project. It appeared to all that the very real probability existed that hospitals would lose access to tax-exempt bond financing in the bond markets as of midnight, December 31, 1985.

Thus, all parties concluded that they had one final opportunity to redefine their enterprise-level business partnership to achieve their strategy to transform the academic medical center enterprise under mutually acceptable terms. With only three and a half months to go before the anticipated deadline, no one in the evolving DHMC leadership group doubted that decision time was at hand.

PLACING THE HEALTH CARE MANAGEMENT ROLE IN A STRATEGIC PERSPECTIVE

Above all else, health care managers (i.e., those in executive leadership positions) must define strategic goals to assure their organization's survival and growth and to guide the organization to achieve these goals. They do this by applying strategic management concepts (see Chapter 14), integrating them with core elements of organizational and systemic management theory, and by adapting and transforming organizational structure, over time. Figure 2.3 presents a model integrating several of these core elements.

The model in Figure 2.3 emphasizes management's role of defining and achieving targeted strategic outcomes (stated in either value or profitability terms). This is their unique role and responsibility within the health care organization. To discharge this role effectively, managers must do four things over time. These include the following:

1. Determining when and how to institute change in organizational structure and priorities (organizational transformation)

2. Determining when and how to institute change in the organization's distinctive competencies and strategic objectives (strategic transformation)

3. Developing and executing specific strategies required to achieve strategic objectives (strategic execution)

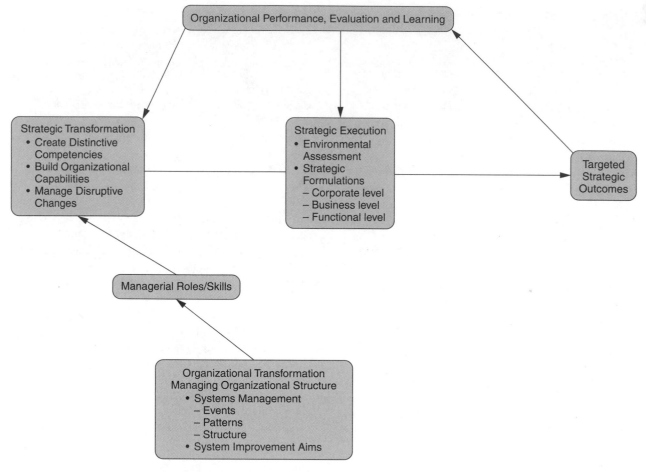

Figure 2.3. Roots of Organizational Effectiveness and the Managerial Role: A Strategic Perspective

SOURCE: Reprinted with permission from William E. Welton, Dr. P.H., M.H.A., University of Washington, 2004. Based on Charles W. L. Hill and Gareth R. Jones, *Strategic Management Theory: An Integrated Approach,* Fifth Edition. Copyright © 2001 by Houghton Mifflin Company. Adapted with permission. Also based on material from the Institute of Medicine, Prahalad & Hamel, Nelson & Winter, Tushman & Romanelli, Mintzberg, Gosling & Mintzberg, and Anderson & Johnson.

4. Assuring appropriate levels of organizational learning so that improvements can be made (strategic transformation)

Each of these elements flows from bottom to top and left to right within Figure 2.3, and each is discussed below, in turn.

Organizational Transformation

Strategically oriented managers assure achievement of targeted strategic outcomes by managing the evolution of their organization's systemic structure, over time (Nelson & Winter, 1982; Anderson & Johnson, 1997). Managers must apply continuous judgment as to whether, when, and how to intervene in ongoing operations, whether by reacting to events or altering such fundamental elements of system structure as routines, processes, or culture (Nelson & Winter, 1982; Anderson & Johnson, 1997; Tushman & Romanelli, 1985).

Most of the time, managers attempt gradual adaptation strategies (dealing with "events" and "patterns" in the Anderson and Johnson model), but occasionally, they decide to make fundamental structural change to accelerate adaptive and transformative processes. Practitioners know this as the "punctuated equilibrium" mechanism of organizational adaptation (Tushman & Romanelli, 1985). Anderson and Johnson (1997) refer to this as "operating at the structural level." The critical management role is determining the intervention level and/or timing of intervention required to achieve organizational transformation.

Others have referred to the need to manage disruptive change (Cristensen & Overdorf, 2000). Organizational managers accomplish all of this through development of specific skills and professional competencies known as "management heuristics" (Nelson & Winter, 1982). This model also incorporates six important recommendations for health system performance improvement put forward by the Institute of Medicine in its watershed report *Crossing the Quality Chasm: A New Health System for the 21st Century* (Institute of Medicine, 2001).

Taken in their totality, the elements required for organizational transformation are at the core of management's adaptation management role.

Strategic Transformation

To achieve the organization's targeted strategic outcomes, the manager must create distinctive competencies within the organization by integrating resources (human and capital), capabilities, and technology (clinical, information, and organizational) (Prahalad & Hamel, 1990). Newly developed distinctive competencies will have a significant relationship to competencies developed in the past. Managers will also identify unique opportunities to integrate these three elements in new ways to form new competencies allowing the organization to create and maintain sustainable competitive advantage. In the health care enterprise, many of these distinctive competencies will be located within individual clinical care systems (see Figure 2.1 and related discussion).

Strategic Execution

Given the manager's assessment of competitive forces and opportunities as well as distinctive organizational competencies and organizational capabilities, he or she must select and execute appropriate strategies to achieve selected goals. **Execution skills** emphasizes the well-known strategic management processes of environmental assessment (internal and external environments), strategy formulation at corporate, business, and functional levels within the organization, decision making required to implement and manage strategies selected, risk assessment and risk management of strategies selected, and strategy evaluation to support the organizational transformation process discussed above.

The final step in the **strategic management** loop is a feedback or learning step. The manager must evaluate strategic performance achieved and adjust organizational capabilities, distinctive competencies, strategic goals, or execution strategies as necessary to assure continuing achievement of targeted strategic outcomes (Porter, 1985; Hill & Jones, 2002). (See Chapter 14 for additional discussion of strategic issues.)

Individual managers may have greater proficiency in one or another role or domain category, but each one must be capable of exercising all roles as well as integrating all of them in various priority mixes required in different situation. A well-balanced integration of these skills is essential to assure that the manager can implement his or her critical organizational adaptation role most effectively, over time. The balance of this chapter will explore the special requirements and challenges facing health care managers focusing on this objective.

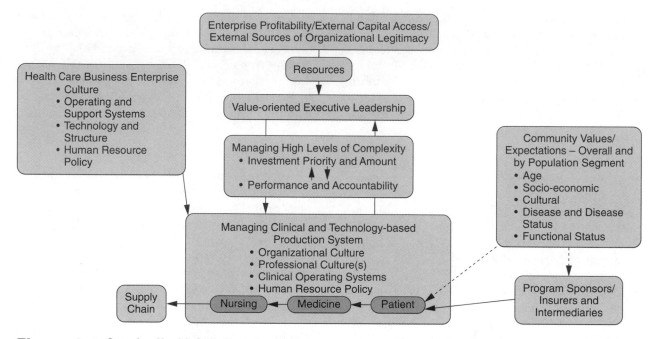

Figure 2.4. Complex Health Care Organization Systems: Leadership and Management Skill Requirements

SOURCE: Reprinted with permission from William E. Welton, Dr. P.H., M.H.A., University of Washington, 2004.

EXPLORING HEALTH CARE'S DISTINCTIVE CONTEXT AND EXECUTIVE LEADERSHIP REQUIREMENTS

While the strategic frame for the executive leadership role discussed above applies in the general case, it is now important to place the frame within a health care context. Executive leadership roles and positions within the health care industry require application of distinctive skills and perspectives, including special skill sets related to:

1. Organizing and managing clinical and technology-based production systems

2. High levels of organizational complexity, working with highly trained professionals

3. The need for providing value-oriented executive leadership

Figure 2.4 shows the interplay of these managerial skills and responsibilities in the health care enterprise. Each of the three special skill sets is discussed, in turn (Welton, 2004).

Managing Clinical and Technology-Based Production Systems

The core "production work" of health care organizations is to provide safe, effective, and efficient clinical services. This work is completed by highly trained and professionally qualified and motivated health care personnel—physicians and nurses with significant contributions from many other categories of health professionals and technicians. All of these professional and technical personnel operate within well-defined but semi-independent professional value systems. Clinical services are provided within organized and integrated clinical care systems, each of which generally includes diagnostic, therapeutic, and rehabilitative components that must be coordinated across inpatient and ambulatory boundaries. Each clinical care system is built around one or more aspects of medical technology, depending on the clinical areas served; the underlying technology within each clinical care system changes rapidly with the development of new interventional and care delivery techniques, new pharmaceutical interventions, and new medical supplies and equipment. The fact that services are organized and delivered within a community, professional, and personal service-oriented context is important to all involved.

Managing High Levels of Organizational Complexity

Health care managers must continuously monitor and evaluate the safety, effectiveness, and efficiency of these systems, intervening when and where necessary to improve these characteristics and assure accountability. Health care managers must accomplish all of this while recognizing the common fact that the clinical team leaders (usually physicians) operate under different economic incentives than the hospital or other organization and have different employers, often with competing strategic objectives (see Debate Time 2.2).

From an overall perspective, the health care business enterprise serves individual patients, and

✣ IN PRACTICE   A Medical Center in Transition (3) . . . Aligning the Players

Within a hectic 30-day period, the hospital, clinic, and college reached agreement on a program and financial plan by mid-October 1985. In this agreement, MHMH committed to make a substantial down payment from its reserves. Dartmouth College agreed to purchase the hospital's existing land and buildings for an equivalent amount, while donating a pristine 225-acre site nearby to the hospital for development of a new medical center campus. The hospital agreed to undertake a substantial capital campaign to complete the equity contribution required to assure financial feasibility. The college agreed to assist in the capital campaign and guarantee a minimum amount, after the two organizations agreed on a joint fund-raising organization and campaign parameters. Importantly, both the clinic and college agreed to terms of rental guarantees for their space within the new integrated medical center campus. Finally, the MHMH trustees agreed to donate the land for the new campus to the DHMC organization. This meant that the DHMC organization could assure that the new facilities would meet the shared goal of creating a modern and completely integrated academic medical center by determining the conditions that the new facilities would have to meet.

After the hospital trustees assured creditors of the quality of the hospital's credit—with strong support from its medical center partners—the bond issue closed at noon on December 31, 1985.

However, the hospital, acting by mutual agreement as project developer, and its medical center partners were only at the beginning of the story. Historical relationships had been transformed into a new skeleton. The partner organizations still had to negotiate the details of their new enterprise relationship and to create the type of business environment required to establish a truly integrated clinical operating organization that would lay the foundation for the clinical operation. While Varnum continued to lead the overall transformational effort, he asked Welton to lead and integrate the program, facilities, and operational planning efforts. He asked his CFO, Richard Showalter, to assume responsibility for financial management of the complex project and to support development of a new set of business relationships among the parties. Both of these supporting roles, properly executed and coordinated, were essential to executing the broader transformational plan.

Over the next two years, the partners operated a joint planning process through which they developed plans for the physical facility. The central agreement among the parties was first to design a facility that would work best for patients and their medical providers, and next, to negotiate the business arrangements required to support this and meet the requirements of the partner organizations. This required exceptional creativity, a commitment to patient service by all, and a willingness to consider all options jointly. The partners agreed to assure a jointly acceptable solution by implementing their plans through joint agreement on overall priorities, by using an integrated planning process, and by committing to the discipline a fixed and unified project budget. These commitments, supported by the contribution of internal planners supported by a cadre of excellent architectural, legal, and financial advisers—allowed the hospital to develop an innovative and coordinated set of clinical operations, facility operations, and business plans.

The facility plan provided for a vertical "stack" of physically and horizontally integrated clinical services by clinical program, that is, groupings of outpatient medical/surgical, outpatient diagnostic and treatment, inpatient diagnostic and treatment, inpatient critical care and inpatient acute services. The major focus of all was the main entrance, which was the entrance to the physician offices, thus reinforcing the purpose of the patient visit. This was reinforced by a central mall, providing physical integration and connection for all activities and organizational units within the new medical center. From a business and operating perspective, it was no accident that the owners developed the new facility as a condominium, operated under management contract by MHMH and under the overall direction of the DHMC.

through its ability to manage, integrate, and coordinate clinical care processes effectively and efficiently at the clinical service level, it is to generate capital through operational profitability. Considerable quantities of capital are needed to support the continuing investments in specialized manpower and new clinical technology required to meet patient and community expectations and to support the professional expectations and standards. Increasingly, the organization's ability to operate profitably depends on management's ability to implement complex information-management strategies (often crossing organizational boundaries).

Although some capital is available through philanthropic donations, the vast majority of needed capital comes from profitable operations. To operate profitably, health care managers and executive leaders must be skilled in making complex internal investment decisions and in managing external relationships with communities, politicians, and regulators.

Providing Value-Oriented Executive Leadership

As noted above, health care delivery organizations are complex and strongly resource-dependent organizations. Largely, the communities they serve (local, regional, state-level, and national) are the source of organizational legitimacy and economic and human resources. But the principal and collective source of these key resources is the local community served.

Health delivery organizations must ultimately strike a balance between investing in their ability to generate economic profits and investing in their commitment (implied or actual) to meet community service needs. Communities have generally supported development of health care delivery organizations as either local monopolies or strongly oligopolistic local market structures, and they generally expect these organizations to provide services to all comers. The strongly dominant nonprofit form of organization for these organizations and the broad range of economic preferences and privileges granted to them by society through tax exemptions and other devices reinforce this expectation.

Executive leadership of health care delivery organizations must exhibit value-oriented decision-making, **human relations**, and priority-setting skills, as illustrated in the challenges facing James Varnum and his colleagues at the Mary Hitchcock Memorial Hospital (see "In Practice," p. 60–61). Executive leadership must communicate effectively with a broad range of community stakeholders, while being aware of different ethical styles and approaches and while making implicit and explicit commitments to meet community stakeholder needs. At the same time, executive leadership must manage the business enterprise effectively to assure continuing community support, while operating profitably.

CROSSING THE QUALITY CHASM: DISTINCTIVE CHALLENGES FOR HEALTH SERVICE MANAGERS

In 2000 and 2001 the Institute of Medicine published two important reports highlighting the distinctive demands health care organizations face as providers of personal health services.

In the first of these reports, *To Err Is Human: Building a Safer Health System* (Institute of Medicine, 2000), the study committee suggested that between 44,000 and 98,000 deaths result annually from preventable medical errors during hospitalization. The report ranked "deaths due to preventable hospital error" as the nation's eighth-leading cause of death. The committee's unavoidable overall conclusion was that "health care is not as safe as it should be" (Institute of Medicine, 2000), and it went on to observe:

> Although all industries face concerns about liability, the organization of health care creates a different set of circumstances compared to other industries. In health care, physicians primarily determine the amount and content of care to be rendered. A hospital or clinic often produces the care directed by the physician. The consumer, purchaser, and health plan share in decisions to determine whether and how treatment decisions directed by the physician are paid, which influences access to care. Although some of these decisions could be under one umbrella, they are often dispersed across different and unrelated entities. Compared to other industries, there is no single responsible organization in health care that is held accountable for an episode of care. The physician, in particular, has a significant responsibility for the well-being of his patients and the decisions made concerning their care. This distinctive arrangement in organization and decision making in health

care creates a unique set of liability issues and challenges in creating an environment conducive to recognizing and learning from errors.

The committee recommended that health care organizations should move immediately to design safe systems of care, incorporating the following principles:

> 1) providing leadership, 2) respecting human limits in process design, 3) promoting effective team functioning, 4) anticipating the unexpected, and 5) creating a learning environment. (Institute of Medicine, 2000) and based on three key design principles: 1) standardizing and simplifying equipment, supplies, and processes; 2) establishing team training programs; and 3) implementing nonpunitive systems for reporting and analyzing errors and accidents within organizations.

In *Crossing the Quality Chasm: A New Health System for the 21st Century* (Institute of Medicine, 2001), the study committee extended its earlier work by proposing adoption of six overall aims to improve functioning of the nation's health care system. The six aims are that "health care should be: 1) safe, 2) effective, 3) patient-centered, 4) timely, 5) efficient, and 6) equitable."

To achieve these outcomes within the context of the systemic challenges described above, the committee recommended that:

> Whatever their form, organizations will need to meet six challenges . . . that cut across different health conditions, types of care (such as preventive, acute, or chronic), and care settings:
> - redesigning care processes;
> - making effective use of information technologies;
> - managing clinical knowledge and skills;
> - developing effective teams;
> - coordinating care across patient conditions, services, and settings over time; and
> - incorporating performance and outcome measurements for improvement and accountability.

Executive leaders and clinical process managers within the health care industry are challenged with organizing care processes to address—in partnership with their medical staff affiliates—the issues and goals discussed above. To accomplish these operating objectives, they must ensure that their organizations perform in a balanced manner, in which customer service (patients and physicians) objectives, internal business process (i.e., clinical

system) objectives, enterprise-level financial objectives, and enterprise-wide organizational learning objectives are simultaneously and synergistically achieved. A commonly accepted tool used by managers to allocate resources and monitor performance is known as the "balanced scorecard" (Kaplan & Norton, 1996).

Figure 2.5 describes a series of relationships and accountabilities within the clinical health care

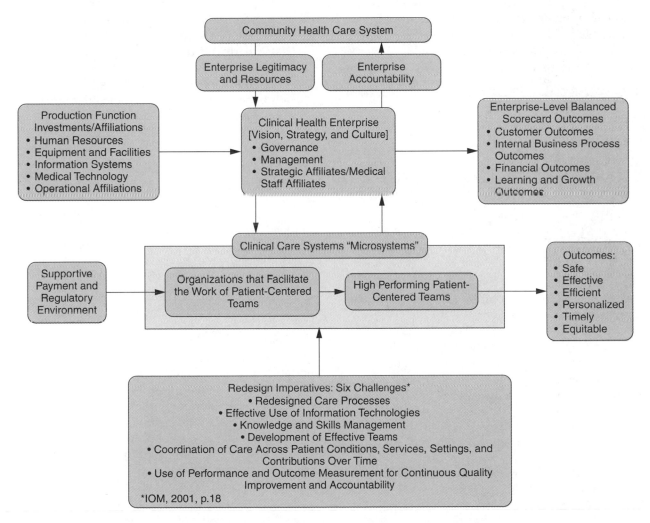

Figure 2.5. Enterprise Strategic Management Model with IOM Care System Redesign Imperatives

SOURCE: Reprinted with permission from William E. Welton, Dr. P.H., M.H.A., University of Washington, 2004.

enterprise that suggests a simultaneous integration of activities and objectives at three organizational levels: the organization's clinical care system or "microsystem" level (Mohr & Batalden, 2002; Nelson et al., 2002); the enterprise or organizational level; and the community health care system level. At the same time, Figure 2.5 suggests an organizational framework for addressing the system development and management recommendations discussed in the two important Institute of Medicine studies described above and within which their interaction can be coordinated to assure and produce positive and measurable outcomes at each level, while assuring each level to meet accountabilities and expectations for improvement.

DEVELOPING A STANDARDIZED KNOWLEDGE BASE FOR PROFESSIONAL LEADERSHIP AND FOR HEALTH CARE MANAGERS WITHIN THE HEALTH CARE INDUSTRY

The central theme of this chapter emphasizes the organizational adaptation and transformation role and responsibilities of managers. Within the context of these complicated and dynamic organizations, adaptation and transformation require development and honing of professional leadership competencies. The following discussion explores this important and developing area of knowledge within the health care management community. Please note the relevance of this discussion to the "Roots of Organizational Effectiveness and the Managerial Role" in Figure 2.3.

Fundamental Behavioral Skills Required for Success in Management Roles

Much work has been done since 1950 to define the set of traits, attributes, and behaviors that will allow

identification of the most successful executive leaders and managers. Katz put one early and particularly useful conceptualization forward in 1955 (updated in 1974). This conceptualization, based on what successful executives do (rather than what traits and characteristics they possess) identified three fundamental skill sets possessed by successful executives. The three fundamental skill sets are (a) technical skills, (b) human skills, and (c) conceptual skills (Katz, 1974).

Katz (1974) defines each as follows:
1. Technical skill: An understanding of and proficiency in, a specific kind of activity, particularly one involving methods, processes, procedures, or techniques.
2. Human skill: The ability to work effectively as a group member to build cooperative effort:
   a. within the team he leads, and/or
   b. in facilitating and managing intergroup relationships.
3. Conceptual skill: Involves the ability to see the enterprise as a whole; it includes recognizing how the various functions of the organization depend on one another, and how changes in any one part affect all the others; and it extends to visualizing the relationship of the individual business to the industry, the community, and the political, social, and economic forces of the nation as a whole.

Katz (1974) also observed that requirements for and reliance on technical skills occurred most frequently at lower management levels (but can be important at every management level to achieve leadership focus in technically specialized areas); human skills were important at every level of management; and conceptual skills become most important (and often critical) in senior executive leadership positions. Elaborating on the nature of conceptual skill sets, he noted that conceptual skills involve: "thinking in terms of: a) relative emphases and priorities among conflicting objectives and criteria; b) relative tendencies and probabilities (rather than certainties); and c) rough correlations and patterns among elements (rather than clear-cut cause and effect relationships)."

Finally, Katz (1974) paid particular attention to CEO role requirements when he noted that the chief executive officer must be:

1. effective in balancing conflicting values within the organization (conflict resolution skills) to create an efficient operating environment;

2. an effective strategist . . . to provide the framework and direction for overall company operations; and

3. must change his management style and strike different balances among his personal skills as conditions change or as his organization grows in size and complexity.

Building on this conceptual foundation many researchers extended these concepts to identify more finely grained models of specific competency sets (characteristics and behaviors requires for success in managerial and executive careers). Of particular note is the extensive and complementary work of competency researchers, including McClelland (McClelland, Atkinson, Clark, & Lowell, 1953; McClelland, 1971), Boyatzis (1982), and Goleman (1995).

Current and Evolving Health Care Professional Leadership Competency Concepts

Since 2001, the health care management field has worked to define a set of core professional leadership competencies for its managers. This work has been led by the National Center for Healthcare Leadership (NCHL) and is intended to provide a model to guide development of formal educational programs and personal career development plans in support of long-term health industry leadership development. Competencies in this model are defined as "the technical and behavioral characteristics that leaders must possess to be successful in positions of leadership across the health professions—administrative, medical and nursing" (NCHL, 2004).

NCHL's Healthcare Leadership Competency Model, version 2.0, contains twenty-six specific leadership competencies organized into the three competency domains. These three competency domains are designated: (a) Transformation, (b) Execution, and (c) People. Each is defined, in turn, and the specific competencies contained therein are described in the following sections (NCHL, 2004).

Transformation

Visioning the changing role of the organization in the local community, region, and national health arena from provider of care to creator of wellness and a "provider without walls." Component competencies include:

1. Achievement orientation
2. Analytical thinking
3. Community orientation
4. Information seeking
5. Innovative thinking
6. Strategic orientation
7. Financial skills

Execution

Focusing on organizational priorities that improve the safety, effectiveness, timeliness, efficiency, and equitability of patient-centered care (definition content first suggested by Institute of Medicine, 2001). Component competencies include:

1. Accountability
2. Change leadership
3. Collaboration
4. Impact and influence
5. Initiative
6. Organizational awareness
7. Performance measurement

8. Information technology management
9. Communication
10. Process management and organizational design
11. Project management

People

Creating an organizational climate that values employees from all backgrounds and provides an energizing environment for them. Also includes the leader's responsibility to understand his or her impact on others and to improve his or her capabilities, as well as the capabilities of others. Component competencies include:

1. Interpersonal understanding
2. Professionalism
3. Relationship building
4. Self-confidence
5. Self-development
6. Talent development
7. Team leadership
8. Human resources management

While this work has been developed collaboratively by NCHL and Hay Group, Inc. (a human resource consulting firm), it is important to know that it is based on work developed in the field of emotional intelligence and particularly on the more recent work of Goleman and others (Goleman, 1998, 2000; Goleman, Boyatzis, & McKee, 2002). The overall objective of this leadership competency work is to articulate a standardized base of behavioral competencies for professional leadership within the field. This work is significant to individual managers and to health care organizations in that it provides guidance for formulation of career-long leadership development programs.

In reviewing this work, it is important to note that the three NCHL competency domains—transformation, execution, and people—seem to link generally and respectively to Katz's conceptual, technical, and human classifications of skills required for successful executive performance discussed earlier. It is important to note, however, that while this is generally true from the perspective of thematic dominance, each of the NCHL competency domains contains a mix of specific individual competencies with some falling in each of Katz's conceptual, execution, and people skill sets.

Integrating NCHL Professional Leadership Competencies within the Managerial Role

In reflecting on the implications of this work, it is important to note that it is consistent with and reinforces the observations contained in earlier sections of this chapter—see Figures 2.1 to 2.5 and associated discussions. In fact, these connections are easily integrated into Figure 2.6 (a synthesized and enhanced version of Figure 2.3, incorporating key elements of the *NCHL Professional Leadership Competency Model*). In undertaking a close examination of Figure 2.6, one easily connects the significance of the transformation, execution, and people competence domains. Moreover, one immediately sees the connection of this work to the world of practice.

Thus, the movement to develop professional leadership competencies complements earlier discussions regarding the distinctive nature of health care organizations, of the leadership roles within them, and of the management challenges they face in meeting strategic goals and community expectations. One should also note that the execution domain of the *NCHL Professional Leadership Competency Model* incorporates the six aims for health system improvement recommended by the Institute of Medicine in its watershed report: *Crossing the Quality Chasm: A New Health System for the 21st Century* (Institute of Medicine, 2001).

Competency Development as a Career-Long Action-Based Reflective Activity, Conducted within an Integrating Framework

Material earlier in this chapter discussed the importance of considering management as an integrating activity. In considering the development of professional leadership competencies, it is equally important to consider an integrative context to support their career-long development. Competency development does not simply occur, competencies are gained through a life-long process (beginning with student educational experiences) of experience-based reflection and growth (Mintzberg, 2004).

Importantly, experience (good or bad) becomes the source of personal learning and development, while a focus is maintained on action-based learning. While action becomes the source of learning, it is also important to assure that adequate time is set aside for reflection. In this case, reflection may take the form of personal reflection, peer-to-peer reflection discussions, or mentor-facilitated reflection. The important thing is that it occurs, not how it occurs. It is also important that reflection periods include opportunities to integrate theory from previous learning or from contemporaneous reading and research. Once managers complete such a process of reflection and theoretical integration, they are better prepared to move to new and more effective management actions within their practice environment and range of responsibilities. Thus, one sees a mechanism for personal and organizational growth and development.

Mintzberg (2004) goes on to note the importance of conducting these activities within an appropriately integrated conceptual framework. In making this observation, he identifies such a framework as containing five "mind-sets."

1. Reflective (about self)
2. Worldly (about context)

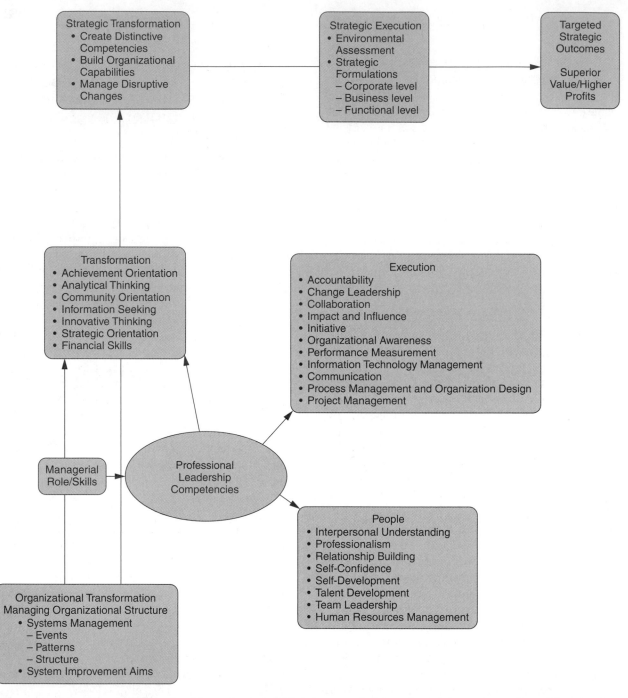

Figure 2.6. Managerial Roots of Organizational Effectiveness: A Strategic and Competency-Based Perspective

SOURCE: Reprinted with permission from William E. Welton, Dr. P.H., M.H.A., University of Washington, 2004. Based on Charles W. L. Hill and Gareth R. Jones, *Strategic Management Theory: An Integrated Approach,* Fifth Edition. Copyright © 2001 by Houghton Mifflin Company. Adapted with permission. Also based on Material from NCHL Health Leadership Model (version 2.0, 2004). Copyright © 2004 by National Center for Healthcare Leadership.

3. Analytical (about organization)

4. Collaborative (about relationships)

5. Action (about change)

In considering the elements of this framework and their integration, one immediately observes the integration of the various elements of the managerial role discussed within this chapter. It is particularly important to note the importance of viewing management as an integrated and integrating activity, the importance of management's central role of environmental scanning and of initiating and managing adaptive responses (action) requiring change in organizational structure and culture. Finally, it is important to note that the importance of doing so through relationship management (often embedded in management of managerial processes).

This then becomes a viable framework for lifelong competency development and improvement. Over the length of a management career, managers who systematically develop and integrate these practices and mind-sets into their personal management practice are likely to see progression to include a broader range of competency development and to higher and higher levels of proficiency in their application. In the final analysis, one must conclude that the development of competencies and associated proficiency levels is as much a part of the managerial role as is the improvement of any one or more technical or scientific aspect(s) of managerial skill(s).

Ultimately, these observations reinforce Mintzberg's (2004) conclusion that "Management is a practice that has to blend a good deal of craft [experience] with a certain amount of art (insight) and some science (analysis), [and that] Managing (organizations) is a difficult, nuanced business, requiring all sorts of tacit understanding that can only be gained in context." (See Debate Time 2.3.)

CONCLUSION

Health system executive leaders and organizational managers, alike, are expected to lead organizational adaptation and transformation to create and maintain sustainable competitive advantage, allowing them to achieve the organization's strategic objectives (see "In Practice," p. 65). They must do this within complicated business organizations that are technologically driven and clinically focused. This requires special capabilities to manage at both of the clinical care system and enterprise-levels, while integrating these perspectives and often-conflicting priorities. As noted throughout the preceding discussion, all of this happens within a strong and highly integrated conceptual, behavioral, and leadership-oriented context. The preceding discussion has emphasized development and integration of all three of these critical areas.

In the final analysis, executives and managerial leaders must develop and demonstrate abilities to lead, apply, and innovate within their managerial roles and assignments (Association to Advance Collegiate Schools of Business, 2004). Within the health care environment, this expectation translates to:

- Leading complex organizations, clinical service delivery organizations, and health care systems

- Applying knowledge in new, challenging, and complex situations

- Innovating by adapting and integrating evidence-based and theoretically sound management concepts with career-long operating experience to cope with challenges caused by unforeseen events and by dynamically changing operating environments

This chapter has explored the distinctive context of the health care system, the characteristics of organizational units operating within the system, and the challenges facing executive leaders and organizational managers within the health care system. This chapter has explored the management role within an overall strategic management frame and context. This chapter has suggested five "mental models" for consideration (i.e., Figures 2.1 to 2.5), which, collectively, allow readers to explore the behavioral context and rationale for management work, for organizational and behavioral processes,

DEBATE TIME 2.3 What Do You Think?

For the past half-century, much emphasis has been given to the importance of master's-level preparation for business and health care managers. The core of this preparation has emphasized the development of highly technical knowledge in a range of functional knowledge areas, including finance, strategy, marketing, organizational behavior, management science, operations management, information technology, and organization management. In this context, the teaching of management has emphasized the so-called hard or scientific analytic skills, and it has emphasized development of analytical skills within each of the relatively narrow functional areas listed above. Yet, Henry Mintzberg (2004) has recently called this strategy into question in his book *Managers, Not MBAs.* In this thought-provoking discussion, Mintzberg observes that the managerial role is an integrated one in which managers must integrate the art, craft, and science of management. Another way of looking at this is that successful managers must continually integrate elements involving vision (art), experience (craft), and analysis (science). Development of management skills thus requires integration of imagination, experience, and logic, as well as the use of inductive, iterative, and deductive decision making, respectively (Mintzberg, 2004).

These observations are important for consideration by the major stakeholders of the management educational community: shareholders, organizational directors or trustees, organizational managers, management educational programs, and potential managers as they contemplate the nature of a successful management career. All of the above stakeholders might be well advised to consider the importance of a balanced development of skills associated with each of Mintzberg's five mind-sets: reflective (about self), worldly (about context), analytical (about organization), collaborative (about relationships), and action (about change) (Gosling & Mintzberg, 2003; Mintzberg, 2004). A balanced approach to management education must emphasize integrated development of skills in each of these areas and must, therefore, encourage integration of the art, craft, and science of management. Moreover, management students must realize that the educational process is lifelong and that their own experience and mentoring relationships are likely to create some of the most significant opportunities for development and integration of knowledge in these important skills areas and mind-sets. What do you think?

and for executive leadership and organizational managerial roles. This chapter also discusses the challenge posed by recent Institute of Medicine studies on challenges inherent in the health care industry's responsibility to ensure the well-being of its patients through a concentration on structural change. Finally, this chapter incorporates discussion of a series of newly emerging professional leadership competencies for executive leaders and managers within the health care management profession. This work has led to presentation of a sixth

mental model (Figure 2.6) in which strategic management and executive leadership concepts are appropriately integrated with newly emerging health care professional leadership competencies.

While the complexities and challenges of executive leadership and organizational management roles were each explored in some detail within the distinctive health care context, the most significant observation may well have been the integrated and integrating nature of executive leadership and organizational management work within a fundamental

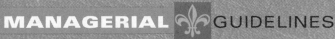

MANAGERIAL GUIDELINES

1. Concept models of organizations and of the managerial role help managers make sense of the complex reality in which they work. No one model provides all the answers; rather different models offer different but useful insights about the context, aims, and functions of management.

2. The environment of health care organizations is increasingly complex, fast changing, and demanding. Managers must design effective processes and structures for keeping up with external changes affecting the organization, determining their implications, and deciding how the organization should respond.

3. Organizations need to adapt to changes in their environment. They must also secure inputs from and sell outputs to external sources. Hence, effective management involves "managing" external interactions, as well as "running a tight ship" internally.

4. Management is a strategically focused and integrating activity. By integrating interpersonal, informational, and decisional management roles in the context of personal characteristics and style, the context of the job, and strategic priorities, the manager assures development of appropriate organizational structure and culture. By integrating executive leadership skills with management process skills, the executive leader assures appropriate organizational adaptation and transformation.

5. Managers should consciously model and act in concert with the behaviors and values they seek to develop in the organizations. Behavior by others consistent with these values should be encouraged and recognized.

6. Building consensus, forming coalitions, and negotiating compromises are activities that are becoming more important for managers as the number of external and internal parties that health care organizations must deal with increases.

7. Translating potential conflicts over desired outcomes into cooperation or collaboration requires that the manager search for common ground among the different interest groups.

8. Managers must understand and then act on the knowledge that power or the ability to get things done in the organization of the future will come more from empowering, inspiring, and supporting others and from teamwork—not so much from the manager's own authority or decisions. Through the sharing of power, the manager's effectiveness will be enhanced.

9. Managers must understand the roles of the business enterprise and of the clinical systems within the enterprise. It is important to understand opportunities to create synergy and assure returns through appropriate investment, relationship management, and maintenance of supportive internal environments and communication systems. Likewise, it is important to understand the need for accountability at three organization levels: community, enterprise-wide, and clinical operating system(s) within the enterprise.

10. Managers should look for opportunities to assess their mastery of the competencies and skills associated with the different management roles, and should consciously seek to improve their weaknesses. Managers should also strive to develop a good

(continues)

MANAGERIAL GUIDELINES *(continued)*

sense of self-awareness, and to be intro-
spective about how they react to different
types of situations.

11. Managers should develop competencies in
three domains—transformation, execution,
and people management. Transformation is
essential to recognizing, selecting, and communicating adaptation opportunities

and/or requirements. Execution is essential
to assure that organizational/systemic
transformation takes place on goal and on
schedule. People management is essential,
since both transformation and execution require the commitment and ongoing support of people within the organizational
system.

---

strategic management frame. The opportunities and
requirements for developing conceptual skills, integrating skills, and communication skills are noted,
as are the special role of management skills, routines
and heuristics, notably those involved with initiation and management of "organizational transformation," and the development, maintenance, and/or
change of "organizational structure, over time." As a
final observation, this chapter notes the importance
of developing an action-oriented set of integrated
competencies and of enhancing them through a
process of action-oriented and reflection-based improvement over a managerial career.

In this context, this chapter becomes an appropriate linkage between the nature of organizations
(Chapter 1) and the broad range of technical organizational skills required to manage within the
range of management activity domains. These include: (a) motivating and leading people and groups
(Chapters 3 through 5); (b) operating the technical
system (Chapters 6 through 9); (c) positioning the
organization for success (Chapters 10 through 13);
and (d) charting the future (Chapters 14 and 15).

DISCUSSION QUESTIONS

1. As you think about the managerial role within
the health care business enterprise, how

would you describe the role in behavioral
terms and from a behavioral perspective?

2. How would you describe the organizational
and managerial implications of aligning
internal organization structure and culture
with the demands of and opportunities
presented by the organization's external
environment?

3. How would you describe the relationship
between core principles of strategic
management and the behavior of enterprise
managers within health care organizations?
In completing this description, what is the
relationship between the managerial role and
the effectiveness of the business enterprise?

4. How would you differentiate and describe the
work that managers do in managing
organizational structure and culture, as
opposed to managing organizational process?
Why is it important to distinguish between
the two aspects of the managerial role?

5. Why is it important to view the managerial
role as an integrating and initiating activity?
Describe the significance of the managerial
role and executive leadership in initiating
and facilitating organizational and cultural
change.

6. Within the health care organization, what is
the relationship between the "business

enterprise" and its "clinical care systems"? How can the two be coordinated and what is the role of health care managers in assuring the effectiveness of this coordination?

7. What are the implications for health care enterprise managers of the enterprise's distinctive operating environment characteristics?

8. Describe the challenges to health care enterprise managers associated with adapting the recommendations of the Institute of Medicine's *Crossing the Quality Chasm: A New Health System for the 21st Century* report. Why are these organizational adaptation challenges particularly challenging in the health care organizational enterprise environment?

9. What is the difference between an executive leader and an organizational manager in health care organizations? Why is it important to consider such distinctions? How do these distinctions relate to the managerial role as described within the chapter?

10. Why is it important for health care managers to develop a strong conceptual perspective and to develop a set of managerial competencies within the transformation, execution, and people domains? How do these perspectives and competencies relate to the work of executive leaders and organizational managers within health care organizations? How would you expect individuals in managerial and leadership roles to develop and refine these competencies over their careers?

REFERENCES

Anderson, V., & Johnson, L. (1997). *System thinking basics: From concepts to causal loops.* Waltham, MA: Pegasus Communication, Inc.

Argyris, C. (1999). *On organizational learning.* Malden, MA: Blackwell Business Publishers.

Association to Advance Collegiate Schools of Business (AACSB International). (2004). *Accreditation standards—Assurance of learning standards, Standard 18: Master's level degree in general management (i.e., MBA programs).* St. Louis, MO. Available from http://www.aacsb.edu/resource_centers/assessment/std-18.asp

Boyatzis, R. (1982). *The competent manager: A model for effective performance.* New York: Wiley-Interscience.

Bridges, W. (1991). *Managing transitions: Making the most of change.* Cambridge, MA: Perseus Books.

Burke, W. (2002). *Organizational change: Theory and practice.* Thousand Oaks, CA: Sage Publications.

Cristensen, C., & Overdorf, M. (2000, March/April). Meeting the challenge of disruptive change. *Harvard Business Review.*

Drucker, P. (1994, September/October). The theory of business. *Harvard Business Review*, 95–104.

Garvin, D. (1998, Summer). The processes of organization and management. *Sloan Management Review*, 33–50.

Goleman, D. (1995). *Emotional intelligence: Why it can matter more than IQ.* New York: Bantam Books.

Goleman, D. (1998). *Working with emotional intelligence.* New York: Bantam Books.

Goleman, D. (2000, March/April). Leadership that gets results. *Harvard Business Review*, 78–90.

Goleman, D., Boyatzis, R., & McKee, A. (2002). *Primal leadership: Realizing the power of emotional intelligence.* Boston, MA: Harvard Business School Press.

Hayes, J. (2002). *The theory and practice of change management.* New York: Palgrave MacMillan.

Hill, C., & Jones, G. (2002). *Strategic management: An integrated approach* (5th ed.). Boston, MA: Houghton-Mifflin.

Institute of Medicine. (2000). To err is human: Building a safer health system. Washington, DC: National Academy Press.

Institute of Medicine. (2001). *Crossing the quality chasm: A new health system for the 21st century.* Washington, DC: National Academy Press.

Kaplan, R., & Norton, D. (1996, January/February). Using the balanced scorecard as a strategic management system. *Harvard Business Review*, 76.

Katz, R. L. (1974, September/October). Skills of an effective administrator. *Harvard Business Review.*

Kotter, J. (2001, December). What leaders really do. *Harvard Business Review, 79,* (11) 85.

Kotter, J. (1996). *Leading change.* Cambridge, MA: Harvard Business School Press.

Luke, R., Watson, S., & Plummer, M. (2004). *Healthcare strategy: In pursuit of competitive advantage.* Chicago, IL: Health Administration Press, and Washington, DC: Association of University Programs in Health Administration (AUPHA), 284 pp.

McClelland, D., Atkinson, J., Clark, R., & Lowell, E. (1953). *The achievement motive.* New York: Appleton-Century-Crofts.

McClelland, D. C. (1971). *Motivating economic achievement.* New York: The Free Press.

Mintzberg, H. (1989). *Mintzberg on management: Inside our strange world of organizations.* New York: Free Press.

Mintzberg, H. (1990, March/April). The manager's job: Folklore and fact. *Harvard Business Review,* 17–30.

Mintzberg, H. (1994, Fall). Rounding out the manager's job. *Sloan Management Review,* 11–26.

Mintzberg, H. (2004). *Managers, Not MBAs: A hard look at the soft practice of managing and management development.* San Francisco, CA: Berrett-Koehler Publishers, Inc.

Mintzberg, H. & Gosling, J. (2003, November). The five minds of a manager. *Harvard Business Review,* 33–41.

Mohr, J., & Batalden, P. (2002, March). Improving safety on the front lines: The role of clinical microsystems. *Quality and Safety in Health Care, 11*(1), 45–50.

Nelson E., Batalden P., Huber, T., Mohr, J., Godfrey, M., Headrick, L., & Wasson, J. (2002, September). Microsystems in health care: Part 1. Learning from high-performing front-line clinical units. *Journal of Quality Improvement (JCAH),* 28(9), 472–493.

National Center for Healthcare Leadership (NCHL). (2004). *NCHL Healthcare Leadership Competency Model, version 2.0.* Developed by the National Center for Healthcare Leadership and Hay Group, Inc., © 2004 National Center for Healthcare Leadership. All rights reserved. Chicago, IL.

Nelson, R., & Winter, S. (1982). *An evolutionary theory of economic change.* Cambridge, MA: The Belknap Press of Harvard University.

Perrow, C. (1984). *Complex organizations: A critical essay* (3rd ed.) New York: McGraw-Hill, Inc., Chapter 4: The Neo-Weberian model: Decision-making, conflict and technology, 119–156.

Porter, M. (1985). *Competitive strategy: Creating and sustaining superior performance.* New York: Free Press.

Porter, M., & Teisberg, E. (2004, June). Redefining competition in healthcare. *Harvard Business Review,* 65–76.

Prahalad, C., & Hamel, G. (1990, May/June). The core competence of the corporation. *Harvard Business Review,* 79.

Sterman, J. (2000). *Business dynamics: Systems thinking and modeling for a complex world.* Boston, MA: Irwin/McGraw-Hill, Chapter 1, 3–39 & Chapter 3, 83–105.

Tushman, M., & Romanelli, E. (1985). Organization evolution: A metamorphosis model of convergence and reorientation. In *Organizational Behavior* (Vol. 7). JAI Press, Inc., 171–222.

Welton, W. (2004). Managing today's complex healthcare business enterprise: Reflections of distinctive requirements of healthcare management education. Washington, DC, Association of University Programs in Health Administration, *Journal of Health Administration Education,* 21, (4).

Zaccaro, S. (2001). *The nature of executive leadership: A conceptual and empirical analysis of success.* Washington, DC: American Psychological Association.

TWO

Motivating, Leading, and Negotiating

THE NATURE OF ORGANIZATIONS: FRAMEWORK FOR THE TEXT

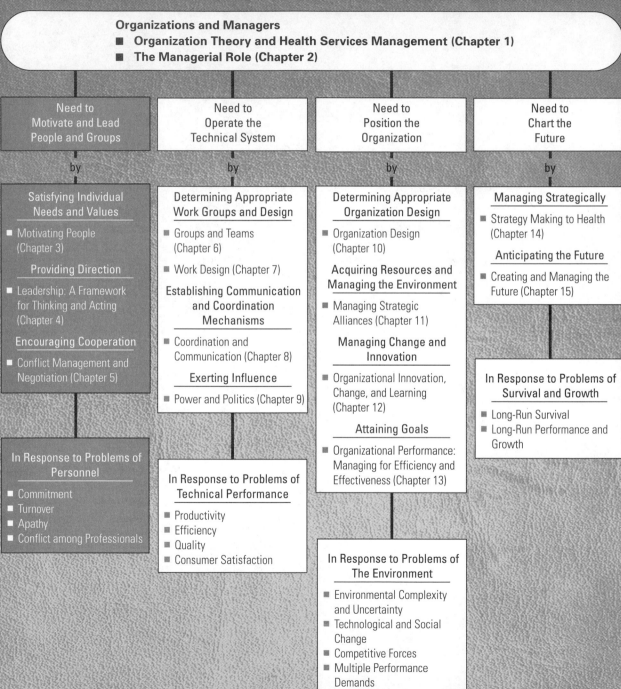

Organizations and Managers
- Organization Theory and Health Services Management (Chapter 1)
- The Managerial Role (Chapter 2)

Need to
Motivate and Lead
People and Groups

Need to
Operate the
Technical System

Need to
Position the
Organization

Need to
Chart the
Future

by

by

by

by

Satisfying Individual
Needs and Values

- Motivating People
(Chapter 3)

Providing Direction

- Leadership: A Framework
for Thinking and Acting
(Chapter 4)

Encouraging Cooperation

- Conflict Management and
Negotiation (Chapter 5)

Determining Appropriate
Work Groups and Design

- Groups and Teams
(Chapter 6)
- Work Design (Chapter 7)

Establishing Communication
and Coordination
Mechanisms

- Coordination and
Communication (Chapter 8)

Exerting Influence

- Power and Politics (Chapter 9)

Determining Appropriate
Organization Design

- Organization Design
(Chapter 10)

Acquiring Resources and
Managing the Environment

- Managing Strategic
Alliances (Chapter 11)

Managing Change and
Innovation

- Organizational Innovation,
Change, and Learning
(Chapter 12)

Attaining Goals

- Organizational Performance:
Managing for Efficiency and
Effectiveness (Chapter 13)

Managing Strategically

- Strategy Making to Health
(Chapter 14)

Anticipating the Future

- Creating and Managing the
Future (Chapter 15)

In Response to Problems of
Personnel

- Commitment
- Turnover
- Apathy
- Conflict among Professionals

In Response to Problems of
Technical Performance

- Productivity
- Efficiency
- Quality
- Consumer Satisfaction

In Response to Problems of
Survival and Growth

- Long-Run Survival
- Long-Run Performance and
Growth

In Response to Problems of
The Environment

- Environmental Complexity
and Uncertainty
- Technological and Social
Change
- Competitive Forces
- Multiple Performance
Demands

Chapters 3 through 5 deal with fundamental issues related to motivation, leadership, and negotiation. These processes are fundamental building blocks for working effectively with individuals and groups. Understanding multiple sources of motivation, different approaches to leadership, and various ways of managing conflict and negotiations are key determinants of successful managerial performance.

Chapter 3, "Motivating People," focuses on a variety of issues related to motivation. The chapter addresses the following questions:

- What are some of the common myths associated with motivating people?

- What are the major content and process approaches to understanding motivation?

- What are some of the more effective ways of dealing with motivational problems?

The chapter emphasizes multiple approaches for dealing with motivational issues.

Chapter 4, "Leadership: A Framework for Thinking and Acting," addresses the multiple ways in which leadership has been defined and various approaches to understanding leadership effectiveness. Specific questions examined include:

- What is known about the different perspectives regarding effective leadership?

- What are the special leadership challenges facing health services organizations?

- What skills are needed to be successful health care leaders?

The chapter sets forth an integrative model of leadership for the reader's consideration.

Chapter 5, "Conflict Management and Negotiation," highlights the major forms of conflict that occur in health services organizations and various approaches for dealing with them. Special attention is devoted to structuring and managing negotiation processes. Among the key questions addressed are:

- What are the major causes of conflict in health services organizations?

- What are the pros and cons of different approaches for managing conflict?

- What are the primary concepts and approaches associated with effective negotiation?

The chapter emphasizes multiple approaches to managing conflict and the importance of preparation for effective negotiation.

Upon completing these three chapters, readers should have a fuller understanding of the relationships among motivation, leadership, and conflict management and negotiation. Readers should have a firm grasp of the various approaches to dealing with these issues and understand which approaches are most likely to be effective under different circumstances.

CHAPTER 3

Motivating People

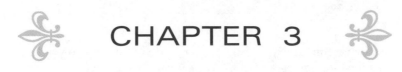

Myron D. Fottler, Ph.D., Stephen J. O'Connor, Ph.D., Mattia J. Gilmartin, RN, Ph.D., and Thomas A. D'Aunno, Ph.D.

CHAPTER OUTLINE

- ❧ Motivation and Management
- ❧ Content Perspectives
- ❧ Process Perspectives
- ❧ Motivating Health Care Professionals and Support Personnel
- ❧ Motivational Problems

LEARNING OBJECTIVES

After completing this chapter, the reader should be able to:

1. Define motivation and distinguish it from other factors that influence individuals' performance.
2. Recognize popular but misleading myths about motivation.
3. Understand that motivation depends heavily on the situations in which individuals work.
4. Understand managers' roles in motivating people.
5. Identify key characteristics of the content of peoples' work that motivates them.
6. Identify important processes involved in motivating people.
7. Assess and deal with motivational problems.

KEY TERMS

Behavior Modification	Hierarchy of Needs	Motivators
Empowerment	Hygiene Factors	Reinforcement Theory
Equity	Instrumentality	Self-actualization
Expectancy	Job Redesign	Valence
Gainsharing	Motivation	

🔱 IN PRACTICE   Dr. Intimidation

If hospitals want to reduce medication errors, one challenge is to get their physicians and other medication prescribers to react without condescension and intimidation to questions and concerns from the professionals charged with carrying out the orders. That's the conclusion reached by the Institute for Safe Medication Practices after a survey it conducted showing that such intimidation contributes to medical errors by preventing nurses and pharmacists from voicing concerns about the correctness or safety of medications.

In a survey of 2,099 health care practitioners, 40% of respondents assumed a prescription was correct at least once during the previous year rather than raise the matter with a physician or other prescribing professional with a reputation for reacting with intimidation. When they did speak up, 49% said they felt pressure to give the medication despite their concerns. Often no harm resulted, but 7% of all respondents said they were involved in a medication error during the past year "in which intimidation clearly played a role," according to the institute. Some 10% of pharmacists reported intimidation-related medical errors.

Hospitals are trying to change their culture to head off medical errors by encouraging caregivers to report errors without fear of sanction and enable everyone to learn from them, said Hedy Cohen, the institute's vice president. Good working relationships among those caregivers are crucial to the effort. "Part of this culture change is working as a team, which will prevent errors," Cohen said.

Often, however, pharmacists and nurses were left to huddle with colleagues or do research on their own to assuage fears about orders. Among pharmacists, 23% said they attempted to clarify the safety of an order themselves at least 10 times during the year rather than interact with a prescriber.

Physicians were more likely to use condescending language or be impatient with requests from nurses rather than pharmacists, but more than 20% of both groups reported such incidents happened at least 10 times in the past year. Nearly half of all respondents said past experiences with intimidations have altered how they handle questions or clarifications.

The experiences sometimes included strong verbal abuse, mentioned by 48%, but subtle expressions of exasperation may be all it takes to throw cold water on communication, Cohen said. "It's like with your spouse," she said. "If every time you ask a question they look at you (derisively) and they put their hands on their hips, you're not going to ask more questions."

For additional information on the Institute for Safe Medication Practices, visit: http://www.ismp.org/.

Source: Morrissey, J. (2004, April 5). Dr. Intimidation; Surly prescribers increase risk of errors: Survey. *Modern Healthcare, 34* (14), 10.

CHAPTER PURPOSE

Interpersonal interaction among health care providers within an organization may have profound implications on medication errors and other adverse events (see "In Practice," Dr. Intimidation). The objective of this chapter is to understand how to motivate individuals to perform effectively in health services organizations. The chapter consists of five major sections. The first section defines motivation and distinguishes it from other factors that can affect performance. This section also describes common but misleading myths about motivation. As antidotes to these myths, we emphasize that motivation is situational. There are several characteristics of individuals and the settings in which they work that managers should take into account in trying to motivate people. The section concludes by examining the role that managers can play to maintain or increase motivation. The next two sections identify the most important factors that managers can influence to improve or maintain the motivation of employees and coworkers. The focus is on those approaches that seem most promising, and we refer readers to more extensive reviews (Ambrose & Kulik, 1999; Jurkiewicz, Massey, & Brown, 1998; Kanfer, 1990; Steers & Porter, 1987; Mitchell & Daniels, 2002). Finally, the last section examines common motivational problems and discusses how to assess them. Several alternatives for dealing with motivational problems are explored.

MOTIVATION AND MANAGEMENT

Motivation is a central topic for health services managers, but it can also be an especially difficult one. The types of workers managers might be ex-

pected to motivate can range from highly educated and professional ones such as physicians and nurses, to minimum wage workers such as nurse's aids in long-term care settings (Vance, 1997).

The environment of health care continues to swiftly change, requiring regular improvements in productivity while simultaneously requiring cost containment. Mergers, layoffs, lower profit margins, increased regulatory demands, cost-cutting pressure, savy purchasers and consumers, and intense competition have combined to squeeze the expense out of this system, making the workforce health care's most expensive resource (Thomas, 1998). The theories and techniques of motivation that will be described in this chapter are excellent tools for making health care's most expensive resource its most valuable asset. Empirical evidence indicates that human resource practices, such as those that improve motivation, can positively influence an organization's financial performance (Huselid, 1995; Pfeffer, 1998). Consequently, a highly motivated workforce can serve as a difficult-to-replicate competitive advantage (Zigarelli, 1996).

A primary task of management is to motivate people to perform at high levels toward meeting organizational objectives (Steers & Porter, 1987), but many managers are unclear as to how this should be accomplished (Kovach, 1995; Medcof & Hausdorf, 1995).

In addition to motivating individuals to improve productivity and efficiency, health care managers may wish to motivate workers to reduce absenteeism and tardiness (Mercer, 1988), to improve problem-solving ability, to promote creativity and innovativeness (Colvin, 1998), to work interdependently and cooperatively as team members, to develop consumer-oriented attitudes and behaviors (O'Connor & Shewchuk, 1995), to reenergize those who no longer feel challenged (Kennedy, 1997), to remotivate following a reduction in force (McConnell, 1996), to get people to take on added responsibilities (Nordhaus-Bike, 1997), to recruit hard-to-find workers such as information technology professionals (Appleby, 1998), and to motivate moral and ethical behavior (Vidaver-Cohen, 1998).

Defining and Distinguishing Motivation

The beginning of wisdom in motivating people is to recognize what motivation is and is not (Mohr, 1982). We define **motivation** as a state of feeling or thinking in which one is energized or aroused to perform a task or engage in a particular behavior (Steers & Porter, 1987). This definition focuses on motivation as an emotional or cognitive state that is independent of action. This focus clearly distinguishes motivation from the performance of a task and its consequences. Notice, too, that motivation can be a state of either feeling or thinking, or a combination of the two. For some individuals, motivation is more a matter of feeling than thinking, while, for others, the reverse is true.

Myths about Motivation— and Some Antidotes

There are several popular but misleading myths about motivating people. Our view is that these myths are more harmful than helpful and, as a result, need to be confronted early in this chapter. Four particular myths are addressed below.

Myth 1: Motivated workers are more productive. To illustrate this myth, consider this conversation (Muchinsky, 1987).

Supervisor: George just isn't motivated any more!
Foreman: How can you tell?
Supervisor: His productivity has fallen off by more than 50%.

Motivation should not be confused with performance. People can be highly motivated but still per-

form poorly. Performance depends not just on motivation but also on ability and a host of situational factors such as the availability of resources needed to perform a job well (Locke & Latham, 2004). Motivation is just one of several factors that managers need to consider in trying to improve or sustain individuals' performance. Nonetheless, it is often a critical factor.

Myth 2: Some people are just motivated and others aren't. This myth is based on the view that motivation is a personality trait or characteristic that remains relatively stable from time to time and place to place. If this view were taken to its extreme, it would suggest that managers should carefully select only those employees who have the trait of motivation, for managers could otherwise do little to influence motivation and behavior.

In contrast, we take the view that motivation is more specific to situations (i.e., influenced by factors in an individual's environment) than it is a stable personality trait or characteristic (Kanfer, 1990). There is strong empirical support for the view that situations significantly shape individual behavior (Davis-Blake). For example, as illustrated in the case of "Dr. Intimidation," if the situational environment is poor (e.g., condescension, intimidation, verbal abuse, and disrespect), it is difficult for people to remain motivated. This demotivation can have a direct impact on patient care and safety.

We argue that, even if motivation were a somewhat stable personality trait, it would still be important for managers to ensure that employees have work conditions that will reinforce their tendency to be motivated or change their tendency to be unmotivated. In short, motivation and behavior are produced by a complex interaction of situational and individual factors.

Myth 3: Motivation can be mass produced. A major myth about motivation is that it can be mass

IN PRACTICE   A Cry for Help

Working and keeping motivated on a busy 24-bed general intensive care unit, a charge nurse tells her story:

ICU nursing is becoming frustrating. It is frustrating to always be there, to work so closely with patients, to do so much to keep them going, and then have someone else get all the credit. The nurses do the work, they act as the eyes and ears monitoring and responding to the patients' condition, but it is always the physician who saves them and gets the accolades.

The ICU is also becoming a more dangerous and scary place to work. In addition to tuberculosis, HIV, and hepatitis, there are more bloodborne and communicable diseases than ever before. Patients who come here are often under the influence of drugs or alcohol. They often react badly to pharmaceuticals we administer to them. Because the atmosphere is unfamiliar, they frequently get violent. Even old people can get violent.

Consumerism is rampant in health care. Everyone is an expert. The families continually remind me to wash my hands. Administration has recently been demanding more consumer-friendly behavior from the ICU nurses. They recently instituted wide open, 24-hour visiting hours. They told us, 'You will tolerate someone being here 24 hours a day as long as there is no bonafide reason that they shouldn't be there.' For the most part this is fine with us. We are part of a very family- and community-oriented health system, and families can really help out. They can reassure their kids or make certain their elderly parents or grandparents don't fall out of bed and are comfortable. In some cases, if a family member is not available, we have to hire sitters for $12 an hour to keep an eye on the patient. Generally, the sitters are unskilled people who can't participate in the patient care process. Usually they knit, eat chips, read, listen to the radio, or sleep.

Although the presence of family members can assist us, more often than not, they impede our ability to do our work. We have one 'frequent flyer' who is in here all the time. His wife will not leave. She insists on doing his care. The husband has severe diabetes, and she insists on doing the glucose monitoring and dressing changes. We can't get rid of her. She makes the nurses very uncomfortable. Sometimes you have to take care of the entire family, not just the member in the bed. Many families are already dysfunctional to begin with; they don't usually function any better in the ICU setting.

People who go into ICU nursing go into it because they are more comfortable working with technology than with people. They do best, and I hate to say this, when the patient is paralyzed, sedated, and ventilated. Those really caring nurses go into oncology or the touchy-feelies, not ICU.

Our system has been restructuring lately, and administration has been trying to focus less on financial rewards and more on nontangible rewards. The ICU nurses do receive a higher pay differential, because the work is more demanding and specialized. However, administration wants to get away from differentials because, as they say, 'Everything is getting to be a specialty.' But believe me, money still talks!

A year ago, administration cut back ICU staffing in an effort to save money. Shortly after that time, we went into a 10-month period of very high census and very high acuity. The highest anyone could ever remember, and we were understaffed! Work became horrible. I didn't want to go. Every time it would be hellish. The 24 ICU beds were always full of seriously ill people.

As the demands and stresses became greater, the necessary ICU 'community behaviors' were just put aside. The nurses weren't motivated to work as a team anymore; they began focusing on 'their' patients only. But we all have to keep watch on the telemetry banks and the arrhythmia alarms. Phones ring that have to be answered. The pneumatic tubes [which transport lab results, blood samples, and pharmaceuticals] need to be attended to. These activities are not assigned, but need to be done as a team.

Often, nurses that were scheduled to work eight hours would have to stay for 12. For a while, we had to work every weekend and holiday. To help ease the staffing void, the hospital began to rely on external agency, pool nurses at a higher wage. When the pool nurses come here, they are not 100%. They might be totally unfamiliar with our environment, and we don't necessarily know their skill level. Naturally, these nurses take a lot of orientation and maintenance time. Furthermore, because pool nurses are not given computer passwords, we have to do their computerized charting, which creates more work for us. The pool nurses are hired guns who are paid about $12 more per hour than we are. They also work whenever they want to.

Although we are a nonprofit, we have a gain-sharing plan. Administration thinks money is not an issue with us. They played with the equations. We worked very hard—all out—for 10 months in a very difficult and understaffed environment. We did receive our gain-share checks, but it was practically nothing. Because of the high patient census and acuity, coupled with staff cutbacks, the external agency pool was used heavily. They are paid a premium. Apparently, that is where most of our gain-share went. We didn't feel that the gain-share checks rewarded us at all. In the end, it had nothing to do with all the extra effort. That was our reward for being full-time, committed, extremely hard working, and concerned for quality.

I can go down to the agency tomorrow and make $12 an hour more than I do now.

For additional information see the website: American Association of Colleges of Nursing, Information about the nursing workforce and labor shortage in the United States,
http://www.aacn.nche.edu/

For Discussion

1. In this case what work-related factors are demotivating the nursing staff? Can the influence of these factors be changed?
2. What role do managers and clinical leaders play to improve staff morale and motivation in this situation?

---

produced (for example, in speeches by charismatic leaders to large groups of people or by placing motivational posters throughout the workplace). Though these approaches sometimes work, most often they do not (Laurinaitis, 1997). Typically, in order to motivate people effectively, managers need to treat them as individuals. Contrary to the myth of mass production, we assert that individuals vary widely from each other in many ways. As a result, it is a central and recurring theme of this chapter that managers must motivate employees and coworkers on an individual basis, taking each person's situation into account. At least three important types of individual and situational differences should be considered:

1. job position or occupation
2. career stage
3. personal factors

Job position or occupation. One of the most distinctive features of health care organizations is the number of different occupational groups and job categories involved. These groups range from nurse's aides and porters to nurses, physical therapists, and physicians. Health care occupations vary along dimensions such as the amount and type of training they require, their power and status, and what types of individuals are attracted to them. Managers should understand how their ability to motivate individuals may vary according to their occupation or job category. For example, union contracts often prohibit certain types of changes in job design and responsibilities; managers need to know what occupational groups are covered by such contracts and how they affect certain approaches to motivation.

Career stage. A second important way in which individuals vary is their career stage. To illustrate, consider a recent graduate of a health services management program. He may be highly motivated by assignments that provide opportunities for learning about the different divisions of a health care organization. In contrast, his colleague who has more experience may wish to work on a single project from start to completion. Managers need to be sensitive to such career stage needs, motives, and values (Kanfer & Ackerman, 2004).

Personal factors. Perhaps more than we recognize, people at work are influenced by a variety of factors from their personal lives. For example, personal factors sometimes parallel career stages. A recent graduate may have few family ties that would limit her interest in work that involved travel, whereas a manager with young children may be less motivated by opportunity for travel on the job. Other important personal influences that can affect motivation include family illness, divorce, substance abuse, health problems, child care, and financial stress. These are clearly delicate areas for managers to tread. Yet, managers need to be aware that such personal factors can affect work motivation. On the one hand, it may be harmful to pry into the personal lives of employees and coworkers. On the

other hand, it may be very helpful to be sensitive to needs at work that stem from their personal lives.

Myth 4: Money makes the world go 'round. We do not deny that many, if not most, individuals care about and are motivated by money (Stajkovic & Luthans, 2001). But too often managers think only of money when trying to motivate people. Unfortunately, money is likely to be in short supply for health care managers, at least in the next several years. Fortunately, money is not always the most important motivator; indeed, it seldom is. In the next sections, the importance of several other factors in motivating people that do not require cash will be discussed.

Manager's Role

The situational perspective described above implies that managers should take an active role in systematically assessing the motivation of their employees and coworkers. Individuals' motivation can vary over time and with the kind of work they are performing. Thus, managers need to periodically assess motivation and performance, taking into account the occupational, career stage, and personal factors discussed above. Such assessments should include informal interviews with employees and coworkers in which open-ended questions are asked about individuals' needs, motives, perceptions, and values (Zima, 1983). These assessments need not be lengthy. What matters more is that they are timely; employees feel comfortable in openly expressing their concerns, and managers use the opportunity to do problem solving and goal setting. In short, managers can play a critical role by not only assessing their employees' motivation but by taking the lead to alter conditions that can increase motivation.

What factors make people energized or aroused to work? Further, what factors influence how individuals' energy is directed and to what tasks, how intense their arousal is, and how long they persist in these states? These are the key questions that managers need to address to motivate people. Research attempts to explain work motivation through two basic types of theories: content and process. *Content theories* are concerned with *what* energizes behavior, while *process theories* focus on *how* behavior is energized.

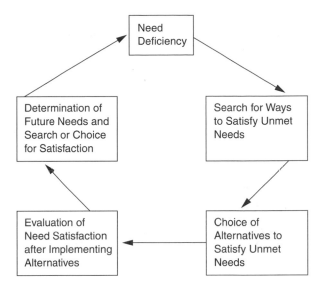

Figure 3.1. A Framework for Employee Motivation

CONTENT PERSPECTIVES

Content perspectives on motivation focus in large part on needs and need deficiencies. According to content perspectives, motivation can be considered a goal-directed, internal drive, which is aimed at satisfying needs. A need can be a physical or psychological deficiency that makes specific outcomes or goals attractive. The need, in turn, stimulates individuals' internal drives, which directs them toward those goals that have the capacity to satisfy the need (O'Connor, 1998). Researchers agree that people have a multitude of needs with varying degrees of intensity. Such needs create a state of disequilibrium within the person, which, in turn, creates a desire to meet the need or needs she is experiencing. Consequently, individuals search the environment for potentially satisfying goals. Once attained, these goals will lead to a reduction in the disequilibrium or the fulfillment of their needs. Motivation can be increased to the degree that peoples' needs can be satisfied on the job.

Thus, content perspectives try to answer the question, What factor or factors motivate people? Some assert that motivation is a function of pay, working hours, and working conditions. Others suggest that autonomy and responsibility are the causes of motivation (Kovach, 1987). Still others believe either or both sets of factors could be important in a given situation.

The motivation framework in Figure 3.1 is a good starting point for understanding how needs

can motivate people. The motivation process often begins with needs that reflect some deficiency within the individual. For example, the employee might feel underpaid or lacking recognition vis-à-vis other employees. In response to these unsatisfied needs, the employee searches for ways to satisfy them. She may ask for a raise or promotion, work harder to try to earn either, or seek another position outside the organization. Next, she chooses one or more options. After implementing the chosen option or options, she then evaluates her success. If her hard work resulted in a pay raise or a promotion, she will probably continue to work hard. If neither has occurred, she will probably try another option.

The Need Hierarchy

Theory Overview

Many theorists advanced the concept of a need hierarchy, but Abraham Maslow (1943) developed the most popular version in the management field in the 1940s. He proposed that people want to satisfy various needs and that these needs can be

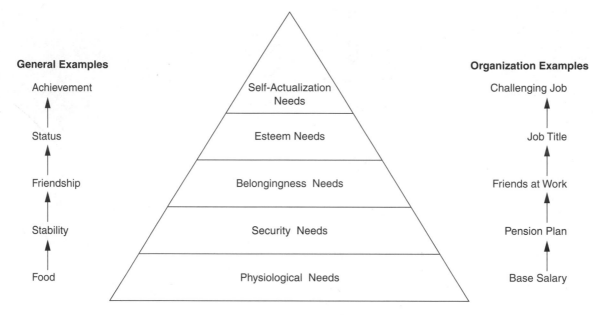

Figure 3.2. Maslow's Hierarchy of Needs

SOURCE: Adapted from Maslow, A. H. (1943), A theory of human motivation. *Psychological Review 50*, 370–396.

arranged in a hierarchy of importance as shown in Figure 3.2.

Maslow's **hierarchy of needs** assumes there are five need levels that must be satisfied sequentially. The *physiological* needs include such things as air, water, food, warmth, shelter, and sex. They represent basic issues of survival and biological function. In organization settings, such needs are generally satisfied by adequate wages and a satisfactory work environment that provides adequate lighting, temperature, and ventilation.

The *security* needs include a secure physical and emotional environment. Examples include the need to be free from worry about money and job security. In the workplace, security needs are satisfied by job continuity (no layoffs), a grievance system (to protect against arbitrary action), and an adequate health insurance and retirement package (for security against illness and eventual retirement). The latter is especially important, because as the health care environment continues to profoundly change,

many employees may fear the loss of their jobs due to mergers, downsizing, or closings.

Because health care organizations have the potential to be fairly hazardous places to work, security needs are frequently important in these settings. The ICU nurses (see In Practice, p. 82) for example, feared being subject to violence or of contracting conditions such as tuberculosis, hepatitis, or HIV.

Belongingness needs involve social processes. They include the need for love and affection and the need to be accepted by one's peers. For most people, they are satisfied by a combination of family and community relationships outside the job and friendships on the job. A manager can promote the satisfaction of these needs by encouraging social interaction and by making employees feel part of a team or work group. Sensitivity to an employee's family problems can also help employees meet this need.

Esteem needs are actually composed of two different sets of needs: the need for a positive self-image or self-respect and the need for recognition and respect from others. For example, the ICU nurses felt they did not receive adequate recognition for what they did on the job. They believed that physicians were getting all the credit. Managers can help address esteem needs by providing signs of accomplishment such as job titles, public recognition, and praise (i.e., extrinsic rewards). They may also provide more challenging job assignments and other opportunities for employees to feel a sense of accomplishment.

Self-actualization needs, at the top of the hierarchy, involve realizing one's potential for continued growth and individual development. These are most difficult for a manager to identify and meet due to individual differences in goals. However, allowing employees to participate in decision making and the opportunity to learn new things about their work may promote self-actualization.

Maslow suggests that the five need categories constitute a hierarchy. People are motivated first to satisfy the lower level needs beginning with physiological needs. As long as these remain unsatisfied, the individual is motivated only to fulfill them. When these needs are satisfied, they cease to motivate people and they move up the hierarchy and become sequentially concerned with each higher level in turn. This process is termed *satisfaction-progression*—as an individual satisfies one set of needs, the next higher-level set of needs will dominate. This process will continue until the level of self-actualization is reached.

Research Support and Evaluation

The need hierarchy has a certain intuitive logic, but research indicates various shortcomings in the theory. While the progression principle suggests a systematic approach to satisfying needs from lowest to highest levels, research provides little evidence that a stepwise hierarchy actually exists. For example, some research shows that the five levels of need are not always present and the order of the levels is not always the same as Maslow proposed (Pinder, 1984; Steers & Porter, 1987).

Nor has research confirmed the deficit principle, in which unmet needs systematically motivate behavior (Schwartz, 1983). Needs do not fall into a neat five-step hierarchy (Mitchell & Mowdgill, 1976; Wahba & Budwell, 1976). There are some rather obvious exceptions to the theory to necessitate caution. For example, outstanding artists have continued their creative work while sacrificing health and security. Soldiers risk death for an ideal. Some employees strive for excellence despite their low-wage, dead-end jobs. Others employed in higher-wage jobs offering numerous opportunities for growth and development fail to take advantage of such opportunities. While their lower-level needs are being met, they do not strive to meet higher-level needs identified by Maslow's need hierarchy.

A major reason why the literature shows little support for Maslow's theory is because the needs are ambiguous and overlap, rather than being distinct and independent (Lee, 1980). In some studies, the lower-level needs formed a cluster, and the higher-level needs formed a cluster.

The major problem with Maslow's need hierarchy is that it cannot be turned into a practical guide for managers who are trying to enhance work motivation. The research evidence is just not there to support such rules of thumb as "If you satisfy employees' physiological and safety needs through job security and a competitive compensation system, then employees will be motivated mainly by needs for affiliation or self-actualization." It would be helpful if the advice were accurate, but it is not.

Application

Though managers cannot apply Maslow's needs hierarchy mechanistically, it is not unreasonable to conclude that unmet needs do motivate *most* employees *most* of the time. Maslow did identify some of the major categories of human needs that *may* motivate different employees at different times. In practical terms, organizations should provide employees with wages sufficient for food and shelter;

reasonable protection of jobs, health, and safety; a satisfactory physical and social environment at work; and rewards or recognition that reinforce individual esteem. Managers should also recognize and support growth needs by providing opportunities for career advancement, encouraging personal self-development, and creating environments in which individuals can explore their individual talents and dreams.

The major implication of Maslow's theory for management is that organization policies and practices must pay attention to all of these needs if the organization hopes to have employees working up to their full potential. For example, allowing understaffing so that registered nurses work such long hours that they do not get enough sleep probably reduces their desires for providing high-quality patient care (achievement) and creativity. During periods of retrenchment, being arbitrary and capricious about employees' job security interferes with cooperation, initiative, and other desirable behaviors. On the other hand, paying exclusive attention to the more basic physiological and security needs while ignoring the needs for achievement and self-esteem would defeat organizational purposes. Maslow's theory keeps managers aware of employees' higher level needs when considering motivation strategies.

It should also be noted that people's needs change over time. The needs, wants, and desires of individuals in their sixties differ from those of individuals in their twenties (Kanfer & Ackerman, 2004). Moreover, all employees have a variety of needs motivating them, and these differ by individual. One study found that the individual's position in the organizational hierarchy affects need satisfaction significantly with lower-level personnel less satisfied with their level of need achievement than higher-level personnel (Hurka, 1980). The manager's task is to develop situations that permit as many employees as possible to satisfy as many wants as possible. The astute manager will recognize what specific needs are important to motivate each individual.

ERG Theory

Theory Overview

As a result of the above criticisms of Maslow's approach to employee motivation, Clayton Alderfer proposed an alternative hierarchy called the ERG theory of motivation (Alderfer, 1972). The letters *E, R,* and *G* stand for existence, relatedness, and growth. The ERG theory collapses Maslow's need hierarchy into three levels. *Existence* needs correspond to the physiological and security needs of Maslow's hierarchy. *Relatedness* needs focus on how people relate to others and encompass Maslow's need to belong and need to earn the esteem of others. *Growth* needs include both the need for self-esteem and self-actualization.

While the ERG theory assumes a hierarchy of needs as suggested by Maslow, there are three important differences. First, the ERG theory suggests that more than one level of need can motivate behavior at the same time. Unlike Maslow, the emergence of relatedness and growth needs does not require satisfaction of the existence needs. For example, people can be motivated by a desire for money (existence), friendship (relatedness), and the opportunity to learn new skills all at once.

Second, while Maslow's hierarchy functions according to the satisfaction-progression principle, whereby essentially satisfied needs progress to a higher level of needs, the ERG theory has a *frustration-regression* element. Maslow maintained that each lower-level need must be satisfied before an individual can progress to a higher need level. In contrast, the ERG theory suggests that if needs remain unsatisfied at higher levels (i.e., growth), the individual will become frustrated, regress to a lower level, and begin to pursue those things again. For example, an employee receiving "adequate" pay (as defined by the employee) may attempt to seek opportunities for personal growth on the job. If these needs are frustrated, the employee may regress to being motivated to earn more money.

Third, the ERG theory suggests that needs are not fixed. The opportunities available in the organization may affect employee needs. Relatedness and growth needs may become more intense in an organization where there is ample opportunity to meet them (Mitchell, 1984).

Research Support and Evaluation

Research suggests that the ERG theory may be a more valid account of employee motivation in organizations than Maslow's needs hierarchy (Alderfer, 1968; Pinder, 1984), but it, too, has received contradictory reviews when empirically examined (Arnolds & Boshoff, 2002; Schneider & Alderfer, 1973). The key insights from both Maslow and Alderfer are that some needs are more important than others and that people may change their behavior after any particular set of needs has been satisfied.

Application

The major managerial implication of the ERG theory is that health care managers should assume that *all* employees have the potential for continued growth and development. This suggests the desirability of offering ongoing opportunities for training and development, transfer, promotion, and career planning to all employees.

Two-Factor Theory

Theory Overview

Another well-known content perspective on employee motivation is the two-factor theory developed by Frederich Herzberg on the basis of 200 interviews with accountants and engineers in Pittsburgh (Herzberg, 1987; Herzberg, Mausner, & Snyderman, 1959). He asked them to describe occasions when they felt especially satisfied and highly motivated and other occasions when they had been dissatisfied and unmotivated. Surprisingly, he found that entirely different sets of factors were associated with satisfaction and high motivation and with dissatisfaction and low motivation. He found that the key factors in satisfaction and motivation were achievement, recognition, the work itself, responsibility, and advancement. He labeled these factors

motivators since their presence increases job satisfaction and motivation but their absence does not lead to dissatisfaction. Herzberg also found that if a second group of factors, **hygiene factors,** were negative or absent, dissatisfaction results. These hygiene factors included company policy and administration, supervision, salary, interpersonal relations, and working conditions. The presence of positive hygiene factors, by themselves, prevents dissatisfaction but does not lead to satisfaction and motivation.

Note that the factors influencing the satisfaction dimension—motivation factors—are specifically related to the work content (i.e., intrinsic factors). The factors presumed to cause dissatisfaction—hygiene factors—are related to the work environment. According to Herzberg, changing the environment alone will not enhance employee motivation.

Research Support and Evaluation

Herzberg's two-factor theory has several limitations and weaknesses. His sample was not representative of the general population. His findings may also have been affected by the fact that people often attribute good outcomes (satisfaction) to themselves, and poor outcomes (dissatisfaction) to others. The findings in his initial interviews are subject to different interpretations, some of which differ from the one he offered. Subsequent research often failed to uphold the theory in that some factors, such as salary, appear to be associated with both satisfaction and dissatisfaction (House & Wigdor, 1967; Pinder, 1984; Vroom, 1964). Research also shows that both categories of factors serve to motivate. In one study of managerial and professional workers, the hygiene factors were as frequently associated with self-reports of high performance as were the motivators (Schwarb, Devitt, & Cummings, 1971).

Other researchers question whether the individual factors are mutually exclusive. For example, salary is defined as a hygiene factor, but for many highly paid executives and professionals, salary may be viewed as a form of recognition. Logic suggests that, in reality, these factors do not operate

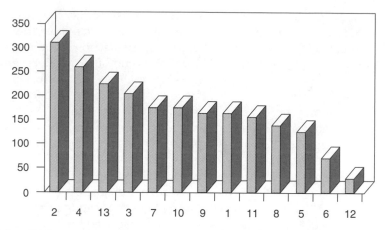

1. Salary (163)
2. Freedom in Decision-Making (311)
3. Opportunities for Advancement (203)
4. Opportunities for Personal Growth (260)
5. Chance to Serve Humankind (124)
6. High Job Profile/Visibility (72)
7. Organization's Reputation (180)

8. Organization's Financial Condition (137)
9. Geographic Location (164)
10. Institutional Mission/Values (177)
11. Corporate Culture (157)
12. Appearance of Physical Work Environment (34)
13. Caliber of the Management Team (223)

Figure 3.3. **Relative Perceived Importance of Retention Variables**

SOURCE: Fottler, M. D., Shewchuk, R. M., O'Connor, S. J. (1998). What matters to health care executives? Assessing the job attributes associated with their staying or leaving. *International Journal of Organization Theory and Behavior, 1*(2), 223–247.

separately from one another in a given person. The desires for advancement and for recognition—both motivators—are connected to feelings and attitudes about salary—a hygiene factor.

Still other researchers criticize the theory for being too simple. Lee (1980) flatly states that "the evidence to date clearly eliminates Herzberg's theory as a general or universal theory of work motivation." Steers and Porter (1987), on the other hand, take a more positive view: "It appears that a fruitful approach to this controversial theory would be to learn from it that which can help us to develop more improved models rather than to accept or reject the model totally."

A study of 522 health care managers examined how 13 variables motivated them to remain (retention) in their current position, or to be recruited (re-

cruitment) into a new one (Fottler, Shewchuk, & O'Connor, 1998). Of these variables, four were consistently observed to be the most important in making a retention or recruitment decision (see Figures 3.3 and 3.4). These four variables were (1) freedom in decision making, (2) opportunities for personal growth, (3) caliber of the management team, and (4) opportunities for advancement. In keeping with Herzberg's theory, the variable least likely to influence health care managers in their decision to stay with, or leave, an organization was appearance of the physical work environment. These observed results and others (Alpander, 1985; Longest, 1974) offer some limited corroboration to the greater importance of motivators and the lesser importance of hygienes in terms of what motivates workers in health care settings.

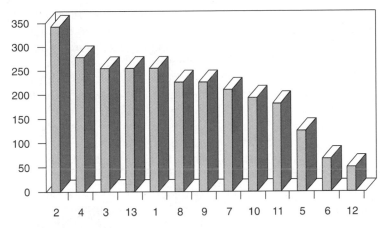

1. Salary (253)
2. Freedom in Decision-Making (344)
3. Opportunities for Advancement (256)
4. Opportunities for Personal Growth (277)
5. Chance to Serve Humankind (127)
6. High Job Profile/Visibility (73)
7. Organization's Reputation (213)

8. Organization's Financial Condition (226)
9. Geographic Location (225)
10. Institutional Mission/Values (194)
11. Corporate Culture (180)
12. Appearance of Physical Work Environment (48)
13. Caliber of the Management Team (255)

Figure 3.4. Relative Perceived Importance of Recruitment Variables

SOURCE: Fottler, M. D., Shewchuk, R. M., O'Connor, S. J. (1998). What matters to health care executives? Assessing the job attributes associated with their staying or leaving. *International Journal of Organization Theory and Behavior, 1*(2), 223–247.

Application

Despite the above criticisms, the two-factor theory has had a major impact by increasing managers' awareness of motivation and its importance. Herzberg argued there are two stages in motivating employees. First, the manager must make sure the hygiene factors are not deficient. Pay and security must be appropriate, working conditions must be safe, and supervision must be acceptable. By providing hygiene factors at an appropriate level, the manager does not stimulate motivation but does avoid dissatisfaction.

The manager should then proceed to stage two—giving employees the opportunity to experience motivation factors such as achievement and recognition. The result is predicted to be a high level of satisfaction and motivation. Herzberg goes a step

further than most theorists and describes exactly how to use the two-factor theory in the workplace. Specifically, he recommends that jobs be redesigned and enriched to provide higher levels of the motivation factors. For example, the jobs of some clinical laboratory workers can become extremely monotonous and boring because the work is often highly standardized, which results in exacting routines. As the standardized task is repeated over and over, the work becomes more tedious and less likely to offer potential motivation. Redesigning a job to be horizontally enlarged so that a worker carries out a greater variety of tasks can help in this regard. By further enriching this job, the worker would now have greater control over a wider variety of tasks.

Herzberg's theory has value for health care managers because it identifies a wide range of factors involved in employee motivation. Consideration of all of these factors is useful in any attempt to enhance motivation and to diminish demotivating factors in an organization. The theory has also had a major influence on job design in many health services organizations because it has made managers more aware of the importance of job challenge and responsibility in motivation (also see Chapter 7). The trend toward the employment of multiskilled health practitioners is one manifestation of this awareness (Blayney, 1992; Vaughan, Fottler, Bamberg, & Blayney, 1991).

Learned Need Theory

Theory Overview

The theories of Maslow, Alderfer, and Herzberg identify a number of individual needs and then attempt to arrange them in some order of importance. Other content views of employee motivation focus more on the important needs themselves without concern for ordering them. The three needs most often discussed are the needs for *achievement, power,* and *affiliation.* Far more importantly, it has been argued that these needs, and the behaviors associated with the efforts to satisfy them, can be learned (McClelland, 1961, 1975).

John W. Atkinson (1961) proposed that everyone enjoys an "energy reserve" that can be released depending upon individual incentives to achieve desired goals. He also proposed the above three basic human drives. David C. McClelland (1961) gave form to these three drives and related them to performance in organizations.

The first basic drive is the need for achievement and refers to the individual's need to accomplish complex tasks, compete, and resolve problems. It reflects the desire to achieve a goal more effectively than in the past. People with a high need for achievement are assumed to have a desire for personal responsibility, a tendency to set moderately difficult goals, a need for specific goals and immediate feedback, and a preoccupation with their task.

The second basic drive, a need for power, refers to the individual's desire to influence or control oth-

ers' behavior. It also represents the desire to control one's environment. Individuals high in power needs are thought to be more suited to management than achievers. In this view, "power" implies being responsible for control of others and for influencing behavior in complex situations (McClelland & Burnham, 1976).

The third drive, the need for affiliation, reflects an individual's desire to associate with others in friendly circumstances. It is similar to Maslow's belongingness need. Those high in affiliation prefer friendly, participative work environments where the quality of group interaction with coworkers is more highly valued than achievements or influence. People with a strong need for affiliation are likely to prefer (and perform better in) a job that entails a lot of social interaction. Few of these individuals manage effectively in most organizations because they tend to emphasize friendship at the expense of organizational productivity and effectiveness. As McClelland and Burnham (1976) state, "[t]he top manager's need for power ought to be greater than his or her need for being liked." However, as teamwork becomes increasingly necessary to carry out administrative functions, somewhat stronger needs for affiliation may be a welcome adjunct for health care managers. By being somewhat more accommodating and cooperative, those managers maintaining slightly greater needs for affiliation may benefit a team-based work setting by reducing dysfunctional conflict and bringing together diverse groups of workers.

Research Support and Evaluation

McClelland concluded that, although the need for achievement is the main motivation for those who wish to start and develop their own small businesses, the need for power is a crucial motivator of top executives in larger, more complex organizations. Most successful managers exercise their power in a controlled and disciplined way on behalf of others and create a strong sense of team spirit among their subordinates. Studies have found that managers as a group tend to have a stronger power motive than the general population and that successful managers tend to have stronger power motives than less successful managers (Holland, Black, & Miner, 1987; McClelland & Burnham, 1976). Other research has shown that people with a strong need for power are likely to be superior performers, have good attendance records, and occupy supervisory positions (Cornelius & Lane, 1984). Chusmir (1986), in a unique study of health related occupations, evaluated 70 health-related job categories relative to the extent they satisfied needs for power, achievement, and affiliation. The health care jobs best able to satisfy needs for power, and least able to fulfill affiliation needs, are predominantly management roles such as nursing school dean or hospital administrator (Table 3.1).

Persons with high achievement needs tend to flourish in very competitive situations, enjoy challenges, and thrive in complex and stimulating environments such as those found in most health care organizations. McClelland argued that these achievers would be best suited to situations where independent responsibility and autonomy prevail. The implication is that, while many achievers are found in professional positions such as physicians, they are not always among the best managers in highly bureaucratic organizations. Since such organizations are based on diffused authority and group activities, achievers are often uncomfortable in situations of group responsibility and control. The health care occupations in Chusmir's (1986) study that appear best able to fulfill the achievement need are those of technician (dialysis, electrocardiographic, surgical, hematology/serology) and technologist (i.e., medical, radiologic, nuclear medicine).

An important aspect of McClelland's theory is that all three needs are acquired. Individuals develop these needs to varying degrees through life experiences. They are learned drives evolving from one's background and environment. Indeed, since a high need for achievement is important for professional and managerial success in nonbureaucratic organizations, McClelland devised a training program for increasing one's need for achievement. Studies found that employees who complete this achievement training tend to make more money and receive promotions faster than other employees (Kiechel, 1989; Nicholls, 1984). Moreover, achievement training may also affect organizational outcomes. In one case, three different groups of small business employees were given 70 hours of achievement training and assistance. Median profits for these businesses increased from $280 per month to $670 per month (Miron & McClelland, 1979).

Application

Other managerial implications of McClelland's work are far reaching. For individuals already set in their ways, matching work environments with their needs is crucial to their motivation and career success. Employees established in health care organizations undergoing rapid change may need counseling or education to help them adapt to the new environment. For example, an affiliation-oriented manager may not fare well in an entrepreneurial environment that emphasizes achievement.

Further, organizations might focus on identifying and selecting individuals with high levels of achievement motivation or other desired values and behavior. Many hospitals, for example, use both psychological testing and structured interviewing in employment selection and promotion decisions. These approaches determine the prospective candidate's service orientation, performance, motivations, and ability to work as a team member. The result has been a collaborative, achievement-oriented culture with shared values among the employees.

An Assessment of Content Theories

It is well accepted that motivation has important origins in human needs. Need theories of motivation assume that people attempt to satisfy such needs and wants. A simplistic view is that all a manager or supervisor has to do to release his or

Table 3.1. Health Care Motivation Profiles of over 70 Health-Related Occupations in Terms of the Degree to Which They Satisfy Needs for Achievement, Power, and Affiliation

Job Title	DOT Code	Need Profile	Ach	Aff	Pwr
Hospital administration and operations					
Hospital administrator, superintendent, coordinator rehabilitation services emergency medical services coordinator, sanitarian	117	Pwr	2	1	4
Coordinator auxiliary personnel	127	Pwr	2	1	5
Supervisor, volunteer services, food service, ward service, tray line, floor housekeeper, manager	137	Ach and Pwr	3	2	3
Executive chef	161	Ach	4	1	2
Central supply supervisor	164	Balanced	2	2	2
Medical services administrator, hospital record administrator, communications coordinator, assistant hospital administrator, executive housekeeper, librarian, director food services, director volunteer services, buildingsuperintendent, laundry superintendent	167	Pwr	3	2	4
Hospital insurance representative	267	Pwr	3	2	4
Hospital collection clerk	357	Ach	4	2	2
Cook	361	Ach	4	2	2
Hospital admitting clerk, cashier, insurance clerk, receiving clerk, ward clerk	362	Ach	4	2	2
Medical record technician, x-ray file clerk, medical service technician	367	Balanced	3	3	3
Ambulance attendant, emergency medical technician	374	Aff	1	4	1
Ward supervisor, ward attendant, psychiatric aide	377	Aff	1	4	1
Linen room attendant, clerk, checker, exchange attendant	387	Aff	2	3	2
Television rental clerk	467	Aff	2	3	2
Food tray assembler	484	Aff	0	3	0
Formula maker, formula room worker	487	Aff	1	3	1
Diet clerk aide	587	Aff	1	2	0
Hospital attendant	674	Aff	0	3	0
Hospital entrance attendant, messenger, admitting office guide, food service worker, tray line worker	677	Aff	1	3	0
Ambulance driver	683	Pwr	1	1	2
Central supply worker, cleaner, clothes room workers	687	Aff	4	0	2
Medical and dental technology					
Medical technologist, teaching supervisor	121	Ach	4	0	2
Medical technologist, chief	161	Ach	5	1	2
Radiologic technologist, chief	162	Ach	5	1	2
Chemistry, microbiology, technologists, orthotist, prosthetist	261	Ach	5	1	2
Cytotechnologist	281	Ach	3	1	1

Table 3.1. (continued)

Job Title	DOT Code	Need Profile	Ach	Aff	Pwr
Medical and dental technology *(continued)*					
Medical, nuclear medicine, hematology serology, tissue technologists, orthotist, prosthetist assistant	361	Ach	4	2	2
Dialysis, electrocardiographic technicians, electroencephalographic, radiology, x-ray technologists	362	Ach	4	2	2
Ultrasound technologist	364	Ach	4	2	2
Surgical technician	374	Aff	1	4	1
Medical and dental technology					
Medical lab assistant or technician, hematology or serology technician	381	Aff	3	2	1
Cephalometric analyst	384	Aff	1	3	1
X-ray developing machine operator	685	Aff	0	1	0
Laboratory assistant	687	Aff	1	2	0
Nursing					
Dean, school of nursing, educational consultant, state board nursing; directors: Community health nursing, educational community health, nursing service, occupational health nursing, school of nursing, executive director nurses association	117	Pwr	2	1	4
Nurse instructor	121	Pwr	4	0	2
School nurse, community health staff nurse	124	Pwr	1	1	3
Head nurse, nurse supervisor, nurse consultant	127	Pwr	2	1	4
Nurse practitioner, nurse midwife	264	Balanced	2	2	2
Nurse anesthetist	371	Ach and Aff	3	3	1
General duty nurse, office nurse, private duty nurse, staff nurse, licensed practical nurse	374	Aff	1	4	1
Therapists					
Coordinator, rehabilitation services	117	Pwr	2	1	4
Occupational, physical, manual arts, recreational therapists	124	Pwr	1	1	3
Art, music therapists	127	Pwr	2	1	4
Hypnotherapists	157	Ach	4	1	1
Industrial therapists	167	Pwr	3	2	4
Physical therapist assistant	224	Pwr	1	1	3
Corrective or respiratory	361	Ach	4	2	2
Assistant therapy aide	377	Aff	2	4	2

SOURCE: Chusmir L. H. (1986). How fulfilling are health care jobs? *Health Care Management Review, 11*(1), 30
© 1986 Aspen Publishers, Inc.

Maslow's Model	Alderfer's Model	Herzberg's Model		McClelland's Model
Self-Actualization Needs	Growth Needs	Motivation Factors	Achievement Recognition Advancement The Work Itself Possibility for Personal Growth Responsibility	Achievement
Ego and Self-Esteem Needs				Power
Social and Belongingness Needs	Relatedness Needs	Hygiene Factors	Status Company Policy and Administration Quality of Supervision Relations with Supervisor Relations with Peers Relations with Subordinates Salary Job Security Personal Life Working Conditions	Affiliation
Safety and Security Needs	Existence Needs			
Physiological Needs				

Figure 3.5. A Comparison of Needs Theories of Motivation

her employees' motivation potential is to identify their needs and then take steps to satisfy them. Unfortunately, there is no simple set of needs and need satisfiers that would be universally applicable. First, as noted above, people differ on the basis of age, gender, race, and other demographic and background characteristics. No one set of motivators is likely to be appropriate for all employees since their needs will be different. Second, organizational context and culture differ both across organizations and within organizations. The learned needs of a given individual may vary depending on the incentives present in his or her organization. Third, for a given individual, needs change over time. This has already been implied by the needs hierarchy theorists. The relative importance of various needs is changing, thus forcing managers to aim at a moving target (Fried & Slowik, 2004). Fourth, employees in different positions in an organizational hierarchy will undoubtedly differ in terms of their configura-

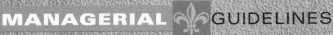

MANAGERIAL GUIDELINES

1. Employees often have unmet needs that they attempt to satisfy through work. These include physiological, security, social esteem, self-control, power, and achievement needs. Such unmet needs will vary from individual to individual based on a wide variety of factors. No two persons will have the same profile of each of these needs.

2. At any given point in time, people attempt to satisfy a wide variety of needs. They exchange their labor for rewards that they value because these rewards respond to their needs. Such rewards may be intrinsic or extrinsic to the job. Intrinsic motivation is particularly important for health care professionals.

3. Health care managers can motivate people by determining what needs and rewards they view as most important. This can be accomplished through formal and informal means of communication.

4. Rewards may be both economic and noneconomic. They should be relevant to the priority needs of particular employees or employee groups. What is a hygiene factor for one person may be a motivator for another. However, satisfied needs are not motivators for anyone.

5. Employees should be selected on the basis of how well their needs, motivations, and qualifications match the requirements of each position. Written examinations and oral interviews may be used to assess the degree of job-applicant match.

6. Redesigning jobs is another alternative for increasing this match. Redesigning offers much potential for increased motivation to the extent that it involves building in responsibility, decision making, control, autonomy, challenge, and opportunities for achievement.

7. Training programs that emphasize enhancement of the achievement motive can enhance motivation.

8. Managers should be concerned with both hygiene factors and motivators as defined by the employees themselves.

tion of needs and potential motivators. Fifth, resource constraints or lack of such constraints may also affect the relative importance of various needs.

Despite these caveats, content theories of motivation help health care managers focus on individual needs in the motivation process. All provide useful insights into factors that may promote motivation in a given situation. Moreover, they are not separate and discrete views of motivation but share much in common with one another. Figure 3.5 compares the needs identified by the four content theories described in this section. It should be noted that, while they do not necessarily agree on whether there is a hierarchy of needs or whether individuals attempt to satisfy multiple needs simultaneously, some of their basic concepts are similar and overlap with one another.

Employees in health services organizations have a variety of needs motivating them. For example, one study of registered nurses found achievement, interpersonal relations, and the work itself to be major motivators (Longest, 1974), another identified autonomy or personal control, promotion opportunities, and work scheduling (Ford & Fottler, 1992), and yet another found interpersonal relations, work itself, and recognition to be most important (Rantz,

Scott, & Porter, 1996). While the specifics differed in all studies, most of the key factors were motivators identified by Herzberg. The task of health care managers is to identify the specific needs of their employees and then develop opportunities that permit these employees to satisfy their needs.

Employees' needs can be identified by attitude surveys and continuous two-way oral communication with various subgroups of employees (Farnham, 1989; Reibstein, 1986). When possible, the manager should also attempt to recognize what needs are important in the motivation of each individual employee and to match those needs to the requirements of positions to which those individuals are assigned (Chusmir, 1986). Studies of job redesign typically find significant increases in motivation and performance over time (Hackman & Oldham, 1980; Griffin, 1991). Needs themselves may also be modified by special motivation training courses (Durand, 1983).

Based on identified needs, astute managers will alter their leadership and communication style, economic rewards, noneconomic rewards, job assignments, training and development emphases, and feedback to maximize the need fulfillment of as many subordinates as possible. For example, some will need to be left alone to work independently. Others will need more structure, goals, and feedback. Since employees have different needs, they must be managed in different ways. Managerial Guidelines (see page 97) provide a convenient summary of the managerial implications of content theories.

Though content theories provide useful insights into motivational factors, they do not constitute a complete theoretical or managerial approach to employee motivation. They do not shed much light on the process of motivation. For example, they do not explain why employees might be motivated by one factor rather than by another at a given level or how their different needs might be satisfied. These questions involve behaviors or actions, goals, and feelings of satisfaction that are addressed by various process theories of motivation. It is to these theories that we now turn.

PROCESS PERSPECTIVES

In this section, we examine five approaches to motivation that, although they differ from each other, share a focus on the processes involved in motivation. In contrast to the approaches examined in the previous section that concern the content of work and its influence on motivation, these approaches attend to the context in which work is done as well as individuals' reactions—especially thoughts and feelings—to work.

Equity Theory

Theory Overview

Adams proposed a theory of work motivation that assumes that individuals value and seek fairness, or **equity,** in their relationships with employers (Adams, 1963, 1965). Relationships are fair when people perceive that their outcomes (e.g., pay) are proportionate to their perceived contributions or inputs (e.g., task performance). Further, people evaluate fairness by comparing themselves to others. In other words, people contrast their perceived inputs and outcomes with their perceptions of others' inputs and outcomes. To the extent that this ratio is seen as unequal, individuals experience tension.

Adams proposed two kinds of inequity. Underpayment refers to the case when someone perceives that she is receiving fewer rewards from a job than another person making a comparable contribution. In contrast, overpayment occurs when someone perceives that she is receiving more rewards than another person making a comparable contribution.

Adams also proposed that people are motivated to reduce tensions that result from perceived inequity. The greater the perceived inequity and resulting tension, the greater the motivation to reduce it. In other words, from the perspective of equity theory, work motivation stems from the need to reduce tensions caused by inequity.

Depending on the magnitude of the perceived injustice and individual as well as situational circumstances, people may use one of several approaches to reduce inequity and restore balance in their relationships with employers. These approaches include altering their perceptions of their own or others' inputs or outcomes, changing their inputs or outcomes, getting others to change their inputs or outcomes, and leaving the inequitable situation altogether (Campbell & Pritchard, 1976).

Research Support and Evaluation

There are a relatively large number of studies testing various aspects of Adams's equity theory. Most of these have concentrated on the effects of perceived inequity in pay on quality and quantity of work performance when people are paid either hourly or on a piece-rate. Results from most studies support equity theory's hypotheses about the effects of underpayment (Greenberg, 1982). The results from studies examining hourly payment are also stronger than results from studies examining piece-rate payment (Muchinsky, 1987). One study found experimental support for the "double demotivation" hypothesis—that pay discrepancies decrease work motivation in both lower- as well as higher-paid groups. "Compared with equitably paid workers, employees who felt they were being under- or overpaid reported lower job satisfaction and greater readiness to change jobs" (Carr, McLoughlin, Hodgson, & MacLachlan, 1996).

Despite the empirical support for equity theory, it has several limitations that managers should consider. The theory does not help to identify which of several approaches to restoring equity an individual will take. In actual work situations, there are typically several ways that perceived inequities can be addressed. One can simply convince oneself that an inequity is not worth worrying about or will be reduced at the next annual review.

Further, the theory does not specify who people are likely to compare themselves with to assess their equity with employers. Do people compare themselves more often with immediate coworkers, or are comparisons with colleagues in other organizations equally or more important? For example, do primary care physicians compare their income to that of specialists such as orthopedic surgeons, or do they only consider the pay levels of other primary care physicians?

Another problem is that studies have not examined how perceptions of equity vary over time and how such variation affects motivation (Kanfer, 1990; Kanfer & Ackerman, 2004). Most studies take a short-term view of equity issues, and the theory provides little guidance about how to deal with variation over time in work situations. Finally, it is not clear how this theory can be used to motivate people who perceive no important inequities in their work. That is, the theory proposes that people are motivated to reduce tensions created by perceived inequities in inputs and outcomes. It provides no guidance for managers once they have addressed perceived inequities other than to try to be as fair as possible.

Application

Despite the limitations just noted, we believe that equity theory provides some useful guidelines for health care managers. First, it is important to note that people compare themselves to others in many situations and in many ways. Such comparisons affect not only their motivation but other aspects of their behavior as well. When people experience uncertainty, they are especially likely to turn to others, consciously or unconsciously, to provide them with cues about what to do. Equity theory would be useful even if its only contribution were to remind us of the importance of social comparison. The case of the ICU nurses (see In Practice p. 82) is a good example of this. The ICU nurses compared themselves to the external pool nurses who worked alongside them. From this comparison, they felt that they earned $12 per hour less and contributed substantially more.

Second, managers need to directly address perceptions of inequities so that individuals are not motivated to reduce their contributions or inputs or to leave their jobs. It may be that perceptions of inequity can be changed simply by explaining differences between jobs or other conditions that

---

IN PRACTICE   Motivating a Primary Care Physician in an HMO

Dennis Ralston, M.D., a primary care physician, is employed by a large, staff model health maintenance organization (HMO). Because such a large proportion of his patients are diabetic, he has been intimately involved in the development of a new, long-term diabetic disease-management program for his HMO. The HMO wants the disease to be managed in such a way that it is kept under control so that patients can maintain a higher quality of life and longer-term costs do not rise as a result of the need for more extensive medical interventions. Dr. Ralston is very confident that between his own ability and the detailed guidelines for managing the disease developed by the HMO, he will be able to do a good job of keeping his diabetic patients' disease under control. The disease-management guidelines require him to get patients to test their blood sugar levels four times per day using testing strips that cost over $100 per month, and to frequently order relatively expensive laboratory tests, glaucoma screenings, and podiatric referrals throughout the course of a year.

The HMO uses financial incentives to motivate primary care physician behavior, primarily through the use of a "holdback," a bonus pool of dollars from which the physicians can share at the end of the year. The more dollars the physicians save the HMO over the course of the year, the bigger the pool—and the bigger the incentive check at year's end. Although the disease-management guidelines recently went into effect, the HMO's financial incentive system for its primary care physicians has not changed in any way. Dr. Ralston realizes that since a large percentage of his patients are diabetic, if he is to vigorously adhere to the guidelines, he may not receive any incentive dollars at year's end.

Adapted from S. J. O'Connor (1998). Motivating effective performance. In: Ginter P., Swayne L., Duncan W. J., eds. *Handbook of Health Care Management.* Cambridge, MA: Blackwell Business Publishing, 431–470.

For Discussion

Instead of the holdback bonus, what other performance-enhancing incentives could the management team at this HMO use to change physician practice patterns?

---

make it necessary to reward or treat people differently. In other cases, managers may need to consider pay raises or increases in other ways to reward people. In still other cases, there may be nothing that a manager can do to restore perceptions of equity. But, if such concerns are not addressed, it is clear that they can be a source of motivational problems.

Finally, we have argued that it is important to motivate people on an individual basis. Equity theory reminds us that even this approach has limits. To the extent that people are treated as individuals, perceptions of inequity are likely to increase because people will be comparing themselves to others who are being treated differently; such differences can trigger perceptions of inequity.

Expectancy Theory

Theory Overview

Expectancy theory has several variations that all trace their roots to cognitive psychology in the early 1950s. Georgopoulos, Mahoney, and Jones and Vroom were the first to apply expectancy theory to work motivation (Georgopoulos, Mahoney, & Jones, 1957; Vroom, 1964). Vroom's expectancy model was particularly influential. Since this early research, expectancy theory has become perhaps the most prominent theory of work motivation. The theory assumes that people are rational decision makers who will expend effort on work that will lead to desired rewards. Further, the theory assumes that people know what rewards they want from work and understand that their performance will determine the extent to which they attain the rewards they value.

Though there are several variations of expectancy theory, they all share four central components (Mitchell, 1982). First, there are *job outcomes*. These include both rewards (e.g., pay raises, promotions, recognition) and negative experiences (e.g., job loss, demotion).

Second, there are **valences.** These are individuals' feelings about job outcomes. Like job outcomes, they can range from positive to neutral to negative, and they vary in strength as well as direction.

The third component is **instrumentality,** which refers to the perceived link between performance and outcomes. In other words, instrumentality is the extent to which individuals believe that attaining a job outcome depends on, or is conditional on, their performance. For example, if a nurse thought that an outcome (pay raise) depended highly on his performance rather than some other factor (hospital patient volume), the instrumentality for the outcome would be high.

Finally, **expectancy** is the perceived link between effort and performance. That is, to what extent do individuals believe that there is a relationship between how hard they try and how well they do?

Using the expectancy theory model, we can illustrate the degree to which the primary care physician described in "In Practice" (see page 100) will be motivated to vigorously adhere to the HMO's disease-management guidelines. Expectancy is the perceived link between effort and performance. This physician is confident that by following the guidelines, he will be able to do a reasonably good job of controlling the disease among his patients. The physician has a high expectancy probability for performing effective diabetes disease management. However, the physician knows that due to the higher short-term costs of effectively managing his patients, there is also a high probability that he will not share in any financial bonuses paid out at year's end. Because this is a job outcome he does not favor, it receives a negative valence. Instrumentality, or the probability that performance will lead to outcomes, is fairly high, but the outcome has a forceful negative valence. Because the outcome (no end-of-year bonus) is not related to performance, the physician's motivation to carry out high-quality diabetes disease management has been substantially reduced.

Motivation is the end product of valence, instrumentality, and expectancy. People are motivated when a combination of factors occurs: They value an outcome (i.e., valence is high and positive), they believe that good performance will be rewarded with desired outcomes (i.e., instrumentality is high), and they believe that their efforts will produce good performance (i.e., expectancy is high). In contrast, motivation is likely to be low if the components of expectancy theory have low values. If people do not care about their job outcomes, then they have less reason to work for them. Or, if organizations do not link outcomes to performance (e.g., pay raises are linked to seniority rather than performance), then people have less reason to care about their performance. Similarly, if effort and performance seem unrelated, then there is less reason to try hard. Each of these factors can decrease motivation, and if all are present, it is improbable that motivation will be high. The HMO administrator from the "In Practice" may improve the linkage between outcomes and performance by placing greater emphasis on quality indicators as a condition of participating in the bonus incentive pool.

Research Support and Evaluation

Empirical support from many studies of expectancy theory is quite good (Hom, 1980; Kennedy, Fossum, & White, 1983; Muchinsky, 1987; Stacy, Widaman,

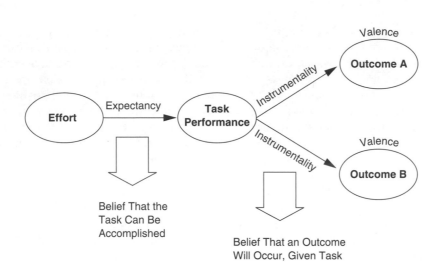

Figure 3.6. Expectancy Theory Process

& Marlatt, 1990; Tsui, Ashford, St. Clair, & Xin, 1995; Wanous, Keon, & Latack, 1983). Nonetheless, the theory seems to receive more support in studies that examine the levels of effort an individual will expend on different tasks than in studies that examine the strength of motivation across different people (Kennedy, Fossum, & White, 1983).

Expectancy theory rests clearly on the assumption that people are highly rational and consciously engage in decisions to work harder on tasks that they believe will maximize their gains while minimizing their losses. Though this assumption works quite well for many people in many situations, it is not universally valid. People have unconscious motives (Locke & Latham, 2004). Moreover, their calculations about the links between effort and performance and performance and reward are not always accurate. In this regard, the HMO physician may be highly motivated to control diabetes disease among his patients, while fully aware that such outcomes will not be financially rewarded. Most likely this is because he can acquire other valued outcomes such as a sense of personal satisfaction and achievement that derive from being able to effectively help people.

Further, some studies indicate that the strength of the theory may vary depending on personality factors (Weiner, 1986). For example, the theory may hold more strongly for people who have a high internal, rather than external, locus of control. Such people tend to believe that their lives are under their own control more than the control or influence of external events. As a result, people with a high internal locus of control believe that there are strong links between their efforts and performance and their performance and outcomes. These beliefs, as noted above, are central to the theory's predictions about motivation.

Application

Despite these limitations, expectancy theory (Figure 3.6) provides very useful guidelines for managerial action (Pritchard, De Leo, & Von Bergen, 1976). These include:

1. Incentives or job outcomes should be chosen so that they are attractive to employees. Perhaps the best way to do this is to ask employees directly about their preferences using surveys or interviews.

2. The rules for attaining incentives must be clear to all involved. For example, expected levels of performance should be spelled out in as much detail as possible. Such rules should be stated in job descriptions and employee orientations. These rules should also be reviewed periodically, both informally and formally. We add here a note from equity theory: The rules should be perceived as fair.

3. People must perceive that their efforts will lead to the desired level of performance.

There are many practical limitations involved here simply because several factors can intervene to weaken the link between effort and performance. For example, people may be trying hard but lack the resources (e.g., equipment) to do well, or as is often the case in health care, there is a great deal of interdependence between people so that performance depends on all their efforts. Work done in groups or teams often has this feature. When this is the case and coworkers' efforts are lacking, an individual's perceptions of the link between their efforts and group or unit performance can be easily diminished. In any case, managers need to make it clear that, insofar as they are able, they will not hold people accountable for performance problems that stem from factors not in their control.

Reinforcement Theory

Theory Overview

Reinforcement theory, also known as operant conditioning or behavior modification, is based on the work of B. F. Skinner. The theory has three components: stimulus, response, and consequence. A stimulus is any condition or variable that elicits a response, such as a request from a supervisor for some information. A response is a behavior performed contingent on a stimulus. A consequence is anything that follows a response that changes the likelihood that the response will occur again following a stimulus.

In turn, there are three types of consequences: rewards (termed *positive reinforcement*), which in-

crease the likelihood of a response; punishments, which decrease the likelihood of a response; and negative reinforcement, which is the removal of a reward or punishment to increase the likelihood of a response.

Further, research shows that four types of connections between responses and consequences can increase the frequency of a response. These include:

1. *Fixed interval.* People are rewarded at a fixed time interval. For example, people paid on an hourly basis are on a fixed-interval reward schedule.

2. *Fixed ratio.* People are rewarded on the basis of a fixed number of responses. For example, physicians who are paid on a fee-for-service basis are rewarded on this schedule.

3. *Variable interval.* Responses are rewarded at some time interval that varies. For example, government safety inspections of hospital oncology units for the proper storage, handling, and documentation of therapeutic radioactive materials such as iridium and cesium generally occur at any time and are unannounced (i.e., at variable intervals) (O'Connor, 1998).

4. *Variable ratio.* Reward is based on behavior, but the ratio of reward to responses varies. Gambling games such as lotteries and blackjack can be extremely addictive, because they reinforce the player on a variable schedule.

In short, from the perspective of reinforcement theory, motivation results when people are rewarded contingent on performance, based on the above schedules. In general, research indicates that responses are maintained best on ratio schedules.

Research Support and Evaluation

Research from a variety of settings indicates that reinforcement schedules work. As noted, the results may vary depending on the type of reinforcement schedule that is used, but performance is better when rewards are given contingently. This result is, of course, consistent with the views of expectancy theory.

Reinforcement theory has drawn sharp criticism since Skinner (1969) published his first work in this area. One critique is that it encourages managers and others to manipulate employees through the design of reinforcement schedules over which employees have no control. Similarly, if employees have no input into selecting rewards, reinforcement may be ineffective. The antidote for these criticisms seems clear: Employees need to have input into the design of reinforcement systems. Again, this guideline is consistent with an expectancy theory perspective.

A second common critique is that reinforcement theory presents a flat, one-dimensional view of human nature and motivation. That is, the theory says little about human emotion or cognition (Seo, Barrett, & Bartunek, 2004). People are often portrayed as somewhat mindless robots in pursuit of rewards. This critique is similar to a critique of expectancy theory; it views people as very rational in pursuit of valued outcomes. The difference here is that critics of reinforcement theory argue that it does not even give people credit for thinking.

Application

The primary lesson from reinforcement theory is that performance, if not motivation, is better when rewards are given contingently. The effectiveness of reinforcement schedules will vary; thus, it is best to take a pragmatic approach and see what works best in a given situation.

Goal Setting

Theory Overview

Locke (1968) proposed a motivation theory that focuses on the role of goals and *goal setting.* He and his colleagues define a *goal* as something that an individual is consciously attempting to attain (Locke & Latham, 1984, 1990a, 2004). Goals are powerful because they direct people's attention, focus effort on tasks related to goal attainment, and encourage people to persist in such tasks. Further, Locke proposed that the more difficult and specific the goal, the greater the motivation will be to attain it. In short, a goal provides guidelines for how much effort to put into work.

Several conditions must be met for goals to have a positive influence on performance. First, people must be aware of goals and know what must be done to attain them. Second, goals must be accepted as something that people are willing to work for. People must be committed to goals. In other words, goals can fail to motivate people if they are seen as too difficult (Sherman, 1995; Tully, 1994) or too easy or if an individual does not know what tasks are required for goal attainment (Muchinsky, 1987).

Research Support and Evaluation

The empirical support for key parts of goal-setting theory is impressive. Nearly 400 studies—mostly experimental—show that specific, difficult goals lead to better performance than specific, easy, vague goals, such as "do your best" or no goals at all (Locke & Latham, 1990a).

There is also support for the view that commitment to goals is critical to effective performance (Erez & Zidon, 1984). In turn, commitment to goals is generally higher when people think they can attain the goals and when they value them (Locke, Latham, & Erez, 1988). Further, monetary rewards increase goal commitment if people value money and the amount is sufficiently large (Stajkovic & Luthans, 2001).

One surprising finding is that assigning goals to individuals generally leads to the same level of commitment and performance as when individuals participate in setting goals or when they set goals for themselves. Perhaps assigned goals work well because they come from authority figures or because assigned goals, if difficult, are more challenging (Locke & Latham, 1990b). We are concerned about applying these results to health care professionals, however, given that many of them are trained and socialized to set their own goals. In this case, managers need to be sure that goals are specific and difficult regardless of who sets them.

Research also shows that goal setting is more effective, and usually only effective, when feedback is given to individuals so that they can monitor their performance in relation to goals. Indeed, goal setting without feedback seems to have little long-term effect on performance (Becker, 1978). On the other hand, feedback without goal setting is also ineffective. People need both goals and feedback on progress toward goals to be motivated. Furthermore, self-created feedback appears to exert a greater effect on motivation than feedback from external sources (Ivancevich & McMahon, 1982). Finally, for goal setting to be effective, people must have the ability to reach or approach the goals (Locke, 1982). Once again, this result is consistent with the expectancy theory.

The strength of this perspective is its simplicity and ease of application. It seems to be generalizable; its principles can be applied in any circumstance. Moreover, as noted above, it has a very strong base of empirical support.

There are, of course, some important unanswered questions. How do people become committed to goals, and why do they select certain goals and not others (Hollenbeck & Klein, 1987)?

Application

The implications for managers are relatively straightforward:

1. Set or encourage people to set goals that are difficult and specific; revise and update goals as necessary. Prompts such as daily, weekly, or monthly "to do" lists are examples of useful techniques.

2. Provide timely and specific feedback to people on their progress toward goals.

3. Build commitment to goals by helping people believe they can attain goals and by selecting goals that are congruent with their values.

4. Consistent with the reinforcement theory, rewards should be given contingent on goal attainment.

5. Make sure that individuals have the ability to achieve goals they or you set.

MOTIVATING HEALTH CARE PROFESSIONALS AND SUPPORT PERSONNEL

One key aspect of health care organizations is that they have large numbers of autonomous professionals working within them. These professionals can include a variety of clinical occupations as well as senior managers, information technology specialists, accountants, and so on. Because so much of the day-to-day work in health care is carried out by clinical professionals, from a management perspective, it is instructive to examine how motivation theories may apply to them.

A profession can be characterized in terms of (1) who its members are (selection, licensure, and cohesion), (2) what it is that they know (knowledge base and standards), (3) why they act as they do (service orientation and code of ethics), and (4) how they direct their activities (occupational autonomy and impact on social policy) (O'Connor & Lanning, 1992). Among the various components, autonomy appears to be a key defining characteristic (Haug, 1988).

Physicians

Health care organizations face pressure to become more productive, innovative, and concerned with quality. Physicians are vitally important to health care organizations because much of the work is carried out at their direction. Managers must be able to motivate physicians to practice high-quality, cost-effective medicine by abandoning detrimental behaviors, such as excessive use of resources (e.g., unnecessary diagnostic testing) and low rates of quality outcomes to resources consumed (O'Connor, 1998).

IN PRACTICE   The M.D. Factor

Manuel Loewenhaupt, M.D., knows doctors. Thousands of them. For nearly a decade, he's been consulting with them, learning from them, and helping them to navigate the troubled waters of change. Now, he's a partner at Deloitte & Touche Consulting Group, Boston. This is his take on changing physician behavior.

Q: How important to population-based health is a change in the ways physicians practice?
A: It's the heart of the whole movement because the bottom line is the way that patient care is delivered. Population-based health is powered by doctors. Without the driver, you have nothing.

Q: In what ways does the relationship between health care organizations and doctors complicate change?
A: Health systems don't have true authority over doctors. If they don't own them, they can't fire them. In some ways, doctors are like high-level programmers in the computer software industry. If they don't like where they are working, they pick up and find a better place. In health care, the incentives for change don't come through a relationship of control and authority.

Q: How does the physician mentality fit in?
A: We're trained not to think of teams or collaboration as an ideal way of working. We're trained to rely on our own independent judgment. I recently read a survey in which doctors were asked to list their fictional heroes. The most popular responses were Superman, the Lone Ranger and Maverick, the combat pilot in the movie *Top Gun.* I can't think of a tougher group of people to try to manage.

Q: How well do doctors respond to business management concepts?
A: Physicians don't work well with an authority model. In fact, most view themselves as artists, not managers or executives. There attitude often is,

"Please don't bother me, please don't irritate me, and please don't try to manage me. Just leave me alone and let me do my thing."

Q: What mistakes do health care organizations make trying to motivate doctors to change?
A: Too often, administrators couch the message in the wrong terms. Telling a doctor that a new way of working will help the health system thrive may have little motivating effect. Few doctors are lying awake at night worrying about the financial well-being of a hospital or health system. In fact, many doctors may actually fear improved performance of a hospital, because in a reimbursement state of mind, a strong hospital may get that way by reducing its payment to doctors.

Q: Are you saying that the best strategy is motivate doctors financially?
A: Not necessarily. Most people's first guess is that doctors are motivated by money, and they wouldn't be completely wrong. When doctors rank their priorities, money is in the top five, but not always number one. There are other key motivators, too. Among them are the increased ability to provide excellent care, more time in which to do it, efficiency, and peer recognition. If you want to influence doctors, you need to look at these elements, too.

Q: What misconceptions do physicians have about the business of running a health system?
A: Most doctors have very little understanding of the way that care is delivered through a system. They view administrators as little more than bean counters. And they don't understand the complicated financial models that drive and influence health care delivery.

Q: Specifically, which behaviors need to change?
A: First, we have to move away from the solo model of practice to a more collaborative model. Second, we need to work toward eliminating inappropriate

variations in care. Most variations are driven not by clinical science, but by a "this-is-the-way-I-was-trained" mentality. And third, we need to get away from reflexive medicine—the kind of medicine that's driven by tradition rather than by scientific evidence. We can no longer rely on the "way it's always been done here."

Q: Are physicians beginning to "get it"?
A: Many are. But there's still a great deal of resistance out there. In some of my meetings with physicians, I do an exercise in which I ask them to describe the ideal practice environment of the future. When I read their responses, I see a lot of descriptions that sound exactly the way things were 10 years ago. People want to turn back the clock. Then I find myself explaining repeatedly that there's probably not going to be a rewind like that.

Q: Whose job is it to change the way that health care is delivered?
A: It's going to take a real collaboration between health system leaders and physician leaders. Many smaller organizations haven't figured out how to build that collaborative piece, and that's where they're struggling. One of the big problems that they are facing is history. There is still a lot of leftover bad feelings from earlier moves. But everyone is going to have to get beyond all that.

Q: What's the first step in moving physicians toward new ways of practicing?
A: Awareness. Often, that comes not from a health system, but from the market. In Detroit, for example, when the Ford Motor Company declared that it is going to reduce its health care expenditures by 30%, it was a wake-up call. Ford got aggressive in its contracting, and everyone realized that business as usual was over. There was this instant awareness that it would be crazy to try to achieve different results by doing the same old thing.

Q: What's your advice to health care organizations that are trying to influence physician behavior?
A: It's a complicated process, and it's not necessarily linear. It's going to happen at a tempo that many business managers will see as too slow. At the same time, doctors are probably going to see it as too fast. But if you work toward a partnership with physicians, and you can achieve a sense of shared investment, shared returns, and shared mission, you can convert physicians from barriers to champions of the cause.

The M.D. factor, *Crossroads: New directions in health management,* a supplement to *Hospitals & Health Networks,* November, 1997, Copyright 1997, American Hospital Publishing, Inc. by Health Forum.

The task of motivating physicians can be a difficult one indeed. Physicians are educated and socialized to think and act with a great deal of individual discretion and autonomy in their day-to-day work. Generally, they resent managerial or organizational forays into their activities (O'Connor, 1996) (see "In Practice," The M.D. Factor). However, their remarkable traditional autonomy has been receding (O'Connor & Lanning, 1992). For example, the determination of physician salaries, fees, and processes of care delivery have been gradually shifting from the physicians themselves, to a system of hospitals, payers, and managed care organizations (Zimberg & Clement, 1997).

The traditional fee-for-service payment system is a direct reward system: The more work the physician does, the more he bills and collects, and thus, the more he is rewarded. As the fee-for-service physician payment method goes the way of the dinosaur, and more intricate compensation methods become the norm, we must be cautious not to exclusively fixate on new financial schemes to modify physician behavior. "[W]hile compensation is as powerful an extrinsic motivator for physicians as it is for anyone, this incentive operates in the context of other powerful motivational resources, routinely underestimated and ignored by management" (Plume, 1995).

For example, merely inverting the fee-for-service economic reward structure such that physicians who use fewer resources receive more economic rewards is probably not a good idea. According to Kongstvedt (1996), such a system—exclusively rewarding reduced resource consumption—ignores other critical activities such as participating in quality improvement programs, complying with organizational policies, and exhibiting concern for patient satisfaction.

Because of their professional socialization and strong achievement needs, physicians want to deliver high-quality excellent care to their patients. However, in order for them to know how well they are doing in this regard, they need to be able to assess how well they are doing with respect to their peers, their own past performance, and to benchmark goals. One way of accomplishing this is to develop high-quality information systems that provide feedback on a frequent basis. Such a system can allow medical professionals to know not only how well they are doing, but to also enhance their confidence that they are doing things right (Kongstvedt, 1996).

Feedback can be a powerful tool to assist managers in motivating physician behavior; however, there are several factors that should be considered in order to maximize the feedback effectiveness. First, in order for feedback to have value, physicians must truly see that their behavior needs to change. Second, feedback needs to be frequent, timely, and given at precise time intervals in order to sustain new behaviors. Third, feedback must be useable, consistent, correct, and of sufficient diversity. It should contain various important utilization, financial, and quality-related data that are valid representations of what is being measured. Otherwise, behavior problems can intensify as rewards flow to improvements based on flawed feedback data (Charns & Smith Tewksbury,

1993). Last, managers should not portray the feedback as "good" or "bad." Professionals, such as physicians, know when they have missed the goal.

Support Personnel

Methods of staff motivation may vary somewhat depending upon the type of personnel. Whereas professionals may exhibit high levels of need for autonomy and control, achievement, and personal growth on the job, support personnel may exhibit lower levels of these higher-order needs. Not all clerical and service employees respond to the same incentives as do professionals.

For example, a manager who assumed such needs among all staff members might be surprised to learn that some support personnel will not respond to opportunities for autonomy and personal growth on the job. Rather, they may view their jobs as a means of providing income and seek various forms of personal fulfillment off-the-job through their families and leisure activities.

Several years ago one of the chapter authors was assigned a new secretary. When he attempted to ask him to do some basic research on the computer and to edit one of his articles, he was told "It's not my job." The author was attempting to broaden the individual's job duties beyond those that were merely clerical, but he resisted because he did not have a need/desire to perform "higher-level" functions. On another occasion, the author hired an assistant to perform program-related administration functions for a master's program in health administration. He attempted to provide broad, general guidance concerning what needed to be done and had hired the assistant because he had indicated that he wanted to be treated "like a professional" during the job interview. After several months, the author concluded that nothing was done unless he specified what needed to be done in great detail, specified a deadline, and followed up. There was a disconnect between the assistant's expressed desire to be treated like a professional and his behavior. He took advantage of the broad supervision and lack of detailed oversight to conduct personal business, "play" on the computer, and only perform those tasks that he enjoyed while "forgetting" those he found distasteful. He also neglected to communicate to his supervisor regarding the status of various activities, thus requiring the supervisor to follow up on all details to make sure they were all done and done well. In sum, the assistant was present physically, but not mentally.

The point is not that individuals in clerical or service positions lack higher-level needs such as autonomy and personal growth. Rather, health care managers need to determine what will motivate various support personnel rather than assuming that what motivates the manager and professional colleagues will also motivate all others. In cases where the individual lacks higher-level needs, the manager might attempt to convince the employee that a broader job scope and more autonomy is in his or her interest. Alternatively, the manager might provide more structure and direction. In the cases cited above, the author opted to provide more structure and direction and the result was higher levels of employee performance.

One should not conclude that support personnel (i.e., clerical and service workers) lack higher-level needs and necessarily need more structure and control. One hospital used two attendants to maintain their school of nursing. Each attendant was responsible for their particular area with no supervision and the facility was always spotless. They were commended verbally and in writing for the high quality of their work. The vice president for Human Resources attributed their motivation and good work to the pride and ownership they felt in what they viewed as "their" area.

When the School of Nursing was closed, the two attendants were transferred to the hospital. In the hospital, they were viewed as new employees, moved around on a regular basis, and no longer had autonomy and ownership of a specific area. The quality of their work suffered and they were written up by supervisors for attitudinal problems, lack of motivation, and inadequate work performance. Even though there was no fault of their own, their job structure and environment had changed and so too had their motivation.

These previously highly motivated employees became accustomed to autonomy, personal control, responsibility, and pride of ownership. All of these had been taken away from them when their jobs were restructured. Even though they were not professional staff members, they had responded positively to opportunities to fulfill their higher-level needs noted above and negatively when these opportunities were withdrawn.

The important point in motivating both professional and support personnel is that various methods of motivation noted in "Managerial Guidelines" in this chapter should be viewed contingently. That is, the manager needs to assess the degree to which his or her employees desire fulfillment of which higher-level needs and then respond to these needs in terms of how the job is structured as well as his or her managerial style. When it comes to managing staff, one size (i.e., style) may not fit all.

An Assessment of Process Theories

Each process theory has limitations that make it incomplete for understanding and motivating behavior. On the other hand, taken together the theories offer a powerful set of guidelines for health care managers (see "Managerial Guidelines"). Process theories share the view that the content of work is often not enough to motivate people; they need reinforcement, expectations, fairness, and goals to be energized to perform their best.

Indeed, taken together, process theories suggest a cycle of managerial action as follows:

1. Goals should be set at the time of hiring and at periodic performance evaluations.

2. Expectations about goal attainment and consequences should also be set at this time.

3. Perceptions of fairness should be checked periodically.

4. Reinforcement should be given contingent on performance.

MANAGERIAL GUIDELINES

1. Check employees' perceptions of the fairness of their work and rewards. Address perceived inequities as best as possible, given resource constraints. Unfortunately, perceptions of inequity are especially likely when managers try to take individuals' different needs into account.
2. Select rewards that are attractive to employees.
3. Make sure that the rules for attaining rewards are clear to everyone.
4. Make sure that people understand that their efforts will lead to the desired level of performance.

5. Reward people contingent on performance; try various reinforcement schedules to see what works best in your setting.
6. Set or encourage people to set goals that are difficult and specific; revise and update goals as necessary.
7. Provide timely and specific feedback to people on their progress toward goals.
8. Build commitment to goals by helping people believe that they can attain them and by selecting goals that are consistent with their values.

This cycle used in concert with the guidelines suggested from content perspectives can go a long way toward increasing motivation in health care organizations.

MOTIVATIONAL PROBLEMS

Nature and Causes

A major challenge for all health care organizations is to avoid employee motivation problems and to remedy such problems if they do occur. Despite their best efforts, most organizations do experience some problems of employee motivation. The symptoms may involve apathy, low-quality work, and complaints from supervisors and patients.

The causes of motivational problems often fall into three categories. First, there may be inadequate performance definition. This means the employees do not fully understand what is expected of them.

There is no clear definition of what is expected of employees nor any continuous orientation of employees toward effective job performance. Symptoms of this problem include a lack of goals, inadequate job descriptions, inadequate performance standards, and inadequate performance assessment.

Second, there may be impediments to employee performance. Among the most important of these may be bureaucratic or environmental obstacles, inadequate support or resources, and a mismatch between the employee's skills and job requirements. An example is a hospital experiencing significant understaffing in nursing. Since the nursing staff is probably overworked, stressed-out, and burned-out, efforts to provide a motivating environment will fail unless and until adequate staffing is provided. Research has shown that inadequate nurse staffing and consequent high workloads are the major problems motivating nurse turnover (Fottler, Crawford, Quintana, & White, 1995). Obviously, it is difficult to motivate overworked and overstressed nurses to high levels of productivity and service quality.

Third, there may be inadequate performance-reward linkages. Rewards may be economic or noneconomic. Symptoms of this problem are inappropriate rewards that are not valued by employees, inadequate rewards for performance, delay in receipt of rewards, a low probability of receiving rewards, and inequity in the distribution of rewards.

Determining the specific causes of a particular employee motivation problem is difficult. The most effective approach is for managers to develop communication skills, interpersonal skills, and interview skills so that two-way communication with employees is effective. The emphasis is on listening and encouraging employees to speak frankly. As a result, the problems and frustrations of particular employees—both individuals and groups—are well-understood by both their immediate supervisors and higher-level managers. Many organizations have found that an upward communication system utilizing interviews has paid off in terms of reduced absenteeism and turnover, increased productivity, and higher profits (Imberman, 1976).

Employee attitude surveys can also be useful in collecting information about employee beliefs and attitudes as long as they are anonymous and there is assurance the results will be acted upon (Fottler et al., 1995; Taglinferri, 1988; York, 1985). First, such surveys are valuable for identifying the problems and impediments to performance that need to be reviewed and modified. Second, they are useful for learning the value that employees attach to a number of different outcomes such as money, recognition, autonomy, and affiliation. Discrepancies between employee and management views provide a basis for exploring ways to modify employee beliefs or job conditions to create a better match of employee values and job attributes. Third, attitude surveys are useful for learning the nature of employee beliefs about contingencies. In particular, surveys should reveal the extent to which employee beliefs about expectancies and instrumentalities (i.e., probability of receiving reward and adequacy in meeting needs) match those that managers believe exist for these employees. Unfortunately, this diagnosis of employee attitudes and needs is deficient in most health services organizations. One survey found only 43% of health care employees felt their organization seeks their opinions and suggestions. Worse yet, only 26% felt their organizations act on their input (Lutz, 1990a).

Potential Solutions

Table 3.2 outlines the three motivational problems discussed in the beginning of this section together with potential solutions. It is important to recognize that most motivational problems have more than one cause and more than one solution. In fact, the latest theory and research suggest that successful employee motivation programs should include several integrated and mutually reinforcing motivational approaches (Locke & Latham, 1990b, 2004). At a minimum, these approaches should include positive reinforcement with behavior modification if necessary, high challenge or difficult goals, valued rewards contingent upon performance expectancy of success, employee feedback, employee involvement or participation, job redesign, and low situational constraints. The long-run goal should be to develop and retain a "culture of performance."

In situations where motivational problems exist, the cause is often an inadequate linkage between performance and rewards valued by the employee (see Problem 3 of Table 3.2). Empirical research on attitudes of registered nurses indicates a trend toward more negative attitudes toward communication, pay, and promotional opportunities over time (Heckert, Fottler, Swartz, & Mercer, 1993). Apparently, as competition has increased, health care managers have reduced labor costs by restraining the growth of pay and the opportunity for advancement. While this policy contains costs and makes the organization more cost-competitive in the short run, it also adversely affects employee morale and motivation. One solution is **behavior modification**, a technique for applying the concepts of reinforcement theory in organizational settings (Luthans & Kreitner, 1985; Stajkovic & Luthans, 2001). First, the manager specifies behaviors that are to be increased or decreased. Then these target behaviors are measured to establish a baseline against which the effectiveness of behavioral

Table 3.2. Common Employee Motivation Problems and Potential Solutions

Motivational Problems	Potential Solutions
1. Inadequate performance definition (i.e., lack of goals, inadequate job descriptions, inadequate performance standards, inadequate performance assessment) 2. Impediments to performance (i.e., bureaucratic or environmental obstacles, inadequate support or resources, poor employee-job matching, inadequate information) 3. Inadequate performance-reward linkages (i.e., inappropriate rewards, inadequate rewards, poor timing of rewards, low probability of receiving rewards, inequity in distribution of rewards)	■ Well-defined job descriptions ■ Well-defined performance standards ■ Goal setting ■ Feedback on performance ■ Improved employee selection ■ Job redesign or enrichment ■ Enhanced hygiene factors (i.e., safe and clean environment, salary and fringe benefits, job security, staffing, time-off-job, equipment) ■ Behavior modification or positive reinforcement (individual or group) ■ Pay for performance ■ Enhanced achievement or growth factors (i.e., employee involvement-participation, job redesign or enrichment, career planning, professional development opportunities) ■ Enhanced esteem or power factors (i.e., autonomy or personal control, self-management, modified work schedule, recognition, praise or awards, opportunity to display skills or talents, opportunity to mentor or train others, promotions in rank or position, information concerning organization or department, preferred work activities or projects, letters of recommendation, preferred work space) ■ Enhanced affiliation or relatedness factors (i.e., work teams, task groups, business meetings, social activities, professional and community group participation, personal communication or leadership style)

modification will be assessed. The manager then analyzes the situation to ascertain what rewards employees value most and how best to tie these rewards to the target behaviors. Next, rewards are given so that desired behaviors have pleasant consequences and undesirable behaviors have unpleasant consequences. Finally, the target behaviors are measured again to determine the value of the program.

One popular extension of behavior modification is *pay for performance*. This links the desired behavior or outcomes to one specific positive employee outcome—higher pay. In most cases, it applies primarily or exclusively to management personnel.

One way to classify such plans is according to the level of performance targeted—individual, group, or total organization. Within these broad categories, literally hundreds of different approaches for relating pay to performance exist. Failure often occurs because the rewards are too small, the links between performance and rewards are weak, and supervisors resent performance appraisal ("Labor letter," 1980; Lawler, 1989; Rollins, 1987). Successful programs establish high standards of performance, develop accurate performance appraisal systems, train supervisors in the mechanics of performance appraisal and the art of giving feedback, and use a wide range of pay increases.

Well conceived and well designed pay-for-performance plans tend to work because they clearly articulate standards of performance and provide a strong motivation for employees to focus on meeting these standards. Health care managers who have launched pay-for-performance plans have generally found them to have high employee acceptance and to be effective management tools for increasing cost-efficiency, productivity, and quality of care (Berger & Moyer, 1991). The goals and performance standards that are rewarded have more intrinsic meaningfulness to employees if they are tied to the strategic goals of the organization (Fottler, Blair, Phillips, & Duran, 1990).

Problems with pay-for-performance may result if the organization uses a forced distribution or forced ranking system. Here the organization places limits on how many employees can be placed into each rating group. Typically rating groups are proportionally distributed according to a normal bell-shaped curve. If every worker cannot attain the highest ranking simultaneously, then a "forced" ranking rating system is in place.

A forced distribution of any kind creates unhealthy competition among employees. One employee's high rating "forces" someone else to get a lower rating since there can only a limited number in the top group. Employees who continue to try to get to the top rating and end up in the next-to-the-highest group eventually quit trying (extinction).

Proponents of this system say if you measure people on almost any variable, you will get a normal distribution (Figure 3.7). In other words, performance is probably normally distributed, so forced rankings should be fair. The problem with

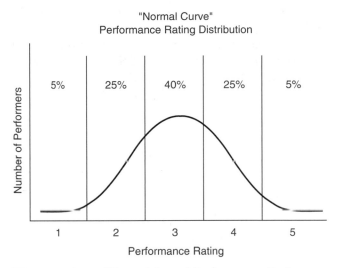

Figure 3.7. "Normal Curve" Performance Rating Distribution

SOURCE: Daniels, A. C. (1994). *Bringing out the best in people: How to apply the astonishing power of positive reinforcement.* New York: McGraw-Hill, Inc. (p. 153, Figure 18-1). Reproduced with permission of The McGraw-Hill Companies.

that logic is that organizations don't hire on the basis of a normal distribution (Daniels, 1994).

Unlike many Wall Street brokers who are motivated primarily by money, many health care workers choose their profession for reasons other than salary. Consequently, health care organizations need to identify and respond to a wide variety of noneconomic needs that may motivate their employees (see Table 3.2). There are a wide variety of employee involvement-participation programs that are based on the belief that employees at all levels in the organization can and will contribute useful insights to the effective functioning of the organization given an opportunity. The most common programs are gain-sharing suggestion systems, union-management committees, and total quality management programs (Cotton, Volrath, Frogett, Lengnick-Hall, & Jennings, 1988; Lawler, 1989). Employee participation in making critical job and organizational decisions is the one common element in all of these programs.

One method of employee participation is to seek employee input into management policies, strategies, tactics, and through written employee attitude surveys. These usually cover such topics as supervision, pay, benefits, communication, and policies. However, merely conducting attitude surveys is not sufficient by itself. The results need to be used in organizational decision making, which responds to problem areas identified by employees (Fottler et al., 1995). Otherwise, employees may become angry and cynical if management fails to act on their comments, complaints, and suggestions. Attitude surveys appear to be more effective than exit interviews in identifying employee concerns and problems that may impede employee motivation.

One approach that encompasses many of the participation strategies discussed above is employee **empowerment.** The empowerment process is one of "directed autonomy" whereby employees are given an overall direction yet considerable leeway concerning how they go about following that direction. It also necessitates sharing information and knowledge with employees, which enables them to understand and contribute to organizational performance, and giving them the autonomy to make decisions that influence organizational outcomes (Ford & Fottler, 1995). It is the issue of power that differentiates empowerment from earlier approaches to employee participation (i.e., delegation, decentralization, and participatory management) that tended to emphasize employee input but made no real change in the assignment of power and authority.

Obviously, empowerment is a matter of degree rather than an absolute (Ford & Fottler, 1995). Health care executives could choose to provide higher degrees of empowerment for some individuals and teams doing certain tasks than for others. He or she could empower subordinates in terms of any or all of the following: problem identification, alternative development, alternative evaluation, alternative choice, and implementation. Employee involvement-participation appears to be highly desired in health care organizations (Blackburn & Rosen, 1993).

Employees also desire participation linked to incentives. **Gainsharing** encourages employees to find ways to increase productivity and to cut costs in exchange for receiving a share of the savings realized. Gainsharing programs are viewed as innovative approaches to bringing about productivity improvements in developed, labor-intensive industries such as hospitals (Barbusca & Cleek, 1994). To be successful, gainsharing programs require top management to start disseminating relevant information and giving employees the time and tools to get involved.

Employee recognition programs offer another method of linking employee participation and rewards. Simple recognition practices may include: random and informal public praise for good work, organizing a departmental gathering to honor achievements of one or more employees, and publishing employee accomplishments and complimentary or thank you letters from patients or visitors in the organization's newsletter (Huseman & Hatfield, 1989; McConnell, 1997). Surveys of nonhealth employees show most believe simple positive feedback from management and recognition for a job well done serve as valued rewards capable of motivating employees (Koch, 1990; Rawlinson, 1988). Such feedback and recognition may also take more tangible forms as noneconomic award programs. Examples include trophies, wall plaques, certificates, letters or handwritten personal notes of thanks, visits or telephone calls by top executives, and luncheon invitations (Huseman & Hatfield, 1989). For such awards to be effective motivators, they must recognize only high-performing employees (Blanchard & Bowles, 1998).

Job redesign is yet another strategy that can lead to increased intrinsic motivation (also see Chapter 7). It is based on the premise that altering certain aspects of the job to satisfy employees' psychological needs will motivate them to exert more effort. According to Hackman and Lawler, satisfaction of higher-order needs (which is the essence of intrinsic motivation) occurs when the employee experiences these psychological states (Hackman &

Oldham, 1980). First, the job allows the employee to feel personally responsible for a significant segment of his or her work outcomes. Autonomy or personal control is the key job dimension contributing to feelings of personal responsibility for job outcomes. Second, the job involves doing something that is perceived as meaningful by the individual. The three core dimensions that can make jobs more meaningful are task identity (i.e., completion of a whole task), skill variety (i.e., utilization of different skills), and task significance (i.e., substantial impact). Third, the job provides the employee with knowledge of results. Feedback from the job itself or from another individual is the core job dimension, which provides knowledge of results.

Job redesign aims to enrich a job so that the employee is more motivated to do the work. It is most appropriate when there is a demonstrated need to redesign jobs—for example, due to employee down-time, and it is feasible to redesign jobs given the present structure of jobs, legal constraints, technological constraints, and the characteristics and values of employees. Job redesign in health care is feasible but may be subject to more legal and professional constraints than most other industries (Blayney, 1992).

One popular approach to job redesign in health services is the multiskilled health practitioner (MSHP). MSHPs are persons who are cross-trained to provide more than one function, often in more than one discipline. These combined functions can be formed in a broad spectrum of health-related jobs ranging in complexity from the nonprofessional to the professional level, including both clinical and management functions. The additional functions or skills added to the original job may be of a higher, lower, or parallel level. This means the concept includes both job enlargement (i.e., addition of parallel or lower-level functions) and job enrichment (i.e., addition of higher-level functions). Research has shown positive results such as higher patient and employee satisfaction, cost savings, reduced lengths of stay, reduced waiting time, improved patient compliance, improved quality of care, and improved employee retention (Fottler, 1996).

Job redesign may apply to either individual positions or to groups of employees. For employees with high growth needs, job redesign can pay off. Research in both nonhealth care organizations and health care organizations has generally supported the validity of the job characteristics model in enhancing employee motivation for employees who strongly value personal feelings of accomplishment and growth (Al-pander, 1990; Guzzo, Jette, & Katzell, 1985). However, the actual success of any job redesign effort is likely to depend on other reinforcing or nonreinforcing factors such as the reward system and top management support (Fried & Ferris, 1987).

One study examined how the level of organizational commitment of nurses and nurse's aides employed in long-term care settings influenced family satisfaction with the quality of services received. The study also examined how the job redesign variables (i.e., autonomy, task identity, skill variety, task significance, and feedback) influenced organizational commitment. Findings indicate that family members' satisfaction with the quality of services received is significantly and positively influenced by organizational commitment, which in turn is significantly and positively correlated with autonomy, task identity, and skill variety. Although feedback and task significance were dropped from the model due to measurement difficulties, this study suggests that redesigning nursing and nurse's aides jobs in long-term care settings can serve to motivate these employees to be more committed to the organization as well as to provide higher levels of perceived service quality (Steffen, Nystrom, & O'Connor, 1996).

Overall Assessment

As we have seen, there are many approaches to dealing with motivational problems among employees. None are foolproof. Whether a particular approach succeeds in a particular setting depends first on whether it was properly matched with the primary causes of low motivation. Second, it depends on how and whether the program was introduced and implemented so that resistance was minimized and commitment maximized. For example, favorable reaction is likely to be greatest if the affected employees have some voice in choosing and implementing a particular motivation program. Third, it depends on whether the program is compatible with other aspects of the organization's culture (Hames, 1991; Mohrmann & Lawler, 1984). The simultaneous introduction of several mutually supportive and mutually reinforcing motivation programs is probably most effective in overcoming motivation problems, assuming they are all relevant to the causes of the problem. An example is the program at Sharp Healthcare (see "In Practice").

Two reviews of the literature have compared the relative effectiveness of several motivation programs. One concluded that financial incentives were most effective, while goal setting was also quite effective (Locke, 1982). Participative decision making and job redesign were relatively less certain to produce significant improvements. The other study suggested that employee training and goal setting were most likely to improve motivation or productivity, followed closely by changes such as carefully designed financial incentives (Guzzo, Jette, & Katzell, 1985). Job redesign is less powerful but still has a significant impact on productivity. This review also suggests that combined interventions are more effective than single-method approaches. Yet almost any of these approaches can be effective if they are matched to the motivational problem, are carefully implemented, involve all parties, and are implemented in a culture that emphasizes employee motivation and performance.

✤ IN PRACTICE   Staff Motivation at Sharp HealthCare

Sharp HealthCare is an integrated, regional health care delivery system based in San Diego, California, serving a population of approximately 3 million. Sharp includes four acute-care hospitals, three specialty hospitals, and three medical groups plus a full-spetrum of other facilities and services. It operates 1,847 beds, has approximately 2,541 physicians on medical staffs, 1,587 physicians in medical groups, and had more than 12,000 employees with $5,852 million in assets and $1.1 billion in annual income. It is San Diego's largest private employer.

Sharp has recently been named "the best company to work for" in the large-employer category by the *San Diego Business Journal* for the second year in a row based on the company's work environment and positive impact on employees. Mr. Michael Murphy, president and CEO, noted:

We are very proud of this honor. It gets to the heart of what we are working together to achieve becoming the best place to work, the best place to practice medicine, and the best place to receive care. Since launching the healthcare experience in 2001, Sharp has dedicated itself to transforming the health care experience for employees, physicians, and customers. The focus on purpose, worthwhile work and making a difference lit a spark with Sharp team members that has led to increased employee, physician, and patient satisfaction, enhanced loyalty, and improved outcomes.

Pillars of Excellence

Since 2001, Sharp has adopted six pillars of excellence as the foundation for its vision of the health care experience, which are the basis for everything from strategic planning, organizational goal setting, priority setting, management performance evaluation, and other agendas. There are measures and targets set under each pillar that align each individual leader's goal with their department, division, and the entire Sharp system. With the pillars as a guide, communications and work planning are made more manageable and various outcomes measurement enhanced.

Of the six pillars, the three most relevant to staff motivation are Quality, Service, and People. A few of the measures used to determine performance targets under each of these three pillars are:

- Quality—accreditation and licensing scores; infection control measures; patient safety
- Service—overall patient and physician satisfaction in Sharp hospitals and medical groups
- People—increased employee satisfaction and retention

Model Behaviors and Scripts

To ensure Sharp is the best place to work, the best place to practice medicine, and the best place to receive care, all employees are required to exemplify the Must Haves, five essential behaviors and actions in the workplace:

- Greet people with a smile and "Hello," using their name when possible.
- Take people where they are going, rather than pointing or giving directions.
- Use key words (scripts) at key times: "Is there anything else I can do for you? I have time."
- Foster an attitude of gratitude and send thank-you notes to deserving employees.
- Round with reason to better commit with staff, patients, family, and other customers.

Employee Forums

In the spirit of a "no secrets" culture, Sharp keeps the line of communication between management and employees open; each unit holds quarterly employee forums led by the entity CEO. The purpose is to share important updates and information and recognize and celebrate the work of Sharp employees. Up to 20 forums are held around the clock over a two-day period to attract as many employees as possible. The agenda for these forums is based on each of the six pillars of excellence. Sample topics include system or entity report cards, patient satisfaction scores, physician satisfaction scores, model behavior standards, facility openings, celebrations, and wins.

Re-recruiting Employees

With most health care organizations nationally approaching and sometimes exceeding 20% turnover, Sharp is enjoying a rate of about 10%. High and increasing levels of employee satisfaction and retention are top priorities for both individuals and managers, as well as the entire system. One of the tools managers to use retain the employees is re-recruitment of current employees rather than new ones. Re-recruiting recognizes employees for their contributions, renews their sense of self-worth and loyalty, and ensures their longevity.

The following four steps are used in Sharp's re-recruiting technique:

- Identify the great, good, and low-performing employees in each department. Great performers are those who always have a positive attitude and take initiative to tackle projects and solve problems. Good performers are those who need help developing in some areas, but are generally reliable employees. Low performers are those who take no initiative to complete tasks and have a negative attitude.
- Meet with your great performers individually to let each of them know they are a valuable asset to your department and company. Let them know

(continues)

IN PRACTICE (continued)

what they are doing right, cite specific examples, and ask them what you can do to ensure their longevity with Sharp.

■ Meet with your good performers individually to let them know how much you value their contribution, provide specific examples, and let them know that you want them to stay with your organization. Be sure to also specify areas in need of improvement.

■ Meet with your marginal performers individually to let them know that their behaviors or actions are not consistent with the organization's standards. Specify areas in need of improvement and let them know the consequences of not taking steps to change negative behaviors and actions.

Employee Opinion Survey

Sharp also surveys its 12,000 employees annually through an online employee opinion survey using a password sent from an outside vendor to the employee's home. The survey asks for team members' opinions on many aspects of their work experience to ensure they feel adequately supported and have the tools, supplies, and training to provide the best health care possible. Results are provided to all Sharp managers and employees. A demo of a results page from a sample employee opinion survey may be viewed at http://www.perceptyx.com/

Each manager reviews the system, entity, and department results with their staff members at a dedicated staff meeting set aside to vote on the top three priorities they would like their department to address. The manager assigns action teams to address each of these priorities. The actionable items and the plan to address them are part of a 90-day action plan that each manager must share with his or her supervisor. Progress toward the top three goals is

addressed in quarterly updates that are reviewed with and turned in to the supervisor. Once the first three priorities are addressed, the manager then addresses additional priorities with his/her team.

Actions and results emanating from employee opinion surveys are reported back to staff at staff meetings. The top actions to address staff needs are then shared and celebrated at Leadership Development for Managers at the end of each fiscal year.

Overview

As a result of the implementation of the six pillars of excellence, including those managerial strategies and tactics that enhance employee motivation, there have been a number of positive impacts on the organization:

■ Employee satisfaction scores increased by 9% in the first year with an additional increase of 3% in year 2.

■ Employee turnover is 10% as compared to industry norms of between 18 and 20%.

■ Patient satisfaction scores are rising steadily with many departments in the top 1% in the United States.

■ A recent independent survey of San Diego residents ranked Sharp HealthCare number one among all San Diego health care systems and number one in providing the very best overall experience.

Sources: http://www.sharp.com and Michael W. Murphy, president and C.E.O. of Sharp HealthCare, "Using Evidenced-Based Management to Transform Health Care." Presentation at the 2004 Annual Meeting of the Association of the Association of University Programs in Health Administration, Loews Coronado Bay Resort, San Diego, June 4, 2004.

Web site: Sharp HealthCare, San Diego, California, http://www.sharp.com

MANAGERIAL GUIDELINES

1. The major reasons for low employee motivation are lack of understanding concerning expectations, organizational impediments to performance, and lack of valued rewards for performance.
2. A variety of upward communication methods are available to assist health care managers in determining the nature and causes of employee motivation problems including direct supervisor communication, interviews, and employee attitude surveys.
3. Expectations can be clarified through well-defined job descriptions, performance standards, goal setting, and feedback on performance

4. Attitude surveys are effective means of identifying and removing motivational impediments as long as management follow-up to concerns occurs.
5. Motivational impediments can be removed by addressing relevant hygiene factors in the environment as well as better matching of employee and job through improved selection and job redesign.
6. Inadequate performance-reward linkages can be addressed through behavior modification, pay for performance, and provision of desired motivators related to achievement or growth or esteem or power needs of employees.

DISCUSSION QUESTIONS

1. How can content and process motivation theories best be combined in practice?
2. How can managers distinguish a motivational problem from other factors that affect an individual's performance?
3. How can motivational theories be used to select the best potential solution for a given individual's needs?

REFERENCES

Adams, J. S. (1963, November). Toward an understanding of inequity. *Journal of Abnormal and Social Psychology, 67,* 422–436.

Adams, J. S. (1965). Inequity in social exchange. In L. Berkowitz (Ed.), *Advances in Experimental Social Psychology, II.* New York: Academic Press.

Alderfer, C. P. (1968). An empirical test of a new theory of human needs. *Organization Behavior and Human Performance, 16*(2), 42–175.

Alderfer, C. P. (1972). *Existence, relatedness, and growth.* New York: Free Press.

Alpander, G. G. (1985). Factors influencing hospital employee motivation: A diagnostic instrument. *Hospital and Health Services Administration, 30*(2), 67–83.

Alpander, G. G. (1990). Relationship between commitment to hospital goals and job satisfaction: A case study of a nursing department. *Health Care Management Review, 15*(4), 51–62.

Ambrose, M. L., & Kulik, C. T. (1999). Old friends, new faces: Motivation research in the 1990s. *Journal of Management, 25*, 231–292.

Appleby, C. (1998). Brain drain. *Hospitals and Health Networks, 72*(8), 41–42.

Arnolds, C. A., & Boshoff, C. (2002). Compensation, esteem valence and job performance: An empirical assessment of Alderfer's ERG theory. *International Journal of Human Resources Management, 13*(4), 697–719.

Atkinson, J. W. (1961). *An introduction to motivation.* New York: Van Nostrand.

Barbusca, A., & Cleek, M. (1994). Measuring gain-sharing dividends in acute care hospitals. *Health Care Management Review, 19*(1), 28–33.

Becker, I. J. (1978). Joint effect of feedback and goal setting on performance: A field study of residential energy conservation. *Journal of Applied Psychology, 63*, 428–433.

Berger, S., & Moyer, J. (1991). Launching a performance-based pay plan. *Modern Healthcare, 21*(33), 64.

Blackburn, R. B., & Rosen, B. (1993). Total quality and human resources management: Lessons learned from Baldridge Award–winning companies. *Academy of Management Executive, 7*(3), 49–60.

Blanchard, K. H., & Bowles, S. M. (1998). Get gung ho. *Success, 45*(5), 30–31.

Blayney, K. D. (Ed.). (1992). *Healing hands: Customizing your health team for institutional survival.* Battle Creek, MI: W. K. Kellogg Foundation.

Campbell, J. P., & Pritchard, R. D. (1976). Motivation theory in industrial and organizational psychology. In M. D. Dunnette (Ed.), *Handbook of industrial and organizational psychology* (pp. 63–130). Skokie, IL: Rand McNally.

Carr, S. C., McLoughlin, D., Hodgson, M., & MacLachlan, M. (1996). Effects of unreasonable pay discrepancies for under- and overpayment on double demotivation. *Genetic, Social, and General Psychology Monograph, 122*(4), 475–494.

Charns, M. P., & Smith Tewksbury, L. J. (1993). *Collaborative management in health care: Implementing the integrative organization.* San Francisco: Jossey-Bass Publishers.

Chusmir, L. H. (1986). How fulfilling are health care jobs? *Health Care Management Review, 11(1),* 27–32.

Colvin, G. (1998). What money makes you do. *Fortune,* 138(4), 213–214.

Cornelius, E., & Lane, F. (1984). The power motive and managerial success in a professionally oriented service company. *Journal of Applied Psychology, 69,* 32–40.

Cotton, J. L., Volrath, D. A., Frogett, K. L., Lengnick-Hall, M. D., & Jennings, K. R. (1988). Employee participation: Diverse forms and different outcomes. *Academy of Management Review, 13*(1), 8–22.

Daniels, A. C. (1994). *Bringing out the best in people: How to apply the astonishing power of positive reinforcement.* New York: McGraw-Hill, Inc.

Davis-Blake, A., & Pfeffer, J. (1989). Just a mirage: The search for disposition effects in organizational research. *Academy of Management Review, 14*(3), 385–400.

Durand, D. E. (1983). Modified achievement motivation training: A longitudinal study of the effects of a condensed training design for entrepreneurs. *Psychological Reports, 52*, 901–911.

Erez, M., & Zidon, I. (1984). Effect of goal acceptance on the relationship of goal difficulty to performance. *Journal of Applied Psychology, 69*, 69–78.

Farnham, A. (1989, December). The trust gap. *Fortune,* 56–78.

Ford, R. C., & Fottler, M. D. (1992). Studies of nurses' attitudes during the 1980's: What have we learned? In D. F. Ray (Ed.), *Proceedings of the annual meeting of the Southern Management Association* (pp. 130–132). Mississippi State, MS: Southern Management Association.

Ford, R. C., & Fottler, M. D. (1995). Empowerment: A matter of degree. *Academy of Management Executive, 9*(3), 21–29.

Fottler, M. D. (1996). The role and impact of multiskilled health practitioners in the health services industry. *Hospital and Health Services Administration, 41*(1), 55–75.

Fottler, M. D., Blair, J. D., Phillips, R. L., & Duran, C. A. (1990). Achieving competitive advantage through strategic human resources management. *Hospital and Health Services Administration, 35*(3), 341–363.

Fottler, M. D., Crawford, M. A., Quintana, J. B., & White, J. B. (1995). Evaluating nurse turnover: Comparing attitude surveys and exit interviews. *Hospital and Health Services Administration, 40*(2), 278–295.

Fottler, M. D., Shewchuk, R. M., & O'Connor, S. J. (1998). What matters to health care executives? Assessing the job attributes associated with their staying or leaving. *International Journal of Organization Theory and Behavior, 1*(2), 223–247.

Fried, Y., & Ferris, G. R. (1987). The validity of the job characteristics model: A review and meta analysis. *Personnel Psychology, 40*(3), 287–322.

Fried, Y., & Slowik, L. H. (2004). Enriching goal setting theory with time: An integrated approach. *Academy of Management Review, 29*(3), 404–422.

Georgopoulos, B. S., Mahoney, B. S., & Jones, N. W. (1957). A path-goal approach to productivity. *Journal of Applied Psychology, 41*, 345–353.

Greenberg, J. (1982). Approaching equity and avoiding inequity in groups and organizations. In J. Greenberg, & R. L. Cohen (Eds.), *Equity and justice in social behavior.* New York: Academic Press.

Griffin, R. W. (1991). Effects of work redesign on employee perceptions, attitudes, and behavior: A long-term investigation. *Academy of Management Journal, 34*(2), 425–435.

Guzzo, R. A., Jette, R. D., & Katzell, R. A. (1985). The effects of psychologically based intervention programs on worker productivity: A meta analysis. *Personnel Psychology, 38*(3), 275–291.

Hackman, J. R., & Oldham, G. (1980). *Work redesign.* Reading, MA: Addison-Wesley.

Hames, D. S. (1991). Productivity-enhancing work innovations: Remedies for what ails hospitals? *Hospital and Health Services Administration, 38*(4), 545–557.

Haug, M. E. (1988). A re-examination of the hypothesis of physician deprofessionalization. *The Milbank Quarterly, 66*(Supplement 2), 48–56.

Heckert, D. A., Fottler, M. D., Swartz, B. W., & Mercer, A. A. (1993). The impact of the changing healthcare environment on the attitudes of nursing staff. *Health Services Management Research, 6*(3), 191–202.

Herzberg, F. (1987). One more time: How do you motivate employees? *Harvard Business Review, 65,* 109–120.

Herzberg, F., Mausner, B., & Snyderman, B. (1959). *The motivation to work.* New York: John Wiley.

Holland, M. G., Black, C. H., & Miner, J. B. (1987). Using managerial role motivation theory to predict career success. *Health Care Management Review, 12*(4), 57–64.

Hollenbeck, J. R., & Klein, H. J. (1987). Goal commitment and the goal-setting process: Problems, prospects, and proposals for future research. *Journal of Applied Psychology, 82,* 212–220.

Hom, P. W. (1980). Expectancy prediction of reenlistment in the National Guard. *Journal of Vocational Behavior, 16*(2), 235–248.

House, R. J., & Wigdor, L. A. (1967). Herzberg's two-factor theory of job satisfaction and motivation: A review of the evidence and a criticism. *Personnel Psychology, 20*(3), 369–389.

Hurka, S. J. (1980). Need satisfaction among health care managers. *Hospital and Health Services Administration, 25*(3), 43–54.

Huselid, M. A. (1995). The impact of human resource management practices on turnover, productivity, and corporate financial performance. *Academy of Management Journal, 38*(3), 635–672.

Huseman, R. C., & Hatfield, J. D. (1989). *Managing the equity factor.* Boston: Houghton-Mifflin.

Imberman, W. (1976). Letting the employee speak his mind. *Personnel, 53*(6), 12–22.

Ivancevich, J. M., & McMahon, J. T. (1982). The effects of goal-setting, external feedback, and self-generated feedback on outcome variables: A field experiment. *Academy of Management Journal, 25*(2), 359–372.

Jurkiewicz, C. L., Massey, T. K., & Brown, R. J. (1998). Motivation in public and private organizations: A comparative study. *Public Productivity & Management Review, 21*(3), 230–250.

Kanfer, R. (1990). Motivation theory and industrial and organizational psychology. In M. D. Dunnette, & L. M., Houghlin (Eds.), *Handbook of industrial and organizational psychology* (pp. 75–170). Palo Alto, CA: Consulting Psychologists Press, Inc.

Kanfer, R., & Ackerman, P. L. (2004). Aging, adult development and work motivation. *Academy of Management Review, 29*(3), 423–439.

Kennedy, C. W., Fossum, J. A., & White, B. J. (1983). An empirical comparison of within-subjects and between-subjects expectancy theory models. *Organizational Behavior and Human Performance, 32*, 124–143.

Kennedy, M. M. (1997). How to put new life into an old job. *Healthcare Executive, 12*(5), 44–45.

Kiechel, W. (1989, April 10). The workaholic generation. *Fortune,* 50–62.

Koch, J. (1990). Perpetual thanks: Its assets. *Personnel Journal, 69*(1), 72–73.

Kongstvedt, P. R. (1996). *The managed care health care handbook* (3rd ed.). Gaithersburg, MD: Aspen Publishers, Inc.

Kovach, K. A. (1987). What motivates employees: Workers and supervisors give different answers. *Business Horizons, 30*, 58–65.

Kovach, K. A. (1995). Employee motivation: Addressing a crucial factor in your organization's performance. *Employment Relations Today, 22*(2), 93–105.

"Labor letter." (1980, February 20). *The Wall Street Journal,* p. A1.

Laurinaitis, J. (1997). Actions speak louder than posters. *Psychology Today, 30*(3), 16.

Lawler, E. E. (1988). Choosing an involvement strategy. *Academy of Management Executive, 2*(3), 197–204.

Lawler, E. E. (1989). Pay for performance: A strategic analysis. In L. R. Gomez-Mejia (Ed.), *Compensation and benefits* (pp. 136–181). Washington, DC: Bureau of National Affairs.

Lee, J. A. (1980). *The gold and garbage of management theory and prescriptions.* Athens, OH: Ohio University Press.

Locke, E. A. (1968). Effects of knowledge of results, feedback in relation to standards, and goals on reaction-time performance. *American Journal of Applied Psychology, 81*, 566–574.

Locke, E. A. (1982). Relation of goal level to performance with a short work period and multiple goal levels. *Journal of Applied Psychology, 67*, 512–514.

Locke, E. A., & Latham, G. P. (1984). *Goal setting: A motivational technique that works.* Englewood Cliffs, NJ: Prentice Hall.

Locke, E. A., & Latham, G. P. (1990a). *A theory of goal setting and task performance.* Englewood Cliffs, NJ: Prentice-Hall.

Locke, E. A., & Latham, G. P. (1990b). Work motivation and satisfaction: Light at the end of the tunnel. *Psychological Science, 1*(4), 240–246.

Locke, E. A., & Latham, G. P. (2004). What should we do about motivation theory? Six recommendations for the twenty-first century. *Academy of Management Review, 29*(3), 388–403.

Locke, E. A., Latham, G. P., & Erez, M. (1988). The determinants of goal commitment. *Academy of Management Review, 13*, 23–39.

Longest, B. (1974). Job satisfaction of registered nurses in a hospital setting. *Journal of Nursing Administration, 4*(3), 46–52.

Luthans, F., & Kreitner, R. (1985). *Organization behavior modification and beyond: An operant conditioning approach.* Glenview, IL: Scott, Foresman.

Lutz, S. (1990a). Hospitals stretch their creativity to motivate workers. *Modern Healthcare, 20*(9), 20–33.

Lutz, S. (1990b). Employee suggestions net $20 million in savings. *Modern Healthcare, 20*(9), 21–22.

Maslow, A. H. (1943). A theory of human motivation. *Psychological Review, 50,* 370–396.

McClelland, D. C. (1961). *The achieving society.* Princeton, NJ: Van Nostrand.

McClelland, D. C. (1975). *Power: The inner experience.* New York: Irvington.

McClelland, D. C., & Burnham, D. H. (1976). Power is the great motivator. *Harvard Business Review, 54*(2), 100–110.

McConnell, C. R. (1996). After reduction in force: Reinvigorating the survivors. *The Health Care Supervisor, 14*(4), 1–2.

McConnell, C. R. (1997). Employee recognition: A little oil on the troubled waters of change. *The Health Care Supervisor, 15*(4), 83–90.

The M.D. Factor. (1997). *Crossroads: New directions in health management,* a supplement to *Hospitals & Health Networks.*

Medcof, J. W., & Hausdorf, P. A. (1995). Instruments to measure opportunities to satisfy needs, and degree of satisfaction of needs, in the workplace. *Journal of*

Occupational and Organizational Psychology, 68(3), 193–199.

Mercer, A. A. (1988). Commitment and motivation of professionals. In M. D. Fottler, S. R. Hernandez, and C. L. Joiner (Eds.), *Strategic management of human resources in health services organizations* (pp. 181–205). New York: John Wiley and Sons.

Miron, D., & McClelland, D. C. (1979). The impact of achievement motivation in small business. *California Management Review, 22*, 34–46.

Mitchell, T. R. (1982). Motivation: New directions for theory, research, and practice. *Academy of Management Review, 7*, 80–88.

Mitchell, T. R. (1984). *Motivation and performance.* Chicago: Science Research Associates.

Mitchell, T. R., & Daniels, D. (2002). Motivation. In W. Borman, D. Ilgen, & R. Klimoski (Eds.), *Comprehensive handbook of psychology. Industrial and organizational psychology,* pp. 225–254. New York: Wiley.

Mitchell, V., & Mowdgill, P. (1976). Measurement of Maslow's need hierarchy. *Organization Behavior and Human Performance, 16*(2), 334–349.

Mohr, L. B. (1982). *Explaining organizational behavior.* San Francisco: Jossey-Bass.

Mohrmann, S. A., & Lawler, E. E. (1984). Quality of worklife. *Research in Personnel and Human Resources Management, 2*, 219–260.

Moore, J. D. (1996). Samaritan's revolution: New pay model aims to overhaul how workers think. *Modern Healthcare, 26*(31), 27, 30, 32–34.

Muchinsky, P. M. (1987). *Psychology applied to work: An introduction to industrial and organizational psychology.* Belmont, CA: Wadsworth, Inc., 341–378.

Nicholls, J. G. (1984). Achievement motivation: Conceptions of authority, subjective experience, task chores, and performance. *Psychological Review, 91*, 328–346.

Nordhaus-Bike, A. M. (1997). Cutting with kindness. *Hospital and Health Networks, 71*(2), 62–63.

O'Connor, S. J. (1996). Who will manage the managers? In A. Lazarus (Ed.), *Controversies in managed mental health care* (pp. 383–401). Washington, DC: American Psychiatric Press.

O'Connor, S. J. (1998). Motivating effective performance. In P. Ginter, L. Swayne, & D. J.

Duncan (Eds.), *Handbook of health care management* (pp. 431–470). Cambridge, MA: Blackwell Business Publishing.

O'Connor, S. J., & Lanning, J. A. (1992). The end of autonomy? Reflections on the post-professional physician. *Health Care Management Review, 17*(1), 63–72.

O'Connor, S. J., & Shewchuk, R. M. (1995). Service quality revisited: Striving for a new orientation. *Hospital and Health Services Administration, 40*(1), 535–552.

Pfeffer, J. (1998). *The human equation: Building profits by putting people first.* Boston: Harvard Business School Press.

Pinder, C. (1984). *Work motivation.* Glenview, IL: Scott, Foresman.

Plume, S. (1995). Redesigning physician compensation mechanisms: A fool's errand. *Motivation & Emotion, 19*(3), 205–210.

Pritchard, R. D., De Leo, P. J., & Von Bergen, C. W. (1976). A field experimental test of expectancy valence incentive motivation techniques. *Organizational Behavior and Human Performance, 15*, 355–406.

Pujol, J. L., & Tudanger, E. (1992). A vision of excellence. *HRM Magazine, 35*(6), 112–116.

Rantz, M. J., Scott, J., & Porter, R. (1996). Employee motivation: New perspectives of the age-old challenge of work motivation. *Nursing Forum, 31*(3), 29–36.

Rawlinson, H. (1988). Make awards count. *Personnel Journal, 67*(10), 139–146.

Reibstein, L. (1986 October 27). A finger on the pulse: Companies expand use of employee surveys. *The Wall Street Journal,* 27.

Rollins, T. (1987). Pay for performance: The pros and cons. *Personnel Journal, 66*(5), 104–107.

Schneider, B., & Alderfer, C. P. (1973). Three studies of measures of need satisfaction in organizations. *Administrative Science Quarterly, 18*(4), 489–505.

Schwarb, D. P., Devitt, W. H., & Cummings, L. L. (1971). A test of the adequacy of the two-factor theory as a predictor of self-report performance effects. *Personnel Psychology, 24*, 293–304.

Schwartz, H. S. (1983). Maslow and the hierarchial enactment of organizational reality. *Human Relations, 36*(10), 933–956.

Seo, M. G., Barrett, L. F., & Bartunek, J. M. (2004). The role of affective experience in work motivation. *Academy of Management Review, 29*(3), 423–439.

Sherman, S. (1995). Stretch goals: The dark side of asking for miracles. *Fortune, 132*(10), 231–232.

Skinner, B. F. (1969). *Contingencies of reinforcement: A theoretical analysis.* New York: Appleton-Century-Crofts.

Stacy, A. W., Widaman, K. F., & Marlatt, G. A. (1990). Expectancy models of alcohol use. *Journal of Personality and Social Psychology, 58*(5), 918–928. Steers, R. M., & Porter, L. W. (1987). *Motivation and work behavior.* New York: McGraw-Hill.

Stajkovic, A. D., & Luthans, F. (2001). Differential effects of incentive motivators on work performance. *Academy of Management Journal, 4*(3), 580–590.

Steffen, T. M., Nystrom, P. C., & O'Connor, S. J. (1996). Satisfaction with nursing homes: The design of employees jobs can ultimately influence family members' perceptions. *Journal of Health Care Marketing, 16*(3), 34–38.

Taglinferri, L. E. (1988). Taking note of employee attitudes. *Personnel Administrator, 33*(4), 96–102.

Thomas, L. (1998). Maximizing the human resource asset. *The Health Care Supervisor, 16*(4), 35–39.

Tsui, A. S., Ashford, S. J., St. Clair, L., & Xin, K. R. (1995). Dealing with discrepant expectations: Response strategies and managerial effectiveness. *Academy of Management Journal, 38*(6), 1515–1543.

Tully, S. (1994). Why go for the stretch targets? *Fortune, 130*(10), 145–158.

Vance, A. (1997). Motivating the paraprofessional in long-term care. *The Health Care Supervisor, 15*(4), 57–64.

Vaughan, D. G., Fottler, M. D., Bamberg, R., & Blayney, K. (1991). Utilization and management of multiskilled health practitioners in U. S. hospitals. *Hospital and Health Services Administration, 36*(3), 347–419.

Vidaver-Cohen, D. (1998). Motivational appeal in normative theories of enterprise. *Business Ethics Quarterly, 8*(3), 385–407.

Vroom, V. (1964). *Work and motivation.* New York: Wiley.

Wahba, M. A., & Budwell, L. G. (1976). Maslow reconsidered: A review of research on the need hierarchy theory. *Organization Behavior and Human Performance, 15*(2), 317–333.

Wanous, J. P., Keon, T. L., & Latack, J. C. (1983). Expectancy theory and occupational/organizational choices: A review and test. *Organizational Behavior and Human Performance, 32*(1), 66–86.

Weiner, B. (1986). *An attributional theory of motivation and emotion.* New York: Springer-Verlag.

York, D. R. (1985). Attitude surveying. *Personnel Journal, 64*(5), 70–73.

Zigarelli, M. (1996). Human resources and the bottom line. *Academy of Management Executive, 10*(2), 63.

Zima, J. P. (1983). *Interviewing: Key to effective management.* Chicago: Science Research Associates, Inc.

Zimberg, S. E., & Clement, D. G. (1997). Physician motivation, satisfaction and survival. *Medical Group Management Journal, 44*(4), 19–20, 22, 24, 26, 63.

CHAPTER 4

Leadership: A Framework for Thinking and Acting

Dennis D. Pointer, Ph.D.

CHAPTER OUTLINE

- ❧ Foundational Concepts
- ❧ Leadership Perspectives and Theories
- ❧ Pulling It All Together
- ❧ Several Distinctive Aspects of Leadership in Health Care Organizations

LEARNING OBJECTIVES

After completing this chapter, you will:

1. Appreciate why leadership skills are so important.
2. Understand what leadership is and what it's not.
3. Understand the distinction between management and leadership.
4. Understand the leadership role and how it is performed.
5. Understand the key features of major leadership perspectives and associated theories.
6. Consider how different perspectives of leadership can be combined into a more integrative framework.
7. Appreciate several distinctive challenges of leading in health care organizations.
8. Possess a solid foundation for continually developing your leadership knowledge, skills, behaviors, and styles.

KEY TERMS

Attributes
Behavioral Perspective
Clinical Mentality
Consideration
Contingency Perspective
Expectancy
Follower
Follower Maturity
Gender

Initiating Structure
Instrumentality
Leadership
Leadership Role
Leadership Style
Managerial Mentality
Managerial Office
Managerial Role
Professional

Relationship-Oriented Leader
  Behavior
Skills Perspective
Task-Oriented Leader Behavior
Trait Perspective
Transactional Leadership
Transformational Perspectives
Valence

> "Think like a ~~man~~ [person] of action.
> Act like a ~~man~~ [person] of thought."
> *Aristotle*

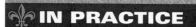 **IN PRACTICE**   We're Searching for a Leader But May Not Fully Understand What Leadership Is

You're on the board of a 250-bed short-term general hospital that is working with a search consultant to recruit a new chief executive officer. The present occupant of the position will be retiring in five months after 23 years of service. The headhunter has a unique background. She holds a Ph.D. in organization behavior and taught this subject in a health administration program for 10 years.

In addition to all of the other types of experience, knowledge, and skills necessary for being a successful hospital CEO, the board wants to recruit someone who is an exceptional leader. The board has expressed this desire to the consultant and selected her because they feel she can help them find such a person.

The consultant is meeting with board members, over dinner, for the first time since being retained. While coffee and dessert are served, she begins talking with the board about why they feel

leadership ability is so important in this search. She observes: "For the search to locate someone with the type of leadership you want, we must have a shared notion of precisely what we're looking for. If you all define leadership in different ways and have varying ideas about what an exceptional leader is, we're in for some difficulties as this process unfolds. I have a few questions that I want you to think about. Take the next 10 minutes to jot down some notes on a piece of paper. Don't feel like you have to compose elegant prose; go for substance. This exercise may seem a bit academic. Indeed, I ask these questions of students taking my leadership course at the university. I've found they are very helpful in getting people to begin thinking more rigorously about leadership. Let me warn you upfront they're not easy to answer. After you're finished, we will spend some time discussing your ideas."

Here are the questions:

- What is leadership? Rough out a one- or two-sentence definition that captures its essence.
- Is leadership synonymous with management or is leading just one of many things managers do? In what ways are they different and how are they the same?
- Think of some individuals you feel are really exceptional leaders. What do they have in common?
- Think of some individuals who are truly lousy leaders. What do they have in common?
- How does leadership affect the performance of individuals, groups, and entire organizations?
- Have you ever known people who were successful leaders in one situation and failures in others? Why is this so?

Pause a few moments, take out a piece of paper, and answer these questions. It's far easier not to expend the effort and just press ahead. However, prior to being exposed to others' thinking about leadership, it's important to clarify your own. You might want to share your answers, and frustrations in composing them, with fellow students. One of the real benefits of this exercise is gaining an appreciation of how varied peoples' notions of leadership are. Save your responses to these questions. You might want to answer them again after completing this chapter.

CHAPTER PURPOSE

This chapter will help you gain an understanding of one of the most fundamental management concepts, leadership; the means by which things get done in organizations. A manager can formulate goals, strategize, interact with others, communicate, collect information, make decisions, plan, organize, monitor, and control; but nothing happens without leadership.

First, the concept "leadership" is defined. As the preceding "In Practice" case demonstrates, this is very difficult to get a firm grip on. Second, what scholars working in the field have learned about leadership is explored, addressing the most important conceptual frameworks and specific theories forwarded in the vast leadership literature. Third, an integrative model of leadership is developed, pulling together major perspectives forwarded in the literature. Fourth, several distinctive aspects of leading in health care organizations are addressed. Finally, suggestions for continually improving your leadership, knowledge, skills, and behaviors are forwarded.

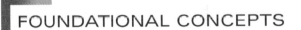

FOUNDATIONAL CONCEPTS

Can you imagine the following advertisement running in the "Help Wanted" section of *Modern Healthcare?*

A major nation-wide health care system undergoing rapid expansion in every region of the country is seeking applicants for executive positions at all levels.
LEADERSHIP ABILITIES ARE NOT REQUIRED
Send resume and salary history to:

Modern Healthcare
Box 554B
740 N. Rush Street
Chicago, IL 60611

Of course not!

Leadership is among the most valued management abilities. Health care organizations are presumed to thrive under great leadership and face difficulty, or even fail, when it's poor. Everyone is looking for leaders. People with good/exceptional leadership skills get hired and promoted. Those without the leadership "right stuff," no matter how good they are at performing other aspects of their jobs, face career stagnation or, worse, find themselves looking for a different position or a new line of work. Think for a moment about yourself. How would you like to be tagged as a nonleader or someone with no leadership potential? How would this affect your ability to get, or keep, a management position in a health care organization?

As important as leadership is, when asked to define and describe it, people have trouble. Perhaps you experienced difficulty when attempting to answer questions in the opening case. Leadership is an elusive concept. Here is a stripped-down definition, including only the essentials with which most scholars working in the field would have little disagreement:

Leadership is a process through which an individual attempts to intentionally influence human systems in order to accomplish a goal.

- *Leadership is a process.* It is a verb, an action word. Leadership manifests itself in the doing; it's a performing art.
- *Only individuals lead.* The locus of leadership is in a person. Inanimate objects don't lead, groups don't lead, organizations don't lead; only people do. When looking for leadership, our subject is an individual.
- *The focus of leadership is human systems*; typically called **followers**. The system might be an individual, members of a group, people in an organization, citizens of a community, or the population of a nation. Leadership can't exist without an interaction among someone who is leading and those who, for whatever reason, choose to follow.

- *Leadership is influencing.* This is leadership's "center of gravity." Who is influenced? . . . followers (people in systems). What is influenced? . . . their thoughts, feelings, and actions—the cognitive, affective, and behavioral targets of leadership.
- *The objective of leadership is goal accomplishment.* Leadership is instrumental; it's done for a purpose.
- *Leadership is intentional,* not accidental. All of us unknowingly influence others many times each day. These are not acts of leadership; they are just "happenings."

This definition of **leadership** is "method neutral." It incorporates a continuum of prescriptive and participative approaches. For example, on the prescriptive end of the spectrum, the leader: (1) recognizes the problem or opportunity, (2) defines it, (3) formulates a solution, and then (4) influences followers to accept it. The approach is leader-centric and emphasizes step 4, getting followers to accept the leader's solution/goal. Using a participative approach, the leader proceeds through the four-step recognizing, defining, formulation, and influence process *with* members of the system; it is follower-centric. The leader influences the *process* of problem solving and opportunity seizing with followers, not the just the outcome of it.

Leadership is exercised in many different places and a wide variety of situations. For example, you lead when attempting to persuade the person sitting next to you in accounting class to join you at the student center for lunch. Keep in mind, all of the key elements are here: you, the locus of leadership, a potential follower, and an act of intentional influence to accomplish a goal. However, the focus of this chapter is on a particular type of leadership, *that engaged in by managers in organizations.*

Organizations exist to accomplish tasks that are so large and/or complex they can't be undertaken by individuals and small groups. They do this by sequentially subdividing work. For example, the delivery of acute inpatient care in a community is a very large and complex task, which a hospital

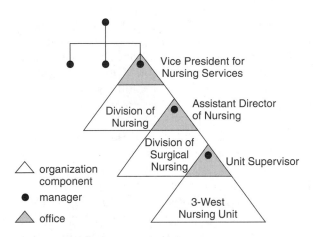

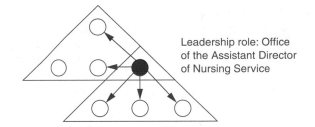

Figure 4.1. Organization Components and Managerial Offices

Figure 4.2. Multiple Directionality of the Manager's Leadership Role

"carves up." Nursing services does some of it, ancillary services does other parts, **professional** services does others, and so on. Work is parceled out to departments, divisions, programs/services, and units. In the process, the hospital creates a series of hierarchically layered components, all of which must be managed.

Figure 4.1 presents a schematic of one vertical slice in an organization composed of three hierarchically layered components. In each there is a **managerial office** and associated sets of expectations called **managerial roles**. Roles are constellations of things managers are expected to do because they hold the office (Katz & Kahn, 1966). They are attached to the office, not the person occupying it. Officeholders come and go, but roles (although not, necessarily, the way they are performed) remain the same. There are a wide variety of ways to describe the roles of a manager; several models were presented in Chapter 2. *The critical point is that leadership is one of many roles managers are expected to perform* because of the office they hold. Leadership and management are not the same thing; they aren't synonyms. This is a terribly important notion. Keep the concepts of *manager* (an individual who holds an office attached to which are multiple roles) and *leadership* (one of

these roles) straight. A lot of people don't, and it leads to considerable confusion. Execution of the **leadership role** (influencing) is how managers get things done. While leadership is not the only role of the manager, it is certainly the central one.

The terms *leadership* and *leader* will be used as a convenience. In doing so, what's meant is:

- *Leadership*—one role of the manager
- *Leader*—a manager performing the leadership role

Put Figure 4.1 under a magnifying glass and you have Figure 4.2. It focuses on one managerial office in the hospital's chain of command, an assistant director of nursing service. This manager is a subordinate in one component of the organization (the division of nursing service) reporting to a vice president, and a peer of assistant directors having the same reporting relationship. Simultaneously, this manager holds a superordinate office in the component for which he/she is responsible. Reporting to the assistant director are other managers (unit supervisors), each of whom is responsible for a different part of the surgical nursing division.

This illustration prompts several important points:

- Leadership is multidirectional. The assistant director leads not only subordinates but also peers and his superior. Only when we conceptualize leadership as intentional influence and when the proper distinction between managing and leadership is made does this become clear. For example, the assistant director of nursing intentionally influences or leads (but does not manage) her peers in chairing a departmental work group to implement a new scheduling system. She also leads her superior in providing direction prior to an upcoming budget review and negotiation session with the hospital's chief financial officer.

- Not only does the assistant director lead in all directions, he is simultaneously led from these same directions—from above by his superior, from the side by peers, and from below by subordinates. Leadership is an interactive "two-way street." The arrow of influence points in multiple directions simultaneously.

- Although leadership is multidirectional, the downward focus has received the greatest amount of attention. When one thinks of leadership, the first thing that comes to mind is the relationship between managers and their subordinates. Most leadership research (which will be reviewed in the next section) has this focus.

- Influencing upward is one of the least recognized and poorly understood areas of management. The literature has very little to say, and makes few recommendations, about this type of leadership.

- When one leads, irrespective of its direction, the focus is typically on individuals who hold managerial offices. For the most part, managers lead other managers.

- The extent to which leadership (attempts to influence) is successful depends on the amount of authority associated with a particular managerial office and power of the person holding it. The concepts of authority and power are addressed in Chapter 9.

LEADERSHIP PERSPECTIVES AND THEORIES

The vast majority of leadership thinking, theorizing, and research can be classified into five perspectives (often called "schools"): trait, skills, behavioral/style, contingency, and transformational. They are described in the sections that follow. This is not a complete and exhaustive review of the literature. Limitations of space prohibit a full exploration of the nuances of different models comprising each perspective, review of empirical results supporting and questioning their validity, and discussion of their strengths/weaknesses. If you are interested in comprehensive and very readable treatments, consider *Leadership: Theory and Practice* by Peter Northouse (Sage Publications, 2004), and *Leadership in Organizations,* 4th edition, by G. A. Yukl (Prentice-Hall, 1998). The objective is to provide you with a brief and introductory tour of the terrain; key original-source references are included if you wish to dig deeper. The basic work on these perspectives focuses on leadership in general, not its execution in particular types of organizations (such as health care).

Keep in mind that scholars are interested in understanding leadership and the factors that effect it. However, the ideas, rules of thumb, principles, models, and tools that can be employed to improve leadership practice are generally (and should be) grounded on this understanding.

Trait Perspective

Because individuals lead, it's natural and reasonable to look at them and their characteristics. The question posed by the **trait perspective** is: What attributes separate successful from unsuccessful leaders and effective from ineffective leadership? People have been looking at the characteristics of "great men" for centuries; scholarship employing this perspective has spanned the entire twentieth century.

Early work focused almost exclusively on military commanders and those holding political office. In the late 1930s psychologists became interested in the relationship between individual characteristics and leadership effectiveness in organizations. Even though critiques of this work in the 1940s suggested that such relationships were weak and not able to be generalized across different situations, the hunt continued.

⚜ DEBATE TIME 4.1   What Matters Most: Nurture, Nature, or Circumstances?

At this point you should have a fairly clear idea of what leadership is and what it's not, in addition to possessing a good feel for the organizational context in which the leadership role is performed. All managers are not equally effective or successful leaders. The question is: What factors explain the variability? There has been a raging debate regarding this issue in the literature over the last 70 years. Here are three different points of view. What's yours?

The Nature Argument

Variability in leadership effectiveness and success is due to traits and dispositions that individuals are endowed with at birth or develop very early in life. By the time a person assumes a management position, these characteristics are set and nearly impossible to change in any significant way. Some people have traits that predispose them to be successful leaders; others don't.

The Nurture Argument

Variability in leadership effectiveness and success is due to abilities, skills, and behaviors that managers can learn. Personal traits/dispositions provide an important foundation, but leaders make themselves, they are not made.

The Circumstances Argument

Differences in leadership effectiveness and success are due to the characteristics of the circumstances in which managers find themselves. Sets of traits and skills/behaviors are important, but their value is context-specific. In one context certain traits, abilities, and behaviors may predispose a manager to be an effective leader; in a different one, the result could be ineffectiveness and failure.

- If you agree with the nature argument, which personal traits and dispositions are most associated with leadership effectiveness and success?
- If you agree with the nurture argument, which abilities and behaviors are most important?
- If you agree with the circumstances argument, which aspects of context are most critical?
- Think back for a moment to the opening case. Let's say that each board member has a different opinion of what matters most. What would be the consequences?
- People often espouse a circumstances argument. However, their actual "theory in use" is generally a blend of the nature and nurture arguments. Do you find this to be the case, and if so, why?

Thousands of studies have examined every imaginable attribute: physical, psychological, and sociodemographic. Major reviews and meta-analyses of the trait literature have been undertaken by Stogdill (1948, 1974), Mann (1959), and Lord, de Vader, and Alliger (1986). These studies have identified a few characteristic clusters that are present in leaders, as compared to followers, and effective, as contrasted to ineffective, leaders. They are:

- *Intelligence*—general perceptual, conceptual, and problem-solving ability
- *Articulateness*—ability to express ideas clearly and powerfully

- *Confidence*—self-esteem and belief in one's competencies/capacities

- *Initiative and persistence*—desire to take on a task and complete it

- *Sociability*—inclination and ability to develop a rich web of interpersonal relationships

Counter to experience, logic, and common sense, it is hard to argue that individual traits have no effect whatsoever. However, scholars began to appreciate that while traits had an impact, they did so not as originally imagined. First, traits are best thought of as predispositions. A particular trait, or set of them, tend to predispose (although not cause) an individual to develop skills and engage behaviors that influence leadership effectiveness. Second, multiple traits are associated with a given set of skills/behaviors. Third, it is one's behavior, and not traits per se that is most related to leadership effectiveness and success. As Van Vleet and Yukl (1989) note, "What seems to be most important is not traits but rather how they are expressed in the behavior of the leader."

Skills Perspective

Traits and skills overlap. For example, is articulateness a trait (inherent attribute of a person) or skill (something that can be acquired/developed)?

The contemporary development of the **skills perspective** can be traced to an article by Katz (1955) in *Harvard Business Review* suggesting that effective leadership is based upon possessing/developing three core skills:

- *Technical*—proficiencies regarding the work of the organization that produces products/services and serves customers (influence over things)

- *Conceptual*—proficiencies dealing with identifying, defining, and manipulating abstractions (influence over ideas)

- *Human*—proficiencies regarding interacting and working with others (influence over/with people)

Katz held that the importance of these skills varied across organizational level as follows:

	Technical	Conceptual	Human
Top management	low	high	high
Mid-level management	moderate	moderate	high
Production-level management	high	low	high

More recently, Mumford and colleagues (2000) developed a skills-oriented leadership model based on research employing a sample of 1,800 military officers. A simplified representation is depicted in Figure 4.3.

Individual **attributes** (cognitive, motivational, and personality) predispose and facilitate a manager developing specific skills that result in effective leadership behaviors. The skills identified by Mumford overlap with those of Katz:

- *Problem solving*—the ability to identify, understand, specify, and solve ill-defined organizational problems

- *Social judgment*—the ability to understand people and how they interact in social systems

- *Knowledge*—the ability to accumulate information and organize it into coherent mental models/maps

These abilities can be acquired/developed through education, training, experience, and coaching.

This perspective, of which Katz (1995) and Mumford and colleagues (2000) are an example, has been criticized because it focuses more on general management, rather than strictly (and more narrowly defined) leadership skills.

Behavioral/Style Perspective

Work undertaken from this perspective has focused on: identifying dimensions that can be employed to describe/categorize specific leadership behaviors, developing models of **leadership style** (a combination of behaviors), and examining how different styles are related to leadership effectiveness. Scholars were looking for the one best way (behaviors or combinations of them) to lead.

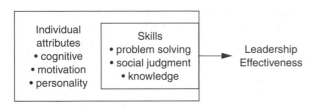

Figure 4.3. Simplified Leadership Skills Model

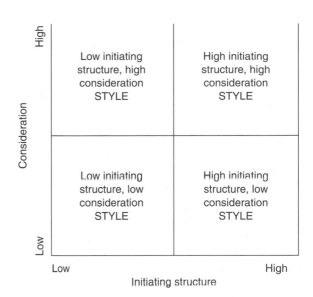

Figure 4.4. The Ohio State Leadership Behaviors and Styles

One of the first behavioral-focused leadership studies was conducted by Lewin, Lippitt, and colleagues (1939) at the University of Iowa. They compared three styles of leadership—autocratic, democratic, and laissez-faire—in groups. Designated leaders were confederates of the researchers and instructed on how to perform the various styles. Democratic leaders coordinated activities of the group and facilitated majority-rule decision making on important decisions; autocratic leaders directed the activities of the group and made important decisions absent input from members; laissez-faire leaders (who accidentally emerged during the course of the study) provided neither facilitation nor direction. This work was significant because it focused on behavior rather than traits, identified and described different leadership styles, and found that variations in style had an impact on followers.

Several major behavioral/style leadership studies were undertaken immediately after the conclusion of World War II. One of the most widely cited was conducted by investigators at the Ohio State University (Stodgill & Coons, 1957). Two dimensions of leader behavior were identified: **initiating structure**, the degree a manager defines and organizes the work that is to be done and the extent attention is focused on accomplishing objectives established by the manager; and **consideration**, the extent a manager exhibits concern for welfare of the group and its members, stresses the importance of job satisfaction, expresses appreciation, and seeks input from subordinates on major decisions. Initiating structure and consideration were not con-

ceptualized as opposite ends of the same continuum, but rather as separate dimensions. A manager's behavior could range from high to low on both. As depicted in Figure 4.4, the two dimensions combine to form four leadership styles. Researchers hypothesized that group performance is maximized when a manager has a leadership style high on both consideration and initiating structure; research results do not support this assertion (Fleishman, 1973; Korman, 1966).

Likert (1961) and colleagues at the University of Michigan identified two leadership behaviors: job-centered and employee-centered. They were defined similar to consideration and initiating structure in the Ohio studies. Initially these two behaviors were depicted as opposite ends of the same continuum; later work reconceptualized them as two independent dimensions.

Throughout the 1950s and 1960s a large number of studies were conducted to investigate the relationship of specific behaviors/styles (using both the Ohio and Michigan models) on follower/group satisfaction and performance. Results were contradictory, weak, and inconclusive (Yukl, 1998). As with the trait research, it appeared that other factors were confounding results.

While the Ohio and Michigan studies provided theoretical underpinnings for the **behavioral perspective**, several other works are frequently referenced in most reviews of this literature. Blake and Mouton (1978), for example, drew upon previous research and formulated the Managerial Grid, popularized in their book of the same name. The model, originally developed as a consulting tool, was extensively employed in leadership development programs during the 1960s and 1970s. The grid has two dimensions: production orientation and people orientation. Using a production orientation, behaviors are directive and focused on accomplishing assigned objectives and tasks. Employing a people orientation, behavior focuses on enhancing the quality of manager-follower and follower-follower interactions. A leader's behavior can range from low to high on both dimensions, resulting in five different styles:

- *High production and low people orientation:* Leadership behavior focuses exclusively on goal and task accomplishment, and maximizes productivity through explicit direction and tight control.

- *High production and high people orientation:* Leadership behavior is goal and task centered but seeks a high degree of follower involvement.

- *Low production and high people orientation:* Leadership behavior focuses on creating fulfilling relationships even if goal and task accomplishment suffer.

- *Low production and low people orientation:* Leadership behavior focuses on neither goal and task accomplishment nor on fulfilling the needs of followers; minimal energy is expended on execution of the leadership role.

- *Moderate production and moderate people orientation:* Leadership behavior balances goal/task accomplishment and follower need fulfillment.

Blake and Mouton (1982) contend that the high production- and high people-oriented style is most effective and results in the best outcomes (group productivity and satisfaction) irrespective of the situation. Little research supports the assertion, but there is some evidence that this style is preferred by managers and perceived by them to be most effective (Yukl, 2006).

Contingency Perspective

In the early 1960s, it became increasingly apparent that variations in leadership effectiveness and success could not be adequately explained by either traits, skills, or behaviors. Attention turned to incorporating situational characteristics, or contingencies, into leadership models.

An initial contingency model was presented by Tannenbaum and Schmidt (1973), which portrayed leadership behavior as a continuum that ranged from manager-centered to follower-centered. In the manager-centered style, considerable authority is exercised, and followers have little opportunity to participate in making decisions affecting them; leadership behavior is directive. In the follower-centered style, the manager exercises a minimum amount of authority, and followers have considerable freedom to set their own goals and determine how tasks should be executed; leadership behavior is participative. Tannenbaum and Schmidt, contrary to previous models, conceptualized behaviors as bipolar. One was either manager-centered, follower-centered, or somewhere in between. The authors explicitly stated there was no one style equally effective in all situations. Additionally, they noted that the effectiveness of a particular style depended upon three factors: characteristics of the leader, followers, and the situation in which leaders and followers interact. This model underscored that leadership effectiveness depended on contingencies and suggested some categories of them. However, the model did not indicate how such contingencies affect the selection of a particular leadership style.

A number of contingency models have been developed and four of them are presented here: leadership match, path-goal, leadership effectiveness/ adaptability (LEAD), and attribution theory. This selection is made because the leadership match and path-goal models have been the subject of considerable empirical research, and the LEAD model has been widely employed as a teaching and leadership development tool. This section concludes with a discussion of attribution theory, which deals with the manager, herself, as a contingency.

Leadership Match Model

The first comprehensive contingency theory of leadership was developed by Fred Fiedler (Fiedler, 1967; Fiedler & Chemers, 1974; Fiedler, Chemers, & Mahar, 1976). The underlying notion is that managers are unable to alter their style to any appreciable degree. Leadership effectiveness depends not on fitting one's style to the situation but rather on selecting a situation that is conducive to one's style.

Based on behavioral studies (Ohio and Michigan), two leadership styles were specified: task-oriented and employee-oriented. Fiedler developed a unique and controversial way to measure them. After completing a 20-item questionnaire, a person was assigned a least preferred coworker (LPC) score. The score reflected the degree of regard a respondent held for the coworker he preferred least. Managers with low LPC scores (disregard for the least preferred worker) were classified as having a task-oriented leadership style. Managers with a high LPC score (favorable evaluations of the coworker they least preferred) were classified as possessing an employee-oriented style.

Fiedler (1967) identified three situational factors: the manager-follower relationship, which could be good or poor; task structure, which could be either high or low; and manager position power, ranging from strong to weak. The combined effect of these three factors produce situations that are favorable, moderately favorable, or unfavorable to the manager.

Based upon studies conducted with hundreds of groups in a variety of organizations, it was determined that managers with a task-oriented leadership style were most effective in situations that were either favorable or unfavorable. Managers with an employee-oriented leadership style did better in situations that were moderately favorable. There have been a number of criticisms of this work, including questions regarding the validity of the LPC questionnaire and concerns that situational factors and leadership style may not be independent of one another (Nebeker, 1975; Stinson & Tracy, 1974).

Path-Goal Model

The path-goal model is based on the expectancy theory of motivation discussed in Chapter 3 (Porter & Lawler, 1968; Vroom, 1964). Expectancy theory is interested in why someone is motivated to do one thing rather than another. The emphasis is on effort, performance, rewards, motivation, and the relationships between them (**expectancies**, **instrumentalities**, and **valences**). *Expectancies* refer to the belief that a given level of effort will result in a particular level of performance; *instrumentality* is the relationships of various outcomes resulting from that effort; and *valence* refers to the individual's preference. While the expectancy theory of motivation describes such relationships, the path-goal model of leadership focuses on factors that affect them. Initial formulation of this model was developed by Evans (1970a, 1970b) in the early 1970s and then refined by House (1971) and House and Mitchell (1974). It has undergone constant revision over the years.

The path-goal model conceives the manager exercising influence to increase the motivation of a follower attempting to accomplish a specific goal, in a

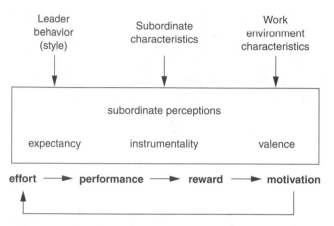

Figure 4.5. Path-Goal Model

particular context, during a finite period of time. As depicted in Figure 4.5, a follower's level of motivation is a result of her perceptions of expectancies, instrumentalities, and valences. The term *expectancies* refers to the belief that a particular level of effort will result in a particular level of performance. *Instrumentality* refers to the relationship of various outcomes resulting from that effort, and *valence* refers to the individual's preference. Such perceptions are affected by three sets of contingencies: leadership behavior or style, features of the work environment, and characteristics of the follower.

In most leadership situations, follower characteristics and features of the work environment are not under the direct control of the manager; in the short run, they are fixed. Follower characteristics include such things as: needs and motives (e.g., the degree to which achievement, power, and affiliation are important to the person); ability (knowledge, skills, and experience) to perform the task; and the extent to which individuals feel they have control over critical contingencies affecting their performance. Features of the work environment include such things as: the extent to which the task is structured or unstructured; the amount of time available to complete the task; the nature and degree of interdependence

among work group members; and a host of organizational characteristics.

The contingency most under a manager's control is her own leadership style. The dimensions that define leadership style are conceptualized as: instrumental behavior (defining objectives and specifying the task to be performed); supportive behavior (providing support to, and fulfilling needs of, followers); participative behavior (seeking followers' input on decisions that affect them); and achievement-oriented behavior (establishing goals and setting expectations that challenge followers).

Given the number of contingencies and the numerous ways in which they can interact with one another, empirical tests have focused only on pieces of the model, and like most leadership research, the results have been conflicting (Schreisheim & von Glinow, 1977). Additionally, because of its complexity, the model is difficult to employ in real-life situations. However, several general observations and suggestions can be forwarded (House & Baetz, 1979).

- One of the most important aspects of leadership behavior is motivation—stimulating the release of, and focusing, follower effort.

- Often the connection between effort, performance, and rewards is unclear to followers. The manager must do everything possible to make these relationships explicit.

- In leading, the manager should appreciate that individuals' valences are heterogeneous; people value various rewards differently. The manager should understand what a follower values and construct rewards accordingly.

- Leadership behavior should help followers define expectancies. Questions that need to be addressed include: How should a follower direct her effort so that it results in high levels of performance? What additional knowledge, skills, and experiences does a follower need to perform assigned tasks?

- Leadership behavior should focus on clarifying instrumentalities. It is important that followers understand the specific type and amount of reward that will flow from a given level of performance.

- The manager should be mindful of how work environment characteristics affect follower expectations, instrumentalities, and valences and the implications of them on the selection of a leadership style. For example, when a task is very unstructured, a follower may not know how to perform the job successfully (e.g., instrumentality is low). In such instances, a higher level of instrumental leadership behavior may be required.

LEAD Model

The LEAD model was developed by Hersey and Blanchard (1977) while they were affiliated with the Center for Leadership Studies at Ohio University. Differing degrees of task- and relationship-oriented behavior (defined in a way similar to the Ohio State, Michigan, and Blake and Mouton studies) produce four different leadership styles: style 1, high task and low relationship; style 2, high task and high relationship; style 3, low task and high relationship; and style 4, low task and low relationship.

Hersey and Blanchard (1977) argued that the single most important contingency in selecting an effective leadership style is follower task-relevant maturity. Maturity is a function of: motivation, having energy and being willing to expend it in order to accomplish the assigned task; responsibility and willingness to plan, organize, and complete the task; and competence, possessing the necessary knowledge, skills, or experience to perform the task proficiently. A mature follower is highly motivated, willing, and able to assume responsibility and possesses the necessary competencies. An immature follower lacks motivation, is not willing to assume responsibility for the task, and doesn't have the necessary competencies. Maturity is situational and task-specific; a follower may be very mature in one situation and immature in another.

Below are two extreme examples of styles that are most effective with followers having varying degrees of task-relevant maturity (Hersey & Blanchard, 1977).

- If the maturity of the follower is very low, the model suggests using a style that is high task and low relationship oriented (style 1). The follower is unmotivated, not willing or able to assume responsibility, and doesn't possess the competencies necessary to perform the task. Therefore, if the task is to get done, leadership must be very directive. A low degree of **relationship-oriented behavior** is recommended so the follower's immaturity is not reinforced.

- If the maturity of the follower is exceedingly high, the model suggests using leadership style 4; a low task and low relationship-oriented behavior. Here the follower is extremely motivated, is very responsible, and possesses all the competencies necessary to perform the task. The follower does not need and, in fact, would likely not appreciate task directiveness; he knows what to do and how to do it. High relationship-oriented behavior is not needed because followers get reinforcement from each other and performance of the task itself. In this case, task and relationship responsibilities are delegated to followers.

This is a highly abbreviated and simplified description of a model that has many more features than can be discussed here. For example, the authors provide a dynamic interpretation that focuses on sequences of leadership behaviors needed to enhance **follower maturity.** They have designed a package of questionnaires that provide feedback regarding: the extent to which individuals perceive themselves employing the four different leadership styles; how others (subordinates, peers, superiors) perceive a manager's leadership style; and how one's selection of different leadership behaviors aligns with the most appropriate style suggested by the model given the maturity of followers in a series of cases.

The conceptualization of follower maturity has been criticized as being unclear, particularly how the factors of motivation, responsibility, and competence combine to produce a unified measure

(Graeff, 1997; Yukl, 2006) and how the maturity of a group can be assessed. There have been only a few published studies conducted to confirm the linkage between follower maturity, execution of the "appropriate" style as suggested by the model, and leader effectiveness (Grief, 1983, 1997). However, managers and students alike find the model simple to use, practical, and intuitively appealing.

Attribution Theory

One important leadership contingency factor is a manager's own frame of reference. Attribution (sometimes referred to as perceptual or cognitive) theory holds that a manager's selection of a leadership style depends on the way follower behavior is perceived and interpreted (Mitchell, Green, & Wood, 1981). Managers notice some things and are unaware of others. Furthermore, what's noticed is always filtered through the manager's unique cognitive frame and reshaped by it. Based on these perceptions, a manager's attributes cause the follower's behavior. There are two general types of attributions: internal (e.g., lack of follower effort or ability) and external (e.g., bad luck, inadequate task design by others, poor supervision).

A manager's choice of leadership behavior is significantly influenced by such attributions (Shaver, 1983). For example, a manager might employ one leadership style if he attributes a follower's poor performance to task overload and use a different one if he feels the cause is laziness. Attribution theorists argue that, in many cases, a manager's choice of leadership style might be due more to his perceptual and cognitive frame than the "reality" of the situation itself; indeed, reality is only what one perceives it to be. The basic notion of attribution theory is a simple one. An important determinant of leadership style is one's perceptions and attributions (Lord, Soto, & de Vader, 1984). The resulting admonition is that managers need to be aware of these inherent biases and develop ways to minimize them.

Contingency Perspective: Selected Implications

Noted below are several implications that transcend the specific models of leadership described in this section.

- The **contingency perspective** helps us appreciate that leadership effectiveness and success depends upon the circumstances. Leadership behaviors and styles focus on influencing specific followers (be they individuals or a group) in a specific context, performing a specific task in order to accomplish a specific objective at a particular point in time. All of these things—contingencies—vary from one circumstance to another. The most effective leadership style in one situation is unlikely to be the most effective in another.

- Leadership behaviors are best described along two dimensions: initiating/tasks and consideration/relationship. These behavioral dimensions combine to produce four leadership styles: high task, low relationship; high task, high relationship; low task, high relationship; and low task, low relationship.

- Three sets of contingencies seem to be most closely related to leadership effectiveness or success:
  - Characteristics of the manager such as his/her traits, skills, knowledge, and experience
  - Characteristics of followers such as their traits, skills, knowledge, experience, working relationships, and level of maturity
  - Characteristics of the situation such as goal clarity, nature of problem/opportunity, and amount of time available

- Leadership effectiveness depends, more than anything else, on a manager: having a broad repertoire of styles and being able to flexibly move among them; possessing the ability to diagnose the most critical contingencies of a given situation; being able to select an effective leadership style for that situation; and possessing the skills and ability to execute the chosen style well.

- The way in which a specific leadership situation is diagnosed depends, in no small measure, on the manager's perceptions and attribution of causes to follower behavior.

- Much of leadership behavior has to do with stimulating, and then focusing, follower motivation.

- Taken to the extreme, contingency-driven leadership—behaving differently toward the same followers in different situations or differently toward various followers in the same situation—may appear erratic and arbitrary. This can be confusing and frustrating for followers unless managers are very explicit about how they are behaving and why.

Transformational Perspective

James McGregor Burns, in his classic work *Leadership* (1978), identified two types of politicians: transactional and transformational. There is a growing body of literature that draws a distinction between these leadership styles in organizations (Tishy & Devanna, 1986). Whereas **transactional leadership** attempts to preserve and work within the constraints of the status quo, the **transformational perspectives** style seeks to upset and replace it.

For the most part, the models of leader behavior that have been examined so far view managers as involved in exchange relationships with followers, the defining characteristic of which is: "I'll provide what you want, if you'll give me what I (or the organization) want." Transactional leadership entails recognizing what followers desire and giving it to them, if their performance warrants. "In these exchanges transactional leaders clarify the roles followers must play and the task requirements followers must complete in order to reach their personal goals while fulfilling the mission of the organization" (Kuhnert & Lewis, 1987). You'll note this sounds very much like the path-goal model of leadership where the manager attempts to influence follower expectancies, instrumentalities, and valences. The objective of leadership is to get followers to comply with the rules of the game as it is currently being played. The result of such transactions, contend proponents of the theory, is ordinary levels of performance (Liden & Dienesch, 1986). Performance improvements, if they occur at all, are marginal and achieved incrementally over a long period of time. Transformational leaders, on the other hand, are more concerned with changes than exchanges. Seeking to alter both the objective and relationships, followers are motivated to take on difficult goals they normally would not have pursued and accept the notion that work is far more than the performance of specific duties for specific rewards. The relationship between the manager and followers is not contractual, but empowering. Advocates of the transformational perspective suggest it produces extraordinary levels of performance that flow from enrollment in a cause rather than compliance with the rules (Bass, 1985).

Transactional and transformational leadership differ across a number of dimensions:

Dimension	*Transactional*	*Transformational*
Goal	Maintain the status quo	Upset the status quo
Activity	Play within the rules	Change the rules
Locus of rewards	Self (maximize personal benefits)	System (optimize systemic benefits)
Nature of incentives	Tit for tat	The greater good
Manager-follower interactions	Mutual dependence	Interdependence
Needs fulfilled	Lower level (physical, economic, and safety)	Higher level (social and self-actualization)
Performance	Ordinary	Extraordinary

Presently, the transformational approach to leadership is a rough framework. Foundational concepts have not been rigorously defined, a comprehensive model has not been developed, and there is virtually no empirical research supporting its primary assertions.

PULLING IT ALL TOGETHER

A century of theorizing and research has identified a number of factors that are related to leadership effectiveness and success. Figure 4.6 provides a summary of these findings. Because the key concepts have been covered in previous sections, the model should be relatively self-explanatory.

Leadership style is a pattern of behavior through which a manager attempts to intentionally influence a system (e.g., individual, group, organization, community, nation) in order to accomplish a goal. Leadership style is defined by three behavioral dimensions.

- *Focus* is the direction of a manager's influence attempts. External leadership focuses outside the boundary of the organizational component for which the manager is responsible (toward superiors or peers). Internal leadership is directed downward toward subordinates.

- *Objective* is what a manager hopes to accomplish in exercising influence. Transformational leadership seeks to alter both the nature of goals sought and manager-follower interactions; the objective is to transcend the status quo. Transactional leadership attempts to optimize the outcome of manager-follower exchange relationships by achieving stated goals in an efficient manner within the "rules" as presently defined.

- *Approach* is the way in which a manager influences followers. In exercising directive (initiating structure, job-centered) leadership, a manager defines the task and specifies how it is to be performed. The focus is on goal accomplishment, and little attention is paid to manager-follower or

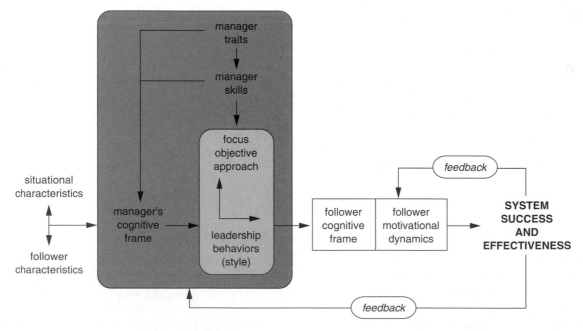

Figure 4.6. Integrated Leadership Model

follower-follower relationships. In exercising facilitative (consideration, employee-centered) leadership, a manager involves followers in making decisions that affect them and pays considerable attention to fulfilling their needs.

A manager's behavior can vary between "high" and "low" on each of these dimensions, the specific combination of which defines a leadership style.

Selection of a leadership style is influenced by two sets of factors: the manager's traits and skills in addition to follower and situation characteristics. These are filtered through the manager's distinctive cognitive frame. The manager's leadership style affects the motivational dynamics (expectancies, instrumentalities, and valences) of followers mediated by their own cognitive frame. The outcomes of leadership attempts include follower efficiency, effectiveness, creativity, and satisfaction. The feedback loops depicted can be either positive (reinforcing a given characteristic) or negative (dampening or extinguishing it).

All models leave out more than they include in addition to overly simplifying complex relationships and dynamics. This one is no exception. The model is admittedly crude and incomplete; but, hopefully, it will stimulate you to continue thinking about how pieces of the leadership "jigsaw puzzle" fit together.

SEVERAL DISTINCTIVE ASPECTS OF LEADERSHIP IN HEALTH CARE ORGANIZATIONS

There are many distinctive aspects of leadership in health care organizations; only two of them are addressed here, professionalism and gender. First, health care organizations are populated by professionals who either perform or directly supervise most of the "real work" done in them. Professionals control the organization's core input, transformation, and output processes. Second, managerial po-

sitions in health care organizations, at all levels, are being increasingly filled by women.

Leading Clinical Professionals

Professionals, because of the complexity and importance of the work they perform, are granted high levels of autonomy regarding what they do and how they do it. Different occupations have varying degrees of autonomy, and hence, possess differing degrees of professionalism. The epitome in health care organizations are physicians. They will be focused on here as a prototypical example, although the notions forwarded can be applied to other clinical professionals such as nurses and pharmacists.

Entertain the notion that physicians possess a distinctly different mentality, cognitive frame, or paradigm than do managers. This mentality, of course, is not "hard wired." Rather, it is mental operating system software programmed through a long/intensive education and socialization process. The programming begins in medical school, continues through residency training, and is reinforced every day by the nature of the work physicians do. Noted below are several critical aspects of this clinical mentality as contrasted to the **managerial mentality** (adapted from Freidson, 1972).

Dimension	Managerial Mentality	Clinical Mentality
Primary allegiance	To the organization	To individual clients
Responsibility	Shared	Personal
Authority relationships	Hierarchical (vertical)	Collegial (horizontal)
Time frame	Long/future	Short/present
Feedback	Delayed and vague	Immediate and concrete
Tolerance for ambiguity	High	Low

In general, the primary allegiance of physicians is to their individual patients for whom they bear personal responsibility. They prefer, and are accustomed to, working in collegial-type relationships where power is symmetrical rather than in those where it flows primarily from the organizational office held. In the practice of medicine, authority relationships are collegial (horizontal and peer-to-peer) rather than hierarchical (vertical and superior-to-subordinate). Dealing with courses of illness that are generally time limited, physicians are trained to focus on the short run; the feedback they receive regarding their performance is generally immediate and concrete (i.e., the patient either improves or gets worse, lives or dies) and their tolerance for ambiguity and uncertainty is quite low. Managers, on the other hand, owe their allegiance to the organization rather than to particular individuals or groups. Because of the high degree of interdependence necessary for accomplishing organizational tasks, accountability is generally diffused or shared, and the power they exercise is defined primarily by the office held. Managerial time frames are long (it takes forever to accomplish anything significant) and feedback is typically delayed and vague. As a consequence, managers have a high tolerance for ambiguity and uncertainty. This is a highly stylized and exaggerated characterization, to be sure.

Two of the most frustrating and vexing aspects of leadership is when one's behavior is misinterpreted by followers and they don't respond as you expected. When the follower is a physician, the notion of **clinical mentality** helps explain why. Refer back to the integrative model of leadership (Figure 4.6). The cognitive frames of managers and physicians are quite different. There are several important implications.

- First, physicians are likely to perceive and interpret a manager's leadership behavior in idiosyncratic ways and quite different than what might be expected or wanted. Remember, the impact registered on physicians comes not from what you intend, or even your behavior, but rather it's a result of what they perceive and the attributions they make.
- Second, physicians have distinctive motivational dynamics. Their expectancies, instrumentalities, and valences differ considerably from those of

managers. Remember, to motivate physicians (influencing to release and focus energy) you have to do so on their terms, not your own.

- Third, managers, because of their mentality and distinctive cognitive frame, are prone to misinterpreting the intentions or behaviors of physicians and attributing negative cause to them (such as not acting in the best interest of the organization). "I just can't understand why Dr. _____ did that." What this generally means is the physician acted differently than the manager would have in that situation. The retort is: "Why would you expect otherwise?" Remember to interpret and attribute the causes of physician behavior from the perspective of their mentality before attempting to understand it from your own.

Most of the work in this area suggests that a style high in consideration, relationship orientation, and participation should be employed in leading professionals (Benveniste, 1987; Raelin, 1986; Shapiro, 1985). The degree of task orientation would depend on the task-relevant maturity of the professional or professional group in that particular situation. If they understand the goal to be achieved, accept and are motivated to undertake it, and possess the competencies to do so (i.e., high maturity), **task-orientated leader behavior** should be low. When this is not the case, a greater degree of directness is warranted. It's important to reiterate that professional task-relevant maturity is situational. A professional might be very mature in one situation (e.g., doing his/her professional work) and quite immature in another (e.g., working on a hospital committee to form an independent practice association).

Leadership and Gender

While issues related to gender and leadership are not unique to health care organizations, they are very important. Females comprise approximately 60% of students in health administration graduate programs and women are occupying senior executive positions in increasing numbers.

MANAGERIAL 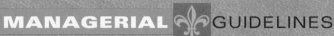 GUIDELINES

1. Identify and work with a mentor during the early stages of your career. Leadership is a performing art; becoming proficient requires coaching from an experienced practitioner who is invested in your development. A growing body of evidence suggests that having an effective mentoring relationship is one of the most important things separating successful from unsuccessful leaders. If you would like to read more about how to work with a mentor, consider *The Mentor Quest: Practical Ways to Find the Guidance You Need* by Betty Southard (Vine Books, 2002).

2. Become a reflective practitioner of leadership. This is the key to really learning from experience. Just as winning sports teams review their game films, so should managers. Get in the habit of replaying and analyzing the leadership situations in which you have been involved sometime before each day ends. It's important you look at both successes and failures. What happened (replay the game film in your mind)? Were the results what you wanted and anticipated? If so, why? If not, why not? What could/should you have done differently? What lessons have you learned from this experience? Such reflection requires considerable discipline; the effort, however, will pay handsome dividends.

3. Seek to better understand yourself. All accomplished artists have a very refined and rich feel for their tools. The primary (some would say, only) tool of leadership is the self. One particularly efficient way to gain enhanced self-understanding is through feedback provided by self-administered questionnaires, instruments, and invento-

ries. There are a lot of different ones available; seek the advice of a faculty member who teaches organization behavior regarding those that may be most helpful.

4. Seek feedback from followers. Rest assured that your intentions and leadership behavior will be perceived by followers in idiosyncratic ways. Our perceptions of self are always somewhat at odds with how others perceive us. To be an effective and successful leader, you must understand those with whom you work (above, sideways, and below). The best way to gain this understanding is by asking and by doing so continually. Some good questions are: How am I coming across? What am I doing that helps you to be as effective, creative, and satisfied as possible? What types of things am I doing that create roadblocks and sap your energy or enthusiasm?

5. It's virtually impossible to lead effectively if you don't have an in-depth understanding of who is following. Invest time and energy in getting to know each follower upon whom your effectiveness and success depends. What are their aspirations? What are their needs and desires? What do they view as their most important competencies (knowledge, skills, experiences) and how could the organization make better use of them? What motivates them?

6. Keep reading and studying. Experience is the single best teacher of leadership. However, there are not enough hours in the day, days in the year, or years in life to acquire all the experience you need. Some of it has to be gained vicariously, and the best vicarious teacher is reading.

The concepts sex and gender are not synonymous. Sex is genetically set as are associated physiological, anatomical, and hormonal differences. **Gender** refers to attributions attached to members of the same sex that are psychologically, socially, and culturally influenced.

Several meta-analyses of gender-focused leadership studies have identified the following consistent results (Dreher & Cox, 1996; Eagly & Johnson, 1990; Eagly & Wood, 1995; Eagly & Karau, S. J. and Makhijani, M. G. 1995):

- Females and males have the same level of motivation to assume leadership roles in organizations.

- The leadership behaviors and style repertoires of males and females are similar; however, women tend to use high relationship-oriented styles more than men.

- Gender is a poor predictor of leadership success and effectiveness.

- The previous finding aside, females are perceived to be less effective than males when two conditions are present: when the setting is male-dominated (particularly the military) and when a high percentage of subordinates are male.

- Individuals who ranked higher in male role orientation (describing themselves as having more masculine characteristics) are perceived to be better leaders than those with feminine, androgynous, or undifferentiated gender roles.

- Women's perceived leadership effectiveness increases as they move up the hierarchy in organizations.

- Female leaders are evaluated differently than males; females and males were assessed equally favorably when they used a democratic, relationship-oriented leadership style; females were evaluated less favorably when they employed an autocratic task-oriented style.

- Women have better developed social skills than men and tend to prefer collaborative, or web-leadership, styles.

Overall, there appears to be a stereotypical view of women as less effective leaders than men. I underscore this is a stereotypical perception, because there is no evidence supporting it. There is a gender gap in leadership, and it seems to be the result of a gender bias on the part of both women and men. The traditional solution is to close this gap by assimilation—helping women managers to think and act more like men. Many management educational and training programs, reinforced by organizational culture, implicitly embrace this approach. But, assimilation may be counterproductive. Irrespective of the trait focused upon (gender, race, ethnicity, sexual orientation), assimilation results in a reduction of diversity at a time when it is needed most in health care organizations. Managerial and leadership heterogeneity is essential for finding different ways to solve new problems and seize emerging opportunities in times of revolutionary change.

The Manager's Essential Leadership Bookshelf

Thousands of books on leadership and hundreds of new ones are published every year; all forward their own recipes for effectiveness and success. No one has the time, energy, patience, or money to consume even a small proportion of what is being written. Here are some favorites; a handful of books that are sound, interesting, challenging, and useful. Although there are clearly many others that warrant inclusion, these (listed in alphabetical order by author's last name) are recommended without reservation. Notice that the copyright dates span more than a decade; but these books have faired well with the test of time.

- Bennis, W. (1989). *Why leaders can't lead: The unconscious conspiracy continues.* San Francisco: Jossey-Bass.

- Covey, S. (1990). *Principle-centered leadership.* New York: Simon and Schuster.

- Gardner, J. (1990). *On leadership.* New York: The Free Press.
- Hessesbein, F., Goldsmith, M., & Beckhard, R. (1996). *The leader of the future: New visions, strategies, and practices for the next era.* San Francisco: Jossey-Bass.
- Kelley, R. E. (1991). *The power of followership: How to create leaders people want to follow and followers who lead themselves.* New York: Doubleday/Currency.
- Kouzes, J. M., & Posner, B. Z. (1993). *Credibility: How leaders gain and lose it, why people demand it.* San Francisco: Jossey-Bass.
- Kouzes, J. M., & Posner, B. Z. (1995). *The leadership challenge: How to keep getting extraordinary things done in organizations.* San Francisco: Jossey-Bass.
- Vail, P. (1989). *Managing as a performing art.* San Francisco: Jossey-Bass.

DISCUSSION QUESTIONS

1. Reread the opening case and answer the questions again. Compare those composed before and after reading this chapter. What are the differences? How have you altered your thinking about the nature of leadership and the factors that contribute to its effectiveness and success?
2. You are interviewing for a position, and your prospective employer asks you to describe your leadership style. How would you do so? This is a fairly typical question asked of candidates for management positions, irrespective of level, so it is a good idea to have a reasonably well-thought-out and articulate answer. Draft a one or two paragraph statement; share it with fellow students.
3. Some contend that leadership is highly romanticized. That is, there's a tendency to ascribe far more to leadership as a cause than

is actually warranted. While leadership certainly makes a difference, it may not make as much difference as either managers, followers, or onlookers generally think it does. Successful performance of a group, organization, or nation is the result of many factors interacting in complex ways. However, it's far easier, and more reassuring, to attribute such success to the leadership abilities of an individual. What do you think?
4. Several distinctive aspects of leading in health care organizations have been discussed. What are some other ones that pose challenges for effectively executing the leadership role?

REFERENCES

Bass, B. M. (1985). *Leadership beyond expectations.* New York: Free Press.

Bennis, W. (1989). *Why leaders can't lead: The unconscious conspiracy continues.* San Francisco: Jossey-Bass.

Benveniste, C. (1987). *Professionalizing the organization.* San Francisco: Jossey-Bass.

Blake, J., & Mouton, R. (1978). *The new managerial grid.* Houston, TX: Gulf Publishing.

Blake, R. R., & Mouton, J. S. (1982). Theory and research for developing a science of leadership. *Journal of Applied Behavioral Science, 18,* 275–291.

Burns, J. M. (1978). *Leadership.* New York: Harper and Row.

Covey, S. (1990). *Principle-centered leadership.* New York: Simon and Schuster.

Dreher, G., & Cox, T. (1966). Race, gender and opportunity: A study of compensation attainment and the establishment of mentoring relationships. *Journal of Applied Psychology, 81,* 297–308.

Eagly, A., & Johnson, B. (1990). Gender and the emergence of leaders: A meta-analysis. *Psychological Bulletin, 108,* 233–256.

Eagly, A., & Karau, S. J. and Makhijani, M. G. (1995). Gender and the effectiveness of leaders: A meta-analysis. *Psychological Bulletin, 111,* 3–22.

Eagly, A., & Wood, W. (1995). Explaining sex differences in social behavior: A meta-analytic perspective. *Journal of Personality and Social Psychology, 17,* 306–315.

Evans, M. G. (1970a). The effects of supervisory behavior on the path-goal relationship. *Organizational Behavior in Human Performance, 5,* 277–298.

Evans, M. G. (1970b). Leadership and motivation: A core concept. *Academy of Management Journal, 13,* 91–102.

Fiedler, F. E. (1967). *A theory of leadership effectiveness.* New York: McGraw-Hill.

Fiedler, F. E., & Chemers, M. M. (1974). *Leadership and effective management.* Glenview, IL: Scott, Foresman.

Fiedler, F. E., Chemers, M. M., & Mahar, L. (1976). *Improving leadership effectiveness.* New York: John Wiley.

Fleishman, F. A. (1973). Twenty years of consideration and structure. In E. A. Fleishman & J. G. Hunt (Eds.), *Current developments in the study of leadership* (pp. 1–37). Carbondale, IL: Southern Illinois University.

Freidson, E. (1972). *Profession of medicine: A study of the sociology of applied knowledge.* New York: Dodd/Mead.

Gardner, J. (1990). *On leadership.* New York: The Free Press.

Graeff, C. L. (1983). The situational leadership theory: A critical review. *Academy of Management Review, 8,* 271–294.

Graeff, C. L. (1997). Evolution of a situational leadership theory: A critical review. *Leadership Quarterly, 8,* 153–170.

Hersey, P., & Blanchard, K. H. (1977). *Management of organizational behavior: Utilizing human resources.* Englewood Cliffs, NJ: Prentice-Hall.

Hessesbein, F., Goldsmith, M., & Beckhard, R. (1996). *The leader of the future: New visions, strategies, and practices for the next era.* San Francisco: Jossey-Bass.

House R. J. (1971). A path-goal theory of leader effectiveness. Administrative Science Quarterly, 16, 321–323

House, R. J., & Baetz, M. L. (1979). Leadership: Some empirical generalizations and new directions. *Research in Organization Behavior, 1,* 385–386.

House, R. J., & Mitchell, T. R. (1974). Path-goal theory of leadership. *Journal of Contemporary Business, 3,* 81–98.

Hummel, R. P. (1975). Psychology of charismatic followers. *Psychological Reports, 37,* 759–770.

Katz, D., & Kahn, R. L. (1966). *The social psychology of organizations.* New York: John Wiley and Sons.

Katz, R. L. (1955, January–February). Skills of an effective administrator. *Harvard Business Review.*

Kelley, R. E. (1991). *The power of followership: How to create leaders people want to follow and followers who lead themselves.* New York: Doubleday/Currency.

Korman, A. K. (1966). Consideration, initiating structure and organizational criteria: A review. *Personnel Psychology, 19,* 349–361.

Kouzes, J. M., & Posner, B. Z. (1993). *Credibility: How leaders gain and lose it, why people demand it.* San Francisco: Jossey-Bass.

Kouzes, J. M., & Posner, B. Z. (1995). *The leadership challenge: How to keep getting extraordinary things done in organizations.* San Francisco: Jossey-Bass.

Kram, K. E. (1985). *Mentoring at work: Developmental relationships in organizational life.* Glenview, IL: Scott, Foresman.

Kuhnert, K. W., & Lewis, P. (1987). Transactional and transformational leadership: A constructive and developmental analysis. *Academy of Management Review, 12,* 649–662.

Lewin, K., Lippitt, R., & White R. (1939). Patterns of aggressive behavior in experimentally created social climates. *Journal of Social Psychology, 10,* 271–276.

Liden, R. C., & Dienesch, R. M. (1986). Leader-member exchange model of leadership: A critique and further development. *Academy of Management Review, 11,* 618–634.

Likert, R. (1961). *New patterns of management.* New York: McGraw-Hill.

Lord, R. G., de Vader, C. L., & Alliger, G. M. (1986). A meta analysis of the relation between personality traits and leadership: An application of validity generalization procedures. *Journal of Applied Psychology, 71,* 402–410.

Lord, R. G., Soto, R. J., & de Vader, C. L. (1984). A test of leadership categorization theory: Internal structure, information processing and leadership perception. *Organizational Behavior and Human Performance, 34,* 343–378.

Mann, R. D. (1959). A review of the relationship between personality and performance in small groups. *Psychological Bulletin, 56,* 241–270.

Mitchell, T. R., Green, S. G., & Wood, R. (1981). An attributional model of leadership and the poor performing subordinate: Development and validation. *Research in Organization Behavior, 3,* 197–234.

Mumford, M. D., & Marks, M., Connelly, M. S., Zaccaro, S. J., Reiter-Palmon, R. (2000). Leadership skills: Conclusions and future directions. *Leadership Quarterly, 11,* 155–170.

Nebeker, D. B. (1975). Situational favorability and perceived environmental uncertainty: An integrative approach. *Administrative Science Quarterly, 20,* 281–294.

Northhouse, P. (2003). *Leadership: Theory and practice.* Thousand Oaks, CA: Sage Publications.

Porter, I. W., & Lawler, E. E. (1968). *Managerial attitudes and performance.* Homewood, IL: Richard D. Irwin.

Raelin, J. A. (1986). *The clash of cultures: Managers and professionals.* Boston: Harvard Business School Press.

Schreisheim, C. A., & von Glinow, M. A. (1977). The path-goal theory of leadership: A theoretical and empirical analysis. *Academy of Management Journal, 20,* 398–405.

Shapiro, A. (1985). *Managing professional people.* New York: Free Press.

Shaver, K. C. (1983). *An introduction to attribution processes.* Hillsdale, NY: Erlbaum Books.

Stinson, J. E., & Trancy, L. (1974). Some disturbing characteristics of LPC scores. *Personnel Psychology, 27,* 77–85.

Stodgill, R. M. (1948). Personal factors associated with leadership: A survey of the literature. *Journal of Applied Psychology, 32,* 35–71.

Stodgill, R. M. (1974). *Handbook of leadership.* New York: Free Press.

Stodgill, R. M., & Coons, A. (1957). *Leader behavior: Its description and measurement.* Columbus, OH: Bureau of Business Research, Ohio State University.

Tannenbaum, R., & Schmidt, W. (1973). How to choose a leadership pattern. *Harvard Business Review, 51,* 162–180.

Tishy, N. M. & Devanna, M. A. (1986). The transformational leader. New York: John Wiley

Vail, P. (1989). *Managing as a performing art.* San Francisco: Jossey-Bass.

Van Vleet, D. D., & Yukl, C. A. (1989). A century of leadership research. In W. E. Rosenbach & R. L. Taylor (Eds.), *Contemporary issues in leadership.* Boulder, CO: Westview Press.

Vroom, V. H. (1964). *Work and motivation.* New York: John Wiley.

Yukl, G. A. (2006). *Leadership in organizations.* New York: Prentice-Hall.

CHAPTER 5

Conflict Management and Negotiation

Jeffrey T. Polzer, Ph.D., Margaret A. Neale, Ph.D., and
Jennifer L. Illes, Ph.D.

CHAPTER OUTLINE

- ⚜ The Importance of Conflict Management
- ⚜ The Causes of Conflict
- ⚜ Levels of Conflict
- ⚜ Managing Conflict
- ⚜ Negotiation
- ⚜ Managing Conflict through Third-Party Intervention

LEARNING OBJECTIVES

After completing this chapter, the reader should be able to:

1. Identify reasons why conflict is prevalent in health care organizations.
2. Understand several different types of conflict and the levels at which conflict occurs.
3. Identify several different conflict-management techniques, based on various concerns of the disputants.
4. Identify the basic concepts and dimensions of negotiation.
5. Appreciate the importance of planning for a negotiation and know the key issues to consider when preparing to negotiate.
6. Identify and understand special types of conflict-management situations, such as multiparty negotiations and third-party intervention.

KEY TERMS

Accommodation
Administrative Conflict
Arbitrator
Aspiration Level
Avoidance
Bargaining Zone
Best Alternative to a Negoti-
    ated Agreement (BATNA)
Compatible Issues

Competition
Conflict
Distributive Dimension
Emotional Conflict
Equality Fairness Norm
Equity Fairness Norm
Inquisitor
Integrative Dimension
Intergroup Conflict

Interpersonal Conflict
Intragroup Conflict
Intrapersonal Conflict
Mediator
Need Fairness Norm
Negotiation
Pressing
Reservation Price
Task Content Conflict

✤ IN PRACTICE Negotiations at Culpeper Medical Associates

In the struggle between health care giants and small independent hospitals, Culpeper Memorial is proof that even the tiny can triumph. Located in rural Virginia about 60 miles from Washington, D.C., the 70-bed hospital recently staved off an attempted takeover of its doctor groups by the mighty University of Virginia. In the process, Culpeper has formed a partnership with its primary care doctors and is finalizing negotiations to bring in Health Care Partners, a for-profit affiliate of the university's foundation.

Culpeper focuses on basic acute care, so its 14 primary care doctors are an important asset, says CEO Lee Kirk. When he came to the hospital about a year ago, the doctors were being courted by outsiders. One internist decided to become an employee of the university's own physician group, and that worried Kirk and others. "We were concerned we'd face a divide-and-conquer strategy and what it might do to the community," he says. "So we decided to circle the wagons."

Culpeper called in Medimetrix, a consulting firm that had helped the hospital form its physician-hospital organization four years earlier. Over several months, the Cleveland company set up a series of sessions to help hospital executives and doctors mull over options to a takeover or merger. They eventually formed Culpeper Medical Associates, a tax-exempt, limited-liability company with a physician-chaired board made up of four doctors and four hospital representatives. Under the agreement, all 14 doctors sold their practices to Culpeper Medical Associates and became its employees, with base salaries calculated from historical earnings and current productivity. Incentives included a bonus tied to performance.

To buy the practices, Culpeper Medical Associates needed big money, so it put out feelers for an equity partner. Three hospital systems came forward, and Health Care Partners was chosen because of Culpeper's longtime relationship with the university, Kirk says. "We also send the majority of our tertiary referrals there," he adds. Two representatives from Health Care Partners are to be added to the board, making the for-profit a minority partner with a 49% equity stake.

For John Ashley, M.D., associate vice president of the university's Health Sciences Foundation, the

(continues)

🔷 IN PRACTICE *(continued)*

arrangement is better than an outright purchase. The doctors didn't want their practices acquired, and the university didn't really want to buy them. "We'd rather form partnerships because they require less investment," says Ashley. "Becoming the minority partner allows us to formalize a long-standing informal relationship in a more comfortable way than if we'd come in and played the heavy."

To boost referrals to the university, Culpeper Medical Associates has developed formal processes for the doctors to confer with specialists and use other resources. It also supports the university's mission by bringing in residents and other medical students more regularly. Morton Chiles, a doctor who heads the Culpeper Medical Associates board, sees several advantages. By sticking together, he says, doctors can pool resources, deliver care more efficiently, and

negotiate contracts more competitively. And they keep their much-prized clinical autonomy. Finally, since the transition has been largely seamless, patients are ensured continuity of care. In fact, Medicare recipients now have better access to care because all of Culpeper's primary care doctors will take them.

Culpeper's solution may not be for everybody, Chiles warns. The new setup required delicate negotiating—and what with legal and consulting fees, it hasn't come cheap. Still, he's sure it's the right choice: "It eliminates the potential for fragmenting the local primary care market and devastating the hospital."

Reprinted from Nordhaus-Bike, A. M. (1997, August 20). Partnering: Unite and conquer. *Hospitals & Health Networks*, Vol. 71, No. 16, by permission, Copyright, 1997, Health Forum, Inc.

CHAPTER PURPOSE

The parties involved in the Culpeper Medical Associates negotiations were able to reach a mutually satisfactory agreement despite their potentially conflicting interests. Other health services organizations have not fared so well in crafting good agreements among parties who disagree over how various issues should be resolved. **Conflict** is pervasive in health services organizations, as in all organizations. Conflict occurs every day in a wide variety of situations ranging from emotional disputes between two colleagues, to disputes between departments about lines of authority, to legal disputes involving several organizations. In this chapter, we will focus primarily on the types of conflict that confront managers on a day-to-day basis.

THE IMPORTANCE OF CONFLICT MANAGEMENT

The field of conflict management has grown dramatically in the last decade, reflected both by the amount of research conducted on this topic and the increased importance placed on teaching conflict-management techniques. This increase in popularity, particularly concerning negotiation, has been fueled by several general environmental trends that are especially noticeable in the health services industry (Neale & Bazerman, 1991). First, the marketplace is growing increasingly global as firms face competition from foreign companies. For example, pharmaceutical firms such as Burroughs-Wellcome, Inc. increasingly find themselves conducting business in different countries as their current markets become more competitive. This increased diversity in potential business partners heightens the need for managers to be able to negotiate effectively with people who have different backgrounds, interests, and values.

Second, at the firm level, there has been a vast increase in corporate restructuring throughout the 1990s. Managers in corporations that are going through structural transformations need negotiation skills to ensure their position within the new organization. At an individual level, the workforce is growing increasingly mobile. Many employees proactively manage their career paths, often within multiple organizations. Increased mobility demands better negotiation skills of those changing jobs and those employing these people.

Finally, the shift from a manufacturing-based to a service-based economy means that typical negotiations are likely to be more difficult, because desired outcomes are more ambiguous and therefore harder to specify in negotiated agreements (Neale & Bazerman, 1991). For example, the primary care doctors who sold their practices to Culpeper Medical Associates agreed to use both historical earnings and current productivity to resolve the ambiguity inherent in calculating "fair" base salaries. Such ambiguity is clearly present in many areas of the health services field, increasing the importance of good negotiating skills as negotiations become more difficult.

THE CAUSES OF CONFLICT

The Role of Resource Scarcity

Conflict arises for many reasons and can be characterized in numerous ways. At a very basic level, most conflict occurs because of a fundamental problem inherent in every organization. Organiza-

tional members desire several types of resources, including power, money, information, advice, and praise (Homans, 1961). However, resource scarcity dictates that the members of an organization will not all be able to receive the level of resources they desire. Therefore, conflict arises between organizational members regarding the distribution of desired resources.

It is useful to distinguish conflict from **competition** because many people confuse the two concepts. While conflict is a typical result of resource scarcity, organizational members also compete for resources. However, conflict and competition are distinct concepts. In both cases, the goals of the parties are incompatible. In situations involving resources, this means that the parties cannot both acquire their desired level of resources. However, competition is characterized by parallel striving toward a goal that both parties cannot reach simultaneously, while conflict is characterized by mutual interference. Conflict occurs when a concern of one party is frustrated, or perceived to be frustrated, by another party (Thomas, 1976). Parties can compete and still remain relatively independent of each other. Conflict, on the other hand, requires some interaction or contact between the parties.

Conflict can also occur for reasons that are less tangible than resource acquisition. People may have conflicting perceptions, ideas, or beliefs as well as conflicting resource-allocation goals. For example, one subordinate may perceive that another subordinate receives more praise, even when both subordinates actually receive the same objective amount of praise; two administrators may have different ideas about what an employee dress code policy should entail, and people may have different beliefs about the appropriateness of a certain medical treatment or procedure. A basic but important point to be drawn from these examples is that conflict always occurs because of the differences between people, even though these differences occur on a variety of dimensions.

DEBATE TIME 5.1 What Do You Think?

POINT: Conflict is a necessary and useful part of organizational life. Not all conflict is unhealthy. Low levels of conflict can often stimulate the parties involved and heighten their attention. Novel or creative solutions frequently result from conflict when people search for ways to satisfy a diverse set of interests. In fact, the absence of conflict can be as indicative of problems as too much conflict. For example, Irving Janis (1982) originated the concept of groupthink, which occurs when too little conflict is expressed within decision-making groups. Very low levels of conflict may indicate that unavoidable differences are being suppressed or that the people involved do not have perspectives that differ enough to contribute to a well-thought-out decision.

COUNTERPOINT: Conflict is dysfunctional. Especially in the United States, most people think of conflict as a negative phenomenon. They are usually correct. High conflict levels are typically detrimental and can be destructive. Instead of allocating resources to the production of the goods or services that are the mission of the organization, conflict requires that managers spend time and energy trying to resolve the conflict. In fact, one study discovered that managers spend almost 20% of their time in activities directly related to the resolution of disputes—time that could be much more productively applied directly to achieving the mission of the organization.

In addition, conflict is associated with higher levels of stress. Such an environment can reduce the psychological well-being of employees and make it difficult for them to develop trusting, supportive relationships within the organizational context. It is for this reason that managers spend so much of their time managing and resolving conflict.

Is conflict always dysfunctional? Is it ever useful? Are there certain types of conflict that are more dangerous than others?

Beneficial versus Detrimental Effects of Conflict

Because differences between people are unavoidable, conflict will always exist in organizations and groups. The question that must be addressed by successful managers is how to handle the conflicts that they will inevitably face. Should managers try to create a work environment in which there is as little conflict as possible or is some important purpose served by having certain levels of ambient conflict? This boils down to the question of whether conflict is good or bad, and therefore, whether it should be encouraged in work groups or discouraged and suppressed. This is the focus of Debate Time 5.1.

In trying to ascertain whether conflict is good or bad, functional or dysfunctional, something to be explored or suppressed, part of the puzzle may lie in differentiating various types of conflict. It may be that some types of conflict are important for successful organizational performance while other forms of conflict are associated with problematic organizational performance. In the next section, we will consider three different types of conflict—content conflict, emotional conflict, and administrative conflict—and their unique impact on organizational functioning.

Jehn's Typology of Conflict

Conflict within an organization can be characterized by type regardless of the level at which it occurs. Karen Jehn (1995) devised a typology that includes three types of conflict. **Task content conflict**, the first type, refers to disagreements about the actual task being performed by organizational members. The focus in this type of conflict is on differing opinions pertaining to the task, rather than the goals of the people involved. For example, everyone in a group medical practice may agree that the group should have a marketing campaign, but members may disagree about the content of the advertisements and whether advertising should be run on radio, on television, or in newspapers.

Emotional conflict is an awareness of interpersonal incompatibilities among those working together on a task. It involves negative emotions and dislike of the other people involved in the conflict. The third type of conflict is **administrative conflict** and is defined as an awareness by the involved parties that there are controversies about how task accomplishment will proceed. Disagreements about individual responsibilities and duties are examples of administrative conflict. For example, members of a group practice may disagree about who should decide what type of advertising to use or who should be responsible for working with an advertising agency.

In general, the research conducted by Jehn and others suggests that a moderate amount of task content conflict is critical to the effective functioning of groups. Groupthink, for example, is probably more likely to occur when there is an implicit avoidance of all conflict, but especially task content conflict. Administrative conflict and, to a greater extent, emotional conflict are likely to be the culprits when groups become dysfunctional or impaired because a high degree of conflict inhibits their ability to interact. All three of these types of conflict may occur between individuals, groups and individuals, or different groups as people perform the tasks that make up organizational life. These various levels at which conflict can occur are the focus of the next section.

LEVELS OF CONFLICT

It is useful to consider the level at which conflict occurs, along with the type of conflict, when trying to decide how to manage it. That is, conflict can occur within an individual (**intrapersonal conflict**), between individuals (**interpersonal conflict**), within a group (**intragroup conflict**), and between groups (**intergroup conflict**). The alternatives available for resolving the conflict may depend on the level in the organization at which it exists.

Individual Level

Individual conflict occurs when the locus of the dispute is the individual. Intrapersonal conflict may occur for a variety of reasons. People are often faced with a choice between two options that may vary in attractiveness. In characterizing conflict at this level, it is valuable to think about the relative attractiveness of each option. When two options are equally attractive, approach-approach conflict occurs within the person. This conflict results from the person's effort to differentiate between the two alternatives. For example, a health maintenance organization (HMO) executive may have two equally viable and attractive plans for expanding enrollment. It is difficult to choose either of the options because selecting one necessarily means the other must be turned down.

On the other side of the coin, avoidance-avoidance conflict occurs when a person has to choose between equally unattractive options. If a nursing home is trying to reduce costs, one of two good nurses may have to be laid off. The decision is made more difficult because the options are equally unattractive.

The most prevalent type of intrapersonal conflict is approach-avoidance conflict, which occurs when multiple options each have favorable and unfavorable features. Conflict that is initially approach-approach conflict often turns into approach-avoidance conflict when the person making the decision looks at the alternatives more critically in an attempt to differentiate them. Unattractive components of each option may be found that were overlooked initially, such as additional costs associated with each option for expanding HMO membership enrollment. A person may arrive at a different decision depending on which features of each option the person focuses. After the decision is made, postdecision regret frequently occurs, as the alternative that the person passed up looks increasingly better as more information is gathered about the chosen option.

Group Level

When most people think about conflict, the examples that first come to mind are at an interpersonal level, between two or more people. Conflict at this level typically occurs because of incompatible goals, ideas, feelings, beliefs, or behaviors, as illustrated by the examples in the first section of this chapter. This level of conflict is usually characterized by interdependence between the parties, whereby the choice of each party affects the outcome of the other party. The choice that is optimal for one party may result in a poor outcome for the other, leading to conflict. This is the most common level of conflict that comes to the surface in organizations.

Paralleling individual conflict, group conflict can occur between members of the same group (intragroup conflict) or between members of different groups (intergroup conflict). Intragroup conflict is similar in many ways to interpersonal conflict, with the former type being more complex because of the higher number of people involved. However, this is not the only difference. When a group is involved that has an identity above and beyond its individual members, several things can occur as a result of the influence of the group on its members. A formal definition of what we mean by a "group" may help to clarify the ideas that follow. In this context, a group is defined as:

> an organized system of two or more individuals who are interrelated so that the system performs some function, has a standard set of role relationships among its members, and has a set of norms that regulate the function of the group and each of its members. (Northcraft & Neale, 1990)

As this definition of a group implies, the interactions of the group members are influenced by their roles within the group and by the norms of the group. Members of the group may not always be amenable to these influences, leading to conflict between the individual member and the group. Conflict between the members of a group may result in decreased coordination, communication, and productivity (Deutsch, 1949). Intragroup conflict will come up again later in this chapter in the section on multiparty negotiations.

Intergroup conflict can have a profound impact on the perceptions and behaviors of people. When acting as a member of a group, people tend to divide others into an ingroup and an outgroup. The ingroup consists of all the other members of the salient group. The outgroup consists of those outside the boundaries of the ingroup. Some examples of the characteristics people frequently use to divide people into in- and out groups include gender, race, religious preference, geographic location, organizational membership, departmental membership, and functional position within an organization. Most people are members of numerous groups based on demographic, organizational, or other demarcations. This creates abundant opportunities for intergroup conflict to arise. Intergroup conflict occurs whenever the disputants identify with or represent different groups that are relevant to the conflict during the conflict episode.

Intergroup conflict may have a variety of causes, many of which are the same as those that cause interpersonal conflict, such as resource scarcity, differing beliefs, or incompatible goals. The distinction is simply that the relevant unit from which the differences stem is the group rather than the individual. Intergroup conflict can have a variety of consequences both within and across the groups involved in the conflict. Within the groups, cohesiveness, task orientation, loyalty to the group, and acceptance of autocratic leadership may increase. Between the groups, distorted perceptions, negative stereotypes of out-group members, and reduced communication may result. A mentality of "us versus them" often forms and grows stronger as the conflict escalates (Sherif, 1977).

MANAGING CONFLICT

It is clear that conflict is commonplace, and that for organizational members to function productively, they must manage conflict effectively. There are many strategies for managing conflict, including those that are planned as well as those that emerge as conflict is experienced. Some conflict-management techniques apply to conflict on all levels, while others are relevant for a limited number of types and levels of conflict. In this section, we will briefly introduce the dual-concern model as a typology of conflict-management techniques, focusing on four ways that people handle conflict—accommodation, pressing, avoidance, and negotiation.

The Dual Concern Model

Kenneth Thomas (1976) has developed a two-dimensional model of conflict-management techniques that reflects a concern for both an individual's own outcomes as well as an opponent's outcomes. Depending on these two dimensions of concern, a negotiator might prefer one of five different strategies for handling conflict. If concern for both self and other's outcomes are low, this model predicts that one might prefer an **avoidance** strategy. If concern for one's own outcome is high and concern for the others' outcome is low, then one should prefer a competing, or **pressing**, strategy. If concern for one's own outcome is low and concern for the other's outcome is high, then **accommodation** or capitulation is probably the preferred strategy. If concern for both one's own outcome and the other's outcome is high, then collaboration is the appropriate strategy. Finally, if one has intermediate concern for both one's own and the other's outcomes, then one is likely to prefer a compromise strategy. The dual-concern model is graphically represented in Figure 5.1.

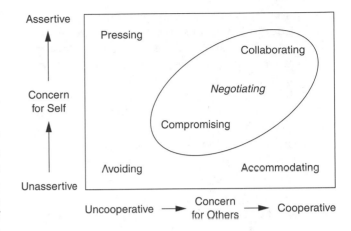

Figure 5.1. Dual Concern Model

SOURCE: Adapted from Thomas, K. "Conflict and Conflict Management," in *Handbook of Industrial and Organizational Psychology*, ed. M. D. Dunnette (Chicago, IL: Rand McNally, 1996), 900. Used by permission of Marvin D. Dunnette.

If we think about how differing preferences for these five strategies might be expressed by an organizational actor in various situations, four different conflict-management techniques can be identified. Accommodation, pressing, avoiding, and **negotiation** (incorporating compromise and collaboration) are described in greater detail in the following sections.

Accommodation

Capitulating to or accommodating the other party is one popular way to deal with conflict. Accommodation does not necessarily require any interaction among the parties and can simply entail giving the other side what they want. It is one of the least confrontational methods for dealing with conflict. Capitulation has the advantage of being efficient in that, by giving the other party what he wants, the conflict ends quickly. Other advantages are that the relationship between the parties may be preserved and that the other party may feel a sense of indebtedness, which may come into play in the future. The adage, "it is better to give than to receive", seems to recommend accommodation, although it is not clear that this advice was meant for organizational members in an increasingly competitive environment. While capitulation may be recommended in some situations, people are unlikely to get what they want by relying on others accommodating them. They may rarely achieve outcomes that are good for them if they use capitulation too often. In most situations, there are better ways to manage conflict.

Pressing

When individuals have as their primary objective the achievement of their interests and are unconcerned about whether other parties get what they want (or even wish to "beat" the other side), they often rely on a series of strategies that are typically described as contentious. These strategies include a variety of tactics such as irrevocable commitments, threats or promises, and persuasive argumentation (Pruitt & Rubin, 1986).

Irrevocable commitments occur when one party credibly guarantees to continue behaving in a certain way that once begun will not be changed. An excellent example of an irrevocable commitment is the game of Chicken. The game involves two participants who are driving their cars at breakneck speed on a direct collision course with each other. The loser in this game is the one who first turns aside—the "chicken"—thereby avoiding a head-on collision and almost certain death for both players. In this game, each side tries to convince the other that they are committed to their course of action—driving straight toward the other car. More generally, irrevocable commitments occur when two parties engage in a test of wills in which neither side is willing to concede. A typical example of the risk of such games and tactics can be seen in the escalation of losses and acrimony that can occur when couples divorce.

Irrevocable commitments are useful because they do not require agreement of the other party to work nor do they require that the committing party be of equal or greater power. In the case of irrevocable commitments, weakness can become strength. Consider Gandhi's power, stemming from his weakness in the face of the other party's strength, to compel the British to modify their policies in India.

Threats and promises are both meant to convey intention. The typical promise is designed to induce some particular behavior by describing what will happen if such an action occurs. For example, one might promise to trade future support on issue A for current support on issue B. Promises do not give information about what will happen if compliance does not occur. Threats, on the other hand, convey what will happen if the preferred behavior does not happen. As such, one might threaten to vote against my interests unless I vote *for* her interests. Threats and promises are designed to have the same effect, but the mechanism by which the effects come about are different. Promises rely on the benefits of compliance while threats work because of the costs of noncompliance. In fact, compared with promises, threats provide more information because they describe how an individual intends to behave in response to a broader variety of actions. Promises tell me only what you will do if I take one particular action. They tell me nothing about what you would do if I take no action or another action.

Compared with threats and promises, persuasive argumentation is a less controlling tactic, although one that requires considerable skill. Through persuasive argumentation, I can influence you to give up something that you hold dear, change a situation you currently enjoy, or lower your aspirations. Consider the difficulty of persuading employees to work fewer hours rather than laying off other organizational members. When undertaking this tactic, one typically appeals to the unattractive alternatives that will ensue if the situation is left unchanged.

Avoidance

The most common response to conflict on any level is to avoid it. In many situations, people avoid conflict when both they and their organizations would benefit if they managed the conflict more proactively.

For example, issues involving quality of care are sometimes ignored because people fear the conflict associated with addressing them. However, avoidance does have its merits. If the issues involved in the conflict are trivial and the parties do not care much about their own outcome or the other party's outcome, avoidance may be the best strategy. The costs incurred by confronting the problem may be greater, at least in the short run, than the benefits that accrue from having the conflict resolved. Avoidance may also be the best way to deal with conflict when someone else can resolve the problem more effectively or when the problem would be better dealt with in the future after the involved parties have cooled down. If avoiding conflict becomes a habit, however, important issues, when they arise, may never get addressed.

Negotiation

Unlike other conflict-resolution tactics, negotiation is a process through which multiple parties work together on the outcome. People negotiate every day, although they do not always think of their activities as negotiations. This becomes clearer, however, when negotiation is defined as the process whereby two or more parties decide what each will give and take in an exchange between them (Rubin & Brown, 1975). This broad definition encompasses a preponderance of activities that people do every day, both within and outside organizations. Negotiations typically, but not always, involve some type of direct interaction between the parties, with the interaction being face to face, verbal, or written. The parties in a negotiation are interdependent in that they both desire something the other party has control over.

An interesting aspect of negotiation that distinguishes it from other forms of conflict resolution is the considerable amount of attention it has received in both applied and scholarly settings. One result of this trend is that we now know more about the behavior of negotiators and the structural factors that influence them than we did in the past. In the next section, we will provide a framework for thinking about negotiations that can be applied equally well to almost any negotiation situation, whether it involves a husband and wife or two nations. By analyzing the structure of a negotiation, negotiators should be able to improve their preparedness for, the process of, and the outcome of the negotiation.

NEGOTIATION

Basic Concepts

A negotiator never *has* to negotiate; there are always alternatives to reaching an agreement through a negotiation. Many were discussed above, such as avoiding the situation or giving the other party what they want. However, when a person in an interdependent situation (i.e., the person desires something the other party has control over and vice versa) does not reach a negotiated agreement with the other party, that person has to settle for another alternative regarding the desired resource controlled by the other party. For example, if a hospital is trying to hire a nurse but does not reach an agreement on an employment contract with a particular nurse, the hospital has to either accept the alternative of not having the position filled or choose the alternative of trying to hire another person for the job. From the nurse's point of view, if an agreement is not reached with the hospital, he will have to settle for another alternative, perhaps accepting a job with another hospital or continuing the job search.

Whether they have thought about them or not, the parties in a negotiation have alternatives that they will implement if the negotiation ends in an impasse. The negotiator will obviously choose her best alternative to an agreement if an impasse is reached, so this alternative will be our focus. Specifically, a negotiator's **Best Alternative To a Negotiated Agreement** (**BATNA**) is an important consideration because it is a source of power in the negotiation (Fisher & Ury, 1981). Being able to walk away from the negotiation if a satisfactory agreement does not appear to be forthcoming can be a valuable negotiating tool. Besides the opportunity to use this information strategically, it is also important to know when you actually should walk away. Knowing your best alternative allows a comparison to be made between the value of your best alternative and the value of various agreements that might be reached, which in turn allows you to know which agreements are desirable and which should be turned down.

A BATNA is put into action by determining a **reservation price.** A reservation price can be thought of as a bottom line, or the point at which you are indifferent between an impasse and an agreement (Raiffa, 1982). A reservation price should be stated in terms of whatever units are being negotiated. In many negotiations, the units of exchange are dollars so that, for example, a negotiator might have a reservation price of $18,000 when buying a car (i.e., the buyer will pay no more than $18,000). A BATNA and a reservation price, although closely related, are distinct concepts. The connection between the two is that a reservation price should equal the value placed on your best alternative *plus* whatever transaction costs you will incur to enact your best alternative (White & Neale, 1994). For example, the expenses that would be involved in hiring another nurse should be taken into consideration in determining a reservation price for a negotiation with a nurse candidate.

An **aspiration level** is what a negotiator would ideally like to achieve in the negotiation. It can also be referred to as a target or goal. An aspiration level should be challenging but attainable. A goal that is too challenging is not motivating because it is not within the realm of possibilities, while one that is too easy also loses its motivating potential once it is surpassed. Typically an aspiration level is stated in the same units as the reservation price (e.g., dollars).

The three concepts just discussed focus on one party rather than the constellation of parties involved in a negotiation. When the parties in a negotiation come together, additional structural features come into play. The most prominent feature is the **bargaining zone.** The bargaining zone is found by combining the reservation prices of each nego-

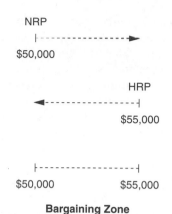

Figure 5.2. Bargaining Zones

tiator and determining whether they overlap, and if so, the extent of the overlap. A positive bargaining zone occurs if a set of agreements exists that both parties prefer over impasse (Neale & Bazerman, 1991). It is easier to understand this concept with the aid of a diagram. Imagine that a nurse and a hospital are negotiating over the nurse's salary. The nurse's reservation price (NRP) is $50,000 and the hospital's reservation price (HRP) is $55,000. This is outlined in Figure 5.2. The bargaining zone is the range of agreements between and including $50,000 and $55,000. If there is no overlap region between the reservation prices of the parties, then a negative bargaining zone exists. Because there are no agreements that are acceptable to both parties, no resolution is possible. It is important for a negotiator to gather information about the size of the bargaining zone during the course of the negotiation.

The Distributive Dimension of Negotiation

Of the two dimensions of negotiation, only the **distributive dimension** is necessarily part of every negotiation. The **integrative dimension,** on the other hand, is never applied in many negotiations. Negotiation always involves the allocation, or distribution, of some set of resources. The distributive dimension is often referred to as that part of negotiation in which value is claimed. In every negotiation, regardless of the amount of resources to be distributed, an integral task for the negotiators is to determine how much each party will take from the "pie" of resources. Single-issue negotiations are the most common example of purely distributive negotiations. The amount of resources is fixed, and whatever one party gains is always at the expense of the other party. Resolving negotiations that are distributive often entails compromise by both parties, as each party concedes a little at a time in a reciprocal manner until they reach an agreement. Negotiators should consider several strategies that may help them claim as large a share of the resources as possible. These strategies are outlined in Table 5.1.

Many negotiators presume that all negotiations are purely distributive and that their task as negotiators is to get as much as they can from the fixed amount of resources to be divided. A common assumption is that the interests of the other party are diametrically opposed to their own interests, and therefore a direct conflict arises over the resources in question. This is called the "fixed-pie bias" (Bazerman, Magliozzi, & Neale, 1985). Based on this assumption, they view negotiation as an adversarial process. The integrative dimension of negotiation is often overlooked because of this bias. Consider the situation at Chiefland Memorial Hospital (see In Practice, p. 160).

Table 5.1. Claiming Value: Distributive Bargaining Strategies

1. Know your BATNA.
2. Determine your bottom line or reservation price.
3. Set a goal or aspiration level that is (a) significantly better than your bottom line and (b) optimistically realistic.
4. Think of what objective standards might be acceptable to the other party.
5. Plan your opening. An initial offer should not be too extreme, but it should prevent the other party from "anchoring" the negotiation.
6. Develop reciprocity. Avoid making unilateral concessions.

The Integrative Dimension of Negotiation

The most basic assumption underlying the integrative dimension of negotiation is that one party can gain without the other party necessarily having to lose. Another way to say this is that there are ways for the parties to mutually benefit. To do this, the parties need to take more of a problem-solving, cooperative approach rather than the contentious, competitive approach that typically characterizes purely distributive negotiations. In effect, the parties try to "expand the pie" of resources, or create value. A key element that should be present for a problem-solving orientation to work is trust between the parties. Trust is crucial because information sharing is at the heart of the negotiation process, and if information is not openly and accurately shared, albeit in a reciprocal manner, it is unlikely that integrative solutions can be found. Negotiating along the integrative dimension, or trying to find mutually beneficial solutions, can be difficult because it frequently requires finding creative or novel solutions that may not have been considered prior to the negotiation.

There are several ways to achieve integrative solutions. Most of them are based on differing interests underlying the conflict on the surface. Although this may sound strange because differences are the reason for the conflict, it is differences *in preferences* that allow integrative negotiation to occur. An example from the Culpeper Medical Associates case at the beginning of the chapter may help to clarify this point (see In Practice, p. 149). Culpeper Memorial Hospital wanted to retain its 14 primary care doctors, but it did not have adequate financial resources to fend off rival employers. The University of Virginia wanted to formalize its relationships with more primary care doctors and had enough money to potentially acquire the practices of Culpeper's doctors. The doctors, on the other hand, did not want the University to acquire their practices and decrease their autonomy. The initial resolution to these conflicting interests was for the university to simply hire away one of Culpeper's internists, with the potential for more such hires to follow. However, a

IN PRACTICE   Conflict at Chiefland Memorial Hospital

James A. Grover, retired land developer and financier, is the current president of Chiefland Memorial Hospital Board of Trustees. Chiefland Memorial is a 200-bed voluntary short-term general hospital serving an area of approximately 50,000 persons. Mr. Grover has just completed a meeting with the administrator of the hospital, Edward M. Hoffman. The purpose of meeting was to seek an acceptable solution to an apparent conflict-of-authority problem within the hospital between Hoffman and the chief of surgery, Dr. Lacy Young.

The problem that concerns Dr. Young involves the operating room supervisor, Geraldine Werther, R.N. Ms. Werther schedules the hospital's operating suite in accordance with policies that she believes to have been established by the hospital's administration. One source of irritation to the surgeons is her attitude that maximum utilization must be made of the hospital's operating rooms if hospital costs are to be reduced. She, therefore, schedules in such a way that operating room idle time is minimized. Surgeons complain that the operative schedule often does not permit them sufficient time to complete a surgical procedure in the manner they think desirable. More often than not, insufficient time is allowed between operations for effective preparation of the operating room for the next procedure. Such scheduling, the surgical staff maintains, contributes to low-quality patient care. Furthermore, some of the surgeons have complained that Ms. Werther shows favoritism in her scheduling, allowing some doctors more use of the operating suite than others.

This situation reached a crisis when Dr. Young, following an explosive confrontation with Ms. Werther, told her he was firing her. Ms. Werther then made an appeal to the hospital administrator, who in turn informed Dr. Young that discharge of

nurses was an administrative prerogative. In effect, Dr. Young was told he did not have the authority to fire Ms. Werther. Dr. Young asserted that he did have authority over any issue affecting medical practice and good patient care in Chiefland Hospital. He considered this a medical problem and threatened to take the matter to the hospital's board of trustees.

As the meeting between Mr. Grover and Mr. Hoffman began, Mr. Hoffman explained his position on the problem. He stressed the point that a hospital administrator is legally responsible for patient care in the hospital. He also contended that quality patient care cannot be achieved unless the board of trustees authorizes the administrator to make decisions, develop programs, formulate policies, and implement procedures. While listening to Mr. Hoffman, Mr. Grover recalled the position belligerently taken by Dr. Young, who had contended that surgical and medical doctors holding staff privileges at Chiefland would never allow a layperson to make decisions impinging on medical practice. Young also had said that Hoffman should be told to restrict his activities to fund-raising, financing, maintenance, and housekeeping—administrative problems rather than medical problems. Dr. Young had then requested that Mr. Grover clarify in a definitive manner the lines of authority at Chiefland Memorial.

As Mr. Grover ended his meeting with Mr. Hoffman, the severity of the problem was unmistakably clear to him, but the solution remained quite unclear. Grover knew a decision was required—and soon.

Source: Adapted from Champion, J. M., & James, J. H. (1980). *Critical incidents in management.* Homewood, IL: Richard D. Irwin, Inc.

deeper analysis of the parties' interests revealed a better solution that made all parties better off. By forming Culpeper Medical Associates and then forming a partnership with Health Care Partners, the university formalized its relationship with the doctors while spending less money to do so, the hospital gained financial resources to retain its group of doctors, and the doctors retained their autonomy.

Additionally, in the Chiefland Memorial Hospital case (see In Practice, p. 160) both hospital administrators and physicians would be in favor of lower costs for the hospital and higher-quality service. However, the two parties differ in the importance they place on these two objectives. Administrators place more importance on lowering costs, while physicians place greater importance on increasing the quality of service. Conflict occurs because increasing quality is thought to require incurring more costs. The underlying interests of both parties may be met, though, if the parties view the problem within the context of a longer time horizon. Increasing quality may raise costs in the short run, but this higher level of quality service may lower costs in other areas, such as malpractice suits, in the future.

There are many techniques for finding integrative solutions. Logrolling entails trading issues that are of differing importance to the two parties (Pruitt & Rubin, 1986). Cost cutting occurs when one party finds a way to make the concessions of the other party less costly. This is often accomplished by one party offering the conceding party some sort of compensation that is related to the issues being negotiated. Cost cutting differs from nonspecific compensation, in which the party that concedes is paid by the other party in some currency that is unrelated to the negotiated issues. Obtaining added resources may sometimes be possible so that both parties can meet their goals. Frequently, the time and effort spent negotiating over a given set of resources may instead be spent finding ways to increase the amount of available resources (Pruitt, 1983). By undertaking one or more of these strategies, the parties in a negotiation may both be better off than if they simply compromised on the issues.

There are many obvious and some not-so-obvious benefits of finding integrative solutions in negotiations. Increasing the amount of resources to be distributed may be necessary for both parties to be able to reach their reservation prices. In these cases, an impasse is likely unless some integrative solution is found. An obvious benefit to finding integrative agreements is that a party's outcomes may be increased because a larger amount of resources is available to be distributed.

Less obviously, a party may also benefit from the opponent receiving a higher outcome. An opponent's satisfaction with the negotiation should increase as the outcome gets better. This should have a positive effect on the relationship between the two parties and should make the agreement more stable. If the other party is required to implement a decision that was reached as part of the negotiated agreement, successful implementation is more likely if the opponent is happy with the outcome, rather than disgruntled. Of course, the importance a party places on an opponent's outcome may vary with the expectation or probability of future interaction or with the types of issues that are being negotiated (e.g., some issues may require implementation, while others may not). The point here is that most people think only of their own outcome when they determine whether they were successful in a negotiation when several benefits, however indirect, may accrue to them if the other party also achieves a good outcome. Several specific strategies for reaching integrative agreements are outlined in Table 5.2.

The Mixed-Motive Nature of Negotiation

When thinking about the distributive and integrative dimensions of negotiation, it is crucial to keep in mind the mixed-motive nature of negotiations. Creating value by finding integrative solutions requires primarily cooperative behavior, while claiming value along the distributive dimension of the negotiation requires primarily competitive behavior. Many people make the mistake of thinking they can segment a negotiation into integrative and distributive components so that, for example, the parties can first integratively expand the pie and then negotiate the distribution of the enlarged pie. In fact, it is very unlikely for these to happen sequentially. Instead, the processes of integration and distribution occur simultaneously.

Negotiators must simultaneously balance cooperative and competitive behavior, so that they enlarge the pie *while* they claim an acceptable share of the enlarged pie. It is this "fundamental tension between cooperation and competition" that is the heart of negotiation, and that makes negotiation both an art and a science. The way that the value is created affects the way it is divided; the process of creating value is entwined with the process of claiming it (Lax & Sebenius, 1986). This is especially true if the motives and behaviors of the other party are unpredictable before the negotiation or are hard to read during the negotiation.

The Role of Information Sharing

Cooperative or competitive orientations are easy to talk about in general terms, but how do they manifest themselves in actual behavior during a negotiation? One of the core behavioral components of negotiation is information sharing. It is through the sharing of information that parties learn about their opponent's preferences on the issues, BATNA and

reservation price, willingness to concede, interest in adding other issues to the negotiation, and in general, their opponent's overall orientation. Although the total amount of information that is shared during the negotiation is likely to affect the quality of the outcome reached by the parties, examining the subtleties of the parties' information-sharing patterns may be more revealing. First, if one party shares much more information than the other party, the party that receives the greater amount of information may have an advantage because they may know more about how far the other party can be pushed or what the chances are of finding an integrative solution. For example, if only one party knows the other's reservation price, the party with this information knows the size of the bargaining zone while the other does not. This could have a profound impact on the outcome of the negotiation.

One clarification here is that sharing information is not the same as talking. One side may talk more than the other party but share a lesser amount of important information. If negotiation is viewed solely as a persuasive process, then the party that talks more may be expected to do more persuading, and thus achieve a better outcome. However, persuasion is typically not included in what we refer to as information sharing. Information that is relevant in this analysis concerns the interests of the party, and thus the side that gives away less of this information may have an advantage.

Even if the amount of information shared by the parties is symmetric, the order in which it is shared may influence the outcomes of the parties. If one party gives away all of his information before the other party gives away any of her information, the party that delays sharing information may have an advantage, knowing more about the issues and the structure of the negotiation than the other party at an earlier point in the negotiation. Ideally, information should be shared in a reciprocal fashion so that one party gives away information incrementally while receiving equivalent amounts of information from the other party.

There are several strategies aimed at getting more information from the other party. Some of them,

Table 5.2. Creating Value: Integrative Bargaining Strategies

---

1. Know your BATNA. Try to ascertain the other side's BATNA.

2. Analyze your own and the other party's reservation prices to determine the bargaining zone.

3. Set priorities on your interests and those of the other party.

4. Construct multi-issue packages of offers that take into account differences between your own and the other party's priorities.

such as asking questions, are simple but often overlooked. These strategies include:

- building trust between the parties so that information is more likely to be shared
- asking questions
- giving away some information unilaterally in the hope that the other party will reciprocate
- making multiple offers simultaneously so the other party's interests can be inferred from the acceptability of each offer
- searching for post-settlement settlements (agreements that occur based on an extended search after an initial agreement is reached) (Raiffa, 1985).

Of course, the accuracy and specificity of information obtained by the other party is crucial. Discerning the accuracy of the information given by the other party is primarily a matter of trust, both on the part of the party giving information (trusting that the other party will not take advantage of true information) and on the part of the party receiving information (believing the information given by the other party).

Compatible Issues

There is one other type of issue we have not yet mentioned that is frequently overlooked when people think of negotiation. **Compatible issues** are those for which the parties have the same preferences. The parties have no conflict over these issues, perhaps making it seem odd that we include them in a chapter about conflict management. However, they are often included in negotiations because the negotiators do not know they have the same preferences on these issues and they make assumptions about the preferences of the other party.

Specifically, as mentioned earlier, many negotiators have a fixed-pie bias, meaning that they systematically assume their task in a negotiation is to split a fixed amount of resources (Bazerman, Magliozzi, & Neale, 1985; Thompson, 1991). The incompatibility bias inhibits negotiators in a re-

lated way, as they assume that the other party's preferences on the issues are necessarily in direct conflict with their own preferences and that they have no common interests (Thompson, 1991). Because of these biases, issues that are included in a negotiation for which the negotiators want the same outcome are often not identified as compatible, and a substantial number of negotiators settle for an outcome on these issues other than the one they both want.

Multiparty Negotiations

Most of the examples that are used to illustrate negotiations are dyadic, involving two parties. Although there are certainly many negotiations that involve only two parties, a substantial portion of negotiations involve three or more parties (which we refer to as multiparty). In health care, frequent examples involve negotiations among state or federal payment agencies, hospitals, and physicians. While many of the concepts of negotiation generalize from dyadic to multiparty negotiations, there are important differences between these types of negotiation.

The biggest difference is the increased complexity that occurs when parties are added to the negotiation. This complexity falls into two categories. First, interpersonal complexity increases as more people become involved in the interaction. For each person, there are more signals, gestures, and other types of communications from others to interpret. The second type of complexity involves the issues themselves. There are now multiple sets of preferences to be worked through rather than just two sets. For example, regarding the same subset of issues, two parties may have compatible preferences, two other parties may have opposite preferences but place a different amount of importance on these issues, while the preferences of two other parties may be diametrically opposed. Sharing the information to determine these preferences becomes much more difficult with multiple parties, and even if perfect information is shared, it is still a complex task to determine an optimal solution that is acceptable to everyone.

The bargaining zone in a negotiation with multiple parties is defined as the set of agreements that exceed every party's reservation price. It can be very difficult to determine whether a bargaining zone exists, much less the size of the bargaining zone. Furthermore, there may be people involved in the negotiation who would prefer that no agreement be reached, so that their purpose at the negotiation table (whether disguised or not) is to impede the process of the negotiation. Building trust may be more difficult between multiple parties, especially if coalitions form within the group of negotiators.

Coalition formation can have a major effect on the negotiation process and outcome. Coalitions may be based on long-standing relationships outside of the negotiation, or they may form during the negotiation based on similarity of preferences. They may form either to try to reach a specific agreement or to try to block a specific type of agreement. What is best for the coalition may not be what is best for the entire group. Negotiators in a multiparty situation should think about who they would like to form a coalition with, who might like to form a coalition with them, and who is unlikely to want to include them in a coalition.

Proactive behavior may be especially helpful in building a coalition because it should be easier to form a coalition initially than to break up an existing coalition and reform another one. However, coalitions, especially those formed around specific preferences in the negotiation, are likely to be unstable. When considering that the typical reason for joining a coalition is to increase your own outcomes, it is not surprising that people readily switch allegiances when they get better offers from other potential coalition partners. As such, coalitions may shift repeatedly during the course of a negotiation. A caveat to this reasoning is that social bonds between people may lend some stability to coalitions (Polzer, Mannix, & Neale, 1998). Whether it is based on an ongoing relationship or a shared group affiliation, such a bond may cause people to forego short-term gains from switching coalitions and instead opt for the longer-term benefits that flow from strong social connections.

Decision rules for reaching agreement may also be necessary in multiparty negotiations. Possible decision rules include unanimity, majority rule, or some other special rule detailing how many people must agree in order to reach a settlement. Some parties may also have veto power, which affects the power balance in the negotiation. These latter considerations may be influenced by the context within which the negotiation takes place. For example, if all the parties are working in the same organization (e.g., physicians employed by the same hospital), there may be hierarchical considerations, existing norms guiding the selection of a decision rule, or pressure from superiors to reach an agreement. Conversely, in a group negotiation in which the parties represent several different organizations (e.g., physicians having their own organizations), many of the parties may have more freedom to withdraw from the negotiation or force an impasse because they may have better alternatives with other sets of organizations. Also, few norms may exist if the negotiation itself is the first time the parties have been together in a group.

The above factors should be considered when preparing for and participating in a multiparty negotiation. If properly managed, the increased complexity inherent in this type of negotiation does not have to be an impediment and can in fact be used strategically if other parties are less prepared for or less able to cope with the complexity.

Fairness and Ethics in Negotiation

Negotiators often make claims about fairness to support their arguments. Fairness is not a unidimensional concept, however, and the application of different norms of fairness can lead to different outcomes. For this reason, it is important to think about which different norms of fairness can be applied in particular situations so that generalized claims for fairness are not used inappropriately. In a negotiation context, fairness will be discussed as it applies to the allocation of resources, which is the typical result of negotiation.

The most prevalent fairness norm in our society is **equality fairness norm**, in which every party gets the same absolute amount of resources (Rawls, 1971). A second fairness norm that is used in most organizations to determine compensation is **equity fairness norm**, whereby each person gets allocated an amount of resources proportional to his inputs (Adams, 1963; Homans, 1961). Defining what relevant inputs consist of and measuring these inputs can often lead to additional conflict, but once norms are in place in organizations regarding these issues, allocating resources equitably is often regarded as fair. Equity can be invoked in many negotiations other than organizational compensation situations as well. A third popular norm of fairness upon which allocations can be based is the need, so that parties receive an amount of resources proportional to their **need fairness norm** for them (Deutsch, 1975). As with inputs in the equity norm situation, determining the relative needs of each party can be tricky. Besides these three pure allocation norms of fairness, people may combine two or three of these norms to determine a fair allocation. Negotiators should consider which of these norms is applicable when they or one of their opponents claims that the negotiated outcome should be "fair."

Many people think of fairness and ethics in negotiation as somewhat entwined. Fairness may not always refer to the norm used for resource allocation, as discussed above, but instead may refer to the process by which people negotiate. For instance, people often say that if a negotiator is "unethical," she is not negotiating fairly. This triggers the same kind of problem that is triggered when determining fair allocations, in that people are not always in agreement about what constitutes ethical behavior. This is especially relevant for negotiation because there are many typical negotiating strategies, such as bluffing or avoiding an answer to a specific question, that fall in a gray area concerning the ethicality of such behavior. Furthermore, many people believe that what is ethical is partially determined by context. For example, in some cultures, bribes are an accepted way of doing business when negotiating. Others adhere to a more absolute form of ethicality, believing that actions are either ethical or unethical regardless of the situation.

We are not going to state any rules about what is ethical or unethical. Instead, our purpose in discussing ethics is to increase the reader's awareness of several issues. First, however it is defined, unethical behavior is typically the result of self-interest (Murnighan, 1992). People act unethically because they benefit from it. When negotiating, regardless of your particular beliefs about ethics, it is important not to assume that the other party has the same beliefs you do or that they will behave (or restrict their behavior) in the same way you will. Also, unethical behavior can have consequences, especially regarding reputations, such that unethical behavior may help negotiators in the short run but may come back to haunt them in the long run. Negotiations can be full of ethical dilemmas. Thinking through and determining your own standards before you get into difficult situations is advised, as is being cautious, especially when making assumptions about the other party's ethical standards.

Preparing to Negotiate

Preparing for a negotiation often has as much to do with achieving a successful outcome as does the actual negotiation. But what exactly should a negotiator do to prepare for the negotiation? In this section, we offer several suggestions for how to increase the probability of a successful negotiation by preparing appropriately.

The least obvious, and perhaps most important, activity that should be worked on before the negotiation is to develop a BATNA, which was discussed earlier. If negotiators can develop a better and more certain alternative to a negotiated outcome, they will have more power in the negotiation and be likely to reach a better outcome. Determining a reservation price, based partially on the BATNA, is the next step to knowing in advance when you will be willing to walk away from the negotiation rather than reach agreement.

Concerning the negotiation more directly, a negotiator should think about what issues are likely to be included in the negotiation if they have not been specified in advance by either party. What additional issues could you bring to the negotiation? What issues might your opponent want to include? Whatever the set of issues includes, the negotiator should determine the importance of each issue relative to the other issues. This facilitates the process of comparing different offers made by the other party and trading low-priority issues for high-priority issues. Collecting information about the other party's alternatives and the importance that party places on each issue is a priority during a negotiation. It follows that negotiators can enhance their position if they can discover some or all of this information about their opponent before the negotiation. Sometimes this information can be gathered directly from the other negotiator prior to negotiating, while in other situations it may be learned from other sources.

Another important piece of information to gather is how many negotiators the other party will be bringing to the table. This question, along with the determination of how many negotiators your party should bring to the negotiation, is the focus of Debate Time 5.2. A negotiator should also determine before the negotiation how important the relationship with the other party is. What future effects are likely to be caused by reputations that are developed in this negotiation? How much is the other party likely to be concerned about the relationship? The extent to which the decisions that are reached during the negotiation need to be implemented by either party after the negotiation is an important factor related to the relationship between the parties. If you have to rely on the other party to implement part of the deal, it is obviously not good to have the other party unhappy with the agreement or with you. Determining the time constraints faced by each party can be useful, as the party who has the longer time before needing to reach an agreement has an advantage, if both parties know about the time constraints of the other.

Even the end of a negotiation requires preparation. If negotiators do not reveal all of their information during the negotiation, they should think about whether they want to share any of this information after the negotiation. It is usually advisable to keep some information confidential even after the negotiation so the other party does not grow concerned about whether she received a good outcome in the negotiation. The better-prepared party in a negotiation is often the most successful during the negotiation. As in school, doing your homework before the negotiation is half the battle when it is time to take the test.

MANAGING CONFLICT THROUGH THIRD-PARTY INTERVENTION

In many conflict situations, the disputants are unable to resolve the conflict. A third party that is not directly involved in the conflict can frequently intervene in one of several different ways to help resolve the conflict. There are many formal, institutional third parties that can be turned to outside of any particular organization. The court system in the United States is a very large example of a third party. Arbitrators are third parties that resolve differences between parties on many different issues, such as professional baseball salaries. The focus of this chapter, however, is on the manager's role as a third party in the day-to-day conflicts that occur in organizational life, rather than on formal third-party systems. To the extent that conflict is disruptive in organizations and hampers productivity, managers can increase the effectiveness of their organizations by intervening in conflict situations. Of course, the time the manager spends trying to resolve the disputes of other people is a cost to the organization, which needs to be balanced with the benefit derived from decreased conflict.

Dispute Intervention Goals

After making the decision to intervene in a conflict, the manager has a wide range of third-party intervention strategies from which to choose. The par-

---

⚜ DEBATE TIME 5.2   What Do You Think?

POINT: The more people I can bring with me to the negotiation table, the better off I will be. There are many benefits to be realized from including several people in a negotiation party. The more people that are at the negotiation, the more ideas they should be able to think of for ways to reach an integrative outcome. If expertise in different areas is helpful during the negotiation, it may be beneficial to have more "experts" on hand. Multiple roles, such as spokesperson, notekeeper, or financial analyst, can be performed more effectively at the table if a different person performs each function. A higher degree of critical thinking may occur when more people apply different perspectives to the problem being negotiated. Finally, if one party has more people at the negotiation than the other party, the bigger party may be perceived as having more power and may achieve better outcomes as a result.

COUNTERPOINT: I am better off negotiating by myself. The most obvious reason to negotiate alone is that time is a valuable resource, and bringing other people to a negotiation that one person can handle is unnecessarily expensive. There are also more subtle reasons, stemming from intergroup conflict, that more people in each party may not result in better outcomes in a negotiation. When there is a team of negotiators on each side of the table, the intergroup boundaries between the parties may be much stronger than if each party consisted of just one person. When an "us against them" mentality occurs in a negotiation, which may be more likely with groups than with individuals, several negative consequences may result, including increased competitiveness, decreased trust, and a decreased level of information sharing. These may in turn result in outcomes that are inferior to those that may have been reached by individual negotiators bargaining in a more cooperative and trusting manner.

Do you feel it is better to negotiate by yourself or with a team? On what conditions might this depend? Can you think of an example from your experience when having more people/fewer people at the negotiating table was beneficial?

---

ticular role the manager plays in the dispute may depend on what he is trying to accomplish and on the constraints imposed by the situation. When intervening in a dispute between subordinates, a manager has a high level of authority, making any type of intervention an option. This is not the case when a manager intervenes in a dispute between two peers. The amount of conflict between the parties may also influence the manager's selection of intervention strategies. The importance of the issues in dispute, the amount of time pressure faced by the manager, the relative power of the disputants, and the relationships between the parties and between the manager and the parties may all affect the manager's choice of intervention strategies (Neale & Bazerman, 1991). The manager may also be con-

cerned with how satisfied the disputants will be with the resolution and their perceptions of fairness regarding the intervention.

Types of Intervention Strategies

The types of intervention strategies a manager can undertake can be usefully categorized along two dimensions—the control the third party has over the process of the dispute and the control the third party has over the outcome of the dispute. Suppose a medical group practice manager is trying to manage the conflict between primary care physicians and specialists involving sharing revenue generated by the group practice. The control the manager desires over the process and outcome is likely to be affected by

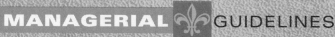

MANAGERIAL GUIDELINES

1. Managers need to analyze the amount and type of both beneficial and detrimental conflicts that currently exist in their organization so that they can focus on eliminating the detrimental conflict.
2. Health care managers should evaluate the level at which conflict usually occurs in their organization. Are there strong group boundaries (e.g., between departments or functional areas) that contribute to conflict, or is most conflict at the individual level?
3. When managers are involved in conflict, they should think explicitly about how much concern they have for the other party, as well as how concerned they are about their own outcomes for the issues involved in the conflict. This should help to determine what conflict-management strategy will be most appropriate.
4. When negotiating, managers need to determine the exact issues that are currently being negotiated and identify any other issues that might be included in the negotiation. Also, the importance of each issue to both the manager and the other party should be compared to determine where mutually beneficial trade-offs might occur.
5. Managers should think carefully about what ethical standards they feel comfortable with *before* they enter situations that involve ethical considerations.
6. Managers should not underestimate the importance of preparing for a negotiation. Failing to adequately prepare is probably the single biggest mistake made by negotiators.
7. If managers are going to intervene in a conflict as a third party, they need to consider how much control they want to have over both the process and the outcome of the dispute. Distinguishing between these types of control will facilitate effective intervention implementation.

the factors discussed in the preceding paragraph. When the manager desires high control over both the process and outcome of the dispute, she may act as an **inquisitor.** In this type of intervention, the manager gathers information on the dispute by asking questions of the physicians, rather than letting them present the information as they would like. The manager then makes a decision about the outcome of the dispute and communicates this to the physicians. As in the court system, a manager acts as a judge or **arbitrator** when he controls the outcome but not the process of the dispute. The parties are free to present their sides of the dispute as they wish, after which the manager makes the decisions necessary to end the dispute. **Mediators** have control over the process of the dispute but have no authority, or do not use their authority, to control the outcome. Acting as mediator, the group practice manager may control the flow of information between the physician groups by separating them and acting as a go-between or may guide the discussion between them when they are together. The outcome, however, will ultimately be decided by the leaders of the respective physician groups.

The manager who chooses not to have high process or outcome control can choose from several options. The most efficient approach from the manager's perspective is to ignore the conflict and hope the disputants will resolve it by themselves. Managers can also delegate responsibility for getting the dispute resolved to someone else. Another option is to threaten the disputants to increase their motivation to resolve the conflict.

Managers have many choices in determining which third-party intervention strategies best fit their needs. It is possible that, for the same dispute situation, a manager may change intervention strategies if the previously chosen strategy does not work. When this happens, a manager will usually progress from strategies involving less control to strategies involving more control.

Although conflict is pervasive, it can be successfully managed through an understanding and application of various conflict-management techniques and negotiation skills. By managing conflict more effectively, health services executives make important contributions to organizational effectiveness while improving the productivity and satisfaction of the people with whom they work.

DISCUSSION QUESTIONS

1. What types of skills do managers need to successfully manage conflict in their organizations? Which of these skills do you possess? What might be your greatest weakness as a conflict resolver? What can you do to strengthen your weak areas?

2. Related to Debate Time 5.1, what are some indications that a health services organization is experiencing dysfunctional levels of conflict? What systems can be put in place to monitor these indicators?

3. What third-party intervention strategies are likely to be favored by managers acting as third parties? What third-party intervention strategies are likely to be favored by the disputants? If these answers are different, what can a manager do to satisfy all the parties involved? What factors may affect your answers to these questions?

4. Regarding intergroup conflict, which groups do you most frequently represent or identify

with in your interactions? How might this change depending on the type of health services organization with which you might be employed?

REFERENCES

Adams, J. S. (1963). Toward an understanding of inequity. *Journal of Abnormal and Social Psychology, 67*, 422–436.

Bazerman, M. H., Magliozzi, T., & Neale, M. A. (1985). The acquisition of an integrative response in a competitive market. *Organizational Behavior and Human Decision Processes, 35*, 294–313.

Deutsch, M. (1949). An experimental study of the effects of cooperation and competition upon group process. *Human Relations, 2*, 199–232.

Deutsch, M. (1975). Equity, equality, and need: What determines which value will be used as the basis of distributive justice? *Journal of Social Issues, 31*, 137–149.

Fisher, R., & Ury, W. (1981). *Getting to yes.* Boston: Houghton-Mifflin.

Homans, G. (1961). *Social behavior: Its elementary forms.* New York: Harcourt, Brace.

Janis, I. (1982). *Groupthink: Psychological studies of policy decisions and fiascoes.* Boston: Houghton-Mifflin.

Jehn, K. A. (1995). A multimethod examination of the benefits and detriments of intragroup conflict. *Administrative Science Quarterly, 40*, 256–282.

Lax, D. A., & Sebenius, J. K. (1986). *The manager as negotiator.* New York: Free Press.

Murnighan, J. K. (1992). *Bargaining games.* New York: William Morrow and Company, Inc.

Neale, M. A., & Bazerman, M. H. (1991). *Cognition and rationality in negotiation.* New York: Free Press, p. 2.

Nordhaus-Bike, A. M. (1997, August 20). Partnering: Unite and Conquer. *Hospitals and Health Network 5*, 7(16).

Northcraft, G. B., & Neale, M. A. (1990). *Organizational behavior: The managerial challenge.* Homewood, IL: Dryden Press.

Polzer, J. T., Mannix, E. A., & Neale, M. A. (1998). Interest alignment and coalitions in multiparty negotiation. *Academy of Management Journal, 41*, 42–54.

Pruitt, D. G. (1983). Achieving integrative agreement. In M. H. Bazerman, & R. J. Lewicki (Eds.), *Negotiating in organizations.* Beverly Hills, CA: Sage.

Pruitt, D. G., & Rubin, J. Z. (1986). *Social conflict.* New York: Academic Press.

Raiffa, H. (1982). *The art and science of negotiation.* Cambridge, MA: Belknap.

Raiffa, H. (1985). Post settlement settlements. *Negotiation Journal, 1,* 9–12.

Rawls, J. (1971). *A theory of justice.* Cambridge, MA: Harvard University Press.

Rubin, J., & Brown, B. (1975). *The social psychology of bargaining and negotiation.* New York: Academic Press.

Sherif, M. (1977). *Intergroup conflict and cooperation.* Norman, OK: University Book Exchange.

Thomas, K. (1976). Conflict and conflict management. In M. Dunnette (Ed.), *Handbook of industrial and organizational psychology.* Chicago: Rand-McNally.

Thompson, L. L. (1991). Information exchange in negotiation. *Journal of Experimental Social Psychology, 27*(2), 161–179.

White, S. B., & Neale, M. A. (1994). The role of negotiation aspiration and settlement expectancies on bargaining outcomes. *Organizational Behavior and Human Decision Processes, 57,* 303–317.

THREE

Operating the Technical System

THE NATURE OF ORGANIZATIONS: FRAMEWORK FOR THE TEXT

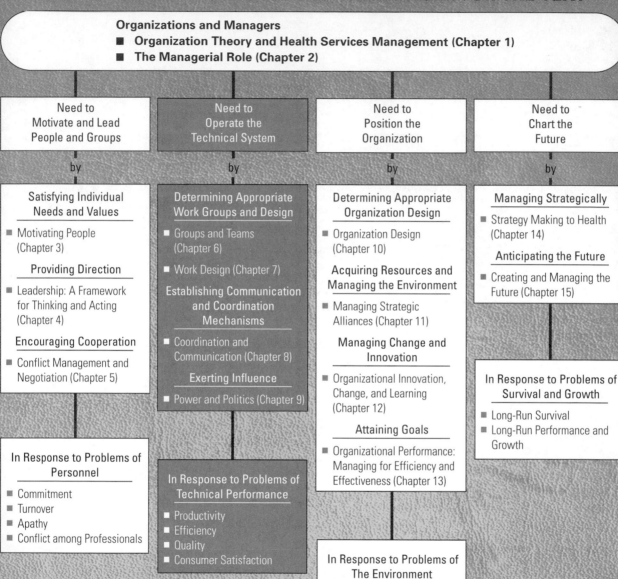

Organizations and Managers
- Organization Theory and Health Services Management (Chapter 1)
- The Managerial Role (Chapter 2)

Need to Motivate and Lead People and Groups	Need to Operate the Technical System	Need to Position the Organization	Need to Chart the Future
by	by	by	by

Satisfying Individual Needs and Values
- Motivating People (Chapter 3)

Providing Direction
- Leadership: A Framework for Thinking and Acting (Chapter 4)

Encouraging Cooperation
- Conflict Management and Negotiation (Chapter 5)

Determining Appropriate Work Groups and Design
- Groups and Teams (Chapter 6)
- Work Design (Chapter 7)

Establishing Communication and Coordination Mechanisms
- Coordination and Communication (Chapter 8)

Exerting Influence
- Power and Politics (Chapter 9)

Determining Appropriate Organization Design
- Organization Design (Chapter 10)

Acquiring Resources and Managing the Environment
- Managing Strategic Alliances (Chapter 11)

Managing Change and Innovation
- Organizational Innovation, Change, and Learning (Chapter 12)

Attaining Goals
- Organizational Performance: Managing for Efficiency and Effectiveness (Chapter 13)

Managing Strategically
- Strategy Making to Health (Chapter 14)

Anticipating the Future
- Creating and Managing the Future (Chapter 15)

In Response to Problems of Personnel
- Commitment
- Turnover
- Apathy
- Conflict among Professionals

In Response to Problems of Technical Performance
- Productivity
- Efficiency
- Quality
- Consumer Satisfaction

In Response to Problems of The Environment
- Environmental Complexity and Uncertainty
- Technological and Social Change
- Competitive Forces
- Multiple Performance Demands

In Response to Problems of Survival and Growth
- Long-Run Survival
- Long-Run Performance and Growth

The four chapters of this section focus on operating critical components of the technical system within health care organizations. This involves determining the appropriate work design, establishing communication and coordination mechanisms, and ensuring and improving performance. The following chapters characterize these functions in order to enhance technical aspects of productivity, efficiency, quality, and consumer satisfaction.

Chapter 6, Groups and Teams, focuses on the effective management of groups and teams. The chapter addresses the following questions:

- Why are groups and teams important?
- How does group structure and process affect performance?
- What are the causes of intergroup conflict, and what strategies are available for its management?

Chapter 7, Work Design, considers the design of work in organizations. The emphasis is on defining different types and components of work and assessing the interconnected nature of work within a variety of health services organizations. The chapter addresses the following questions:

- What is work? Is it different from working?
- How does work design affect individual motivation and productivity?
- How does the interconnectedness of work affect individuals and work groups?

Chapter 8, Coordination and Communication, deals with the essential means through which managers link the various people and groups within the organization and link the organization to other organizations. The following questions provide the major focus of this chapter:

- What is the role of intraorganizational coordination? How is it similar or different from interorganizational coordination?
- What are the major components and barriers of effective communications?

The last chapter in this section, "Power and Politics," discusses the means by which power distributions can be identified, the conditions under which conflict among groups may result, the uses of power to resolve conflict, and the strategies and tactics that are commonly employed to do so. The chapter addresses the following questions:

- What are the sources of power?
- What are the conditions that promote the use of power, politics, and informal influence?
- What approaches are available for consolidating and developing power by managers, physicians, and other groups of health care providers?

Upon completing these four chapters, the reader should be able to understand the nature of work and the processes affecting work within health services organizations.

CHAPTER 6

Groups and Teams

Bruce J. Fried, Ph.D., Sharon Topping, Ph.D., and
Amy C. Edmondson, Ph.D.

CHAPTER OUTLINE

LEARNING OBJECTIVES

After completing this chapter, the reader should be able to:

1. Describe the importance of groups and teams in health care organizations.

2. Distinguish between different approaches to assessing team performance.

3. Understand the factors associated with high-performing teams.

4. Analyze the effects of a work group's composition and size on team performance.

5. Explain the relationship between work group norms and team productivity.

6. Understand the role that cohesiveness plays in determining team performance.

7. Describe key aspects of group process including leadership, the communication structure, decision making, and stages of group development.

8. Explain how a team's task can have a significant effect on team process and productivity.

9. Define the major causes and consequences of intergroup conflict.

10. Explain how available resources, management support, and reward systems can affect teams.

KEY TERMS

Behavior Norm
Boundary Spanning
Communication Structure
Delphi Technique
Environmental Context
Formal and Informal
    Leadership
Formal Groups
Groupthink

Informal Groups
Intergroup Conflict
Management Teams
Nominal Group Technique
Performance Norm
Psychological Safety
Social Capital
Social Loafing
Stages of Team Development

Status Differences
Task Interdependence
Team Cohesiveness
Team Composition
Team Processes
Team Productivity
Team Size

⚜ IN PRACTICE

Improving Preventative Services in a Pediatrics Practice: A Less Than Successful Team

Glendale Pediatrics is a nine-clinician pediatric group practice. The practice serves a largely middle-class suburban population and prides itself on the provision of preventive services. One of the physicians recently attended a continuing medical education program on preventive services. Upon her return, she decided to assess the practice's performance in this area. She and the other physicians were surprised when she distributed the results. Among the findings were:

- Sixty percent of children were behind schedule in at least one immunization.
- Vision screening was conducted and recorded for only 15% of children.
- Fifty percent of children were screened for anemia.
- Twenty-five percent of children had their blood pressure recorded in the patient record.
- Thirteen percent of children were screened for lead.

While the pediatricians were bewildered by these findings, the medical record and nursing staff

found them consistent with their impressions. The findings were presented and discussed at the monthly staff meeting. Two physicians who together saw about 40% of all patients were adamant that their patients were current in their preventive services, so there was no need for a practice-wide effort to improve their preventive service rates. Unfortunately, the data were not linked to individual physicians, so there was no way to verify their claim. Nonetheless, it was agreed that staff, including the two reluctant physicians, work as a team to address the problem. The first meeting was scheduled over the noon hour. One of the physicians arrived at 12:20 P.M., while two others left early, at 12:45. One of the nurses was out sick. No decisions were made and the entire meeting was spent attempting to find a date and time for follow-up meetings.

At the next meeting, one physician stated that during an acute visit, physicians don't have time to go through the medical record to determine if a patient was behind on any preventive services. The other physicians agreed and decided that a form should be

(continues)

IN PRACTICE (continued)

developed listing all preventive services and this should be attached to the medical record. The nurses worked together after the meeting to design the form known as the Preventive Services Chart (PSC).

Three thousand copies of the PSC were printed. When the physicians saw the form, they indicated that it was poorly designed. All relevant services and immunization schedules were not included. The forms were destroyed and the physicians asked the nurses to redesign the form. The nurses consulted with the physician who attended the continuing education seminar to obtain information on the recommended preventive protocols. Based on this information, the form was redesigned with the immunization schedule and other information added. Confident that this was the right form, three thousand copies were again printed. When presented to the physicians, it was discovered that there was little agreement among the physicians and an argument broke out at the next meeting about the immunization schedules and protocols for screening.

After this meeting, one of the nurses in consultation with two physicians develop yet another form with separate columns for each physician's preventive services preferred protocol. The medical records staff, hearing about this new procedure informally over lunch, were skeptical about its feasibility. Moreover, when one of the nurses asked a physician when nurses would record this information, she was told that "nurses have it too easy in this practice. You have a great deal of down time and you certainly can find time to prepare charts for the next day's patients."

During the following three weeks, the following events transpired:

1. Nurses complained to the physicians that medical records staff were not making records available to them in time to do the preventive services review.
2. Medical records staff complained to the physicians that nurses were unrealistically requesting the next day's charts at 9 A.M. so they could spend the day preparing for the next day's patients. They also reported that nurses were rude in their requests.
3. Physicians complained among themselves that preventive services information was absent for almost half of the patients, and they suspected that the information was inaccurate for a significant number of cases for which information was provided.
4. Nurses were spending an additional 1 to 2 hours in the office preparing the next day's files. They complained that the medical records were very hard to decipher. They requested, and were denied, overtime pay.
5. Confusion was rampant when files were prepared for one physician, but another physician ended up seeing the patient. An even more difficult problem was caused by drop-in patients for whom record reviews were not prepared. Nurses spent up to 30 minutes looking over these drop-in charts and recording the information on the PSC.
6. Two weeks after the system was implemented, one nurse quit abruptly at 3 P.M. and walked out.
7. One physician gave each parent the PSC and asked parents to record preventive services themselves since the physicians were "too busy to keep track of this."

After a month, the team met again. The physicians decided that the "solution" caused more problems than it solved. They decided to disband the team and work on the preventive services problem individually.

CHAPTER PURPOSE

As illustrated in the Glendale Pediatrics case, groups and teams are a mainstay of organizational life and will become more important in coming years. The work of health services organizations is increasingly being carried out by groups and teams, and we simply cannot escape the necessity of working in teams. Almost all clinical and managerial innovations are dependent to some degree on effective team performance (see Chapter 12). For example, as patient care technology becomes more specialized, there will be increasing need for team structure to coordinate the work of individual specialists. Quality improvement methods, such as continuous quality improvement, are highly dependent upon well-functioning cross-functional teams.

Teams are pervasive within health services organizations. When managed well, teams can be highly creative and productive and contribute in a positive way to organizational effectiveness. When poorly managed, the organization and its patients or clients can face disastrous consequences.

Most organizational members participate in a variety of teams such as:

- Boards of directors and their committees and subcommittees
- Nursing teams
- Operating room teams
- Research and development teams
- Strategic planning teams
- Treatment teams
- Interorganizational coordinating teams

Members of organizations may assume numerous **task oriented roles** depending on the team and their personal role in the group. An awareness of team concepts is key to organizational performance.

This chapter focuses on the effective management of groups and teams in organizations. It does this by building on Chapters 3 through 5, dealing with issues of motivation, leadership, and conflict management, respectively, and also touches on issues of work de-

sign, power communication and coordination, and organization design, which are subsequently discussed in Chapters 7 through 10, respectively. Following a discussion of the types of groups found in health services organizations, attention is given to issues of team cohesiveness, status differences, team size and composition, communication structure, and task characteristics, including task interdependence and complexity. The following section deals with the question of team productivity and why certain teams are more productive than others.

THE IMPORTANCE OF GROUPS AND TEAMS IN HEALTH SERVICES ORGANIZATIONS

The Glendale Pediatrics case illustrates the variety of ways that teams can run into difficulty. Nonetheless, teams are a mainstay of life in health care, and can be useful vehicles for improving quality—if they are organized and managed in an effective manner.

The use of teams is not unique to health services organizations. It has been found, for example, that 82% of companies with 100 or more employees use teams (Gordon, 1992). The work of health care organizations is increasingly being carried out by teams, and we simply cannot escape the necessity of working in teams. In a study of 56,000 production workers, it was found that one of the most common skills required of employees is the ability to work in a team environment (Capelli & Rogovsky, 1994). Almost all clinical and managerial innovations are dependent to some degree on effective group performance. For example, as patient care technology becomes more specialized, there will be increasing need for team structures to coordinate the work of individual specialists. Quality improvement methods, such as continuous quality improvement, are highly dependent upon well-functioning crossfunctional teams (Fargason

& Haddock, 1992). Given the importance of teams to organizational performance, it is surprising how little systematic attention organizations give to improving team performance, productivity, and efficiency, particularly when decades of research and experience have provided us with a clear understanding of the factors associated with high-performing teams (Cohen & Bailey, 1997).

TYPES OF GROUPS AND TEAMS

There are many different types of groups and teams in all organizations, and in health services organizations in particular. In this chapter, primary attention will be given to formally organized work groups and teams. However, in understanding organizations, it is essential that we understand informal as well as formal structures and processes (Mechanic, 1962). Thus, in addition to formally sanctioned teams, anyone working in an organization needs to be aware of informal groups and their influence on the organization. The importance of informal work group structure and group processes has been recognized for at least 50 years. The Hawthorne experiments firmly established the proposition that an individual's performance is determined in large part by informal relationship patterns that emerge within work groups (Roethlisberger & Dickson, 1939). The work group has a pervasive impact on individual behaviors and attitudes because it controls so many of the stimuli to which the individual is exposed in performing organizational tasks (Hasenfeld, 1983).

Informal Groups

Informal groups are groups that are not directly established or sanctioned by the organization, but often form naturally by individuals in the organization

to fill a personal or social interest or need. There are a variety of types of **informal groups** found in and between organizations. Informal groups can have high motivational value for individuals. A simple, though valid, example of an informal group is a car pool. Car pools meet individual needs by economizing on commuting costs and creating an opportunity for social interaction. They may also be viewed positively by the organization in that they may lead to decreased absenteeism and lateness as well as higher employee morale.

There are a number of circumstances under which informal groups can have a negative impact on an organization. Groups may become overly exclusionary and lead to interpersonal conflict. In other cases, informal groups can become so powerful so as to undermine the formal authority structure of the organization. Consider Etzioni's (1961) classic description of the role of informal groups in factories:

> The workers constituted a cohesive group which had a well-developed normative system of its own. The norms specified, among other things, that a worker was not to work too hard, lest he become a "rate-buster"; nor was he to work too slowly, lest he become a "chiseler" who exploited the group (part of the wages were based on group performance). Under no condition was he to inform or "squeal." By means of informal social control, the group was able to direct the pace of work, the amount of daily and weekly production, the amount of work stoppage, and allocation of work among members. In this instance, informal groups of employees were able to maintain social control as well as control over the pace of work through the imposition of informal, though well-enforced, rules of behavior.

Finally, informal groups can assume a change agent role. Informal groups are often responsible for facilitating improvements in working conditions; such informal groups sometimes evolve into formal groups. A current example is the emergence of physician unions. These often begin informally, perhaps as a group focused on professional interests, but may evolve over time into union status (Erickson, 1997). Informal groups may also emerge to deal with a particular organizational problem or to work toward changes in organizational policies and procedures. Such groups may, in fact, initiate action against a corrupt manager or supervisor.

In sum, informal groups play a unique role in organizations. To the extent possible, managers should be aware of the roles informal groups play in the organization. Where they play a positive role, they may be encouraged by management; when they appear deleterious, managers might consider a variety of alternative options, such as developing a formal employee involvement process to ensure that such attitudes receive a fair hearing in the organizations. Negatively oriented informal groups may be a sign of dissatisfaction among employees.

Formal Groups

In the remainder of this chapter, we focus almost exclusively on **formal groups** and teams. Formal groups arise out of the direct actions or structuring of an organization, and are intentionally established, recognized, and sanctioned by the organization. Because of the difficulties involved in distinguishing between groups and teams, we use these terms interchangeably. We do, however, place certain boundaries on this construct. To distinguish organizational groups from large population-based groups (for example, an ethnic group in a city), we limit our attention to those groups or teams that are authentic organizational-based social systems. Such teams are intact social systems with boundaries, interdependence among members, and differentiated member roles. Organizationally based teams are task-centered: They have one or more tasks to perform and produce measurable outcomes. Finally, they operate within an organizational context and interact with a larger organization or organizational subunits (Hackman, 1990a). This approach is consistent with the following definitions:

> A group is defined as two or more persons who are interacting with one another in such a manner that each person influences and is influenced by each other person (Shaw, 1976).
>
> A team is a collection of individuals who are interdependent in their tasks, who share responsibility for outcomes, who see themselves and who are seen by others as an intact social entity embedded in one or more larger social systems, and who manage their relationships across organizational boundaries (Cohen & Bailey, 1997).

We include groups that are established for a relatively short period of time, such as project task forces, as well as more permanent groups. Cohen and Bailey (1997) provide a useful scheme for classifying teams in organizations. We adopt this scheme in this chapter and provide health care examples of each type of team:

- Work teams are continuing work units responsible for producing goods or providing services. These teams may be directed by supervisors or may be self-managing. In the health care environment, these include treatment teams, research teams, and home care teams. They tend to be ongoing and relatively permanent in nature. As with other teams, membership may be stable or unstable over time, and may be multi- or unidisciplinary. One particular type of work team receiving a great deal of attention are termed "microsystems"—a small group of people who work together on a regular basis to provide care to discrete patient subpopulations (Nelson et al., 2002). These are freestanding units with both clinical and business aims designed to maximize performance outcomes (Batalden, Nelson, Edwards, Godfrey, & Mohr, 2003).

- Parallel teams pull together people from different work units or jobs to perform functions that the regular organization is not equipped to perform. They usually have limited authority and generally make recommendations to individuals higher up in the hierarchy. These include quality improvement teams, employee involvement groups, and task forces. In the health care system, parallel teams may be involved in such activities as continuous quality improvement (CQI) and process improvement, community health needs assessment, and staff search committees. By their nature, they are often multi-disciplinary. As suggested by the diversity of teams falling into this category, these teams may be temporary or permanent features of the organization.

- Project teams are time-limited, producing one-time outputs such as a new product or service or a new information system. In health care, such teams may exist for purposes of planning a new hospital, developing a new asthma drug, or selecting a new human resources information system.

- **Management teams** coordinate and provide direction to the subunits under their jurisdiction. Management teams may exist at the board level, senior management level, or departmental level.

It is important to understand that all personnel are members of a variety of formal and informal groups, and as such, may assume many different team roles and various personas. A surgeon, for example, may play a strong and influential leadership role in the operating room, but when working on a physician staff subcommittee with her peers, may have relatively little power or influence. Roles may vary dramatically with respect to power and normative and behavioral expectations. As team members, it is critical to understand where individuals fit within the context of a particular team. At times, the demands of multiple roles—particularly among professionals—may compete with one another for time and commitment, leading to feelings of role ambiguity, role conflict, and stress.

Notwithstanding the importance of teams in organizations, there is likely no other aspect of organizational life that causes as much ambivalence, and at times disdain and cynicism. Many teams achieve far less than their potential because of coordination, communication, or motivational problems among group members, collectively known as process losses (Steiner, 1972). While many of us enjoy the interactions and synergies associated with working on teams, groups may often create misunderstandings and bring out latent conflicts between individuals. Interprofessional rivalries and status differences are often played out in groups causing anger, dissatisfaction, lower productivity, and frequently, a sense that individuals' knowledge and skills are underutilized. Anyone who has spent time in teams is aware of the destructive potential of personality clashes and of the impact of "toxic managers" (Lubit, 2003) and team leaders. The impact of conflict and psychologically destructive managers is often severe in the relatively intimate environment of work groups and teams. **Social loafing**, a situation in which individuals may exert less effort when they work in a group than when they work alone (also known as "free-riding" and "shirking"), is certainly not uncommon in many teams (George, 1992; Latane, Williams, & Harkins, 1979; Liden, Wayne, Jaworski, & Bennett, 2004).

UNDERSTANDING AND IMPROVING TEAM PERFORMANCE

In understanding team performance, it is important to disentangle two separate questions about performance.

- Is a team approach (or a particular team approach) more effective than nonteam (or alternative team) approaches? In this question, we are asking, for example, if a team nursing approach produces better patient outcomes than traditional nonteam-based methods.

- Assuming that a team approach will be used (for example, a basketball team), what factors account for different levels of team performance? In this chapter, the perspective generally taken is that teams are a mainstay of organizational life and that we need to seek ways of making them more effective. However, we need to be cognizant of the fact that novel team-based approaches are not necessarily superior to traditional methods (Cassard, Weisman, Gordon, & Wong, 1994).

We have all been members of many teams and have had the opportunity to observe other teams in action. From these observations, it is apparent that teams vary in their effectiveness and efficiency. Why is there such variation in the performance of teams? Some variation may be due to differences in the skills of individual members, an explanation that may be salient in certain types of teams, such as sports teams. On the other hand, there are many situations where individual team members may be highly talented, but produce poor decisions or other poor outcomes. Later in this chapter, the concept of "groupthink" is presented in which sometimes disastrously poor advice may be generated by a team of highly talented and skilled individuals because of dysfunctional group and communication processes.

Team improvement is a key aspect of team performance. Even the most high-performing teams continuously seek to improve. In fact, the drive to improve and having the mechanisms to facilitate improvement are mainstays of effective teams. In health care, improvement goes hand in hand with adaptation to change. For teams to maintain their effectiveness in a changing environment, they must be sufficiently flexible to adapt and find new ways to improve their level of performance (Edmondson, 1996; Edmondson, Bohmer, & Pisano, 2001). One of the most important mechanisms to facilitate team improvement is the capacity of teams to learn. High-performing teams critically reflect on their performance, and use their experience to identify areas for improvement and set goals (Edmondson, 1999, 2003).

A MODEL OF TEAM EFFECTIVENESS

What makes teams effective? What can leaders do to help teams become more productive and satisfying? To address these questions and others, team performance is considered dependent upon a host of factors related to team characteristics, team processes, work characteristics, and the larger environment within which the group is embedded. A multidimensional model is necessary because team performance is not a simple phenomenon and is influenced by factors at a variety of levels. While these factors cannot always be controlled, an understanding of their potential impact on team performance should provide leaders with appropriate strategies for team management. Figure 6.1 provides an overview of these factors. At the team characteristics level, the following are included: team composition and size, team relationships and status differences, psychological safety, team norms, and team cohesiveness. At the task level, team goals and task interdependence are discussed. The team context refers to the environment within which the team functions, and includes the level and type of intergroup relationships and conflict the organizational culture and the natural environment. At the team processes level, leadership, communication, decision making, the capacity of the team to learn, the network and interaction patterns that occur in the team, and stages of team development are considered.

Before embarking on a detailed discussion of these factors, several points are in order. First, the purpose in adopting a particular model of team performance is to provide a framework for organizing a large amount of research spanning several decades. Similar models have been developed, with varying strengths and drawbacks (Hackman, 1982; Kolodny & Kiggundu, 1980; Arrow, McGrath, & Berdahl, 2000; Steiner, 1972). The model developed here includes most of the variables considered

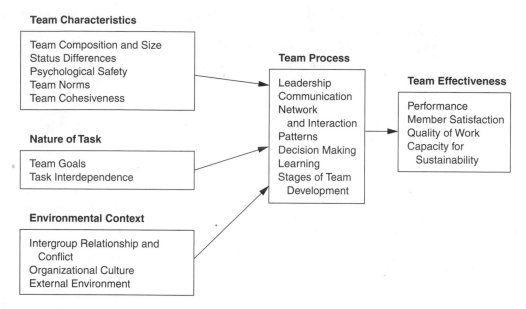

Figure 6.1. A Model of Team Effectiveness

in other models; further, the variables contained in this model have been subjected to empirical tests with a large sample of groups and teams. The second point concerns the nature of research that has led to our conclusions about group performance. Team effectiveness research is frequently inconclusive, due in part to problems with generalizability, small sample sizes, as well as the general problems encountered in testing complex multivariate models. Conclusions and recommendations, therefore, are based on empirical research as well as the qualitative and cumulative experiences of managers.

Team Effectiveness

Team effectiveness goes beyond meeting performance goals to include team member learning and satisfaction, and team sustainability (Hackman, 1982). What does it mean to talk about team performance? In the most general sense, a team performs well when it accomplishes its goals. For some teams, goals are clear, as in a sports team. Other teams, however, are faced with multiple and some-

times conflicting goals (Brodbeck, 1996). A medical group practice, for example, likely has a goal of providing high-quality health services. It may also have efficiency and revenue goals that may conflict with quality goals. Further, the medical practice may seek to position itself as the employer of choice in its community. This may require paying higher than average wages and maintaining a reasonable workload for its employees. While not necessarily conflicting with its quality and revenue goals, they present tensions. Defining performance and performance objectives for most health care teams is thus not straightforward, but it is critically important for team members to understand and agree upon team goals, and to find ways to manage conflicting goals.

Team productivity—the amount of work produced with a given set of resources, such as time, people, money, and expertise—is an important aspect of performance. Assessing the quality of a team's work is more difficult than assessing productivity. Like an organization, a team can be effective in achieving its mission but do so in a highly inefficient manner. Sometimes, of course, efficiency and quality go hand-in-hand. A strategic planning team may eventually produce a well-developed plan, but may take so long to complete the process that it is no longer relevant or useful to the organization. A cardiac surgery team that keeps procedure time as low as possible is attending to efficiency in the use of scarce operating room and staff time and to the quality of care, by reducing a patient's time on bypass (Edmondson et al., 2001). Alternatively, efficiency and quality can be at odds, such as when a team is efficient in decision making but produces poor decisions.

Team member learning and satisfaction, or the degree to which each person finds the experience of working on the team to be helping him or her achieve individual personal and professional goals for satisfying, skill-enhancing work, constitute another important team outcome. If a team performs its tasks well but its members suffer unduly or fail to gain knowledge and skills in the process, the team is, in an important sense, less effective than it would be if these member needs were met. Thus, effective groups are those that not only fulfill the task requirements that serve the organization but also the *social* needs and goals of group members (Cummings, 1978; Guzzo, 1990).

Team member satisfaction can also have a substantial impact on current and future group functioning. In the process of working together, a team can become a more—or less—viable work unit. Optimally, the team will continually refine its processes to facilitate future functioning. When we consider team effectiveness, therefore, we usually consider (1) productivity, (2) quality of work, (3) team member satisfaction, and (4) the capacity of the group for continued cooperation. The following types of questions represent indicators of these dimensions of performance:

- Does the cardiac surgery team produce successful surgeries?
- Does the aged care assessment team increase continuity of care for older persons discharged from the hospital?

- Does the research team produce a proposal that generates funding?
- How quickly is an operating room prepared for the next surgical procedure?
- To what extent does the Alzheimer drug development team stay within its R & D budget?
- Do self-managing nursing units have a positive impact on patient post-discharge outcomes?
- What is the level of satisfaction among patients seen by a physician group practice?
- To what extent are members satisfied with the manner in which a team operates?
- Do team members feel the team is effective? Do team members trust each other?

Considerable research and the framework presented in Figure 6.1 indicate that team effectiveness is dependent upon team processes, including how team members interact, communicate, coordinate their work, and make decisions (Hackman 1982; McGrath, 1984).

Team Processes

Team processes involve the actions and interactions that take place in the team through which decisions are made, problems are solved, and work is accomplished. Thus, team processes refers to the methods of interacting and performing work by team members alone and in interaction with each other. In our description of team processes, we include leadership, communication (both within and outside the team boundaries), decision making, and learning. The end of this section comments on stages of team development, to help team members and managers anticipate some of the predictable events and experiences of a team's life.

Leadership

Leadership in groups refers to the ability of individuals to influence other members toward the achievement of the team's goals. Leadership in groups has been studied extensively. In one study, leadership in intensive care units (ICUs) was positively related to efficiency of operation, satisfaction, and lower turnover of nurses (Shortell, Zimmerman, Rousseau et al., 1994). Successful leaders adopted a supportive **formal** or **informal leadership** style, emphasizing standards of excellence, encouraging interaction, communicating clear goals and expectations, responding to changing needs, and providing support resources when possible. In another study, surgeon leadership was critical to the successful implementation of a new technology (Edmondson, 2003). Successful leaders communicated a compelling rationale for the change, motivating others to exert the necessary effort, and also minimized the status difference between themselves and other members of the operating room team, to facilitate others' ability to speak up with questions, observations, and concerns.

Some teams have multiple leaders. For instance, there may be a formal leader as well as several informal ones. Examples of formal leaders are head nurses, department managers, and project committee chairs. Formal leaders have legitimate authority over the team (i.e., the organization has granted these individuals power along with some ability to use formal rewards and sanctions to support that authority). The formal leader may not be the most influential person on the team. The extent to which team members accept the formal leader's wishes is, in large part, determined by the reaction of the informal leader(s) to those wishes. Note that there is a difference between ad hoc groups, such as parallel and project teams, and formal work teams. In a parallel or project team, an informal leader may be selected as the group's formal leader. This is the rationale for appointing high-profile individuals to chair significant CQI teams or to serve as "honorary chairs" of important search committees. In work teams, however, there is no opportunity for choice. It may be that the formal leader is not the person on whom the teams depend, but it is the "informal leader who embodies the values of the group, aids it in accomplishing objectives, facilitates group maintenance, and usually serves as team spokesperson" (Hunsaker & Cook, 1986).

In deciding upon a leadership style, therefore, group leaders need to consider in realistic terms their formal and informal authority within the group. Use of a coercive or forceful style may backfire when the individual does not have the power to back up decisions. Such a leader may find that the informal leader is able to veto, modify, or sabotage demands. Webster, Grusky, Young, and Podus (1998), using case-management teams, found that "powerless leaders" were faced with the formation of cliques and competition from more influential members. It is best, therefore, for the formal leader not only to consider the views of informal leaders, but also to collaborate with them if possible. Related issues of leadership are discussed further in Chapter 4.

Communication Network and Interaction Patterns

A group cannot function effectively as a team unless members can exchange information. Team leaders are usually best positioned to help manage communications within a team and between the team and external groups (Hackman, 1982). Consider the case of a nurse in a neonatal intensive care unit who has just met with a patient's physician and must pass on vital information to the nurse on the next shift as well as to the parents who will visit during the next shift. How does information get conveyed? Without workable **communication structures**, important information may be lost or inaccurately communicated. In fact, the evaluation and design of communication structures are important components of many quality improvement projects (see Chapter 8).

Communication speed and accuracy in a team are influenced both by the nature of the group's communication network and by the complexity of the group's task. When a task is simple and communication networks are centralized (e.g., a wheel and spoke structure), both speed and accuracy are higher. When tasks are relatively complex, centralized communication networks lower both speed and accuracy, because people serving as network hubs (i.e., information disseminators) may suffer from information overload. In this situation, communication networks are best decentralized (e.g., a star-shaped structure), relieving a manager from the need to filter (and possibly distort) information before it is passed on. In the example of the neonatal intensive care unit, it would be inefficient and risk error to have a nurse on the earlier shift communicate needed information to a head nurse first, who would then pass it on to the next shift's nurse. Timeliness and accuracy are both served by direct communication between the two nurses on the front lines of care. The team should thus use a communication structure that encourages direct interaction between nurses on sequential shifts.

The team communication network can be best described in terms of process behavior and interaction strategies (Coopman, 2001; Stewart & Barrick, 2000). This involves the type of interaction that occurs between members (Stewart & Barrick, 2000). Most measurement of this behavior is based on the work of Bales (1950), who separated group process into either maintenance behaviors or task behaviors. The maintenance category includes interpersonal activities that lead to open communication, supportiveness, and reduction of interpersonal conflict. Task behaviors are those that relate directly to the team's work on its task. Using such a classification system, it should be possible to determine how group interaction develops and to assess the effectiveness of the process (Hackman, 1987). In a study of multidicisplinary, interagency teams coordinating services to youth with serious emotional disturbances, it was found that new teams engaged in more maintenance behavior than older, more experienced teams (Topping, Breland, & Fowler, 2004). Moreover, the focus on maintenance interactions occurred throughout the meeting indicating that teams in the forming stage do interact differently. As a result, the new teams had less task-oriented interaction; therefore, they reviewed fewer cases and engaged in less task-oriented behavior.

Although most of the focus in teams is on internal communications, many teams also rely on external relationships to perform well (Gladstein, 1984). **Boundary-spanning** activities help teams

coordinate with other teams in the organization and ensure that team activities serve the needs of the organization as a whole. Nadler and Tushman's (1988) research found that successful groups matched their information-processing capacity to the information-processing demands of the task environment.

New product or new technology teams, for example, use a diverse array of members, including researchers from the marketing department, physicians from the medical staff, and administrators from the top management team. Each member serves in a boundary-spanning role, because he or she is responsible for representing and communicating with their external function, while also working interdependently with other members of the team. Clearly, it is not just the amount of the external communication but also the type of communication that occurs between a team and its outside boundaries. Ancona and Caldwell (1992a) use the following classification to describe the range of boundary-spanning activities observed in their research:

- *Ambassador activities*—Members carrying out these activities communicate frequently with those above them in the hierarchy. This set of activities is used to protect the team from outside pressures, to persuade others to support the team, and to lobby for resources.

- *Task-coordinator activities*—Members carrying out these activities communicate frequently with other groups and persons at lateral levels in the organization. These activities include discussing problems with others, obtaining feedback, and coordinating and negotiating with outsiders.

- *Scout activities*—Members carrying out these activities are involved in general scanning for ideas and information about the external environment. These differ from the other two in that these activities relate to general scanning instead of specific coordination issues.

Generally, effective teams engage in high levels of ambassadorial and task-coordinator activities and low levels of prolonged scouting activities. Other "isolationist teams" neglected external activity alto-gcthcr, and thus tcndcd to do quitc poorly, proba-bly due to being out of touch with the environment in which they work. In addition, some groups such as R&D teams use boundary spanning as an effec-tive means of communication, but have found that stakeholder (customer) ratings were highest when the project leader—not the team—was the source of information (Hirst & Mann, 2004).

In sum, the increasing reliance on teams in health care organizations and the expanding responsibili-ties placed on them require strong communication structures both within the team and between the team and other groups outside the boundaries.

Decision Making

Most teams are involved in making decisions at some point. This does not mean that all team mem-bers are involved in making all decisions. To illus-trate, for a particular decision, a hospital president may ask for the opinions of his or her senior man-agement team, but retain the right to make the final decision. Similarly, a physician may obtain input from a variety of professionals but make the final determination on treatment. Managers can decrease the probability of misunderstandings by clarifying the role of the team and the role of each member in a particular decision. Team members can generally deal with limitations on their influence as long as the boundaries of their influence are clear initially.

In contrast, decision making in a multidiscipli-nary research team—set up to produce high-quality research by leveraging diversity of inputs—calls for a highly participative approach, with considerable dialogue and discussion prior to coming to a deci-sion, and decisions can be based on consensus and compromise (Edmondson, Watkins, & Roberto, 2003). A third scenario considers the need for speed, reducing the opportunity for extensive par-ticipation in certain teams, for example, decision making in an emergency triage team, where time is critical and decisions must be made quickly and of-ten by a single individual. Clearly, we would not want to use the team decision-making style used by the multidisciplinary research team above in an

emergency department. Conversely, given the ambi-guities faced in research and the need for multiple perspectives (and few urgent time constraints), we would not want one individual making unilateral decisions in this context.

Leaders also can clarify the difference between problem solving and decision making. Some groups, such as many CQI teams, are established to solve problems, or seek methods for improving a particular organizational process. They may not be given authority to implement decisions, however, particularly when substantial resources are required.

The process by which information is exchanged and decisions made is of central importance. Teams naturally attempt to make correct decisions, apply-ing all available information to the issue at hand. One common problem that prevents complete shar-ing of information among members of a team is that of the "free rider". The term *free rider* refers to a member of a team who obtains the benefits of group membership but does not accept a proportional share of the costs of membership (Albanese & Van Fleet, 1985). The free rider is seen as someone who promotes self-interest (the personal acquisition of benefits) over the public interest (the need to con-tribute to the activity that produces those benefits). It is often observed that the larger the group, the greater the free-rider effect (Roberts & Hunt, 1991).

What can managers do to minimize free riding? Through effective use of power, design of organiza-tions (including the size of the organizational units), and control of access to rewards and punishment, management influences the incentive system of group members (Albanese & Van Fleet, 1985). At a routine level, this influence may be achieved by offering fi-nancial incentives or special forms of recognition to particular group members. In the longer run, it is im-portant for managers to deal with the free-rider prob-lem by attempting to broaden the individual's concept of self-interest by creating, communicating, and maintaining a group culture that views effort ex-pended on team processes as contributing to a shared goal that is meaningful to him or her.

Effective use of information in the group deci-sion-making process does not always occur. First, unique information (known by only one member) tends not to surface in group discussions (Stasser, 1999). Experimental studies have demonstrated that groups tend to dwell on common information (that held by all members), such that privately held information fails to surface; further, when it does surface, its impact is often muted (Larson, Christensen, Abbott, & Franz, 1996).

Second, groups can become polarized on an issue in ways that do not reflect the full range of information and opinion in the group. First, as team members compare their positions on the issue with those of others on the team, pressures emerge to accept one position or the other as the *team* position. Second, when one position is more forcefully argued than another, it gains support, despite initial discussion that revealed no clearly favored argument (Cartwright & Zander, 1968).

Third, a phenomenon known as **groupthink** can lead to premature convergence on a poor decision (Janis, 1972). The concept emerged from Janis's studies of high-level policy decisions by government leaders including decisions about Vietnam, the Bay of Pigs, and the Korean War. Groupthink occurs when the desire for harmony and consensus overrides members' rational efforts to appraise the situation. In other words, groupthink occurs when maintaining the pleasant atmosphere of the team implicitly becomes more important to members than reaching a good decision. Some or all of the following symptoms may indicate the presence of groupthink (Janis, 1972):

1. *The illusion of invulnerability.* Team members may reassure themselves about obvious dangers and become overly optimistic and willing to take extraordinary risks.

2. *Collective rationalization.* Teams may overlook blind spots in their plans. When confronted with conflicting information, the team may spend considerable time and energy refuting the information and rationalizing a decision.

3. *Belief in the inherent morality of the team.* Highly cohesive teams may develop a sense of self-righteousness about their role and make them insensitive to the consequences of decisions.

4. *Stereotyping others.* Victims of groupthink hold biased, highly negative views of competing teams. They assume that they are unable to negotiate with other teams, and rule out compromise.

5. *Pressures to conform.* Group members face severe *pressures* to conform to team norms and to team decisions. Dissent is considered abnormal and may lead to formal or informal punishment.

6. *The use of mindguards.* Mindguards are members who withhold or discount dissonant information that interferes with the team's current view of a problem.

7. *Self-censorship.* Teams subject to groupthink pressure members to remain silent about possible misgivings and to minimize self-doubts about a decision.

8. *Illusion of unanimity.* A sense of unanimity emerges when members assume that silence and lack of protest signify agreement and consensus.

The consequences of groupthink are that teams may limit themselves, often prematurely, to one possible solution and fail to conduct a comprehensive analysis of a problem. When groupthink is well entrenched, members may fail to review their decisions in light of new information or changing events. Teams may also fail to consult adequately with experts within or outside the organization, and fail to develop contingency plans in the event that the decision turns out to be wrong.

Team leaders can help avoid groupthink. First, leaders can encourage members to critically evaluate proposals and solutions. Where a leader is particularly powerful and influential (yet still wants to get unbiased views from team members), the leader may refrain from stating his or her own position until later in the decision-making process. Another strategy is to assign the same problem to two separate work teams. Most importantly, groupthink can be avoided by proactively engaging in a process of *critical appraisal* of ideas and solutions, and by understanding the warning signs of groupthink. Managers might also consider alternative systematic methods of decision making that emphasize member participation. **Nominal group technique** and **Delphi technique** elicit group members' opinions prior to judgments about those opinions. These techniques and other approaches help generate ideas, and facilitate objective debate (Delbecq, Van de Ven, & Gustafson, 1975; Edmondson et al., 2003).

Learning

In a changing and uncertain world, a team's ability to learn is essential to its ongoing effectiveness (Edmondson, 1999). In the organizational literature, some discuss learning as an outcome, others as a process (Edmondson, 1999). This chapter joins the latter tradition in treating team learning as a process, and we describe the behaviors and activities through which teams learn. Team learning is defined as an iterative process of reflection and action through which teams may discover and correct problems and errors in their work processes.

Learning processes consist of activities carried out by team members through which a team obtains and processes data that allow it to adapt and improve. Examples include seeking feedback on how well the team's outputs meet its customers' needs, talking about errors, and experimenting. It is through these activities that teams detect changes in the environment, better understand customer requirements, develop members' collective understanding of the situation, or discover unexpected consequences of previous team actions.

A study of cardiac surgery operating room teams learning to use a new technology for minimally invasive surgery found that the teams that were successful did a great deal more reflecting aloud on what they were learning, on how the process was going, and what changes might be made going for-

ward than other teams (Edmondson, 2003). The learning for these teams involved acquiring knowledge and skill related to technical aspects of the new technology. It also involved practicing new interpersonal behaviors, such as speaking up in the operating room in new ways.

The behaviors through which teams learn involve interpersonal risk for individuals. For instance, other team members may think less of an individual for raising a concern, admitting an error, or asking a question for which the answer seems obvious to some. For this reason, learning in teams is greatly enabled by a climate of **psychological safety**, in which people believe that others will not think less of them for well-intentioned risks. This is an element of team climate, and is described further later in this chapter.

In health care, team learning is particularly important for two reasons. First, medical knowledge is constantly developing; individual providers must keep up with new care protocols, medications, and technologies. Physicians keep up with new developments in biology and medical technology by scanning the medical literature, attending conferences, and consulting with trusted colleagues. In fact, developments in science and medicine have always required continuing education for physicians and nurses. At the same time, however, the organizational context of health care delivery has changed in ways that increase the interdependence of the care delivery process, so that groups must learn how to better coordinate their activities to reflect changes in care protocols and to adjust to the unexpected.

Another vital element of team learning in health care is the detection and correction of error. One way this learning occurs is through Morbidity and Mortality (M&M) rounds; however, physicians are often uncomfortable openly discussing errors with their colleagues, such that much learning about error remains private and individual. The current medicolegal environment, which holds the individual accountable for medical outcomes, together with the ethic of professional conscientiousness, serves to reinforce a model of learning focused on private learning by individual practitioners (Bohmer & Edmondson, 2001). Yet, team learning where new insights are rapidly shared among providers is a critical part of the new environment of health care, and increasingly, health care organizations are learning how to learn from their own failures. For example, Children's Hospital and Clinics of Minneapolis instituted "blamefree reporting" and safety action teams to encourage the reporting of mistakes and near misses to learn how to prevent them, and Intermountain Health Care in Utah uses an integrated system that blends information technology and behavioral norms to allow the hospitals to learn from error and continuously improve the quality of care (Edmondson, 2004; Bohmer & Edmondson, 2002). In these cases, managers have worked hard to help people overcome the stigma of error, for the purpose of continuous, collective learning.

Stages of Team Development

Although all teams will not proceed through the same **stages of team development**, the following sequence of development is widely known and has been found to occur in many groups (Tuckman, 1965; Whetten & Cameron, 1998):

1. *Forming.* During the first stage, members become acquainted with each other and with the team purpose. Members attempt to discover what behaviors are acceptable and unacceptable, while establishing trust and familiarity. This early stage is characterized by polite interactions and tentative interactions. Establishing a clear direction is critical.

2. *Storming.* At this stage, the team is faced with disagreement, counter-independence, and the need to manage conflict. Members may attempt to influence the development of group norms, roles, and procedures; therefore, the stage has high potential for conflict. Focusing on process improvements, team achievement, and collaborative relationships can help overcome emergent conflicts.

3. *Norming.* During this stage, the team grows more cohesive and aligned in purpose and actions. Agreement on rules and processes of decision making, roles and expectations, and commitment emerges. Emphasizing the team's direction or goals is essential for forward progress.

4. *Performing.* Once team members agree on the purpose and norms of the group, they can move forward to the task of defining separate roles and establishing work plans. The team is faced with the need for continuous improvement, innovation, and speed. Leaders must be ready to sponsor new ideas, orchestrate their implementation, and foster extraordinary performance from members.

5. *Adjourning.* For temporary teams, the adjournment stage is characterized by a sense of task accomplishment, regret, and increased emotionality.

Not all teams pass through all stages. Some teams may begin at a norming or performing stage (e.g., members that have worked together before), while some may never move beyond the storming stage. Moreover, teams may not move in a linear fashion through the stages, but exhibit long stable periods in which little occurs interspersed with relatively brief periods of drastic progress—a "punctuated equilibrium" model (Gersick, 1989). Finally, some teams may revert to earlier stages of development, as a result of new tasks or responsibilities given the team, a change in formal or informal leadership, the addition of a new member, or the loss of a valuable member. Managers may wish to consider the stage of team development in establishing expectations for a group. For example, research has shown that managers of virtual teams need to know the challenges associated with each stage of the life cycle and time appropriate intervention strategies accordingly (Furst, Reeves, Rosen, & Blackburn, 2004). An example of such a strategy is the active involvement of a senior sponsor in clarifying team mission and goals during the early stages of team development.

Team Process as an Intermediary

Team processes are thus the intermediary between team structures and the outcome of team effectiveness. Through ineffective processes, teams composed of highly talented individuals can be dysfunctional. Conversely, effective processes allow the team to achieve its potential. Team processes are thus important because unlike relatively unchangeable inputs, such as the team's composition and task described below, team processes can be altered and improved upon by team members and leaders. Teams can learn how to better communicate, leaders can improve their ability to manage meetings and coach other team members, team members can experiment with different types of decision making, and teams can learn and improve. The extent to which these and other processes are appropriately used can have a profound impact on team outcomes. Finally, what constitutes effective team processes is contingent on the context. As noted above, saving lives in an emergency department requires extraordinary and rapid communication, and a unilateral decision-making style, while a medical research team can benefit from a participative consensus-seeking approach. In sum, no single set of team processes meets every team's needs; team processes are dependent upon structural aspects of the team, including team size, the nature of team tasks, and the larger context within which the team operates

Team Characteristics

Teams are more than a collection of individuals. Every team has certain characteristics that influence and determine the way members interact with each other. These characteristics include team composition and size, status differences, psychological safety of the team, team norms, and team cohesiveness. The manner in which these are understood and managed will affect the performance of a team. Remember that it is just as important to set the team up correctly as to run it correctly.

Team Composition and Size

Team membership is an important factor in understanding group performance. For certain types of teams, it is easier to control the membership of the group than in others. The CEO of a hospital can select from a wide variety of employees to sit on a strategic planning task force, while the director of nursing may be highly constrained in the nurses chosen for a self-managed nursing team in the pediatric oncology unit. In the latter situation, the director of nursing is limited by the pool of nurses in the unit or trained in such a specialty area. However, an awareness of likely problems related to membership helps, at least, to identify potential problems and to develop strategies to manage them. In our examination of **team composition**, we consider the following diagnostic questions (Hackman, 1990b):

- Is the team appropriately staffed? Is the diversity of members appropriate?

- Do members have the expertise required to perform team tasks well?

- Are the members so similar that there is little for them to learn from one another? Or, so heterogeneous that they risk having difficulty communicating and coordinating with one another?

- Is the team composed of members who have worked together before, or if not, will they need time to get to know each other?

Group composition may vary along a number of dimensions such as age, occupation, gender, tenure, abilities, personality, and experience of members and is an important factor affecting team process and effectiveness. Diversity, or the distribution of personal attributes among interdependent members, is likely to affect the way individuals perceive each other in the group and how well they work together (Jackson, Joshi, & Erhardt, 2003). This, in turn, affects team performance. Most research on group composition concludes that overall diversity of group members is desirable when the task is complex and has a limited time span (Campion, Medsker, & Higgs, 1993). This is especially true when members are heterogeneous in terms of abilities and experiences (Athanasaw, 2003; Gist, Locke, & Taylor, 1987). One study found, however, that a balance between different levels of managerial experience was needed in teams used in entrepreneurial firms from the medical and surgical instruments industry (Kor, 2003). That is, the more effective teams were composed of members with a balance between industry and team experience; too much of either created conflict and decreased the ability of the team to seize new growth opportunities.

The issue of diversity has become a very important concern in health care organizations. Diversity can help to promote quality and competitive advantage by including staff that can best understand diverse cultures. From a legal perspective, diversity is a concern in compliance with equal employment opportunities. Diversity has become so important that the Joint Commission on Accreditation of Healthcare Organizations (2005) has instituted several requirements for staff diversity and cultural competence.

It also seems that when teams have long life spans, effectiveness may be related more to personal compatibility among members (Sundstrom, DeMeuse, & Futrell, 1990). Although diversity brings many advantages, it also comes with problems, such as an increase in conflict and a loss of cohesiveness (Alexander, Jinnett, D'Aunno, & Ullman, 1996; Arrow, McGrath, & Berdahl, 2000). Researchers, finding a negative relationship between diversity and performance in new product development teams, suggest that group heterogeneity might prevent social integration and cohesion from occurring (Ancona & Caldwell, 1992b). As a result, conflict begins in the initial stages of group formation and affects performance throughout the team's existence. In multidisciplinary teams in health care, this is especially prevalent due to the differences between disciplines in basic philosophy and values, treatment modality, and terminology and jargon (Brown & Keyes, 2000; Weist, Lowie, Flaherty, & Pruitt, 2001).

Tenure diversity (i.e., the length of time members have been on the team) can be detrimental to member relations and team performance as well (Owens,

Mannic, & Neale, 1998). New members coming into an already functioning team have to be socialized by the remaining members, taking valuable time away from the task at hand (Dyer, 1984; Moreland & Levine, 1988). Although continuity of staffing is important, boundaries of some groups are, by necessity, more permeable than others. For example, hospital teams often include different physicians and nurses corresponding to the needs of the patients at certain points in their treatment and recovery. Having a clear mission and set of task priorities will decrease many problems associated with tenure diversity (Shaw, 1990), while the use of core and peripheral members and full-time and alternate members will increase team continuity and stabilize the process (Ancona & Caldwell, 1998; Topping, Norton, & Scafidi, 2003; Walsh & Hewitt, 1996). Furthermore, the diversity liability can be alleviated to some extent if members have previous experience working in groups or have been given training in team-building techniques (Athanasaw, 2003; Dailey, Young, & Barr, 1991; Horak, Guarino, Knight, & Kwodor, 1991; Stoner & Hartman, 1993; Thyen, Theis, & Tebbitt, 1993; Topping et al., 2003). Katzenbach and Smith (1993) point out that successful teams don't just happen, but become effective when members have certain skills that permit them to function positively in a group situation. Training and previous group experience, especially if members have worked together before, provide these skills and reduce the potential for conflict.

Given the multidisciplinary nature of health care, diverse groups are very common in health services organizations, and they present unique management challenges (Brown & Keyes, 2000). Oncology treatment teams, for example, may include a variety of physician specialists (e.g., medical oncologists, radiation oncologists, surgical oncologists, pediatric oncologists, pathologists, surgeons, psychiatrists, hematologists, gynecologists, radiologists), physicists, nurses, social workers, psychologists, pharmacists, and nutritionists (Fried & Nelson, 1987). While these types of teams tend to be fluid (i.e., not all team members will be involved in all cases), the multidisciplinary nature of the team raises many questions about leadership, status differences, and the manner in which decisions are made. For example, a nurse who is present at all meetings may be the *formal* leader, but in all likelihood decisional power will reside with the physician most directly involved in treating the patient, even if he or she is an intern or resident. Thus, the role of formal leader may be reduced to that of coordinator rather than decision maker.

Perhaps no other aspect of group and organizational functioning has been studied as much as **team size**. In general, it is believed that size has a U-shaped relation to effectiveness so that too few or too many members reduce performance (Cohen & Bailey, 1997). As teams become larger, communication and coordination problems tend to increase, while a climate of fairness and cohesiveness decrease (Colquitt, Noe, & Jackson, 2002; Liberman, Hilty, Drake, & Tsang, 2001); however, teams have to be large enough to accomplish the task assigned. In other words, groups need to be staffed to the smallest number to accomplish the work (Hackman, 1987). There is some indication that the U-shaped relationship may not hold for all situations or types of teams. In treatment teams, in which boundaries may be permeable, performance is negatively affected by size (Alexander et al., 1996; Vinokur-Kaplan, 1995b). Probably, smaller groups are less cumbersome, having fewer social distractions. Smaller teams also have lower incidences of social loafing (Liden et al., 2004). Individuals in large teams are able to maintain a sense of anonymity and gain from the work of the group without making a suitable contribution.

More often than not, team size is out of the control of the manager, particularly when democratic representational norms pervade an organization. In these situations, constituencies may demand to be represented, and the leader may need to design strategies to make the group more manageable (e.g., forming subcommittees). Otherwise, teams may be overstaffed. Overstaffed teams may tend to perform work in a perfunctory, lackadaisical manner. Large size may also lead to competition and

jealousy among group members, with individuals guarding their particular domain. Some members may remain aloof from the team's efforts and be less willing to help others improve their performance. On the other hand, breaking a team into subgroups (e.g., subcommittees) has its own set of problems. When large teams are divided into smaller ones, each subgroup may become cliquish, and while cohesive within themselves, they may become isolated from the rest of the team.

Although the empirical evidence on the relationship between team composition and size and effectiveness is less than definitive, it still provides information that can be valuable in managing teams. It may be useful to keep in mind the potential problems and benefits that may emerge as a result of group size and diversity. On one hand, managers may have some degree of control over composition and size; conversely, they may not. In the former situation, the decision maker will want to consider the type of task and resources available for training before determining the size and heterogeneity of the team. In the latter, managers have many strategies and interventions to choose from that can help increase team's effectiveness.

Status Differences

Status is the measure of worth conferred on an individual by a group. **Status differences** are seen throughout organizations, and serve many useful purposes. Differences in status motivate people, provide them with a means of identification, and may be a force for stability in the organization (Scott, 1967).

Status differences have a profound effect on the functioning of multidisciplinary teams. Research findings are fairly consistent in showing that high-status members initiate communication more often, are provided more opportunities to participate, and have more influence over the decision-making process (Owens et al., 1998). Thus, an individual from a lower-status professional group may be intimidated or ignored by higher-status team members. The group, as a result, may not benefit from this person's expertise. This situation is very likely in health care, where status differences among the professions are well entrenched (Topping et al., 2003). Often, multidisciplinary teams are idealistically expected to operate as a company of equals, yet the reality of the situation makes this impossible. In a study of end-stage renal disease teams, in which the equal participation ideology was accepted by most team participants, it was clear that the physicians, who had higher professional status than other groups, had greater involvement in the actual decision-making process (Deber & Leatt, 1986). The mismatch between expectations and reality made many team members, particularly staff nurses, feel a sense of role deprivation, with accompanying implications for morale and job satisfaction. This problem is exacerbated in teams characterized by sex diversity. In one study, men were more likely to want to exit teams that were female-dominated for those that were male-dominated or homogenous. Following from this, men have historically been perceived as having higher status in managerial roles in organizations, thereby affecting the men's satisfaction with the team (Chatman & O'Reilly, 2004).

Status differences may have very significant impacts on patient outcomes. According to the recent report, *Keeping Patients Safe: Transforming the Work Environment of Nurses,* "counterproductive hierarchical communication patterns that derive from status differences" are partly responsible for many medical errors (Institute of Medicine, 2003, p. 361). Further, a review of medical malpractice cases from across the country found that physicians (the higher-status members of the team) often ignored important information communicated by nurses (the lower-status members of the team). Nurses in turn were found to withhold relevant information for diagnosis and treatment from physicians (Schmitt, 2001). In this status-consciousness environment, opportunities for learning and improvement can be missed because of unwillingness to engage in quality-improving communication.

Some teams develop norms of equality. However, these democratic norms may run counter to the formal or informal status of individual group members in the larger organization. Within a hospital, a physician may have considerable formal and informal power. Within a CQI team, the same physician may be expected to serve as an equal in analyzing problems and recommending solutions. This discrepancy between outside status and inside status may make management of these teams difficult.

If status inequality exists, it is advisable to build a trust-sensitive environment in which members can disagree with the leader and others on the team without repercussions. Often, CQI teams use training along with nonmember facilitators early in the team development process to cope with the problems brought about by status differences (LaPenta & Jacobs, 1996). In well-managed multidisciplinary groups, lower-status individuals should feel elevated by being part of such high-profile, effective teams.

Psychological Safety

Psychological safety describes individuals' perceptions about the consequences of interpersonal risks in their work environment—largely taken-for-granted beliefs about how others will respond when one puts oneself on the line, such as by asking a question, seeking feedback, reporting a mistake, or proposing a new idea in the team context. In psychologically safe teams, people believe that if they make a mistake, other team members will not penalize or think less of them for it. This belief fosters the confidence to experiment, discuss mistakes and problems, and ask others for help. Psychological safety is created by mutual respect and trust among team members, and leader behavior is a powerful influence on the level of psychological safety in teams (Edmondson, 1999; 2003).

Management research on psychological safety started with studies of organizational change, when Schein and Bennis (1965) discussed the need to create psychological safety for individuals if they are to feel secure and capable of changing. Psychological safety helps people overcome the defensiveness, or "learning anxiety," that occurs when people are presented with data that disconfirm their expectations or hopes, which can thwart productive learning behavior (Schein, 1985). However, the need for a team climate conducive to learning does not imply a cozy environment in which people are close friends, nor does it suggest an absence of pressure or problems. Team psychological safety is distinct from group cohesiveness; as noted, team cohesiveness can reduce willingness to disagree and challenge others' views, creating groupthink (Janis, 1972); this represents a *lack* of interpersonal risk-taking. Psychological safety describes instead a climate that focuses on productive discussion enabling early prevention of problems and accomplishment of shared goals, because people feel less need to focus on self-protection.

Although few of us are without concern about others' impressions, our immediate social context can mitigate—or exacerbate—the reluctance to relax our guard. Research in hospitals and other organizations has found differences across teams in people's willingness to engage in behavior for which the outcomes are uncertain and potentially harmful to their image. When psychological safety is high, teams are much more likely to engage in learning, which in turn promotes team performance (Edmondson, 1999). Just as compelling goals are necessary to motivate learning, psychological safety enhances the power of such goals by facilitating less self-conscious interpersonal interactions. Without a goal, there is no clear direction to drive toward and no motivation to exert the effort; without psychological safety, the risks of engaging wholeheartedly in learning behaviors and other key team processes in front of other people are simply too great.

Team Norms

A norm is defined as a standard that is shared by team members and regulates member behavior. **Behavior norms** are rules that standardize how people act at work on a day-to-day basis, while **performance norms** are rules that standardize employee output. Behavioral norms in teams are far

reaching and may vary substantially from one group to another in the same organization. Norms may govern how much participation is required by each individual, how humor is to be used, the use of formal group procedures (e.g., Robert's Rules of Order), and rules related to absence and lateness. In their study of operating room nurses, Denison and Sutton (1990) describe their surprise at the behavioral norms present in the operating room:

> At first we were surprised by the norms of emotional expression in the operating rooms. The first time we entered the room where a coronary bypass operation was being done, for example, we were surprised by the loud rock music blaring from the speakers, the smiles on the faces of the surgical team, and the constant joking. Denison observed one surgeon who joked and told a series of funny stories as he performed the complicated task of cutting the veins out of a patient's leg that would be used to bypass clogged coronary arteries. Similarly, one reason that Sutton almost passed out during a tonsillectomy was that he became very upset when the surgeon laughed, joked, and talked about "what was on the tube last night" while blood from an unconscious child splattered about.

Performance norms, on the other hand, govern the amount and quality of work required of individuals, as well as the amount of time they are expected to work. Some performance norms require that workers not work too hard so that standards for the group as a whole are kept at a given level. Mullen and Baumeister (1987) use the term *diving* to describe situations in which norms play an important role in motivating individual team members to perform at less than optimum levels. One example of diving results from a team norm that discourages excellence in performance by any team member. Group members socialize other members as to the norm and will punish if violated (Cannon-Bowers, Oser, & Flanagan, 1992). Thus, "rate busters" would be subject to serious sanctions by the other team members. Researchers have documented the practice of "pinging," which involved a periodical punch on the suspected rate buster's arm until he or she reduced the level of effort (Roethlisberger & Dickson, 1939).

Norms are powerful influences in organizations and teams, and the existence of norms is necessary for effective group functioning. Hackman (1976) suggests that norms have the following characteristics:

1. Norms summarize and simplify team influence processes. They denote the processes by which teams regulate member behavior.

2. Norms apply only to behavior, not to private thoughts and feelings. Private acceptance of norms is not necessary, only public compliance is required.

3. Norms are generally developed only for behaviors that are viewed as important by most team members.

4. Norms usually develop gradually, but members can quicken the process. Norms usually are developed by team members when the occasion arises, such as when a situation occurs that requires new ground rules for members in order to protect team integrity.

5. All norms do not apply to all team members. Some norms apply only to newer members, while others may be applied to individuals based on seniority, sex, race, economic status, or profession.

Because of the significance of norms in effective group functioning, it is important to clarify norms publicly so members will know what is expected. This is especially the case for multidisciplinary teams in hospitals and other health care settings (Deeter-Schmelz & Ramsey, 2003). If acceptable norms are established as part of the group process, there is less chance of a so-called interdisciplinary team functioning as cross-disciplinary, with one discipline dominating (Vinokur-Kaplan, 1995a).

Team Cohesiveness

There are a variety of definitions for **team cohesiveness**, many of which focus on the degree to which members of a group are attracted to other members and, thereby, are motivated to stay in the group. Another, more narrow definition that may better fit the purpose of this chapter is used by Goodman, Ravlin, and Schminke (1987): "cohesiveness is the extent that members are committed to the group task." In this definition, the focus is on the decision to produce and acknowledge that members can be committed to a common task but not necessarily be attracted to each other. This is a pragmatic view of cohesiveness that is particularly important for focusing on the management of teams in which members, like nurses, physicians, psychologists, and social workers, are already highly committed to professional standards.

Cohesion is an important component in understanding group process and effectiveness. Highly cohesive teams may have higher performance, improved satisfaction, and lower levels of turnover (Gully, Devine, & Whitney, 1995; Hoegl & Gemuenden, 2001; Yang & Tang, 2004). The relationship between cohesion and effectiveness is stronger when the task requires coordination, communication, and mutual performance (Cannon-Bowers et al., 1992). Specifically, research focusing on treatment teams in psychiatric hospitals, engaged in highly interdependent work, found that cohesive teams had higher performance levels than less cohesive ones (Vinokur-Kaplan, 1995a). Similarly, research examining the effectiveness of geriatric rehabilitation has found that interdisciplinary teams play an important role in improving the quality of care (Wells, Seabrook, Stolee, et al., 2003). Collaboration and cohesion among team members is a key determinant of team effectiveness. Cohesiveness can also promote better enforcement of group norms and general control over group members; however, taken to extremes, this can lead to groupthink-like situations of undue conformity. For instance, there are circumstances under which high levels of cohesiveness can lead to *lower* levels of productivity. If a group's norms favor low productivity, then having a highly cohesive group will likely lead to high levels of conformity to the norm and lower productivity. Similarly, a highly cohesive group may work against a manager's efforts to involve new members in a group, or to have the group interact with other groups. Cohesiveness, therefore, should be viewed in context. In most situations, it is a positive force, while in others, it can lead to conformity to counterproductive norms and practices (McGrath, 1984).

What are the sources of cohesiveness? A central tenet of social psychological theory is that individuals are attracted to others who are similar to them; therefore, homogeneous groups should be more cohesive than heterogeneous ones. Teams composed of all females, for instance, tend to be more cohesive than all male and mixed sex groups (Bettenhausen, 1991). The lack of conflict, team training, a positive predisposition for teamwork, and the presence of trust among members also lead to increased cohesiveness (Bettenhausen, 1991; Deeter-Schmelz & Ramsey, 2003; Pinto & Pinton, 1990). To complicate matters, some research suggests that conflict may be beneficial to group performance, particularly when a group is dealing with complex problem-solving tasks (Cosier, 1981; Janis, 1972; Schwenk, 1983). In this sense, multidisciplinary groups and groups composed of culturally diverse individuals, while likely to exhibit higher levels of conflict and less cohesiveness, may also be more creative and innovative in their approach to problem solving (Jackson, 1992).

Additionally, cohesiveness is influenced by the goal orientation or reward structure of the team. Let's consider two conditions. First is the situation of goal interdependence in which members are evaluated and rewarded (i.e., equal reward structure) as a group. Here, progress to each member's professional/personal goals is the same as progress to the group goals. Conversely, the second condition is one in which group members are judged and rewarded

(i.e., unequal reward structure) as individuals. In essence, one member reaches his or her goal at the expense of another member. In general, the findings support the first or cooperative condition (Parker, McAdams, & Zielinski, 2000; Sundstrom et al., 1990; Yang & Tang, 2004). Team members in the second situation are more likely to be highly competitive, leading to lower cohesiveness due to:

- Less intermember influence and acceptance of other's ideas
- Greater difficulty in communication and understanding
- Less coordination effort, less division of labor, and less productivity (Deutsch, 1949)

Following from this, cohesive groups tend to have levels of interaction that are greater and more positive (Shaw, 1990). This is strengthened by conditions of high interdependency (Gully et al., 1995). That is, groups that have equivalent reward structures not only perform more efficiently, but also develop cooperative strategies such as teamwork and pooling of information that facilitate achievement of jointly shared goals.

Nature of the Task

One of the underlying themes throughout the research on teams and groups is the notion that group tasks can be classified according to their critical demands; that is, certain features of a task dictate the specific group behaviors critical to successful performance. These specific behaviors include not only individual effort but also cooperative and interdependent endeavors (see Chapter 8). This means that effective performance is a function of matching the team process to the task demands (see Chapter 7). In this section, we identify key aspects of the tasks confronting teams and the manner in which they adapt to differences in task design characteristics.

Team Goals

Team goals and their accompanying tasks can be categorized according to goal clarity, complexity, and diversity. Each of these dimensions has implications for the manner in which a team is organized and managed. Some teams work towards goals that are repeated over time; the work of such teams and the manner in which communication and coordination is conducted can be routinized. Although they face variations and some uncertainty, obstetrical teams face a defined set of goals, namely the safe delivery of newborns and the health and well-being of mother and child. The goals and accompanying tasks for such teams and for individual team members are well structured and understood by team members. Where goals and tasks are predictable, and where team members understand exactly what is to be done, the work of a team can become highly routinized.

Contrast this situation with teams facing ambiguous, ill-structured goals. A disaster-preparedness team is perhaps the epitome of this type of uncertainty. In such a situation communication is of paramount importance. Team members must be prepared to adapt to new circumstances, and adjust their work according to the situation. Ongoing coordination and mutual adjustment among team members are essential since routinization is possible only up to a point.

Goal and task clarity was a significant variable in determining the performance of hospital treatment teams, allowing them to meet the hospital's standards of quality, quantity, and timeliness (Shaw, 1990; Vinokur-Kaplan, 1995a). Task complexity is related to team interaction (Shaw, 1976); the more complex the task, the greater the need for interaction, so that it is important that managers plan for enhanced communication among the team members under conditions of complexity. Others have found that an increase in task diversity, as defined by the number of different conditions treated within ICUs, challenges caregivers since their expertise and knowledge can be applied across a wider range of conditions and lead to better outcomes (Shortell et al., 1994).

Task Interdependence

Another form of task diversity focuses on interdependence, which is generally the reason why teams form in the first place. **Task interdependence** refers to the interconnections between tasks, or more specifically, the degree to which team members must rely on one another to perform work effectively. A useful way of classifying this is to use a hierarchy of task interdependence based on exchange of information or resources (Thompson, 1967; Van de Ven, Delbecq, & Koenig, 1976):

- *Pooled interdependence.* A situation in which each member makes a contribution to the group output without the need of interaction among members. Since each group member completes the whole task, team performance is the sum of the individual efforts. Standardized rules and procedures are needed to enhance coordination of team outputs.

- *Sequential interdependence.* A situation in which one group member must act before another one can. Group members have different roles and perform different tasks in some prescribed order with the work flowing in only one direction. There is always an element of potential contingency since readjustment is necessary if any member fails to meet expectations. Coordination using schedules and plans is needed to keep the team on track.

- *Reciprocal interdependence.* A situation in which the outputs of each member become inputs for the others, causing each member to pose a contingency for the other. Group members often are specialists with different areas of expertise and have structured roles; therefore, they perform different parts of the task in a flexible, "back-and-forth" order. Leaders must provide for open communication between members and schedule meetings as necessary.

- *Team interdependence.* A situation in which team members diagnose, problem solve, and collaborate as a group while performing work or work-related activities. The workflow is simultaneous and multidirectional. Coordination requires mutual interactions with group autonomy to decide the sequencing of inputs and outputs among members. Leaders should plan frequent meetings, while also encouraging unscheduled ones.

Interdependence increases uncertainty; therefore, as the degree of interdependence increases, so does the need for information processing along with the necessity for more coordination, communication, and cooperation. Implicit in this is the need for matching the information-processing requirements with interaction or coordination patterns that facilitate information exchange. If team members perceive low interdependence when high interdependence actually exists, then too little effort will go toward coordination. On the contrary, when interdependence is perceived as higher than it really is, too much effort will be expended in coordination behavior at the expense of performance. For this reason, interdependence and coordination must be appropriately matched. Some researchers go so far as to suggest that successful teams are the ones that match interdependence in terms of task, goal, and feedback. That is, a successful team would be one in which reciprocal work is matched with group goals and group feedback. Group goals and feedback mean that rewards would be based on the group goal and feedback given on the group's performance as a whole. Conversely, pooled interdependence should be matched with a situation of individual goals and feedback (Salvedra, Earley, & Van Dyne, 1993).

Regardless of the task characteristic, the important point for the manager to remember is the need to match team task with process and structure. One study demonstrating this matching described the reengineering effort in a large urban hospital system that used teams for overcoming care delivery problems, particularly fragmentation and discontinuities in delivery (Schweikhart & Smith-Daniels, 1996). Focused teams, or relatively autonomous operating units, were formed by merging multidisciplinary clinicians into patient care units, so that pharmacists, respiratory therapists, nurses, and other caregivers were integrated through shared governance and cross-training. The teams were given high levels of autonomy and accountability, while sharing responsibility for both care production work, execution of the patient's care plan, care-management work, planning, and coordinating the

care. In this case, high levels of task complexity and interdependence were matched with a team structure that allowed increased levels of communication and interaction.

A relatively new type of team is known as the virtual team, in which team members may be not only separated by geography and time, but also by culture and language. In this situation, managers faced with the dual challenges of coordinating work among individuals from different disciplines, and from different cultures (Barczak & McDonough, 2003). In health care, this type of team is most common in product development (e.g., pharmaceuticals and medical equipment) and in clinical research.

The Environmental Context

Teams do not exist and function in a vacuum. They are constantly affected by pressures and events from outside of the immediate team. In this section, we examine a range of external factors that may affect team performance. These consist of organizational factors, such as organizational culture and intergroup relationships, conflict, and factors in the external environment that include resource scarcity, collaborative history, and urban/rural context.

Intergroup Relationships and Conflict

In the context of teams, the term *intergroup relationships* has two distinct meanings. One stream of research (e.g., Alderfer, 1987) studies how identity group boundaries affect within team processes; we cover these issues in our discussion of diversity and status in health care teams. The other stream pertains to boundary crossing that takes place when teams must coordinate their efforts with other teams in their own and other organizations.

In many situations, effective team performance is dependent upon a team's ability to interact with other teams in a positive and productive manner. In complex organizations, one of the central tasks of many teams is to interact with other teams whose work is related to theirs (Edmonson, 2002). For example, consider the myriad intergroup interactions among teams that must occur in the merging of two hospitals (Dooley & Zimmerman, 2003; Sidorov, 2003; Yang & Tang, 2004).

Teams assembled to deal with staffing issues, technology, finances, architectural concerns, and countless other factors must work with other teams in both their own and the merging organization to implement desired changes. One could imagine the confusion if each individual team chose to work without the advice and input of other teams.

What happens when teams must coordinate their efforts? What are the factors responsible for effective and ineffective intergroup relationships in this context? Intergroup relationships are often lateral, or peer, relationships, rather than hierarchical ones. As health care organizations move away from rigid hierarchical structures to manage work and become more specialized, the need for new coordination mechanisms has increased (see Chapter 8).

In the process of working out challenging coordination issues, **intergroup conflict** is perhaps inevitable (see Chapter 5). It is virtually impossible to design all work processes in advance, given the uncertainty and heterogeneity of inputs in health care, in ways to ensure that the work of groups meshes perfectly with the work of other groups. When conflicts or disagreements occur among groups, it is important that team members possess a repertoire of conflict resolution strategies. In some cases, the interfaces among teams require only fine-tuning; in others, the worst situations, work processes may need to be overhauled to achieve functional intergroup relationships.

While intergroup conflict can occasionally result from interpersonal differences or animosities, most conflict emerges because of factors related to the interdependence among work groups. This is especially true for health care organizations, which have high levels of interaction and greater opportunities for the emergence of conflict. Conflict between groups cannot usually be addressed at an individual level; one member of a group can rarely resolve an intergroup conflict in a unilateral manner. If intergroup conflict is viewed as resulting from problems in the *interface* between groups, then the analysis of the causes and sources of conflict should examine the nature of intergroup relationships.

First, intergroup conflict is more likely to occur when there is ambiguity about teams' respective task responsibilities and roles (Cheser, 1999). This situation largely explains conflicts that occur between professional groups with overlapping practice domains (e.g., between psychologists and psychiatrists) (Brown & Keyes, 2000; Weist et al., 2001). Task and role ambiguity may also be common in organizations undergoing rapid growth or change. In these situations, the nature or implications of the change may be understood differently among different groups. Consider the degree of conflict that occurs when an organization is in the midst of a merger (Dooley & Zimmerman, 2003). This type of conflict points to the need to clearly articulate team roles and distinguish precisely the responsibilities of similar groups. Conflict also arises from intergroup differences in work orientation. Every group has its own set of norms regarding the manner in which work is accomplished. In many organizations, teams have different perspectives on *time*. This difference in time orientation was identified and managed when strategic planning was attempted with a group of family physicians (Fried & Nelson, 1987):

> By its nature, the activity of planning is at odds with the role orientation of most physicians. Planning is a long-term process in which the results of strategic decisions appear over time. The outcomes of planning are often intangible in the short term. By contrast, physicians are trained to be action oriented.
>
> It was discovered early in the planning process that physician attendance at meetings decreased when the pace of work lagged. Therefore, whenever possible, the pace of work was increased to a level more acceptable to physicians. A work plan with specific deadlines was followed.

Related to differences in work orientation is the problem of intergroup goal incompatibility. Sometimes groups must work together when their goals are in conflict, or perceived to be in conflict. This may be the case between teams whose orientation is primarily cost-containment and those whose orientation is focused more on quality concerns. At other times, differences in group culture may cause conflict between teams. Each group develops its own unique norms, communication network, and values, which collectively is referred to as a team culture. When these vary between teams, conflict often occurs. Last, intergroup conflict may occur when there is competition for resources. Teams may have much in common and be oriented toward the same goals, yet still be in conflict because they are competing for the same financial, human, or physical resources. In hospitals, the change to product or program management would tend to increase the likelihood of intergroup conflict as product-line teams develop internal competitive thrusts.

Perhaps of greatest importance for the organization as a whole, as conflict emerges between groups, cooperative relationships are replaced by a win-lose mentality in which victory becomes more important than solving the problem that may have caused the conflict in the first place. Because of this, it is important to develop strategies that can be used in managing and reducing intergroup conflict. Some of these are (see Chapter 5):

- Intergroup training, which uses team-building techniques to improve the work interactions of different functions or divisions in an organization (George & Jones, 1999).

- Structuring the relationship between teams around superordinate goals, or mutually important goals that neither team can achieve without cooperation from the other.

- Examining the interfaces between teams to determine where change is necessary to decrease the conflict (Blake & Mouton, 1978).

- Establishing self-contained teams, which involves the regrouping of conflicting groups into new teams that perform work independently of each other.

Similar to self-contained teams, focused teams are being used more and more in large hospitals to over-

come fragmentation and discontinuities in delivery of care while also decreasing conflict (Schweikhart & Smith-Daniels, 1996). Pharmacists, respiratory therapist, nurses, and other caregivers are assigned to individual care units instead of reporting to overall departments, such as pharmacy, as before.

Organizational Culture

To use teams effectively in organizations, it is extremely important that a suitable culture exists—one that values and emphasizes teamwork and participation (Zarraga & Bonache, 2003). One of the most common complaints heard about teams in organizations is that they do not receive adequate support from the organization as a whole. While many organizations claim to want to move to a team-based organization, they often lack effective culture and strategies for accomplishing this transition. What do managers need to do to implement the change to a team-based organization? A number of important points have been suggested. It is important for top management to ensure that a team culture is consistent with its overall strategy. Senior management needs (1) to believe that employees want to be responsible for their work, (2) to be able to demonstrate the team philosophy, (3) to articulate a coherent vision of the team environment, and (4) to have the creativity and authority to overcome obstacles as they surface (Moorhead & Griffin, 1998; Orsburn, Moran, Musselwhite, & Zenger, 1990).

As with other aspects of organizational life, teams require strong support from senior management to be effective (Liberman et al., 2001). By support, we refer to philosophical backing and resource support. Resource support includes money, human resources, training, and time. Once senior management has made a commitment to teams, it may be necessary to develop a detailed implementation plan. This plan might include a clarification of the organization mission to focus on such things as continuous improvement, employee involvement, and customer satisfaction; selecting sites for teams; preparing a design team to assist with team staffing and operation; planning the transfer of authority from management to teams; and drafting a preliminary plan for implementation. In addition, to be successful, teams need a champion who can provide motivation, encouragement, and work to acquire the resources and support required (Cohen & Bailey, 1997; Shortell et al., 2004).

Training represents a key part of implementing and supporting teams, and to be effective, the organizational culture must support this (Liberman, 2000). No one would ever consider the possibility of a soccer team being successful without substantial training or practice. Based on the experience of countless nonsports teams, the need for continuous training is very apparent. There is vast literature on selecting and training individuals to work in teams, and the knowledge, skills, and abilities necessary for effective teamwork. Such training may include cognitive concerns, such as the rationale or raison d'etre of a team, through affective concerns such as the roles and responsibilities of team members and team norms, as well as logistical issues dealing with meeting management and compensation (Moorhead & Griffin, 1998). Other examples include team interaction training, which can lead to shared mental models (Marks, Zaccaro, & Mathieu, 2000); problem-solving and decision-making training, which can enhance interdisciplinary team interactions (Doran et al., 2002); and newcomer training, which can speed the socialization process (Chen & Klimoski, 2003). Overall, for team training to be comprehensive, it optimally should include requisite technical, administrative, and interpersonal skills.

Also, the type of organizational culture is reflected by the reward system implemented in the organization. Thus, a particular dilemma facing managers in team-oriented organizations is the question of type of reward system. To what extent should the organization bestow team, as opposed to individual, rewards? Do team-based rewards improve team and/or individual performance? Despite the equivocal nature of the literature in this area, there seems to be a natural tendency for team-oriented organizations to at least consider the idea of team-based rewards. In a team-based environment, a variety of mechanisms may be employed to reward team member performance. In some situations, team members are rewarded for mastering a range of skills needed to meet team performance goals. In others, rewards are based on actual team performance. Skill-based pay may reward employees for acquiring specific skills needed by an employee's team. In these situations, team members may increase their compensation by acquiring value-added skill sets. Team bonus plans reward particular teams based on the performance of the team. Finally, gain-sharing plans (usually considered an organization-wide incentive system) typically reward all team members from all teams based on the performance of the organization as a whole (Moorhead & Griffin, 1998).

It should be stressed that while there are many options for rewarding team performance, the number of organizations that actually use team-based incentives is relatively small. A 1996–1997 survey of 2,500 corporations found that the number of companies with group incentives grew from 16% in 1995 to 19% in 1996 (Pascarella, 1997). While this growth is notable, the majority of organizations have yet to implement team-based incentive systems. Part of the reason for this lack of movement is the complexity of such schemes and the lack of agreement on the link between incentives and performance. While there is an intuitive appeal for performance-based compensation, there exists substantial dissent regarding the whole premise of pay-for-performance. Many managers and scholars believe that such schemes are highly destructive to individual, team, and organizational performance (Berwick, 1995). In addition, a number of critical questions need to be resolved to ensure that a team payment system does not yield unintended negative consequences, including (Pascarella, 1997):

- Does the team as a whole receive rewards, or do individuals on the team receive rewards for outstanding team performance?

- If rewards are not uniformly distributed among team members, how does management assess the relative contributions of different team members?

- Should team members be compensated for results, behaviors, or both?
- How should people be rewarded when they have membership on multiple teams?

These are critical questions, the answers to which depend upon the particular manner in which teams are used in the organization as well as the culture of the organization (Beersma et al., 2003).

However, several hybrid compensation structures have been successful in simultaneously motivating low-performing team members to improve while encouraging high-performing members to help in this process (Katz, 2001). An example of a hybrid plan involves a team threshold where once the team as a whole reaches this level, pay increases are based on individual performance. This is especially successful when there are enough highly skilled workers on the team to teach their less-skilled or less-knowledgeable colleagues.

External Environment

Besides the organizational environment, teams are affected constantly by influences from the external environment as well. This makes it important to understand how external factors influence team process and effectiveness (Ancona, 1990; Arrow et al., 2000). Most research has involved organizational factors that affect teams (e.g., support from senior levels of the organization), so there is little known about the effect of external environment (Lacey & Gruenfeld, 1999). For many groups, the greater external environment may exert influence equal to or greater than the internal organizational environment (Hackman, 2003; Salas, Burke, & Cannon-Bowers, 2000). This is particularly true for multidisciplinary, interagency groups that interact with and depend on not only member organizations but also the community environment and local service network for critical resources and support. These teams often are used in resource-deficient rural areas to extend services, making it critical to understand how these conditions affect teams and how to develop strategies to override the effects.

In several studies (Fried, Johnsen, Starrett, Calloway, & Morrissey, 1998; Topping & Calloway, 2000), the findings indicated that resource scarcity was an important issue in the development of mental health delivery systems in rural environments. In areas with high levels of resource scarcity, only a few core providers took a central or gatekeeper role, thereby implying that organizations in that system act more autonomously than a system with more resources. This, in turn, will affect the collaborative behavior or **social capital** existing in the provider network and community as a whole. Social capital can be best defined as a web of cooperative relationships between providers in a service system that involves interpersonal trust, norms of reciprocity, and mutual aid (Veenstra, 2000). In situations of scarce resources where social capital may be low since organizations tend to interact less, there will be little impetus to use teams to solve interorganizational problems. For instance, teams including acute care hospital nurses and community providers are used to provide care to older people discharged from the hospital (Robinson & Street, 2004). Collaboration among team members would be much more difficult in areas characterized by scarce resources where social capital is low.

Another contextual factor influencing collaboration between team members is the collaborative history of the provider network or community. Interagency teams, whose members have a long history of service coordination, tend to report a remarkably easy process of forming and becoming a cohesive, effective group (Topping et al., 2003). There are also rural and urban differences. Many rural areas report that, "everyone knows each other and have worked together before." Thus, a sense of "teamness" is there from the beginning. In addition, urban communities tend to include a larger number of service organizations, so that interagency teams usually are composed of many professionals, while rural areas have to depend on nontraditional groups such as the YMCA, churches, and Boys and Girls Clubs for

✣ DEBATE TIME 6.1   Do We Reward Individuals or Groups?

Traditional methods of compensation reward individuals for individual performance. Theories of motivation focus on linking rewards to performance, facilitating individual performance through coaching and training, and setting challenging yet realistic goals. While there are some exceptions to this individualistic approach to rewards, such as gainsharing plans where employees are rewarded for overall increased productivity, generations of managers have been inculcated with the need to reward individuals based on the merits of individual performance.

We are now in an era where groups and teams are becoming increasingly important. Teams are expected to work together to solve problems, care for patients, and engage in quality improvement and planning activities. Continuous quality improvement efforts are based on effective team functioning. However, our reward systems are still almost entirely focused on the individual. Efforts to implement group reward systems are often met with hostility and suspicion. Many people fear the free-rider syndrome, where some members of the team do not perform up to standard yet receive the same reward as productive team members for group performance. Other people worry that group rewards dilute the motivational potential in rewards. With financial resources growing increasingly scarce, managers want to ensure that the impact of merit pay is maximized. There is therefore a reluctance to deviate from traditional merit pay systems. Finally, where employees are unionized, formally rewarding employees for team performance may be viewed as a breach of contract.

Is it possible to combine merit pay systems with team reward systems? If efforts continue to implement team rewards, will we eventually see a deterioration in individual motivation and commitment?

---

members. This, of course, increases diversity, which may also increase team conflict (Jackson, 1992; Kor, 2003).

CONCLUSION

One of the most important managerial tasks is the development and management of teams. It is now common wisdom that organizations as a whole, as well as individuals, are dependent upon strong and well-functioning teams. As noted, however, teams do not naturally develop and improve. In fact, their level of performance may erode and become dysfunctional over time without deliberate and continuous supportive efforts. Effective managers understand that improving a team's performance is a complex endeavor and that improvement strategies need to encompass team structure and process factors, at the same time recognizing the contribution of individual members of the team (see Debate Time 6.1). Finally, while we can make general theoretical statements about teams, each team develops a distinct personality, and develops in its own way and at its own pace. There is both a science and an art to managing and working with teams.

DISCUSSION QUESTIONS

1. The recently hired director of a new ambulatory care center in a hospital has been instructed to begin holding weekly management team meetings. The

MANAGERIAL GUIDELINES

Managing teams is both an art and a science. In this chapter, we set forth several principles of group process and performance. The management of teams requires knowledge of these concepts and considerable skill and practice. The following managerial guidelines provide specific ideas for developing skills as a group leader:

1. To increase the performance of a team, it is important for managers to ensure the reward structure of the organization that rewards team accomplishments and individual performance.
2. The manager should identify those group norms that are dysfunctional or obsolete and take steps to eliminate those norms.
3. The assignment of tasks among interdependent work groups should be clarified to avoid misunderstandings, conflict, and ambiguity.
4. Managers should be aware of their own conflict management tendencies and seek to broaden their repertoire of conflict-management strategies.
5. Managers should be aware of how team members communicate with each other inside and outside the team environment.
6. Managers should be aware of status differences among team members, and how these differences affect individual participation, group decision making, and productivity.
7. Managers should apply a variety of structured group decision-making techniques, such as nominal group technique, brain-

storming, the Delphi technique, and understand when each is most appropriate.
8. Managers should be clear that group members understand the purpose and authority of the team, the role of the team in the organization, and the specific contributions expected of each individual.
9. Managers should be conscious of the symptoms of groupthink and develop strategies for preventing and dealing with groupthink.
10. Managers should be aware of the group development, the limitations and strengths associated with each stage, and manage the group accordingly. Group leaders should also try to move the group forward to more mature stages.
11. In managing meetings, group leaders should be aware of the following principles (Huber, 1980):
    a. At the beginning of the meeting, review the progress made to date and establish the task facing the group.
    b. Help group members feel comfortable with one another.
    c. Establish ground rules governing group discussions.
    d. As early in a meeting as possible, get a report from each member who has been preassigned a task.
    e. Sustain the flow of the meeting by using informational displays.
    f. Manage the discussion to achieve equitable participation.
    g. Close the meeting by summarizing what has been accomplished and reviewing assignments.

management team is to consist of several physicians, nurses, physician assistants, and a social worker. What advice would you give the director to help promote the team's effectiveness?

2. An interorganizational community task force has been formed to identify obstacles facing the elderly in obtaining needed health and social services. Given the large number of agencies involved in providing services to the elderly and the need for consumer representation, how would you balance the need for full representation with the need to keep group size at a manageable level?

3. Under what circumstances are noncohesive groups more productive than cohesive groups? What strategies can a group leader employ to increase the probability that a cohesive group will be productive?

4. What strategies can a team leader use to increase the commitment of team members? How does a team leader know if members are motivated and committed to the group?

5. If you were just appointed leader of a previously existing team of which you were not an original member, how would you determine its stage of development? Based on that stage, what strategies would you use to make the team effective?

REFERENCES

Albanese, R., & Van Fleet, D. D. (1985). Rational behavior in groups: The free riding tendency. *Academy of Management Review, 10*, 244–255.

Alderfer, C. P. (1987). An intergroup perspective on organizational behavior. In J. W. Lorsch (Ed.), *Handbook of organizational behavior.* Englewood Cliffs, NJ: Prentice-Hall.

Alexander, J. A., Jinnett, K., D'Aunno, T. A., & Ullman, E. (1996). The effects of treatment team diversity and sex on assessments of team functioning. *Hospital & Health Services Administration, 41*, 37–53.

Ancona, D. G. (1990). Outward bound: Strategies for team survival in an organization. *Academy of Management Journal, 2*, 334–365.

Ancona, D. G., & Caldwell, D. F. (1992a). Bridging the boundary: External activity and performance in organizational teams. *Administrative Science Quarterly, 37*, 634–665.

Ancona, D. G., & Caldwell, D. F. (1992b). Demography and design: Predictors of a new product team performance. *Organization Science, 3*, 321–341.

Ancona, D. G., & Caldwell, D. F. (1998). Rethinking team composition from the outside in. In D. H. Gruenfeld (Ed.), *Research on managing groups and teams* (pp. 21–37). Stamford, CT: MAI Press.

Arnold, H. J., & Feldman, D. C. (1986). *Organizational behavior.* New York: McGraw-Hill.

Arrow, H., McGrath, J. E., & Berdahl, J. L. (2000). *Small groups as complex systems.* Thousand Oaks, CA: Sage Publications.

Ashforth, B. E., & Mael, F. (1989). Social identity theory and the organization. *Academy of Management Journal, 32*, 20–39.

Athanasaw, Y. (2003). Team characteristics and team member knowledge, skills, and ability relationships to the effectiveness of cross-functional teams in the public sector. *International Journal of Public Administration, 26*, 1165–1204.

Bales, R. F. Interaction Process Analysis. Cambridge, Mass: Addison-Wesley, 1950.

Barczak, G., & McDonough, E. F. (2003, November–December). Leading global product development teams. *Research Technology Management, 46* (6), 14.

Batalden, P. B., Nelson, E. C., Edwards, W. H., Godfrey, M. M., & Mohr, J. J. (2003, November). Microsystems in health care: Part 9. Developing small clinical units to attain peak performance. *Joint Commission Journal on Quality Improvement, 29* (11), 575–585.

Beckhard, R. (1967). The confrontation meeting. *Harvard Business Review, 43*, 159–165.

Beersma, B., Hollenbeck, J. R., Humphrey, S. E., Moon, H., Conlon, D. E., & Ilgen, D. R. (2003). Cooperation, competition, and team performance: Toward a contingency approach. *Academy of Management Journal, 46*, 572–591.

Benne, K., & Sheats, P. (1948). Functional roles of group members. *Journal of Social Issues, 2*, 42–47.

Berwick, D. M. (1995). The toxicity of pay for performance. *Quality Management in Health Care, 4* (1), 27–33.

Bettenhausen, K. L. (1991). Five years of group research: What we have learned and what needs to be addressed. *Journal of Management, 17,* 345–381.

Blake, R. R., & Mouton, J. S. (1978). *The new managerial grid.* Houston, TX: Gulf.

Blake, R. R., & Mouton, J. S. (1984). *Solving costly organizational conflicts.* San Francisco: Jossey-Bass.

Bohmer, R., & Edmondson, A. (2001, March–April). Organizational learning in health care. *Health Forum Journal,* 32–35

Bohmer, R., & Edmondson, A., (2002). Intermountain Health Care. Harvard Business School Case (#9-602-145). Boston: HBS Press.

Brodbeck, F. (1996). Work group performance and effectiveness: Conceptual and measurement issues. In M. A. West (Ed.), *Handbook of Work Group Psychology* (pp. 285–315). Chichester: Wiley.

Brown, B., & Keyes, M. (2000). Blurred roles and permeable boundaries: The experience of multidisciplinary working in community mental health. *Health and Social Care in the Community, 8* (6), 425–435.

Burchard, J. D., Burchard, S. N., Sewell, R., & VanDenBerg, J. (1993). *One kid at a time.* Juneau, AK: State of Alaska Division of Mental Health and Mental Retardation.

Campion, M. A., Medsker, G. J., & Higgs, A. C. (1993). Relations between work group characteristics and effectiveness: Implications for designing effective work groups. *Personnel Psychology, 46,* 823–850.

Cannon-Bowers, J. A., Oser, R., & Flanagan, D. L. (1992). Work teams in industry: A selected review and proposed framework. In R. W. Swezey, & E. Salas (Eds.), *Teams: Their training and performance.* Norwood, NJ: Ablex Publishing.

Capelli, P., & Rogovsky, N. (1994). New work systems and skills requirements. *International Labour Review, 133* (2), 205–220.

Cartwright, D., & Zander, A. (1968). *Group dynamics: Research and theory* (3rd ed.). New York: Harper & Row.

Cassard, S. D., Weisman, C. S., Gordon, D. L., & Wong, R. (1994). The impact of unit-based self-management by nurses on patient outcomes. *Health Services Research, 29,* 415–433.

Chatman, J., & O'Reilly, C. (2004). Asymmetric effects of work group demographics on men's and women's responses to work group composition. *Academy of Management Journal, 47* (2), 193–208.

Chen, G., & Klimoski, R. J. (2003). The impact of expectations on newcomer performance in teams as mediated by work characteristics, social exchanges, and empowerment. *Academy of Management Journal, 46,* 591–607.

Cheser, R. (1999). When teams go to war—against each other! *Quality Progress, 32,* 25–29.

Cohen, S. G., & Bailey, D. E. (1997). What makes teams work: Group effectiveness research from the shop floor to the executive suite. *Journal of Management, 23,* 239–290.

Colquitt, J. A., Noe, R. A., & Jackson, C. L. (2002). Justice in teams: Antecedents and consequences of procedural justice climate. *Personnel Psychology, 55,* 83–100.

Coopman, S. J. (2001). Democracy, performance, and outcomes in interdisciplinary health care teams. *The Journal of Business Communication, 38* (3), 261–281.

Cosier, R. A. (1981). Dialectical inquiry in strategic planning: A case of premature acceptance? *Academy of Management Review, 6,* 643–648.

Cummings, T. (1978). Self-regulating work groups: A socio-technical synthesis. *Academy of Management Review, 3,* 625–634.

Dailey, R., Young, A., & Barr, C. (1991). Empowering middle managers in hospitals with team-based problem solving. *Health Care Management Review, 16,* 55–63.

Deber, R. B., & Leatt, P. (1986). The multidisciplinary renal team: Who makes the decisions? *Health Matrix, 4* (3), 3–9.

Deeter-Schmelz, D. R., & Ramsey, D. R. (2003). An investigation of team information processing in service teams: Exploring the link between teams and customers. *Journal of the Academy of Marketing Science, 31* (4), 409–425.

Delbecq, A., Van de Ven, A., & Gustafson, D. (1975). *Group techniques for program planning.* Glenview, IL: Scott, Foresman.

Denison, D. R., & Sutton, R. I. (1990). Operating room nurses. In J. R. Hackman (Ed.), *Groups that work (and those that don't): Creating conditions for effective teamwork.* San Francisco: Jossey-Bass.

Deutsch, M. (1949). An experimental study of the effects of co-operation and competition upon group process. *Human Relations, 2,* 199–232.

Dooley, K. J., & Zimmerman, B. J. (2003). Merger as marriage: Communication issues in postmerger integration. *Health Care Management Review, 28,* 55–68.

Doran, D., Baker, R., Murray, M., Bohnen, J., Zahn, C., Sidani, S., & Carryer, J. (2002). Achieving clinical improvement: An interdisciplinary intervention. *Health Care Management Review, 27,* 42–57.

Dyer, J. L. (1984). Team research and team training: A state-of-the-art review. In F. A. Muckler (Ed.), *Human factors review* (pp. 285–323). Santa Monica, CA: Human Factors Society.

Edmondson, A. C. (1996). Learning from mistakes is easier said than done: Group and organizational influences on the detection and correction of human error. *Journal of Applied Behavioral Science, 32* (1), 5–28.

Edmondson, A. C. (1999). Psychological safety and learning behavior in work teams. *Administrative Science Quarterly, 44,* 350–383.

Edmondson, A. C. (2002). The local and variegated nature of learning in organizations. *Organization Science, 13* (2), 128–146.

Edmondson, A. C. (2003). Speaking up in the operating room: How team leaders promote learning in interdisciplinary action teams. *Journal of Management Studies, 40* (6), 1419–1452.

Edmondson, A. C. (2004). Learning from failure in health care: Frequent opportunities, pervasive barriers. *Quality and Safety in Health Care, 13,* 3–9.

Edmondson, A. C., Bohmer, R. M., & Pisano, G. P. (2001). Disrupted routines: Team learning and new technology implementation in hospitals. *Administrative Science Quarterly, 46,* 685–716.

Edmondson, A. C., Roberto, M., & Watkins, M. (2003) A dynamic model of top management team effectiveness: Managing unstructured task streams. *Leadership Quarterly, 219,* 1–29.

Erickson, J. (1997). Turmoil in Tuscon. *American Medical News, 40* (34), 1–23.

Etzioni, A. (1961). *A comparative analysis of complex organizations* (p. 114). New York: Free Press.

Fargason, C. A., & Haddock, C. C. (1992). Crossfunctional, integrative team decision making: Essential for effective QI in health care. *Quality Review Bulletin, 7,* 157–163.

French, W. L., & Bell, C. H. (1990). *Organizational development.* Englewood Cliffs, NJ: Prentice Hall.

Fried, B. J., Johnsen, M. C., Starrett, B. E., Calloway, M. O., & Morrissey, J. P. (1998). An empirical assessment of rural community support networks for individuals with severe mental disorders. *Community Mental Health Journal, 34* (1), 39–56.

Fried, B., & Nelson, W. (1987). Strategic planning with family physicians. *Canadian Family Physician, 33,* 1309–1312.

Furst, S. A., Reeves, M., Rosen, B., & Blackburn, R. S. (2004). Managing the life cycle of virtual teams. *Academy of Management Executive, 18,* 6–20.

George, J. F., & Jones, G. R. (1999). *Understanding and managing organizational behavior* (2nd ed.). Reading, MA: Addison-Wesley.

George, J. M. (1992). Extrinsic and intrinsic origins of perceived social loafing in organizations. *Academy of Management Journal, 35,* 191–202.

Gersick, C. J. (1989). Marking time: Predictable transitions in task groups. *Academy of Management, 32,* 274–309.

Gist, M. E., Locke, E. A., & Taylor, M. S. (1987). Organizational behavior: Group structure, process, and effectiveness. *Journal of Management, 13,* 237–257.

Gladstein, D. (1984). Groups in context: A model of task group effectiveness. *Administrative Science Quarterly, 29,* 499–517.

Goodman, P. S., Ravlin, E., & Schminke, M. (1987). Understanding groups in organizations. *Research in Organizational Behavior, 9,* 121–173.

Gordon, J. (1992, October). Work teams: How far have they come? *Training,* 59–65.

Gordon, J. R. (1999). *Organizational behavior: A diagnostic approach.* Upper Saddle River, NJ: Prentice Hall.

Gully, S. M., Devine, D. J., & Whitney D. J. (1995). A meta-analysis of cohesion and performance. *Small Group Research, 26,* 497–520.

Guzzo, R. A. (1990). Group decision making and group effectiveness in organizations. In P. S. Goodman (Ed.), *Designing effective work groups.* San Francisco: Jossey-Bass.

Hackman, J. R. (1976). Work design. In J. R. Hackman & J. L. Suttle (Eds.), *Improving life at work.* Santa Monica, CA: Goodyear.

Hackman, J. R. (1982). *A set of methods for research on work teams* (Technical Report No. 1). School of Organization and Management. New Haven, CT: Yale University.

Hackman, J. R. (1987). The design of work teams. In J. Lorsch (Ed.), *Handbook of organizational behavior.* New York: Prentice-Hall.

Hackman, J. R. (1990). Introduction. Work teams in organizations: An orienting framework. In Hackman, J. R. (Ed.) (1990a). *Groups that work (and those that don't): Creating conditions for effectiveness teamwork.* San Francisco: Jossey-Bass.

Hackman, J. R. (2003). Learning more by crossing levels: Evidence from airplanes, hospitals, and orchestras. *Journal of Organizational Behavior, 24* (8), 905–1013.

Hackman, J. R., & Oldham, G. R. (1980). *Work redesign.* Reading, MA: Addison-Wesley.

Hasenfeld, Y. (1983). *Human service organizations.* Englewood Cliffs, NJ: Prentice-Hall.

Hirst, G., & Mann, L. (2004). A model of R&D leadership and team communication: The relationship with project performance. *R & D Management, 34,* 147–161.

Hoegl, M., & Gemuenden, H. G. (2001). Teamwork quality and the success of innovative projects: A theoretical concept and empirical evidence. *Organization Science, 12,* 435–449.

Horak, B. J., Guarino, J. H., Knight, C. C., & Kweder, S. L. (1991). Building a team on a medical floor. *Health Care Management Review, 16,* 65–71.

Huber, G. (1980). *Managerial decision making.* Glenview, IL: Scott, Foresman.

Hunsaker, P. L., & Cook, C. W. (1986). *Managing organizational behavior.* Reading, MA: Addison-Wesley.

Institute of Medicine. (2003). *Keeping patients safe: Transforming environment of nurses.* Washington, DC: National Academics Press.

Jackson, S. E. (1992). Team composition in organizational settings: Issues in managing an increasingly diverse work force. In S. Worchel, W. Wood, & J. A. Simpson (Eds.), *Group process and productivity.* Newbury Park, CA: Sage.

Jackson, S. E., Joshi, A., & Erhardt, N. L. (2003). Recent research on team and organizational diversity: SWOT analysis and implications. *Journal of Management, 29* (6), 801–830.

Janis, L. (1972). *Victims of groupthink.* Boston: Houghton-Mifflin.

Joint Commission on Accreditation of Healthcare Organizations. (2005). *2005 comprehensive accreditation manual for hospitals: The official handbook (CAMH).* Oakbrook Terrace, IL: JCAHO, 2005.

Katz, N. (2001). Getting the most out of your team. *Harvard Business Review, 79,* 22.

Katzenbach, J. R., & Smith, D. K. (1993). The discipline of teams. *Harvard Business Review, 71,* 111–120.

Kirkman, B. L., & Rosen, B. (1997). A model of work team empowerment. In R. Woodman & W. Pasmore (Eds.), *Research in organizational change and development* (pp. 131–167). Greenwich, CT: Jai Press.

Kolodny, H., & Kiggundu, M. (1980). Towards the development of a sociotechnical systems model in woodlands mechanical harvesting. *Human Relations, 33,* 623–645.

Kor, Y. (2003). Experience-based top management team competence and sustained growth. *Organization Science, 14* (6), 707–720.

Knaus, W. A., & Duffy, J. (1994). The performance of intensive care units: Does good management make a difference? *Medical Care, 32,* 508–525.

Lacey, R., & Gruenfeld, D. (1999). Unwrapping the work group: How extra-organizational context affects group behavior. *Research on Managing Groups and Teams, 2,* 157–177.

LaPenta, C., & Jacobs, G. M. (1996). Application of group process model to performance appraisal development in a CQI environment. *Health Care Management Review, 21,* 45–60.

Larson, J., Christensen, C., Abbott, A., & Franz, T. (1996). Diagnosing groups: charting the flow of information in medical decision making teams. *Journal of Personality and Social Psychology, 71,* 315–330.

Latane, B., Williams, K. D., & Harkins, S. (1979). Many hands make light the work: The causes and consequences of social loafing. *Journal of Personality and Social Psychology, 37,* 822–832.

Liberman, R. P., Hilty, D. M., Drake, R. E., & Tsang, H. (2001). Requirements for multidisciplinary teamwork in psychiatric rehabilitation. *Psychiatric Services, 52* (10), 1331–1342.

Liden, R. C., Wayne, S. J., Jaworski, R. A., & Bennett, N. (2004). Social loafing: A field investigation. *Journal of Management, 30,* 285–305.

Lubit, R. H. (2003). Coping with toxic managers, subordinates . . . and other difficult people: Using emotional intelligence to survive and prosper. *Financial Times,* Prentice Hall.

Marks, M. A., Zaccaro, S. J., & Mathieu, J. E. (2000). Performance implications of leader briefings and team-interaction training for team adaptation to novel environments. *Journal of Applied Psychology, 85,* 971–987.

McGrath, J. E. (1984). *Groups: Interaction and performance.* Englewood Cliffs, NJ: Prentice-Hall.

McGregor, D. (1960). *The human side of enterprise.* New York: McGraw-Hill.

Mechanic, D. (1962). Sources of power of lower participants in complex organizations. *Administrative Science Quarterly, 7*(4), 349–364.

Moorhead, G., & Griffin, R. W. (1998). *Organizational behavior: Managing people and organizations.* Boston: Houghton Mifflin.

Moreland, R. L., & Levine, J. M. (1988). Group dynamics over time: Development and socialization in small groups. In J. E. McGrath (Ed.), *The social psychology of groups* (pp. 151–181). Beverly Hills, CA: Sage.

Mullen, B., & Baumeister, R. F. (1987). Group effects on self-attention and performance: Social loafing, social facilitation, and social impairment. In C. Hendrick (Ed.), *Review of personality and social psychology.* Beverly Hills, CA: Sage.

Nadler, D. A., & Tushman, M. L. (1988). *Strategic organization design: Concepts, tools, and processes.* Glenview, IL: Scott, Foresman.

Nelson, E. C., Batalden, P. B., Huber, T. P., Mohr, J. J., Godfrey, M. M., Headrick, L. A., & Wasson, J. H. (2002). Microsystems in Health Care: Part 1. Learning from High-Performing Front-Line Clinical Units. *Joint Commission Journal on Quality Improvement, 28* (9), 472–493.

Nelson, R. E. (1989). The strength of strong ties: Social networks and intergroup conflict in organizations. *Academy of Management Journal, 32,* 377–401.

Orsburn, J. D., Moran, L., Musselwhite, E., & Zenger, J. (1990). *Self-directed work teams: The new American challenge.* Homewood, IL: Business One Irwin.

Owens, D. A., Mannic, E. A., & Neale, M. A. (1998). Strategic formation of groups: Issues in task performance and team member selection. In D. H. Gruenfeld (Ed.), *Research on managing groups and teams* (pp. 149–165). Stamford, CT: MAI Press.

Parker, G., McAdams, J., & Zielinski, D. (2000). *Rewarding teams: Lessons from the trenches.* San Francisco: Jossey-Bass Publishers.

Pascarella, P. (1997, February). Compensating teams. *Across the Board,* 16–22.

Pinto, M. B., & Pinton, J. K. (1990). Project team communication and cross-functional cooperation in new program development. *Journal of Product Innovation Management, 7,* 200–212.

Roberts, K. H., & Hunt, D. M. (1991). *Organizational behavior.* Boston: PWS-Kent Publishing Co.

Robinson, A., & Street, A. (2004). Care of older people: Improving networks between acute care nurses and an aged care assessment team. *Journal of Clinical Nursing, 13* (4), 486–497.

Roethlisberger, F. J., & Dickson, W. J. (1939). *Management and the worker.* Cambridge, MA: Harvard University Press.

Rundall, T. G., Starkweather, D. B., & Norrish, B. A. (1998). *After restructuring: Empowerment strategies at work in America's hospitals.* San Francisco: Jossey-Bass.

Salas, E., Burke, C. S., & Cannon-Bowers, J. A. (2000). Teamwork: Emerging principles. *International Journal of Management Reviews, 2* (4), 339–356.

Salvedra, R., Earley, P. C., & Van Dync, L. (1993). Complex interdependence in task performing groups. *Journal of Applied Psychology, 78,* 61–72.

Schein, E. H. (1985). *Organizational culture and leadership.* San Francisco: Jossey-Bass Publishers.

Schein, E. H., & Bennis, W. (1965). *Personal and organizational change through group methods.* New York: Wiley.

Schmitt, M. H. (2001). Collaboration improves the quality of care: Methodological challenges and evidence from health care research. *Journal of Interprofessional Care* (15), 47–66.

Schweikhart, S. B., & Smith-Daniels, V. (1996). Reengineering the work of caregivers: Role redefinition, team structures, and organizational redesign. *Health Care Management Review, 41,* 19–36.

Schwenk, C. R. (1983). Laboratory research on illstructured decision aids: The case of dialectical inquiry. *Decision Sciences, 14,* 140–144.

Scott, W. G. (1967). *Organization theory.* Homewood, IL: Irwin.

Seashore, S. (1954). *Group cohesiveness in the industrial work group.* Ann Arbor, MI: Institute for Social Research, University of Michigan.

Shaw, M. E. (1976). *Group dynamics: The psychology of small group behavior.* New York: McGraw-Hill.

Shaw, R. B. (1990). Mental health treatment teams. In J. R. Hackman (Ed.), *Groups that work (and those that don't)* (pp. 320–348). San Francisco: Jossey Bass.

Sherif, M., & Sherif, C. W. (1953). *Groups in harmony and tension.* New York: Harper.

Shortell, S. M., Marsteller, J. A., Lin, M., Pearson, M. L., Wu, S., Mendel, P., Cretin, S., & Rosen, M. (2004). The role of perceived team effectiveness in improving chronic illness care. *Medical Care, 42* (11), 1040–1048.

Shortell, S. M., Zimmerman, J. E., Rousseau, D. M., et al. (1994), The performance of intensive care units. Does good management make a difference? *Medical Care* 32, 508–525.

Sidorov, J. (2003). Case study of a failed merger of hospital systems. *Managed Care, 12* (11), 56–60.

Stasser, G. (1999). The uncertain role of unshared information in collective choice. In L. Thompson, J. Levine, & D. Messick (Eds.), *Shared cognition in organizations* (pp. 49–69). Mahwah, NJ: Lawrence Erlbaum Associates.

Steiner, I. D. (1972). *Group Process and Productivity,* New York, Academic Press.

Stewart, G. L., & Barrick, M. R. (2000). Team structure and performance: Assessing the mediating role of intrateam process and the moderating role of task type. *Academy of Management Journal, 43* (20), 135–148.

Stigler, G. J. (1974). Free riders and collective action: An appendix to theories of economic regulation. *Bell Journal of Economics and Management Science, 5,* 359–365.

Stoner, C. R., & Hartman, R. I. (1993). Team building: Answering the tough questions. *Business Horizons, 36,* 70–78.

Sundstrom, E., DeMeuse, K. P., & Futrell, D. (1990). Work teams: Applications and effectiveness. *American Psychologist, 45* (2), 120–133.

Thompson, J. D. (1967). *Organizations in action.* New York: McGraw-Hill.

Thyen, M. N., Theis, R., & Tebbitt, B. V. (1993). Organizational empowerment through self-governed teams. *Journal of Nursing Administration, 23,* 24–26.

Topping, S., Breland, J., & Fowler, A. (2004). *Interagency teams: The nature of collaboration, interaction, and effectiveness in serving children and youth with SED* (Working Paper).

Topping, S., & Calloway, M. (2000). Does resource scarcity create interorganizational coordination and formal service linkages? A case study of a rural mental health system. *Advances in Health Care Management, 1,* 393–419.

Topping, S., Norton, T., & Scafidi, B. (2003). Coordination of services: The use of multidisciplinary, interagency teams. In S. Dopson & A. L. Mark (Eds.), *Leading Health Care Organizations* (pp. 100–112). New York: Palgrave Macmillan.

Tuckman, B. W. (1965). Developmental sequences in small groups. *Psychological Bulletin, 63,* 384–399.

Van de Ven, A. H., Delbecq, A. L., & Koenig, R. (1976). Determinants of coordination modes within organizations. *American Sociological Review, 41,* 322–338.

Veenstra, G. (2000). Social capital, SES and health: An individual-level analysis. *Social Science & Medicine, 50,* 619–629.

Vinokur-Kaplan, D. (1995a). Enhancing the effectiveness of interdisciplinary mental health treatment teams. *Administration and Policy in Mental Health, 22* (5), 521–530.

Vinokur-Kaplan, D. (1995b). Treatment teams that work (and those that don't): An application of Hackman's group effectiveness model to interdisciplinary teams in psychiatric hospitals. *Journal of Applied Behavioral Science, 31,* 303–327.

Wagner, J. A. (1994). Participation's effects on performance and satisfaction: A reconsideration of research evidence. *Academy of Management Review, 19,* 312–330.

Walsh, J., & Hewitt, H. (1996). Facilitating an effective process in treatment groups with persons having serious mental illness. *Social Work with Groups, 19,* 5–18.

Webster, C. M., Grusky, O., Young, A., & Podus, D. (1998). Leadership structures in case management teams: An application of social network analysis. *Research in Community and Mental Health, 9,* 11–28.

Weist, M. D., Lowie, J. A., Flaherty, L. T., & Pruitt, D. (2001). Collaboration among the education, mental health, and public health systems to promote youth mental health. *Psychiatric Services, 52* (10), 1348–1351.

Wells, J. L., Seabrook, J. A., Stolee P., et al. (2003). State of the art in geriatric rehabilitation. Part I: Review of frailty and comprehensive geriatric assessment. *Archives of Physical Medical and Rehabilitation, 84* (6), 890–897.

Whetten, D. A., & Cameron, K. S. (1998). *Developing management skills* (4th ed.). Reading, MA: Addison-Wesley.

Yang, H., & Tang, J. (2004). Team structure and team performance in IS development: A social network perspective. *Information & Management, 41,* 335–350.

Zarraga, C., & Bonache, J. (2003). Assessing the team environment for knowledge sharing: An empirical analysis. *International Journal of Human Resource Management, 14* (7), 1227–1246.

CHAPTER 7

Work Design

Martin P. Charns, D.B.A. and Jody Hoffer Gittell, Ph.D.

CHAPTER OUTLINE

- Changes in the Design of Health Care Work
- Contrasting Approaches to Work Design
- Dividing Work into Jobs
- Job Requirements
- Psychological Approach
- Technical Approach
- Summary of Contrasting Approaches
- Applying the Framework

LEARNING OBJECTIVES

After completing this chapter, the reader should be able to:

1. Identify the range of approaches to work design, including the psychological and technical approaches.

2. Understand the relationships between work design and individuals' motivation and productivity.

3. Discuss the differences between work and working.

4. Identify tasks, their characteristics, and their performance requirements.

5. Analyze the interconnectedness of tasks among individuals and among work groups.

6. Understand how to approach the design of individual jobs and of work units.

7. Understand the benefits of drawing on both the psychological and the technical approaches to work design, and how the concept of relational coordination helps to do so.

KEY TERMS

Analyzing the Work

Approaches to Work Design

Coordinating Mechanisms

Designing Individual Jobs

Direct Work

Feedback Approaches to
   Coordination

Horizontal Division of Labor

Interconnectedness of Work

Management Work

Motivating Potential of a Job

Multiskilled Employees

Programming Approaches to
   Coordination

Psychological Approach to
   Work Design

Relational Coordination

Scientific Management

Support Work

Task Inventory Approach to
   Work Design

Technical Approach to Work
   Design

Vertical Division of Labor

Work Requirements

IN PRACTICE   A Tale of Two Units

Unit A, an orthopedics unit in a major Eastern teaching hospital, is characterized by high dissatisfaction among the nursing staff and is the target of frequent complaints from residents and attending physicians. Communication among the nurses, therapists, social workers, residents, and attending physicians regarding patient care is poor, and relationships among them are strained.

The unit generally appears to be in a state of chaos. Patients and their families seek information about their status from physicians, nurses, and other staff, and frequently complain that they receive conflicting information from the medical and nursing staffs. At the same time, lengths of stay are unacceptably long due to poor communication among the staff rather than due to unique patient needs.

The organization of the hospital is similar to that of most major teaching facilities, with the major departments representing professional (nursing, social service, dietary) and nonprofessional (housekeeping, security, transportation) functions.

Unit A has two case managers, RNs by training, whose caseloads are typically 32 patients each. They are responsible for reviewing resource utilization, for ensuring that all staff members adhere to care paths, and for planning patient

discharges. Care paths—protocols specifying the sequence and timing of tasks for patients with particular routine conditions—have been introduced over the past five years to streamline communication among the staff. Unit A staff stopped holding interdisciplinary rounds several years ago on the belief that these meetings consume too much valuable staff time, and have chosen to manage care primarily through care paths instead.

Unit B is an orthopedics unit in a different Eastern teaching hospital. It has a reputation for quality care and responsiveness to both patients and their families. Nurses and other staff express high satisfaction about their work. Communication between nurses, therapists, social workers, residents, and attending physicians is said to be frequent, timely, and accurate, and relationships among them appear to be strong. In general, the unit runs smoothly and responds well to routine situations as well as unusual cases. Patients are routinely discharged on the anticipated day, except when their health status dictates a longer stay.

Unit B differs from Unit A in several ways. Case managers work in four teams made up of one RN and one social worker. Each team has a caseload of 16 patients, giving each team member an

(continues)

IN PRACTICE *(continued)*

effective caseload of only eight patients. Along with their smaller caseloads and their broader set of skills, Unit B case managers have a broader range of tasks than their counterparts on Unit A. Like Unit A's case managers, they are responsible for monitoring resource utilization and adherence to care paths and for planning discharge, but they are also responsible for attending and leading interdisciplinary patient rounds, for attending physician rounds, and for coordinating clinical care. Case managers also follow patients after discharge, to assess any follow-up needs they might have.

Each case-management team is assigned to a small number of orthopedic surgeons, and follows the patients of those surgeons exclusively. The dedication of case managers to a small number of physicians allows them to attend physician rounds and report the physician perspective back to the rest of the staff through interdisciplinary rounds. As a result of their multiple roles and assignment to physicians, case managers on Unit B are the nexus of communication regarding orthopedic patients.

Unit B patients with routine conditions are assigned to care paths, as on Unit A, but their care is still actively managed through interdisciplinary rounds. Interdisciplinary rounds are held twice weekly on Unit B, and are attended by a broad range of functions—the nurse manager, the nurse and social work case managers, primary nurses, physical therapists, and a radiologist. Also attending patient rounds are representatives from the rehab facilities and home care agencies to which patients are referred for follow-up care, facilitating communication and continuity of care across settings.

CHAPTER PURPOSE

Differences between the effectively functioning orthopedic Unit B and the chaotic Unit A are seen by many administrators and health care professionals as arising from differences in leadership or staff competence. Others attribute the differences in unit performance to differences in work design. But they disagree whether Unit B's work design is more effective because it leads to more job satisfaction and a more motivated staff, or because it better supports the flow of information across interconnected jobs. Is Unit B's superior performance due to the psychological or technical benefits of its work design? (See In Practice, page 213.)

The purpose of this chapter is to provide a framework for the design of individual jobs and organizational work groups, and to describe the relationships between work design, motivation, and information flow. Two major approaches to job design are discussed along with their inherent assumptions, strengths, and limitations. An integration of the concepts and a framework for their managerial application are then presented.

Work design concepts can be applied at several levels in an organization. In fact, they can be applied to analyze and design the work of two or more related organizations, such as integrated delivery systems, an organization and its suppliers, or referral networks. In this chapter, the concepts are applied in a single organization. Attention is directed to the design of work contained within single jobs (i.e., job design) and the design of work within organizational units consisting of several jobs (i.e., work unit design).

But in reality, the design of a single job cannot be separated from the design of the work unit. Because jobs on a work unit are interrelated, the design of a single job must be carried out with a view to how it fits with other related jobs. Otherwise, we risk having unintended overlaps between jobs, resulting in inefficiency and confusion, or worse, gaps between jobs such that critical tasks may not be completed in a reliable way. Indeed, work design is closely related to the problems of teamwork (Chapter 6), coordination (Chapter 8), and overall design of the organization (Chapter 10). In this chapter, we discuss both the vertical division of labor and the horizontal division of labor, and how work can be designed to facilitate teamwork and coordination between those who are caring for the same patients.

CHANGES IN THE DESIGN OF HEALTH CARE WORK

Health care has undergone major transitions in the past 10 years. Work arrangements that made half-hearted attempts at efficiency in the fee-for-service health care system are no longer viable. Coordination and the management of care have become primary tools for controlling health care costs. The caregiver—physician, nurse, or other provider—cannot choose the course of treatment, or the equipment or supplies used to provide that treatment without considering the cost implications of these decisions on the patient, themselves, or their related organization. Where once a provider's convenience in scheduling a procedure was dominant, patient-centered services in today's leading organizations often dictate care be given at a time and location preferred by the patient and the insurer. No longer do we assume without question that providers always know or do what is "right" for their patients. Patients, health care organizations, and the benefits provided a patient through their insurance are limiting the discretion of physicians and other providers.

Through direct efforts, such as utilization management and tying financial considerations to patient care practices, as well as more indirect efforts,

such as creating a cost-conscious culture for the organization, managers are influencing physician decision making. The combination of organizational pressures and national efforts to define practice guidelines and outcomes of care are working together to force change. Although it is difficult for physicians to change practice styles developed over many years, to varying degrees they are changing their behavior. Whether the changes will improve or reduce the quality of care or the risk associated with it is still uncertain, but it is a question that will accompany the health care system over the next decade and help drive the quest for quality improvement, as further discussed in Chapter 12 and 13.

Like physicians, nurses are facing challenges to their practice. In the first decade of the twenty-first century we have experienced a severe shortage of nurses and other health professionals. This was caused by many factors including increased acuity of hospitalized patients, increased numbers of jobs in ambulatory settings and case review for insurance approval, women's increased professional opportunities outside of health care, and the drop in the number of nurses needing to work when other family income earners are doing well in a strong economy. In fact, the health care industry has experienced workforce shortages that have been cyclical but generally increasing in severity for many years before the beginning of the new millennium. Over this time the shortage led many hospitals to rethink the design of professional and nonprofessional jobs both to match the availability of lower skilled workers in the labor force and to create more stimulating jobs that workers would not leave. In addition, some organizations used this as an opportunity to redesign their patient care delivery systems to emphasize the patient as the raison d'etre. Even though the nursing shortage ameliorated with the downturn in the world economy in the late 1980s, many organizations continued their redesign efforts (Donnelly, 1989; *Strengthening hospital nursing*, 1992; Tonges, 1989). Many rural hospitals, characterized by a highly variable patient census, have found **multiskilled employees** and cross-trained staff to be effective ways to meet their highly fluctuating demand. It has become a critical element to their survival and is increasingly seen as important in the efforts to efficiently manage larger urban hospitals (Brider, 1992).

However, there is also an opposite trend, toward new job roles that increase the degree of specialization. New job roles are being used to extend the time of physicians, nurses, and therapists and thus to achieve lower costs of care. Physicians themselves continue to become increasingly specialized. One role that has grown dramatically in recent years is the hospitalist, or hospital specialist physician, a physician who specializes in inpatient care in order to become more efficient and effective in hospital-based medicine. This follows other recent trends, such as the emergency room physician and the intensivist. Implications of these new job designs for the coordination of care are addressed in this chapter and chapter 15.

Coordination of patient care continues to be a major challenge for the design of work (Institute of Medicine, 2001). An analysis of Controlled Risk Insurance Company (CRICO) claims showed that the most costly claims stem from failures to coordinate (Martin, 1996). In particular, there is a growing need to coordinate care across organizational boundaries, as more care is being provided outside of the hospital. As a result of shorter hospital stays mandated by managed care, patients are leaving hospitals in more vulnerable condition and are therefore more likely to receive follow-up care in other settings, such as rehabilitation hospitals, skilled nursing facilities, nursing homes, or at home with the help of home care providers. The careful handoff of information is critical to ensuring that patient recoveries continue on course and without error. Evidence shows that health care organizations can take the coordinating mechanisms developed for coordinating care inside their walls, such as clinical pathways, team meetings, case management, and information systems, and adapt them for coordinating care with external organizations (Gittell & Weiss, 2004).

CONTRASTING APPROACHES TO WORK DESIGN

The individual job is the basic element of any organization. As such, job design has been a focus of attention in the literatures of organizational behavior and health management. Contrasting **approaches to work design**, however, are found both in the literature and in practice. The **technical approach to work design** emerges from the tradition of scientific management, which recommends extracting maximum efficiency from workers by designing narrow, repetitive jobs. This approach has broadened beyond its roots in scientific management but still focuses on how job design affects skill and information requirements. The **psychological approach to work design** focuses instead on how job design affects worker motivation. This approach recommends motivating workers by designing jobs that are broad and relatively autonomous from supervisors and other workers. Both approaches argue that job design affects organizational performance, but they disagree about whether job design does so primarily through its effect on technical or psychological factors. (See Debate Time 7.1, p. 217).

In many health care organizations, jobs that are designed and managed from these differing perspectives exist side by side. For example, professionals (e.g., physicians, nurses, social workers) generally determine for themselves both what work to do and how to do it. Technical workers often have more narrowly defined jobs. The psychological approach suggests that professionals should therefore be more highly motivated than technical workers. Yet problems of low productivity, low morale, and dysfunctional individual behaviors, such as alcoholism

DEBATE TIME 7.1   What Do You Think?

The technical and psychological approaches to work design were developed by different groups of scholars based on different sets of premises. When applied to the design of any particular job, the two approaches yield very different outcomes.

The **scientific management** school as one technical approach prescribes breaking down work into discrete, repetitive components, and training workers to be expert in their narrow areas of responsibility. Proponents of this approach argue that simplifying work allows development of expertise, and through repetition of tasks, workers become highly proficient. Developed through this form of job engineering, highly skilled workers contribute to organizational productivity.

The psychological school argues that people should be provided with work that represents whole tasks with which they can identify. This provides the opportunity for people to feel that their work is meaningful, and they are more highly motivated to do it well. Workers' high motivation, in turn, is critical to organizational productivity. From the perspective of the psychological school, repetitive tasks are not rewarding to individuals. Without interest in their work, workers' motivation is low, and so is productivity.

How do you reconcile these different perspectives? What different assumptions form the underpinnings of the two different approaches? What situational factors have to be considered in applying the different theories?

and drug abuse, exist among both professional and technical workers. The technical approach suggests that information flow should be more problematic among those with narrowly defined jobs, but that the benefits of specialization override these costs of co-ordination. Yet complaints about the lack of timely, accurate communication are endemic in health care organizations. To solve problems of motivation and information flow, it is necessary to address both the technical and psychological elements of jobs.

One of the prime reasons for poor management and less than optimal performance in health care and other organizations is that managers confuse "work" and "working" (Charns & Schaefer, 1983; Drucker, 1973) and inappropriately manage the relationship between them. Work is objective and impersonal. It is energy directed at organizational goals, identifiable separately from the person who does it. It is analyzable. Working, on the other hand, is a worker's affective response to work. Far from to-

tally analyzable, it is individual, personal, and subjective.

Managers of technical, nonprofessional workers tend to follow the technical approach to job design. They focus on work and largely ignore working. The workers' affective responses are seen as extraneous elements to be controlled so that they do not interfere with work. In contrast, managers of professional workers tend to follow the psychological approach. Their attention is almost exclusively on working, to the neglect of work. The result is that work is directed at goals chosen by the professional, which may or may not be organizational goals. Similarly, managerial efforts to improve working conditions or to humanize work are often pursued with working in mind and with insufficient and inappropriate consideration for the work requirements. Yet work affects working, and working affects work. Both are important elements in efforts to manage patient care in a way that produces high-quality and efficient outcomes.

In the next two sections, we lay the groundwork for exploring the technical and psychological approaches in greater depth. Regardless of which approach one takes, one must address how work is to be divided into jobs, and what qualities are required of the people who perform them.

DIVIDING WORK INTO JOBS

Work is divided into jobs along two dimensions—horizontal and vertical. The horizontal dimension determines how broad a particular job is—how many related tasks are included in that job. The vertical dimension determines how deep a particular job is—whether that job includes direct work, managerial work, and support work, or just one of the above. (See Figure 7.1 for a depiction of job breadth and depth.) These dimensions are relevant to both the technical and psychological approaches to job design. The two approaches suggest different criteria, however—skill and information requirements rather than motivational requirements—for determining how broad or deep a particular job should be.

In addition, both the vertical and the horizontal division of labor create specialization, and specialization in turn increases the challenge for teamwork and coordination.

Vertical Division of Labor

All organizations perform three different types of work in the **vertical division of labor**: **management work**, **direct work**, and **support work**. Direct work is effort that directly contributes to the accomplishment of an organization's goals. In health care organizations, clinical work performed by doctors, nurses, and other care providers is direct work. In organizations that have multiple

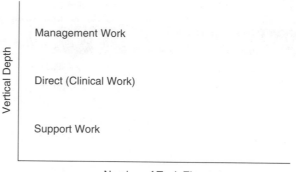

Figure 7.1. Dimensions of Work

goals, such as teaching hospitals, there is a set of direct work activities for each goal (e.g., teaching, research, and patient care). Although an individual may perform more than one type of direct work, the work itself is identifiable and analyzable separate from the person performing it (Charns & Schaefer, 1983; Stoelwinder & Charns, 1981).

Management work includes providing the resources and context within which direct work can be performed effectively and maintaining an alignment between an organization and its external environment. Management work is decision making about the organizational context within which other work is performed (Charns & Schaefer, 1983). For example, it includes determining what services to provide, what services to develop or reduce, what resources to make available to whom, and what systems will perform various functions. Since the primary method of influencing decision making is to influence its premises—the information that is considered in making a decision—management work affects all other work because it influences the premises on which other decisions are made (Simon, 1976).

Support work does not directly result in achievement of an organizational goal, but it is needed for effective accomplishment of other work. For example, support work for clinical work includes such things as maintaining medical records, transporting patients, maintaining the physical surroundings in which care is delivered, and performing laboratory tests. Support work for management work includes providing legal counsel, clerical assistance, data on both internal operations and the external environment, and planning and analytical assistance, as well as personnel support.

These three types of work can be divided into distinct jobs, or combined in the same job. Jobs that encompass two or more of these types of work are considered to have more depth than jobs that encompass only one type of work.

For example, physicians, nurses, and physical therapists have traditionally been responsible for determining a plan of care, as well as delivering that care; but increasingly, these tasks are being carried out by others in the division of labor. Physicians, nurses, and therapists are still responsible for determining the plan of care, while physician assistants, nursing aides, and therapy assistants are increasingly employed for carrying out the plan of care. These job roles are lower paid and, by enabling the physician, nurse, and therapist to manage larger patient loads, they are intended to lower the costs of care.

These additional roles in the vertical division of labor can make coordination more difficult to achieve, by increasing the number of people involved in the care of a given patient. In addition, because these new roles are subordinate, people who fill them often face licensing restrictions that prohibit them from coordinating care directly with other functions or disciplines (e.g., a nursing aide may not have the authority to coordinate with a physical therapy assistant). As a result, those who have less immediate contact with the patient (the physician, nurse, or therapist) are responsible for coordinating a patient's care with each other, even though they are less directly informed about the patient's condition. This pattern of coordination between those *in charge* of the work rather than between those who are *performing* the work is considered an outmoded form of work design that other industries have sought to eliminate.

Horizontal Division of Labor

The best approach for identifying tasks in the **horizontal division of labor** is to assess the natural boundaries in work that occur along the dimensions of time, technology, and territory (Miller, 1959). When different work is or can be performed at different points in time, such as on different days or at different times of the day, distinct tasks can be identified. For example, patient care given during one office visit is distinguishable from that given during another visit, as is patient care delivered to a patient during different hospital admissions. Similarly, discrete tasks can often be identified by the fact that they are performed in different places (territories), such as in hospital, ambulatory, and home care settings. Finally, tasks can be identified by the technology involved.

Technology should be considered broadly to include not only hardware, but also skills and training, personality characteristics and interpersonal orientations, and different practices associated with performing different work. Such different practices may result from tradition, from regulation of government, licensing agencies, or accrediting bodies, or from professional norms of accepted practice. Thus, for example, the work performed by different professional groups is a natural place to look for inherent boundaries (Charns & Schaefer, 1983). In doing so, however, analysis must determine whether differences are real and inherent in the work or are maintained only by tradition.

By taking a broad perspective of technology, we can also ask what differences in work are associated with different parts of an organization's environment. For example, do different patients represent different types of work? Do treating different diseases or preventing illness in contrast to treating it represent the use of different technologies and therefore different work? Often differences in technology overlap with differences in time or territory, but together they help identify discrete tasks.

The more discrete tasks included in a particular job, the broader that job is considered to be. Health care professionals have typically performed broad jobs.

It is interesting to consider the impact of this increased specialization on the challenge of coordinating patient care. On the one hand, these additional roles can make coordination more difficult to achieve, by increasing the number of people involved in the care of a given patient. In addition, because these new roles are subordinate to the existing roles, people filling these roles may face status barriers and licensing prohibitions when they attempt to coordinate care directly with others. For example, certified nursing aides in nursing homes are often discouraged or even prohibited from communicating directly with other disciplines about the care of their patients. According to some reports, this is because no one would listen to them anyway, given the lack of respect they garner from their colleagues in some settings. Others argue that nursing aides are discouraged from communicating directly with other disciplines regarding the care of their patients because all communication must be channeled through the nurse who is responsible for the patient's care. Regardless of the rationale, this practice makes the new job design less effective from a coordination standpoint—the nurse remains responsible for the patient's care and must coordinate with others even though he or she may not have the most immediate contact with the patient in question.

Another area of work design innovation has been in the explosion of case-management jobs, specifically designed to improve the coordination of care. Case managers are now employed by private practice physicians, by hospitals, and by managed care organizations, to manage both inpatient and outpatient care. The rapid growth of the case-management role has led to an unexpected problem, namely the overlapping jurisdictions of case managers and the resulting potential for confusion by patients about who is in charge of coordinating their care.

Finally, physician specialization has continued to increase, particularly in the area of hospital-based specialties. Experience has suggested that private practice physicians are not ideally equipped to treat patients in the hospital setting, due to the distinctive routines and communication patterns that exist in that setting. By specializing in hospital-based care, physicians can become increasingly expert in working within that setting. This trend has led to the rise of "intensivists" who specialize in intensive care medicine, to the rise of emergency room specialist physicians, and more recently to the rise of "hospitalists" who specialize in the delivery of care on hospital medical units. Recent findings suggest that patient care teams led by hospitalists achieve significantly better risk-adjusted outcomes, including shorter lengths of stay, lower total costs, lower likelihood of readmission and lower rate of mortality, relative to patient care teams led by private practice physicians (Gittell, Weinberg, Bennett, & Miller, 2004). Furthermore, these teams report significantly higher levels of coordination, particularly between the physician and other team members, than do patient teams led by private practice physicians. Here then is an example where an increase in specialization has actually contributed to an improvement in the coordination of care, because hospitalist physicians have the opportunity to focus on the delivery of care to a particular type of patient, thus becoming familiar with other members of the patient care team who work with that type of patient.

The hospitalist physician represents a different form of specialization than the work design literature typically addresses. Rather than further splitting up the work involved in caring for a given patient, which makes coordination more challenging to achieve, this form of specialization occurs around the type of patient served. The impact of this form of specialization is to focus the time of care team members around a particular set of repeated interactions, thus improving the coordination of care.

Job Requirements

Once a job has been defined as a set of tasks in the horizontal and vertical divisions of labor, several approaches exist for determining the personal attributes needed to perform well in that job. Galbraith (1977) has provided a set of categories for determining the behaviors required for effective task performance. Galbraith's five categories in cumulative order are:

1. decisions to join and remain in an organization

2. dependable role performance

3. effort above minimum levels

4. spontaneous and innovative behavior

5. cooperative behavior

In general, all jobs require the first two categories of behavior. Organizations require that people join and remain employed in their jobs and that they perform dependably. These two minimum levels of behavior, however, are often not completely met. Where the work itself or the working conditions do not provide a worker with an acceptable level of rewards—including satisfaction—turnover and absenteeism result. Dependable role performance also does not occur when people do not know what is expected of them or they feel that the work that is expected of them is not equitably balanced with the rewards of the job.

When jobs require more than the first two minimum categories of behavior, the design of the job itself becomes a greater concern. When all elements of the work cannot be anticipated, spontaneous and innovative behavior is required. This requirement can be distinguished from behavior above minimum levels by the frequency with which unanticipated events occur and the degree of innovative behavior required. It is characterized by an individual needing to recognize that spontaneous and innovative behavior is required and having the skills and willingness to act. When, in addition, the work requires an individual to recognize and be willing and able to work with others to achieve the desired outcome, it requires cooperative behavior.

The five categories of behavior are cumulative and form a scale directly related to the inherent uncertainty of the work. Thus, work that is highly certain and predictable generally requires only the first two categories of behavior. The uncertainty inherent in work requires cooperative behavior in addition to all four other categories of behavior.

Regardless of whether one takes the psychological or technical approach, one must address how work is to be divided into jobs, and what qualities are required of the people who perform them. Each approach suggests a different criterion, however—motivation versus information—for thinking about these job design issues.

PSYCHOLOGICAL APPROACH

The psychological approach, rooted in psychology and organizational behavior, focuses on worker motivation. This approach assumes that, when individuals perform work that meets their needs for growth, and jobs themselves are intrinsically rewarding, substantial motivation results (also see Chapter 3). Professional jobs, in which there generally is a strong relationship between an individual's self-concept and her work, are examples. On the other hand, routine, repetitive jobs that encompass only a small portion of a larger task or jobs that are strictly and narrowly delineated are difficult for anyone to identify with. Such jobs limit the extent of an individual's involvement in the work and the motivation to perform well; therefore, productivity suffers. The psychological approach therefore argues that well-designed jobs are broad rather than narrow.

Sometimes, however, when individuals have total discretion over the way they do their work and what work they perform, their motivation may be directed toward other than organizational goals. In fact, they may work against the organization's goals. The assumption that motivation will result in organizationally desirable productivity does not necessarily hold. Even so, professional workers are often given complete discretion over what they do and how they do it. This, in fact, is one of the attributes of a profession. In medicine, generally regarded as the prime example of a profession, professional work is typically off limits to organizational job design analysis.

The autonomy of health care professionals, however, is being challenged. The issues of cost control, quality, competition, and responsiveness to customers have come to dominate the health care system of the 1990s. Health care managers have responded to these issues and to the challenges of a market-driven health care system by moving to make their organizations more price sensitive; cost effective; and patient, family, and client centered.

Assumptions Underlying the Psychological Approach

Underlying the design of any job are assumptions about individuals and the relationship between individuals and their work. These assumptions may be formally stated (as in a labor contract) or not, and they may be recognized by managers or not. The psychological job design approach is based upon the general assumptions that people work to satisfy a broad range of needs and that the design of a job affects the person's ability to meet those needs. Two perspectives can be taken to consider in greater detail the relationship between job design and motivation.

First, consider that people are motivated by unfulfilled needs and that they exert effort to satisfy those needs. If opportunities for meeting a person's needs are provided by the work itself, the person will be motivated to perform the work. Where work itself does not provide opportunities to satisfy individual needs, the person will seek other outlets and may not be motivated to perform the work. Thus, it is important to match people and their needs to jobs and their inherent **work requirements**. For example, if work requires an individual only to join and remain in the organization and to perform dependably, these behaviors can often be obtained by matching the job to people with economic needs and rewarding them monetarily. When such jobs are held instead by peo-

ple whose needs are for achievement or other forms of personal growth, the individuals most likely will not respond only to monetary rewards and will direct their efforts away from the dependable role performance required by the organization (McClelland, 1975). These people are better matched to jobs that require spontaneous and innovative behavior.

A second perspective on individual motivation is based upon the assumption that people evaluate courses of action for the purpose of choosing among them. The expectancy model of motivation posits that individuals exhibit behavior that they perceive will result in outcomes that yield valued rewards (Porter & Lawler, 1968; Vroom, 1961). In its simplest form, the model indicates that people subjectively evaluate possible behaviors in terms of three elements: the probability that a behavior will yield a desired outcome, the probability that the outcome will yield rewards, and the value of those rewards to the individual. These three elements combine multiplicatively in a person's assessment so that, if any one element is low, it is unlikely that the person will choose the associated behavior. Where that behavior is required to perform work effectively, we must ask how the elements of the model of motivation are affected by the job.

When work is intrinsically rewarding to individuals—that is, when effectively performing the work itself is inherently rewarding—we can see that there is a direct connection between behavior and rewards. This is likely to occur with the following psychological conditions (Hackman, Janson, Oldham, & Purdy, 1975):

- *Experienced meaningfulness.* The job is seen as important, valuable, and worthwhile.
- *Experienced responsibility.* Individuals feel personally responsible and accountable for the results of their efforts.
- *Knowledge of results.* Individuals understand how effectively they are performing the job.

These three aspects of working have a major impact on a person's motivation and are themselves affected both by characteristics of the individual and by the content of the work itself.

Three characteristics of a job contribute to its experienced meaningfulness: skill variety, task identity, and task significance. Skill variety refers to the variety of different skills and talents required of an individual in performing a job. A job that has task identity represents an identifiable piece of work that an individual can perform from beginning to end and that has a visible outcome. Task significance refers to the impact a job has on the lives of other people. In general, because health care organizations perform work that directly affects other people, great potential exists for designing jobs with high task significance. Yet by designing isolated jobs in which people cannot see how their work is an important part of a whole effort that helps other people, one can create jobs low in all three core dimensions.

Experienced responsibility for work outcomes is directly affected by the degree of autonomy in a job. The components of autonomy are freedom and discretion in scheduling work and in determining procedures to be used in performing it. A considerable degree of autonomy is present in jobs falling into Galbraith's (1977) categories of "effort above minimum levels," "spontaneous and innovative behavior," and "cooperative behavior."

Feedback on work performance provides an individual with the third psychological dimension, knowledge of results. The most direct feedback is from the work itself, available primarily in situations in which an individual has responsibility for a whole and identifiable element of work. Where job design itself cannot provide direct feedback, it is important to obtain feedback from supervisors or peers.

An additional potential source of feedback is an organization's performance evaluation system. In some organizations, performance evaluation is based solely on the subjective appraisal of an employee's supervisor. In others, however, it is based upon achievement of measurable goals. To the extent the goals for assessment of an individual align with the organization's goals, the individual's efforts can be directed at achievement of the organization's goals, in addition to serving as a feedback mechanism. In some organizations, the goals used for performance evaluation are goals of the program or department for which the individual has a major share of responsibility (Kotch et al., 1986).

To some degree, skill variety, task identity, and task significance can substitute for one another because they all contribute additively to experienced meaningfulness. Together they combine multiplicatively with autonomy (experienced responsibility) and feedback (knowledge of results) in contributing to the overall **motivating potential of a job**. A job's motivating potential score (MPS) can be expressed as follows (Hackman et al., 1975):

$$\text{MPS} = 1/3 \text{ (Skill Variety + Task Identity + Task Significance)} \times \text{Autonomy} \times \text{Feedback}$$

Whether a job with a high MPS will actually result in high individual motivation depends upon the characteristics of the jobholder. People with high growth needs—strong needs for achievement, self-actualization, and personal development—will be most motivated by jobs with high motivating potential. It is also possible for people who do not have high growth needs to find their growth needs stimulated by jobs with a high MPS. On the other hand, not all people react positively to challenging jobs, and the autonomy and challenge may result instead in anxiety and low performance. Individuals also differ in their preferences for working individually versus working in groups, or for routine versus innovative work. Fit between an individual's preferences for work and the organization's preferred mode of working results in greater job satisfaction (Chatman, 1991).

When people successfully accomplish work that satisfies their needs, job satisfaction is experienced. This in turn contributes to the expectation that future performance will result in satisfaction, and high levels of motivation generally result. Satisfaction, however, can result from meeting other needs, either within or outside of the workplace, but without contributing to motivation or to job performance. For example, satisfaction results from meeting one's social needs in the work setting. Although meeting the social needs of one's staff may increase satisfaction and even reduce turnover, it will not necessarily result in high motivation or performance.

TECHNICAL APPROACH

The technical approach is based on the scientific management school of thought developed by Taylor (1911) and Gilbreth (1911). Scientific management had its genesis in manufacturing organizations and led to the development of industrial engineering. Through examination of job activities in time-and-motion studies, industrial engineers design jobs to most efficiently utilize technology and to minimize wasted human effort. Within a technologically driven work setting, workers most suitable to the jobs are selected and trained. Through experience, workers become more proficient at their jobs, and thus specialization and routinization of work activities attempt to take advantage of the individual's learning curve. Since an objective of this approach is elimination of extraneous activities, its success depends on ensuring that people perform the job as designed.

Scientific management has made important contributions to management, especially in heavy industries such as the U.S. automobile industry. Scientific management approaches have gone beyond manufacturing settings, however, and have made contributions to both inpatient and ambulatory health care settings.

There are three assumptions underlying the scientific management approach to job design:

1. Work can be divided into repetitive routine elements.

2. Workers can be trained and motivated to perform dependably.

3. Workers' motivation derives primarily from economic rewards that can be associated with reliable performance of the work, rather than from job design itself.

Although these assumptions have face validity in many situations, they are also inherently limiting. Often the work cannot be divided into elements that can be repetitively performed. In addition, workers frequently seek more than economic rewards from their work and react to routine repetitive jobs by not performing dependably or by quitting the job. From a purely economic perspective, the cost of repeated recruiting and training often exceeds the benefits believed to be gained from technological efficiency. In human terms, the inefficiency and potential for errors that might harm patients are increased.

The routine nature of many jobs in support services in hospitals and other care settings, such as transport, laboratory, laundry, and radiology, allows job activities to be studied from a scientific management perspective. However, systems designed in this manner are tailored to meet specific conditions and are inherently unresponsive to change or uncertainty. Since patient needs and emergencies are not always subject to specification, employees at *all* levels of a health care organization are frequently required to use their own judgment, which limits the usefulness of scientific-management principles.

The **task inventory approach to work design** is a more flexible version of the technical approach and is often used in studies of jobs of health professionals, especially nurses, physicians, and physician assistants. In the mid-1960s, a shortage of health workers was predicted in the United States. In response, the task inventory methodology was developed in order to categorize job activities and determine whether parts of a professional's job might be performed by other workers (Braun, Howard, & Pond, 1972; Nelson, Jacobs, & Breer, 1975; *The utilization of manpower,* 1975). Kane and Jacoby (1973), for example, demonstrated the feasibility of using physician assistants (Medex) for job activities not requiring a fully trained physician. The same methodology is currently the basis for

(1)	(2)	(3)	(4)
Task	Who Now Performs Task	Knowledge and Skills Required	Alternative Performers and Their Training Needs
1.			
2.			
3.			
4.			
5.			

Continue as needed.

Figure 7.2. Task Inventory

studies seeking to determine the costs of nursing and other care activities in response to hospital prospective payment, managed care, and continuing changes in health care financing.

In this tradition Gilpatrick (1977), for example, conducted the Health Services Mobility Study, identifying and analyzing tasks of health care workers and determining job skills and knowledge needed to perform each task. This approach specified the required job skills and knowledge of health care workers, thereby providing a basis for defining their educational needs. Common educational needs for various jobs and career ladders were developed by which individuals could advance not only upward but also across traditional disciplines. Curricula in many schools of allied health have been modified to produce multicompetent health professionals to work in health care settings (Beachey, 1988; Blayney, Wilson, Bamberg, & Vaughn, 1989; Hedrick, 1987; Russell, Richardson, & Escamilla, 1989).

In applying the task inventory approach, it is helpful to develop a table similar to that in Figure 7.2. Elements of work, or tasks, are listed in the first column. Then for each task, who currently performs the task is (are) listed in column 2, the knowledge and skills required are listed in column 3, and other individuals who perform the task or other jobs in which the task could be incorporated are listed in column 4. Additionally, the training required for the individuals is noted in column 4. The task inventory method provides a helpful approach to identifying tasks. When using this method, it is important not to overlook significant but difficult to observe aspects of work. Furthermore, this approach starts with a description of the status quo. To the extent that a set of jobs does not include important aspects of work that should be present, the analysis will be incomplete.

Unlike scientific management, the task inventory methodology does not assume that jobs are better if narrowly defined. The methodology could yield the recommendation that a given job should be either more narrowly or more broadly defined, based on skill and information requirements.

The Interconnectedness of Work

Once tasks have been identified, it is necessary to determine how they fit together to form a coherent whole. While the psychological approach considers how tasks should be combined to improve worker motivation, the technical approach is to determine for each task the other tasks essential to its effective performance. Some tasks are more interconnected than others. At one extreme are tasks that can be performed independently of each other. For example, feeding one patient and performing laboratory tests on a specimen from another patient are independent tasks. In contrast, successful performance of other types of work requires that different tasks occur in sequence or that one element affects a second task that, in turn, acts upon the first task. For example, in medical diagnosis, initial diagnosis determines what laboratory and radiologic procedures are required. The results of those studies refine the original diagnosis. At the most complex level, tasks affect each other simultaneously. Van de Ven, Dethecq, and Koenig (1976) have called this "team interdependence," while Thompson (1967) called it "reciprocal interdependence," exemplified by the administration of anesthesia and the performance of surgery on a patient.

The concept of **interconnectedness of work** is critical to effective work design. When interconnected elements of work are performed by different people, components must be coordinated to ensure effective performance. Coordination requires resources from the organization, such as development and use of plans and protocols, supervision of people responsible for interconnected elements, or discussion among those people. Where possible, therefore, it is most effective to design jobs to minimize spreading interconnected elements over several people. This model is not always feasible because elements are often too numerous for a one-person assignment; because elements are so different from one another that no one individual has the skills, training, desire, or inclination to do them all; or because technological advantages outweigh costs of coordination. When the interconnected elements cannot reside within one single job, it is best to organize work to contain the interconnected elements within a single work group (Charns & Schaefer, 1983; Thompson, 1967).

It is often the interconnectedness of work that health care organizations fail to address as they attempt to respond to the pressures of a competitive health care system. Efforts to improve institutional responsiveness through reorganization, continuous quality improvement, and other measures must address how the elements of work fit together and how they influence job design and performance.

Coordinating Interconnected Work within Units

Coordination of work has been the subject of considerable research. How to achieve coordination among interconnected tasks within a single unit is the subject of this section. Additional aspects of coordination are considered in Chapter 8.

Much research has shown, in health care and other settings, that coordination affects organizational performance (Argote, 1982; Duncan, 1973; Georgopoulis & Mann, 1962; Shortell et al., 1994; Van de Ven et al., 1976). Knaus, Draper, Wagner, and Zimmerman (1986) found that variations in mortality in critical care units were related to the level of coordination in the units. With the development of more refined measurement tools, this line of work continues to be advanced (Shortell, Rousseau, Gillies, Devers, & Simons, 1991). Recently Young et al. (1998) found the pattern of coordination among nurses, surgeons, and anesthesiologists to be related to risk-adjusted rates of postsurgical complications. In addition to clinical outcomes, some studies have found a link between coordination and outcomes such as greater patient satisfaction and shorter lengths of stay

(Gittell et al., 2000). These performance outcomes are increasingly relevant in a more cost-conscious, patient-centered health care environment.

But research also shows that the most effective way of achieving coordination varies with the characteristics of the work performed. Duncan (1973), for example, provided one of the first empirical studies of variation in coordination within work units, finding that work units change their patterns of interaction in response to differing levels of task uncertainty. Building upon the theoretical work of March and Simon (1958), Van de Ven et al. (1976) found variations in patterns of coordination among units facing different levels of task uncertainty.

Charns, Stoelwinder, Miller, and Schaefer (1981) and Charns and Schaefer (1983) extended the findings of Van de Ven et al. (1976) and the theoretical writings of Mintzberg (1979) to suggest that work groups use two primary approaches to coordination—programming and feedback—and that the use of these approaches is related to the effectiveness of patient care units. Charns and Strayer (1981) replicated these findings in a residential school for severely emotionally disturbed children.

The set of **programming approaches to coordination** includes three ways of standardizing the performance of work that are most effective when the work is well understood and programmable.

- Standardization of work processes is the use of rules, regulations, schedules, plans, procedures, policies, and protocols to specify the activities to be performed. Included are care plans and multi-disciplinary clinical critical paths, which specify for a particular patient condition the interventions required and anticipated results at various times.

- Standardization of skills is the specification of the training or skills required to perform work. Often this is achieved through specification of minimum levels and types of education, certification as evidence of meeting minimum qualifications, or on-the-job training.

- Standardization of output specifies the form of intermediate outcomes of work as they are passed from one job to another.

In situations of high uncertainty, programming approaches alone cannot provide the needed coordination. Exchange of information and feedback is needed. **Feedback approaches to coordination**, which facilitate the transfer of information in unfamiliar situations, include the following:

- Supervision is the basis for coordination through an organization's hierarchy. It is the exchange of information between two people, one of whom is responsible for the work of the other.

- Mutual adjustment is the exchange of information about work performance between two people who are not in a hierarchical relationship, such as between two nurses, between a nurse and a physician, or between a case manager and other care providers.

- Group coordination is the exchange of information among more than two people, such as through meetings, rounds, and conferences.

Feedback approaches to coordination are more time consuming and require more effort than programming approaches. However, they are needed in situations characterized by high levels of uncertainty.

One feedback approach is case management. There has been an explosion of case-management jobs in health care, employed by hospitals, health maintenance organizations, and physician groups, specifically to improve the coordination of care. Case managers play the role of boundary spanners, helping to facilitate handoffs and helping the patient negotiate the boundaries between different members of the care provider team. Like boundary spanners more generally, case managers play an information-processing role within organizations (Galbraith, 1977) and between organizations (Aldrich & Herker, 1977). Organizational scholars have learned that boundary spanners are most successful when they not only process information, but also read contextual clues (Tushman & Scanlan, 1981), build trust (Currall & Judge, 1995), and build shared goals, shared knowledge, and mutual respect across boundaries (Gittell, 2002). However, to play these multiple roles effectively is time-consuming. Research in both airlines and health care shows that case managers are more effective in coordinating work when they are responsible for a relatively small number of flights (Gittell, 2003) or a relatively small number of patients (Gittell, 2002). Smaller caseloads for case managers can allow other participants to use their time more efficiently, therefore reducing overall resource utilization.

Evidence indicates that higher-performing patient care units in teaching hospitals differ from lower-performing units in their greater use of all six types of **coordinating mechanisms** (Charns et al., 1981). High-performing units utilize plans, rules, procedures, and protocols not as constraints and organizational red tape but as guidelines for routine work. Contrary to previous research findings, effective use of programming approaches actually allows staff—especially nurses—greater discretion in their work.

Similarly, one programming approach that has become increasingly prevalent—clinical pathways (Bohmer, 1998)—has the potential to increase the quality of communication and the quality of working relationships, rather than replace the need for them, as earlier theory would have predicted. A nine hospital study of care coordination for surgical patients showed that clinical pathways that included greater numbers of the relevant clinical functions led to higher levels of relational coordination among clinical staff, as well as higher quality and more efficient patient outcomes (Gittell, 2002). Faraj and Xiao (forthcoming) showed that even in the high-velocity environment of trauma units, programming in the form of trauma protocols plays an important role in the coordination of care. Like clinical pathways that are used for surgical patients, these protocols take the form of a standard operating procedure where roles, decision points, and event sequences are specified. These programmed approaches appear to improve coordination across different members of the patient care team even when actions cannot be fully prespecified, because above all, they provide a shared cognitive framework of the task. Both studies show, however, that these programmed approaches do not diminish the need for informal, relational forms of coordination. Rather they provide a context within which relational forms of coordination can more effectively occur.

In addition, when faced with unfamiliar situations, the higher-performing units increase their use of feedback approaches to a greater extent than the lower-performing ones. This result is consistent with findings from an earlier study of emergency rooms that nonprogrammed approaches to coordination were more effective under conditions of high uncertainty (Argote, 1982). Other feedback approaches help to improve coordination and patient outcomes. For example, in a study of joint replacement surgery, more inclusive team meetings and smaller caseloads for case managers predicted higher levels of relational coordination among clinical staff, as well as more efficient and higher-quality patient outcomes (Gittell, 2002).

Taken together with the findings about clinical pathways, these findings suggest that even relatively straightforward procedures benefit from using feedback approaches in addition to programming approaches. Consistent with previous findings, feedback approaches to coordination have an even stronger impact on outcomes as the uncertainty in patient conditions increases. What is new is that *both* programming and feedback approaches to coordination work by improving the quality of communication and the quality of working relationships among clinical staff, and that these communication and relationship ties—known as relational coordination—improve outcomes even for relatively simple procedures.

Feedback and programming approaches to coordination can both be designed to help to strengthen working relationships, but there are many practices in health care organizations that work in the opposite direction. Nursing staff turnover and rotation, house staff rotation, and limited physicians' and other professionals' involvement in a unit of a remote care setting greatly hinder the development of such relationships and can prevent full use of feedback approaches to coordination. Working relationships are also undermined by the professional identities of health care workers (Abbott, 1988) and by the occupational communities that tend to grow up around those professional identities (Van Maanen & Barley, 1984). Work design can be used to counteract these divisive tendencies and to strengthen key working relationships. As noted earlier, physician job design has large and highly significant effects on relational coordination between the physician and other clinicians, and on patient outcomes (Gittell, Weinberg, Bennett & Miller, 2004). Physician job design can be changed to foster physicians who specialize in hospital-based care, giving them the opportunity to focus on the delivery of care for a particular type of patient and to become familiar with the staff and routines of a particular hospital. This specialization improves coordination rather than increasing the challenge of coordination, because it is specialization around type of patient, rather than further splitting up the work involved in caring for a given patient.

Feedback mechanisms in particular rely on strong relationships among physicians, nurses, and other health care providers who must coordinate their efforts; but such relationships are not often achieved in health care organizations. Nursing staff turnover and rotation, house staff rotation, and limited physicians' and other professionals' involvement in a unit or a remote care setting greatly hinder the development of such relationships and can prevent full use of feedback approaches to coordination. But other aspects of organization design can strengthen these relationships. One study found that staff relationships are better in hospitals where staff are selected for their teamwork skills, and where processes are established for resolving conflicts among staff members involved in the care of a given patient population (Gittell, Weiss, & Wimbush, 2005).

To summarize, coordination affects both the quality and efficiency of organizational performance. Second, the types of coordinating approaches that can be used effectively depend somewhat upon the nature of the work of the unit. Greater advantage can be taken of programming approaches when the work of the unit is limited in scope and uncertainty, though even then programming appears to work better in tandem with feedback approaches. It should be noted that people with greater experience in a particular job will encounter fewer unfamiliar situations than people with less experience. The people with

less experience, therefore, need to use feedback approaches to a greater extent than do highly experienced people. This is typically reflected in their greater reliance on discussions with their manager or peers. Finally, feedback approaches require trust and understanding among people, which in turn requires organizational practices such as consistency in working together, conflict-resolution processes, or selection of staff members who are skilled at teamwork.

SUMMARY OF CONTRASTING APPROACHES

Both approaches to job design explored in this chapter—psychological and technical—reflect the belief that job design affects organizational performance; but they have different views on how job design affects organizational performance. According to the psychological approach, design can improve organizational performance by increasing worker motivation. According to the technical approach, job design can improve organizational performance by improving the flow of information among interconnected jobs. Figure 7.3 depicts this essential difference between the two approaches.

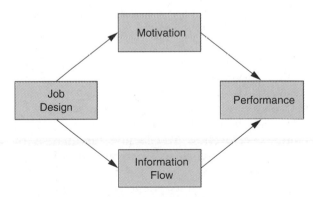

Figure 7.3. Assumptions of Causality in Psychological and Technical Approaches to Work Design

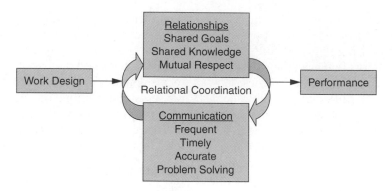

Figure 7.4. Assumption of Causality in Relational Coordination Approach to Work Design

In reality, job design may improve performance through both paths. When coordination is not fully achieved, work performance is hindered due to both technical and psychological factors. In addition to having a direct negative effect on patient care, the failure to coordinate precludes people who perform the work from attaining the levels of achievement or obtaining the sense of competence that would satisfy their needs. Professionals often feel that they are prevented from effectively carrying out their professional work by the ineffective way their organization functions. Where organizational factors hinder work accomplishment, people come to believe that hard work will not result in the desired outcome of good patient care. Using the expectancy model of motivation, the probability that effort will result in the desired outcome is low, and thus the motivation to work hard is reduced. Despite the satisfaction derived from their broadly defined, autonomous jobs, professionals may be dissatisfied by the difficulty of coordinating their work with others to achieve good patient care.

Effective work design therefore requires taking multiple perspectives based upon the analysis of work itself. In **designing individual jobs**, the work requirements should be matched to each workers' needs. To the extent possible, interconnected elements of work should be combined into individual jobs that possess high levels of skill vari-

ety, task identity, task significance, autonomy, and feedback. The design of individual jobs must be done within a framework that considers other related jobs, including that of the supervisor.

A new perspective has emerged in recent years, called **relational coordination**, which captures aspects of both the technical and psychological approaches to work design. Relational coordination encompasses technical concerns with information flow and task interdependence (or the interconnectedness of work), as well as psychosocial concerns with relational interdependence (or the quality of working relationships). Coordination is not seen as a mechanical process of information exchange, but rather as a relational process involving a network of communication and relationship ties among people whose tasks are interdependent (Weick & Roberts, 1993; Gittell, 2002; Faraj & Xiao, forthcoming). Figure 7.4 shows how work design affects relational coordination and performance. Compare with Figure 7.3 to see how the relational coordination approach to work design captures aspects of both the technical and psychological approaches.

Relational coordination takes account of the work itself, but also the process of working. Often the two have been disconnected. Relationships of shared goals, shared knowledge, and mutual respect tend to be weakest between people who carry out different jobs in the same work process—like

DEBATE TIME 7.2   What Do You Think?

In applying the work design concepts to the redesign of patient care delivery systems, two conflicting perspectives typically are raised. On the one hand, heads of existing support departments such as dietary, environmental services, and patient transport argue that staff efficiency can be maximized when staff performing similar activities are organized into separate functional departments. The staff can then be assigned to different patient care units in response to the varying needs of those units. This provides both the most efficient utilization of staff and responsiveness to fluctuations in need for services among patient care units. In addition, when organized in this manner, staff can best maintain proficiency in their particular skill area, thereby assuring the quality of their services.

On the other hand, nurse managers and directors of clinical units argue that multiskilled employees, cross-trained in several functional areas, should be permanently assigned to individual units. Having a broad range of skills reduces fragmentation of delivery of care and allows for flexibility in meeting the varying needs of each unit. By working consistently with the same group of other employees, the multiskilled workers can become part of the patient care team and be most responsive to the unique needs of their units.

Which of these perspectives is correct? If you choose to implement one of these approaches, how do you address the needs expressed by proponents of the other approach? Can you incorporate both perspectives in another creative work design? If so, how?

doctors, nurses, and social workers—even though this is where the task interdependencies tend to be strongest (Gittell, 2004). To achieve the quality and efficiency outcomes that health care organizations are striving for, managers must invest in relationships where they are hardest to build—between people with distinct, competing professional identities, whose work is highly interconnected.

Given the pressure to achieve both efficient and high-quality health care, it is more important than ever for managers to examine work design. How a health care manager chooses to do this is influenced by the range of approaches to work design and their conflicting underlying assumptions. But the failures of job redesign too often have been caused by taking too narrow and restrictive a focus. When managers become believers in one or another approach to job design, they limit their effectiveness and the

opportunity to integrate a variety of approaches for maximum advantage. In the multifaceted health care system of today, no one approach can guarantee success.

APPLYING THE FRAMEWORK

Work design concepts introduced in this chapter provide a framework for analyzing Units A and B (see In Practice, page 213) and determining options for change.

Components of patient care performed by different staff on a unit are highly interconnected. In different ways and with different success, both units used coordinating mechanisms to address these interconnections. Both utilized patient care paths, although on Unit B they were used in conjunction with, rather than as substitutes for, feedback mechanisms such as interdisciplinary rounds. Unit A had eliminated interdisciplinary rounds on the belief that they consumed too much staff time, but more staff and patient time was wasted as a result. Exceptions to the care path were not addressed and resolved in a timely, systematic way, requiring staff to spend much unnecessary time resolving these issues on the unit. Meanwhile, patients were left wondering about their status, and target discharge dates were missed.

Unit B continued to hold interdisciplinary rounds even after adopting care paths, on the belief that exceptions would arise even for patients undergoing routine treatments, and would require a dependable forum for their resolution. Holding rounds twice weekly and involving a broad range of staff members was costly in staff time, but was believed to save more staff time on balance. Unit B administrators also felt patients were better informed as a result of interdisciplinary rounds, therefore reducing patient complaints about conflicting information, and were more likely to be discharged on their target date, therefore satisfying payor needs for efficient resource utilization.

On Unit A, the administration thought that, since primary nurses had total responsibility for their patients, case managers could handle larger patient loads. On Unit B, both the primary nursing patient load and the case-management patient load were significantly smaller, allowing primary nurses and case managers to allocate more of their time to coordinating information flow on a personal basis with physicians and other members of the hospital staff. In addition, the broad range of responsibilities included in the Unit B case manager's job, and the combination of nursing and social work skills achieved through team staffing, made Unit B case managers the lynchpin for coordination of patient care on the unit.

Hospital administrators for Unit A also believed that supervision could be reduced. Thus, the nurse manager's responsibilities were expanded to cover several units. Physically removed from the unit, the nurse manager gave insufficient attention to professional development of new and junior staff. The nurse manager did not effectively orient new nursing and medical staff to the unit's routines, and standardized approaches to coordination broke down. Due to her wide span of control, the nurse manager was also unable to effectively coach Unit A nurses on coordinating exceptions to the care path with other staff members.

It was expected that nurses would coordinate their work with other members of the nursing and medical staffs, but Unit A's organizational arrangements hindered coordination. Nursing assignments were arranged almost randomly, so that a consistent pattern of interactions among staff members that would encourage strong working relationships did not develop. This hindered use of feedback approaches to coordination among nurses. It also made it difficult for a nurse providing care for another's patient to be involved or to identify with the patient, thereby limiting the motivating potential inherent in those efforts. Interactions with house staff also did not follow any consistent pattern, and each house officer had patients cared for by many different nurses. Over time the trust between the nursing and medical staff members on Unit A deteriorated.

On Unit B, the internal organization of nursing into two groups provided a basis for facilitating coordination both among nurses and between nurses and physicians. The small size of each nursing group and the arrangement for associates to cover for nurses within their group allowed nurses to identify with their group's patients. This contributed to the motivating potential of their jobs. Furthermore, the work interconnections among nurses were contained within each group. This facilitated management of these interconnections and contributed to development of trust needed among nursing staff for effective personal coordination. Each group included a mix of experienced and less-experienced nurses, and together with the nurse manager, the formally designated group leader had responsibility for staff development. By aligning teams of house staff and case managers with the nursing groups, the organization facilitated coordination.

As physicians, nurses, and case managers worked together on Unit B, trust among the groups developed, adding to their ability to use mutual adjustment to coordinate their efforts. All of the staff experienced a greater sense of accomplishment, contributing to their satisfaction and motivation. Because of the closeness and commitment of the personnel to other members of their group, they felt a sense of responsibility for the unit. Absenteeism was therefore low, and the more stable staffing in turn contributed to the unit's smooth functioning. The nurse manager considered house staff orientation to be a critical responsibility, and this further contributed to the unit's ability to coordinate its work. Staff and physicians were chosen explicitly for their willingness to work as part of a team, and conflicts were regularly addressed in a weekly problem-solving meeting involving all key disciplines.

In the late 1980s, Unit B introduced multiskilled employees to perform routine work that had been done by staff from several departments. To utilize these staff efficiently, they cared for patients of both teams, which did not allow them to be fully integrated into the teams. By being assigned to a single unit, however, they did feel a part of that unit. Performing many tasks for each patient, the multiskilled employees were responsive to patient needs. They saw the results of their efforts and gained much greater satisfaction from their work than had been the case when many people from different departments did those tasks. Multiskilled workers also contributed to patient satisfaction by reducing the number of staff going into each patient's room. Overall, Unit B addressed its work requirements more effectively than Unit A.

As the examples demonstrate, several factors must be considered to design productive work units consisting of inherently motivating and rewarding jobs. The basis for this design is **analyzing the work** itself. The content of individual jobs, the organization of work units, and the coordination of work both within and between units can be designed effectively only when the work requirements are understood. Just as the framework presented in this chapter was used to analyze the jobs of health professionals on two different patient care units, it can be used to design work in other settings (see Debate Time 7.2, p. 231).

DISCUSSION QUESTIONS

1. Under what conditions does a job with a high motivating potential lead to high job-holder motivation? To high satisfaction? To frustration?
2. What are the potential pitfalls in job redesign?
3. Give examples of highly motivated people who do not contribute greatly to organizational outcomes.
4. What is the relationship among individual motivation and satisfaction and an organization's ability to coordinate work?
5. How do relationships among work group members play a role in effective coordination?
6. Give examples of situations in which dependable role performance is required in a job, but effort above minimum levels is not. What happens when individuals in such jobs innovate? Give examples of jobs requiring cooperative behavior. What happens when people in such jobs are willing to give only dependable role performance?
7. Under what conditions are programming approaches to coordination constraints to effective performance? Under what conditions are they facilitating? When are feedback approaches to coordination inappropriate?
8. Explain how even programming coordinating mechanisms such as clinical pathways or information systems may help to facilitate effective communication and strengthen working relationships.

MANAGERIAL GUIDELINES

1. Jobs should be designed with both technical (information) and psychological (motivation) considerations in mind, taking account of the work itself as well as the subjective experience of working. These design considerations are relevant for both technical and professional jobs, and for jobs involving high or low uncertainty.

2. To enhance motivation, individual jobs should be designed to provide opportunities to satisfy the needs of the person performing a given job. People with high growth needs are more highly motivated by jobs providing experienced meaningfulness, experienced responsibility, and knowledge of results.

3. Work should be designed so that the most highly interconnected elements are contained within individual jobs to the extent that is possible, given considerations of size, limitations imposed by technology, and separation of job elements in time and space. Interconnected work elements that cannot be self-contained within single jobs should to the extent possible be placed within single work groups.

4. Coordination of interconnected work elements that are not contained within a single job directly affects work performance. This coordination generally can be facilitated most effectively through a combination of programming (standardization) and feedback (personal) approaches. Feedback approaches require strong relationships among those who use them.

REFERENCES

Abbott, A. (1988). *The system of professions: An essay on the division of expert labor.* Chicago: University of Chicago Press.

Aldrich, H. and Herker, D. (1977). Boundary spanning roles and organization structure. *Academy of Management Review, 2*(2): 217–230.

Argote, L. (1982). Input uncertainty and organizational coordination in hospital emergency units. *Administrative Science Quarterly, 27,* 420–434.

Beachey, H. W. (1988, November). Multi-competent health professionals: Needs, combinations, and curriculum development. *Journal of Allied Health,* 319–329.

Blayney, K. D., Wilson, B. R., Bamberg, R., & Vaughn, D. (1989, Winter). The multiskilled health practitioner movement: Where are we and how did we get here? *Journal of Allied Health,* 215–226.

Bohmer, R. (1998). Critical pathways at Massachusetts General Hospital. *Journal of Vascular Surgery, 28,* 373–377.

Braun, J. A., Howard, D. R., & Pond, L. R. (1972). The physician's associate: A task analysis. *Physician's Associate, 2*(3), 77–82.

Brider, P. (1992). The move to patient-focused care. *American Journal of Nursing, 9,* 26–33.

Charns, M. P., & Schaefer, M. J. (1983). *Health care organizations: A model for management.* Englewood Cliffs, NJ: Prentice-Hall.

Charns, M. P., Stoelwinder, J. U., Miller, R. A., & Schaefer, M. J. (1981, August). *Coordination and patient unit effectiveness.* Presented at the Academy of Management Annual Meetings, San Diego, CA.

Charns, M. P., & Strayer, R. G. (1981, August). *A socio-structural approach to organization development.* Presented at the Academy of Management Annual Meetings, San Diego, CA.

Chatman, J. A. (1991). Matching people and organizations: Selection and socialization in public accounting firms. *Administrative Science Quarterly, 36,* 459–484.

Currall, S. C. and Judge, T. A. (1995). Measuring trust between organizational boundary role persons.

Organizational Behavior and Human Decision Processes, 64(2): 151–170.

Donnelly, L. (1989, March/April). NME's caregiver system: 21st century patient care delivery. *Healthcare Executive, 4*(2), 25–27.

Drucker, P. F. (1973). *Management: Tasks, responsibilities, practices.* New York: Harper & Row.

Duncan, R. B. (1973). Multiple decision-making structures in adapting to environmental uncertainty: The impact on organizational effectiveness. *Human Relations, 26*(3), 273–291.

Faraj, S., & Xiao, Y. (forthcoming). *Coordination in fast response organizations.* Management Science.

Galbraith, J. R. (1977). *Organization design.* Reading, MA: Addison-Wesley.

Georgopoulis, B. S., & Mann, F. C. (1962). *The community general hospital* New York: Macmillan.

Gilbreth, F. B. (1911). *Motion study.* New York: Van Nostrand.

Gilpatrick, E. (1977). *The health services mobility study.* Springfield, VA; National Technical Information Service.

Gittell, J. H. (2002). Coordinating mechanisms in care provider groups: Relational coordination as a mediator and input uncertainty as a moderator of performance effects. *Management Science, 48*(11), 1408–1426.

Gittell, J. H. (2003). *The Southwest Airlines Way: Using the Power of Relationships to Achieve High Performance.* New York: McGraw-Hill.

Gittell, J. H. (2004). *The strength of weak ties: A relational perspective on task interdependence, coordination and performance.* Unpublished manuscript.

Gittell, J. H., Fairfield, K., Bierbaum, B., Head, W., Jackson, R., Kelly, M., Laskin, R., Lipson, S., Siliski, J., Thornhill, T., & Zuckerman, J. (2000). Impact of relational coordination on quality of care, post-operative pain and functioning, and length of stay: A nine hospital study of surgical patients. *Medical Care, 38*(8), 807–819.

Gittell, J. H., Weinberg, D., Bennett, A., & Miller, J. A. (2004). *Is the doctor in?* Impact of physician job design on relational coordination and patient outcomes. Unpublished manuscript.

Gittell, J. H., & Weiss, L. (2004). Coordination networks within and across organizations: A multi-level framework. *Journal of Management Studies, 41*(1), 127–153.

Gittell, J. H., Weiss, L. and Wimbush, J. (2005). Linking Organization Design and Networks to Improve the Coordination of Work. Unpublished manuscript.

Hackman, J. R., Janson, R., Oldham, G. R., & Purdy, K. (1975). A new strategy for job enrichment. *California Management Review, 17*(4), 57–71.

Hedrick, H. L. (1987, August). Closing in on cross-training. *Journal of Allied Health,* 265–275.

Institute of Medicine. (2001). *Crossing the quality chasm: A new health system for the 21st century.* Washington, D.C.: National Academy Press.

Kane, R., & Jacoby, I. (1973, November). *Alterations in tasks in the physicians office as a result of adding a Medex.* Presented at American Public Health Associates Meeting, San Francisco, CA.

Knaus, W. A., Draper, E. A., Wagner, D. P., & Zimmerman, J. E. (1986). An evaluation of outcome from intensive care in major medical centers. *Annals of Internal Medicine, 104,* 416–418.

Kotch, J. B., Burr, C., Toal, S., Brown, W., Abrantes, A., & Kaluzny, A. (1986). A performance-based management system to reduce prematurity and low birth weight. *Journal of Medical Systems, 10*(4), 375–390.

March, J. G., & Simon, H. A. (1958). *Organizations.* New York: John Wiley & Sons.

Martin, P. B. (1996). *Review of coordination of care issues in CRICO claims* (Forum). Risk Management Foundation of the Harvard Medical Institutions, Inc.

McClelland, D. C. (1975). *The achievement months* (2nd ed.). New York: Halsted Press.

Miller, E. J. (1959). Technology, territory and time: The internal differentiation of complex production systems. *Human Relations, 12*(3), 243–272.

Mintzberg, H. (1979). *The structuring of organizations.* Englewood Cliffs, NJ: Prentice-Hall.

Nelson, E., Jacobs, A., & Breer, D. (1975). A study of the validity of the task inventory method of job analysis. *Medical Care, 13*(2), 104–113.

Porter, I. W., & Lawler E. E., III. (1968). *Managerial attitudes and performance.* Homewood, IL: Irwin-Dolsey.

Russell, D. D., Richardson, R. F., & Escamilla, B. (1989, Spring). Multicompetency education in radiologic education. *Journal of Allied Health,* 281–289.

Shortell, S. M., Rousseau, D. M., Gilles, R. R., Devers, K. J., & Simons, T. L. (1991). Organizational assessment in intensive care units (ICUs): Construct development, reliability, and validity of the ICU nurse-physician questionnaire. *Medical Care, 29*(8), 709–727.

Shortell, S. M., Zimmerman, J., Rousseau, D., Gillies, R., Wagner, D., Draper, E., Knaus, W., & Duffy, J. (1994). The performance of intensive care units: Does good management make a difference? *Medical Care, 32*(5).

Simon, H. A. (1976). *Administrative behavior* (3rd ed.). New York: Free Press.

Stoelwinder, J. U., & Charns, M. P. (1981). A task field model of organization design and analysis. *Human Relations, 34*(9), 743–762.

Strengthening hospital nursing. A program to improve patient care—gaining momentum: A progress report. (1992). St. Petersburg, FL: National Program Office of the Strengthening Hospital Nursing Program.

Taylor, F. W. (1911). *The principles of scientific management.* New York: Harper & Row.

Thompson, J. D. (1967). *Organizations in action.* New York: McGraw-Hill.

Tonges, M. C. (1989). Redesigning hospital nursing practice: The professionally advanced care team (ProACT) model, Part 1. *Journal of Nursing Administration, 19*(7), 31–38.

Tushman, M. L. and Scanlan, T. J. (1981). Characteristics and external orientations of boundary spanning individuals. *Academy of Management Journal, 24*(1), 83–98.

The utilization of man power in ambulatory care: Development of a study methodology. (1975). Bureau of Health Manpower Education. Report of a Cooperative Study.

Van de Ven, A. H., Dethecq, A. L., & Koenig R., Jr. (1976). Determinants of coordination modes within organizations. *American Sociological Review, 41,* 322–338.

Van Maanen, J., & Barley, S. R. (1984). Occupational communities: Culture and control in organizations. In B. M. Staw & L. L. Cummings (Eds.), *Research in Organizational Behavior, 6,* 287–365. Greenwich, CT: JAI Press.

Vroom, V. H. (1961). *Work and motivation.* New York: John Wiley & Sons.

Weick, K. E., & Roberts, K. (1993). Collective mind in organizations: Heedful interrelating on flight decks. *Administrative Science Quarterly, 38,* 357–381.

Young, G., Charns, M., Desai, K., Khuri, S., Forbes, M., Henderson, W., & Daley, J. (1998, December, Part I). Patterns of coordination and clinical outcomes: A study of surgical services. *Health Services Research, 33*(5), 1211–1236.

CHAPTER 8

Coordination and Communication

Beaufort B. Longest, Jr., Ph.D. and Gary J. Young, J.D., Ph.D.

CHAPTER OUTLINE

- Interdependence
- Coordination
- Communication

LEARNING OBJECTIVES

After completing this chapter, the reader should be able to:

1. Differentiate between pooled, sequential, and reciprocal interdependence.

2. Differentiate between intraorganizational and interorganizational coordination.

3. Know a variety of coordination mechanisms used in intraorganizational and interorganizational settings.

4. Understand the importance of applying various coordinating mechanisms to a given situation using a contingency approach.

5. Know how to diagram the communication process and discuss its components.

6. Know ways to make communication more effective.

7. Know the environmental and personal barriers to communication, and ways to overcome them.

8. Understand the flows of intraorganizational communication, and know their uses.

9. Understand important aspects of communicating with two external stakeholders: the public sector and the community.

10. Understand the relationship between conducting stakeholder analysis and effective communication with external stakeholders.

KEY TERMS

Clinical Guidelines or
    Protocols
Communication
Communication Channels
Communication Networks
Contingency View of
    Coordination
Coordination
Critical Pathways
Environmental Barriers to
    Communication

Feedback
Informal Communication
Integrators
Interdependence
Linking Pins
Outcomes Assessments
Personal Barriers to
    Communication
Pooled Interdependence
Programming

Project-Management Design
Reciprocal Interdependence
Sequential Interdependence
Standardization of Work
    Outputs
Standardization of Work
    Processes
Standardization of Worker
    Skills

❧ IN PRACTICE

Press Release: May 13, 2004 CDC Announces New Goals and Organizational Design

Centers for Disease Control and Prevention (CDC) director Dr. Julie Gerberding announced today new goals and integrated operations that will allow the federal public health agency to have greater impact on the health of people around the world. Today's announcement evolved from an ongoing strategic development process called the Futures Initiative, which began a year ago at CDC and has included hundreds of employees, other agencies, organizations, and the public.

The integrated organization coordinates the agency's existing operational units into four coordinating centers to help the agency leverage its resources to be more nimble in responding to public health threats and emerging issues, as well as chronic health conditions. The new coordinating centers and their directors are:

- Coordinating Center for Infectious Diseases—includes the National Center for Infectious Diseases, the National Immunization Program, and the National Center for STD, TB, and HIV Prevention. Dr. Mitchell Cohen will lead this coordinating center.
- Coordinating Center for Health Promotion—includes the National Center for Chronic Disease Prevention and Health Promotion and the National Center for Birth Defects and Developmental Disabilities. Dr. Donna Stroup will lead this coordinating center.
- Coordinating Center for Environmental Health, Injury Prevention, and Occupational Health—includes the National Center for Environmental Health, the Agency for Toxic Substances and Disease Registry, the National Center for Injury

Prevention and Control, and the National Institute for Occupational Safety and Health. Dr. Henry Falk will lead this coordinating center.

■ Coordinating Center for Health Information and Services—includes the National Center for Health Statistics, a new National Center for Health Marketing, and a new National Center for Public Health Informatics. Dr. James Marks will lead this coordinating center.

Dr. Gerberding congratulated and thanked the thousands of employees and partners who have participated in the process and she reminded them all that they really are the cornerstone of CDC's future. She said the time is right to move forward with these changes. "CDC is very strong and credible agency that has—and will always—base its decisions on the best of science. The time for change to enhance your impact is when you're at your best and for CDC that time is right now."

For more information on Centers for Disease Control and Prevention, visit http://www.CDC.gov.

CHAPTER PURPOSE

As demonstrated by the reorganization of the Centers for Disease Control and Prevention, **coordination** and **communication** are closely related strategies through which managers link together the various people and units within their organization and link their organization to other organizations and agencies. Central to understanding the importance of communication and coordination strategies is an appreciation of the high level of interdependence exhibited by health care organizations. Interdependencies exist in both their internal structure and external relationships. Because health care organizations have become increasingly complex internally and have established a wide variety of external relationships, the establishment and maintenance of effective linkages are significant managerial challenges. If linkages are not effective, organizations may become fragmented, fractionated, and isolated with concomitant declines in performance.

The purpose of this chapter is to explore the managerial challenges associated with coordination and communication and to examine effective strategies for meeting these challenges. As demonstrated by the reorganization of the Centers for Disease Control and Prevention (see In Practice, p. 238), a number of approaches are available to achieve effective communication and coordination.

INTERDEPENDENCE

The need for both coordination and communication arises from interdependencies among the people and units within an organization or among organizations pursuing a common goal. Such interdependencies exist within and among organizations whenever work activities are interconnected in some manner physically or intellectually (Charns & Tewksbury, 1993). The degree of **interdependence** varies with the nature of the work requirements as well as the relative roles, responsibilities, and contributions of those performing the work itself (Van de Ven, Delbecq, & Koenig, 1976). Thompson (1967) has identified three forms of interdependence: pooled, sequential, and reciprocal.

Pooled interdependence occurs when individuals and units are related but do not bear a close connection; they simply contribute separately in some way to the larger whole. For example, a group of geographically dispersed nursing homes owned by a single corporation may be viewed as linked largely in the sense that each contributes to the overall success of the corporation, but they have very little direct interdependence. Their activities are pooled to make the corporation more effective.

Sequential interdependence occurs when individuals and units bear a close, but sequential, connection. For example, patients admitted to an acute care hospital become the focal points for extended chains of sequentially interdependent activities. The admitting office checks them in and schedules them in the operating room or other diagnostic and treatment units, notifies the dietary department of special needs, notifies the laboratory of the need for tests, and so on. Most of what is done for the patients until they are discharged occurs in a sequential manner.

Reciprocal interdependence occurs when individuals and units bear a close relationship, and the interdependence goes in both directions. For example, a vertically integrated health care system with acute care and long-term care capacity exhibits reciprocal interdependence. The long-term care beds are occupied by patients referred from the acute care beds. The acute care unit releases certain patients to the long-term care unit and suffers if long-term care cannot accept a patient. Conversely, the long-term care unit suffers if patients are not discharged to it from the acute unit. Further, the long-term care unit may need to transfer patients back to the hospital when acute episodes of illness occur. The interdependence between these units is reciprocal.

The level of interdependence intensifies as its form moves from pooled to sequential to reciprocal. In general, the higher the level of interdependence, the greater the need for managerial attention to effective linkages. Health care organizations generally exhibit very high levels of interdependence among their component parts, usually of the sequential or reciprocal forms. In highly interdependent health care organizations, coordination and communication are critical tasks for managers. These tasks are examined in depth below.

COORDINATION

Coordination is a means of dealing with interdependencies by effectively linking together the various parts of an organization or by linking together two or more organizations pursuing a common goal. This conscious activity is aimed at achieving unity and harmony of effort in pursuit of shared objectives, either within an organization or among organizations participating in a multiorganizational arrangement.

Coordination has long been viewed as one of the most important functions of management. One study found that "coordinating interdependent groups" was rated highly important by middle managers and executives and increased in importance as one moved into higher management positions (Kraut, Pedigo, McKenna, & Dunnette, 1989). Lawrence and Lorsch (1967), in a seminal study carried out more than 30 years ago with manufacturing firms, found that the effective coordination of interdependent units contributed substantially to better firm performance.

Much research also indicates that coordination plays an important role in the performance of health care organizations. Specifically, several studies of intensive care units indicate that effective communication and coordination among clinical staff results in more efficient and better quality of care (Baggs, Ryan, Phelps, Richeson, & Johnson, 1992; Knaus, Draper, Wagner, & Zimmerman, 1986; Shortell et al., 1994). More recent studies of other health care delivery settings also indicate that effective coordination of staff leads to better clinical outcomes (Gittell et al., 2000; Young et al., 1997; Young et al., 1998). Additionally, research suggests that ineffective coordination and communication among hospital staff contributes substantially to adverse events. For example, one study of the care of 1,047 patients in a large tertiary care hospital found that approximately 15% of the 480 adverse events identified (e.g., failure to order indicated tests, misplaced test results) had causes related to the interaction of staff, such as the failure of a consultant team to communicate adequately with the requesting team (Andrews et al., 1997).

For many types of health care organizations, staff coordination is also relevant to their ability to comply with the requirements of accrediting bodies. In particular, both the Joint Commission on the Accreditation of Health Care Organizations (http://www. jeaho.org) and the National Committee on Quality Assurance (http://www.hcqu.org), two leading accrediting bodies in the health care industry, have adopted standards that address coordination among professional groups, patient care units, and service components within health care organizations. While setting standards obviously cannot ensure good coordination, it does symbolize the growing recognition among accrediting and other oversight bodies that coordination is highly important to the performance of health care organizations.

Much of the general literature on coordination pertains to coordination within an organization, an intra-organizational perspective. An interorganizational perspective has become increasingly important within the health care industry with the rise of a wide variety of multiorganizational arrangements for providing patient care (also see Chapter 11). While much of what is known about intraorganizational coordination also applies to interorganizational coordination, there are important differences, and these will be discussed in a subsequent section.

Intraorganizational Coordination

From an intraorganizational perspective, coordination is a necessary response to the internal differentiation of organizations. Differentiation, in this context, is defined as "the state of segmentation of

the organizational system into subsystems, each of which tends to develop particular attributes in relation to the requirements posed by its relevant environment" (Scott, 1982). Organizational units are typically differentiated based on functions or disciplines relative to the organization's overall work activities. Organizations differentiate their units in these ways to handle the complexity of the work itself (Charns & Tewksbury, 1993). That is, through internal differentiation, staff can focus on a particular set of work activities for which they develop expertise. Thus, health care organizations create specialized units for dealing with, for example, finance and human resources on the administrative side, and medicine, surgery, pediatrics, and so forth on the clinical side.

Within health care organizations, the degree of differentiation is particularly great, often reflecting the structure (discipline-based) of American medicine as a whole (Charns & Tewksbury, 1993). For instance, in a hospital there are the primary clinical departments of medicine, surgery, and neurology, each of which may be further differentiated into various subspecialities (e.g., cardiology within the department of medicine). Nursing homes and other institutional providers also tend to be differentiated based on either traditional clinical disciplines or functions.

However, the internal differentiation of health care organizations has also been undergoing some change to accommodate economic pressures and new developments in medical technology. For example, some hospital and physicians organizations are differentiated in part based on the practice setting of staff physicians (Diamond, Goldberg, & Janosky, 1998; Averland, et al., 2000; Hoff, Whitcomb, Williams, Nelson, & Cheesman, 2001). Physicians are either based in a hospital and thus responsible for managing inpatient care services for patients (i.e., hospitalists) or based in ambulatory settings and thus responsible for managing outpatient care services for patients. This type of inpatient/outpatient specialization for physician services reflects a growing need for health care organizations to manage inpatient care

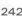
efficiently and at the same time maintain strong outpatient capabilities.

Clearly, the internal differentiation of an organization leads to substantial coordination requirements. For example, consider a hospital that is differentiated based on traditional clinical disciplines. If a patient's needs fit within a single clinical specialty (e.g., cardiology), this form of differentiation does not generate coordination requirements. However, when a patient's needs span two or more clinical specialties and the needs are interrelated (e.g., cardiology and pulmonary medicine), effective coordination between clinical specialties becomes necessary.

Similarly, consider the example of a physician organization where physicians have specialized roles in relation to practice setting—inpatient or outpatient. To the extent that a patient requires only outpatient care, this form of differentiation does not in and of itself entail coordination requirements. But if a patient should require hospitalization, mechanisms for coordinating inpatient and outpatient care must be in place. These mechanisms are necessary to manage the hospital admission process and to ensure the effective and efficient exchange of clinical information between the physician responsible for the patient's in-patient care and the physician responsible for the patient's outpatient care.

It is thus important to recognize the interaction between the need for differentiated units and requirements for coordination. The more differentiation and specialization of labor, the greater the need for coordination.

Intraorganizational Mechanisms of Coordination

Managers use a variety of mechanisms to coordinate work activities. Several different conceptual frameworks have been developed for classifying these mechanisms. March and Simon (1958) identified two primary types of coordination: **programming** and **feedback**. Programming approaches to coordination seek to clarify work responsibilities and activities in advance of the performance of work, as well

as to specify outputs of the work process and skills required. Programming approaches essentially standardize work activities for all expected requirements. By contrast, feedback approaches to coordination entail the exchange of information among staff, usually while the work is being carried out. These approaches permit staff to change or modify work activities in response to unexpected requirements and rely extensively on effective communication, which is discussed in the second half of this chapter.

Mintzberg (1992) elaborates on the March and Simon framework by identifying five coordination mechanisms. They are mutual adjustment, direct supervision, standardization of work processes, standardization of work outputs, and standardization of worker skills. Mutual adjustment and supervision are forms of feedback, while standardization of work processes, standardization of work outputs, and standardization skills are forms of programming. Figure 8.1 illustrates these coordinating mechanisms, which can be summarized as follows:

1. Mutual adjustment provides coordination by informal communications among individuals who are not in a hierarchical relationship to one another. Two physicians sharing information about a patient's clinical condition is an example of mutual adjustment.

2. Direct supervision is a way of coordinating work that occurs when someone takes responsibility for the work of others, including issuing them instructions and monitoring their actions. Direct supervision entails some form of hierarchy within the organization. An example of direct supervision would be a nurse manager providing patient care instructions to a staff nurse.

3. **Standardization of work processes** is an alternative coordinating mechanism that programs or specifies the contents of work. Health care organizations standardize work processes when possible, such as standard admission and discharge procedures or standard methods of performing laboratory tests.

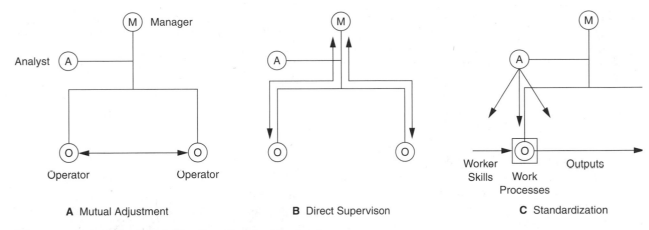

A Mutual Adjustment   B Direct Supervison   C Standardization

Figure 8.1. Mintzberg's Five Coordinating Mechanisms

SOURCE: *Structure in Five: Designing Effective Organizations*, Henry Mintzberg, © 1983. Reprinted by permission of Prentice-Hall, Englewood Cliffs, NJ.

4. **Standardization of work outputs** specifies the product or expected performance, with the process of how to perform the work left to the worker.

5. **Standardization of worker skills** occurs when neither work processes nor output can be standardized. If standardization is to occur in such situations, it must be through worker training. This form is often found in health care organizations where the complexity of much of the work does not allow standardization of work processes or outputs. In such situations, standardization of worker skills and knowledge is an excellent coordinating mechanism. "When an anesthesiologist and a surgeon meet in the operating room to remove an appendix, they need hardly communicate; by virtue of their respective training, they know exactly what to expect of each other. Their standardized skills take care of most of the coordination" (Mintzberg, 1979, pp. 6–7).

Other conceptual frameworks for coordination are similar to Mintzberg's, though some offer additional perspectives as well. For example, Hage

(1980) has developed a framework that includes customs as a coordination mechanism. Many managers rely heavily upon the history and customs of their organizations as coordination mechanisms. For example, it may be customary in a particular nursing home to use the holiday season as an occasion to invite the families of residents into the facility for a meal and social interaction. Knowing this custom permits the various departments to begin their preparations for this event well in advance and facilitates the coordination of their various contributions to its success.

While organizations typically have some combination of these various coordination mechanisms in place, a critically important question for managers is which combination of mechanisms to use or emphasize in a given situation. Indeed, a particular mechanism or combination of mechanisms will achieve different levels of success depending upon characteristics of specific situations. This **contingency view of coordination** is very important for the reader to keep in mind; no single approach to coordination is best for all situations. A contingency approach to intraorganizational coordination requires that managers match the most appropriate coordinating mechanism or mechanisms to a given situation.

In general, programming approaches are relatively efficient to use, as they require little time for personal interaction. However, several factors reduce the utility of programming approaches in favor of greater emphasis on feedback approaches. *Task uncertainty* is perhaps the most important factor to consider. Task uncertainty refers to the variability of the work. As noted by Charns and Schaeffer (1983), if the work methods or processes are largely the same from day to day, most things can be planned for in advance. Different units can perform their work with only a few exceptions that require changes in the methods or processes. For example, the methods by which laboratory tests are ordered and carried out can be largely standardized. However, if work requirements are unpredictable, there will be greater need to establish feedback mechanisms to enable staff to modify or change methods as necessary.

The *degree of interdependency* among organizational units is also a relevant factor. Some research suggests that as interdependencies among units move from pooled to reciprocal, the ability of programming approaches to coordinate work becomes increasingly strained (Van de Ven et al., 1976). This limitation of programming approaches reflects the difficulty of anticipating and specifying all of the work activities in advance in situations of reciprocal interdependence. Accordingly, effective coordination may require a relatively heavy emphasis on feedback approaches.

Managers also need to consider the *size* of the organization. Larger organizations tend to be more differentiated internally; thus, the interdependencies among units are also likely to be greater. To the extent this is the case, coordination may require a substantial emphasis on feedback approaches (Van de Ven et al., 1976).

In recent years, health care organizations have been moving toward increased standardization of direct patient care activities. While health care managers have long relied heavily on the standardized skills of their staff, historically, they have not attempted to standardize the processes or outputs of direct patient care. This orientation to coordination reflects a long-standing sentiment that patient care is not amendable to such standardization (Flood, 1994; Kapp, 1990). Several considerations underlie this sentiment. First, task uncertainty in patient care is considered to be relatively high due to variability among patients' responses to medical interventions. Second, patient care also entails high levels of interdependencies because it requires input from a variety of clinical disciplines. Third, standardizing the outputs of patient care is difficult because the outputs themselves are not easily defined. Is the output, for example, the treatment of a patient's clinical condition? the prevention of a reoccurrence of the condition? or an improvement in the patient's quality of life?

This orientation to coordinating direct patient care appears to be changing. Today, efforts are being put forth to standardize work activities and outputs of direct patient care. This change in orientation is in large part a response to growing pressures on health care organizations to reduce resource utilization and to demonstrate the value of their services.

There are several approaches to standardizing the processes and outputs of patient care activities. One important approach is the use of **critical pathways**. Critical pathways, also known in health care circles as *clinical pathways, care maps,* and *critical paths,* originated in the manufacturing sector, where they have been used for identifying and managing steps in production processes. Applied to health care settings, "[c]ritical pathways are management plans that display goals for patients and provide the corresponding ideal sequence and timing of staff actions to achieve those goals with optimal efficiency" (Pearson, Goulart-Fischer, & Lee, 1995). Thus, for a given diagnosis or condition, a critical pathway specifies the work activities in advance. Critical pathways are most often used for high-volume, high-cost conditions, such as coronary bypass graft procedures and dementia. The development of critical pathways (an example of which is shown in Figure 8.2) may entail a comprehensive review of the scientific literature to identify best practices for managing a clinical condition.

M – Met
U – Unmet
N – Not applicable   Expected LOS: _____   DRG: _____   Date: _____

Shift/Day/Week	Days 5-8	M	U	N	Days 9-12	M	U	N	D/C Outcomes	M	U	N
Consults	• Psych test complete with verbal report (MD) • OT cognitive testing complete (AT)				• Psych test written report back				• Pt/Family will verbalize understanding of results of consult evaluations (T)			
Measurements/ Treatments					• Assessments for depression Possible psychosis, substance abuse Medical status, elimination pattern ADLs & Nutritional status complete (T)							
Tests					• Tests to R/O reversible cause complete (MD) • Appropriate lab work complete (MD)							
Activity/ Safety					• Sleep pattern stable (RN)				• Pt/Family will demonstrate knowledge of patient needs regarding mobility, self-care, and safety factors (T)			
Diet/ Hydration					• Nutrition/Hydration stable (RN)				• Pt/Family able to demonstrate knowledge of patient's nutritional needs (T)			
Medication					• Medication education complete • Establish D/C pharmacy needs				• Pt has stabilized on meds (T) • Pt is compliant w/ meds (T)			
Discharge Planning (Education, Psych/Soc, Homecare, etc.)					• Disposition finalized (3W) • Guardian eval complete (SW) • Support agency referrals complete (HHC, MOW) (T) • Output f/u in place (T) • D/C instructions given (T)				• Pt/Family demonstrates knowledge of f/w plan (T) • Pt/Family demonstrates knowledge of financial coverage (T)			
Special Needs: TX of conc med probs	• Problematic behaviors stable (T)								• Pt/Family demonstrates knowledge of advanced directive (T)			
Variance Facts/ Analysts												
Plan												
Signatures & initials												

Suicide Attempts: _____   Transfer to/from a med/surg unit _____   Re-admits: _____

Patient Falls: _____   Treatment of concurrent medical problems/diagnoses _____

Figure 8.2. Dementia Critical Path—Excerpt
SOURCE: Medical Center Hospital of Vermont.

Clinical guidelines or protocols are also being used to standardize patient care processes. Clinical guidelines address the appropriateness of care by specifying the indications for either tests or treatments (Pearson et al., 1995). Thus, whereas critical pathways standardize the treatment approach for a given clinical condition, clinical guidelines standardize the decision process for adopting a treatment approach. Various government agencies and professional associations have been involved in the development of guidelines. These efforts often involve a comprehensive review of relevant literature.

Another effort to standardize direct patient care is **outcomes assessments**. This is an effort to standardize the outputs of patient care through systematically collecting, monitoring, and reporting performance results. Through such assessments, managers from different organizations or units can detect and attend to undesirable variation in outputs (over time or relative to competitors) by changing or modifying work activities as needed. The selected outcomes essentially define the outputs. Thus, for example, outcomes assessments for inpatient care may focus on mortality and complication rates. For managed care organizations, outcomes assessments may include the percentage of enrollees who receive basic preventive services such as cholesterol screening. Outcomes assessments can also focus on the larger community for which a health care organization is considered accountable. Such outcomes might include the general health status of the population or the incidence of specific clinical conditions such as heart disease. In recent years, a number of government and private oversight bodies for the health care industry have developed profiles of the outcomes of health care organizations that are commonly called report cards (Marshall, Shekell, Leatherman, & Brook, 2000). In addition, many health care organizations have their own internal outcomes assessment programs.

How are these efforts to standardize direct patient care affecting the quality of services health care organizations provide? Certainly there are concerns that efforts to standardize patient care will compromise quality by limiting the flexibility of providers to adapt to unexpected patient care requirements (Kapp, 1990). However, a study by Young et al. (1997) suggests that standardization efforts can improve patient care if they are accompanied by well-developed feedback mechanisms. They studied 44 surgical departments and found that departments that combined a relatively high emphasis on standardizing patient care activities with a relatively high emphasis on feedback-type approaches had better surgical outcomes than their counterparts. Better-performing surgical departments standardized patient care activities when work requirements were well understood. For example, one surgical department developed and implemented a protocol to assist nurses in identifying patients at risk for pressure sores. Nurses would then hold a conference with the attending surgeon and a consulting physician from the department of medicine to consider appropriate prevention strategies. The protocol is a form of standardization of work, while the conference is a feedback mechanism.

Organizations can also establish various structural arrangements for facilitating coordination. For example, Lawrence and Lorsch (1967) found that well-coordinated organizations often rely upon individuals, whom they term **integrators**, to achieve coordination. Successfully playing an integrator role depends more on having professional competence than occupying a particular formal position. People are successful integrators because of specialized knowledge and because they represent a central source of information. Examples of effective integrators are found among all health professionals. In most health care organizations, individual nurses, regardless of formal position, often function as integrators linking physicians to the organization's formal administrative structure. These integrators often provide significant coordination among various departments and subunits, particularly as they relate to patient care.

Along similar lines, organizations may have people serve formally as "**linking pins**" between various units in the organization (Likert, 1967, p. 156). Horizontally, there are certain organizational participants who are members of two separate groups and serve as coordinating agents between the groups. On the vertical axis, individuals serve as linking pins between their level and those above and below. Thus, through this system of linking pins, the coordination necessary to make the dynamic system operate effectively is achieved. This forms a multiple overlapping group structure in the organization. Likert (1967, p. 167) notes:

> To perform the intended coordination well, a fundamental requirement must be met. The entire organization must consist of a multiple, overlapping group structure with every work group using group decision-making processes skillfully. This requirement applies to the functional, product, and service departments. An organization meeting this requirement will have an effective interaction-influence system through which the relevant communications flow readily, the required influence is exerted laterally, upward, and downward, and the motivational forces needed for coordination are created.

The use of a **project-management design** is a structural means for coordinating a large amount of talent and resources for a given period on a specific project (Cleland & King, 1997). For example, a health care organization may wish to organize services into a comprehensive home health care program for the chronically ill by establishing a team organized around the focus of the program—home services for the chronically ill. Team members would be drawn from nursing, social services, respiratory therapy, occupational therapy, pharmacy, and physicians specializing in chronic disease. To market the program and to handle finance and reimbursement issues, expertise would be provided by team members drawn from the organization's administration. A project manager would be responsible for coordinating the activities of team members. In this situation, project organization would permit flexibility and facilitate coordination.

Health care organizations can use the project-management design by superimposing it on an existing functional departmental design. This can be done in a few selected areas or for the whole organization. As discussed in Chapter 10, when the entire organization is structured in this way, it is called a *matrix design*. Figure 10.6 is a matrix design for a psychiatric hospital in which functional managers head departments, and program or product-line managers head major clinical programs or product lines. Notice that the individual worker depicted is a member of nursing *and* the Alzheimer's program. This coordination mechanism is very important when health care organizations move toward a product-line management orientation.

Health care organizations can also move completely to a program or service-line design (also known as product-line design and centers of excellence) for some or all of their activities (Charns & Tewksbury, 1993). This design replaces the traditional functional departmental design with specialized departments or units that focus on a program, service, or a type of patient population (see Chapter 10) . For example, a cancer center will bring together organizationally oncologists, nurses, social workers, other professional and technical staff whose roles and responsibilities focus on the care of cancer patients. Similarly, a women's health center will bring together organizationally relevant professional and technical staff who specialize in providing a range of clinical services for women. In the case of integrated delivery systems, a service-line structure may be used to coordinate patient care activities among multiple health care organizations such as hospitals and physician organizations in such specialized areas as cancer care, women's health, and mental health (Parker, Charns, & Young, 2001). Although a service-line design potentially reduces some of the coordination requirements associated with a functional or discipline-based design, it also can create new coordination problems among the programs or service line structures. The end result may be little more than the replacement of one set of silos replacing for

248

another set. Moreover, because service-line structures usually lead to the dismantling of some or all of the discipline-based departments such as nursing, this type of design raises concerns about the professional development of those clinicians who lose their own departments (Charns & Tewksbury, 1993).

Several studies have been undertaken recently to examine the effects of service-line structures on the functioning and performance of hospitals relative to functional designs (Young, Charns, & Herren, 2004; Greenberg, Rosenbeck, & Charns, 2004; Byrne, Charns, Parker, Meterko, & Ray, 2004). In general, these studies suggest that the service-line design may be more likely to have negative than positive effects on a variety of measures concerning staff coordination, service efficiency, and patient care quality, though the results may be somewhat sensitive to both the type (e.g., mental health) and age (i.e., number of months since first implemented) of a service line. Additionally, one of the studies points to the problems of implementing service lines without various changes in a hospital's infrastructure to support the new design, particularly information systems. This observation that may help explain to some degree the overall disappointing results for service lines (Young, Charns, & Herren, 2004). That is, for service lines to improve staff coordination and be generally effective, those involved in their management presumably must have access to financial, operational, and clinical data regarding their service line. While more research may be needed to fully understand the potential benefits and limitations of the service-line design, the existing research does caution us from setting our expectations too high for any one type of organizational design to resolve coordination problems in complex health care organizations.

Other management approaches such as quality circles and cross-functional quality improvement teams also promote coordination. They rely on nominal group process, multicriteria decision making, cause-and-effect diagrams, and related problem-identification and problem-solving tools to improve communication, coordination, and ultimately the quality of work.

The range of coordination mechanisms available to managers can be seen in the challenges facing the president and vice president of a large teaching hospital as presented in Debate Time 8.1.

Interorganizational Coordination

As noted, interdependence is not limited to situations *within* organizations. Increasingly, health care organizations experience interdependencies with other health care organizations, as in the case of vertically integrated delivery systems (Longest, 1998; Shortell, Gillies, Anderson, Erickson-Morgan, & Mitchell, 1996). Such organizations require patient care to be coordinated across different settings and among health care providers with different educational backgrounds and training. Health care organizations also experience interdependencies with other elements in their external environments, such as various regulatory bodies, suppliers, third-party payors, and so on.

While many of the mechanisms discussed for managing intraorganizational coordination requirements also can be used to manage interorganizational coordination requirements as well, interorganizational coordination does raise special circumstances that must be considered. First, interorganizational arrangements bring together organizations that do not operate, at least not initially, under common ownership, such as in the case of alliances and joint ventures. Accordingly, a structural hierarchy (supervision in the previously discussed Mintzberg framework) for coordinating activities is not readily available. This presents a potentially significant barrier to effective coordination and, at a minimum, requires careful consideration of other available coordination mechanisms. Second, the interorganizational arrangement itself by design may be temporary, anticipating that the participating organizations will separate once a specific, mutual goal has been achieved. Kanter (1990) refers to such arrangements as opportunistic alliances and observes that they are often used as a means for the participating organizations to access new markets or develop new technological capabilities. But the

---

🙣 DEBATE TIME 8.1   What Do You Think?

As we have seen, there are a number of intra-organizational coordination mechanisms, including supervision, standardization of work, customs, integrators, linking pins, and matrix organization. Utilizing a contingency approach, managers in health care organizations use various combinations of these mechanisms to achieve coordination; usually a number of them are used concurrently. Depending upon situations, various packages of these mechanisms might be appropriate.

  Assume you are the president of a large teaching hospital and are concerned about coordinating the responsibilities and roles of the hospital's departments. Choose several coordination mecha-

nisms discussed above that you would emphasize in ensuring good coordination among the departments in your hospital. Be prepared to explain and defend why you think these are the most appropriate mechanisms.

  Now, assume that you are the vice president for nursing services in the same hospital and are concerned about the level of coordination *within* nursing service. Again, choose several coordination mechanisms that have been discussed thus far that you would emphasize in ensuring good coordination within the nursing service. Be prepared to explain and defend why you think these are the most appropriate mechanisms for this purpose.

---

ephemeral nature of these arrangements may be relevant to the types of coordination mechanisms that are appropriate.

  Given these distinctions, it is important to consider the types of linkages and coordination mechanisms for managing interorganizational interdependencies specifically. These can range from straightforward buying and selling of goods and services between organizations as they seek to manage their interdependencies through market transactions, to the buying and selling of organizations themselves. In between is a number of more subtle strategies for managing interorganizational interdependencies. For example, Thompson (1967) developed a categorization of interorganizational linkages including contracting, coopting, and coalescing. Pointer, Begun, and Luke (1988) have applied the concept of the quasifirm to the health care sector. Zuckerman and Kaluzny (1991) have examined interorganizational linkages from the construct of strategic alliances. Longest (1990) incorporates many of these categorizations into a typology of three general classes as follows.

Market Transactions

Market transactions involve focal organizations entering into relationships with other organizations in order to access product markets or obtain operational resources. This is perhaps the simplest form of linkage between organizations. It may entail nothing more than establishing an acceptable contract to purchase some needed item of supply or service or to provide services to a defined population as in an agreement with an HMO. At the more complex level, contracts permit a health care organization to establish stable and predictable (albeit interdependent) relationships with the federal government for reimbursement for Medicare patients, with state governments for reimbursement for Medicaid patients, and with commercial insurers and health plans for their subscribers or members. Contracts are formal agreements, usually negotiated, which define parameters of exchanges between two or more parties. Thus, they are widely used as a mechanism of coordination in a great variety of interorganizational relationships. Negotiation ability as discussed in Chapter 5 is the most important managerial skill for market transactions.

Voluntary Interorganizational Relationship Transactions

A second category of interorganizational linkages is distinguished by the voluntary dimension of the transactions. Horizontal and vertical systems, joint ventures, partnerships, various affiliations, consortia, and confederations are examples of voluntary interorganizational relationships. They can be further categorized as follows:

Co-opting. This form of linkage involves the absorption of leadership elements from other organizations into the focal organizations. In the health care industry, this coordination mechanism often takes one of two forms: management contracts and the placing of representatives of interdependent organizations on the focal organization's governing body.

Management contracts permit one organization to supply to another day-to-day management by agreement (Starkweather, 1981). Management includes at least the CEO, who reports to the governing body of the managed organization and to the managing organization. This is in contrast to the practice prevalent in many health care organizations of using outside contractors to manage individual departments and programs such as housekeeping, food service, or respiratory therapy.

The second co-opting mechanism for achieving interorganizational coordination is by appointment of significant representatives from external organizations to positions in the focal organization, usually the governing body. For example, a hospital system interested in access to capital may find considerable advantage in placing a banker on its governing body. Similarly, an HMO may find it advantageous to place members of its medical group on its board.

Coalescing. This linkage mechanism includes such forms as joint ventures, partnerships, consortia, and federations that occur when two or more organizations *partially* pool resources to pursue defined goals. This is often referred to as "loose cou-

pling" and is characterized by interorganizational relationships in which interdependent and mutually responsive organizations are linked while preserving their legal identities and autonomies and much of their functional autonomy (Weick, 1976). Such linkages are stronger than those in market transactions, but less binding and less extensive than in a merger or acquisition.

Joint ventures, which have become increasingly common among health care organizations, stem from considerations of resource interdependence, competitive uncertainty, and other conditions that make various forms of interdependence more or less problematic (Pfeffer & Salanick, 1978). Among the many types of joint ventures that exist in the health care industry, those between hospitals and physician organizations are especially common, particularly arrangements to provide on an outpatient basis either diagnostic or surgical services. For physicians these joint ventures are often an important source of financial capital, whereas for hospitals the arrangements protect existing sources of revenue for outpatient services from being captured entirely by would-be physician competitors (Jaklevic, 2004; Kocher, Kumar, & Subramanian,1998). Hospitals have also formed joint ventures with each other to provide outpatient services and to combine their purchasing needs for certain supplies and equipment for which volume discounts can be obtained (Bazzoli, Chan, Shortell, & D'Aunno, 2000).

Trade associations are a particularly prevalent form of loosely coupled or coalesced structure in the health care industry. For example, the American Hospital Association has over 5,000 member organizations and has developed a sophisticated political/lobbying activity on behalf of its member hospitals. Similarly, there are regional and state hospital associations that base affiliation on a geographical or state community of interests. As states have become increasingly involved in regulation of the health care sector and in its reform, state hospital associations have increasingly undertaken important lobbying efforts. Associations serve other functions that help member organizations deal with their interdependencies; centralized information, research, and product definition are examples.

Quasifirm.

Defined as "a loosely coupled, enduring set of interorganizational relationships that are designed to achieve purposes of substantial importance to the viability of participating members" (Luke, Begun, & Pointer, 1989), the quasifirm lies between market transactions and ownership arrangements. Quasifirms are similar to a true firm in relation to shared goals, mutual dependency, task subdivision and specialization, bureaucratic structures, and formal coordinating and control mechanisms. However, they are critically distinguished by their absence of ownership linkages.

The collaboration of an acute care general hospital, a large multispecialty group practice, a skilled nursing facility, and an insurance carrier for the purpose of designing, producing, and marketing a managed care product is an example of a quasifirm configuration. This arrangement, which might also be thought of as a virtual integrated delivery system, may be strategically important to the survival of the participants, but allows each to pursue independently other objectives as well (Pointer et al., 1988, p. 171).

Ownership.

Critical to this category of interorganizational relationships is the voluntary nature of the ownership transaction. In recent years, there has been a growing number of cases when hospitals *voluntarily* engage in mergers or acquisitions. Although hostile acquisitions and takeovers are also possible and foreseeable in the future, even under conditions of bankruptcy, most ownership transactions involving health care organizations to date have been voluntary.

One form of ownership transaction is to create a new organization, sometimes called an "umbrella" organization, to span but not to replace the original organizations. Starkweather (1981, pp. 37–38) describes two important subtypes of the umbrella corporation in regard to hospitals. One subtype gives the umbrella corporation limited authority within which its decisions are final. In the other, the um-

brella corporation has more general authority that is usually exercised through unified management, policy, and fiscal control.

Another organizational response to interdependence is merger or consolidation. Consolidation is a formal combination of two or more organizations into a single new legal entity that has an identity separate from any of the preexisting institutions. Merger is a formal combination of two or more institutions into a single new legal entity that has the identity of one of the preexisting organizations. Both forms of consumption, as interorganizational coordinating mechanisms, involve an essential restructuring of organizational interdependence. The restructuring can be in the form of vertical integration (a nursing home merges with a hospital in which the hospital gains the ability to discharge patients to a less intensive level of care, and the nursing home gains a source of referrals), horizontal expansion (two hospitals merge with a resulting larger capacity), or diversification (a hospital absorbs a retail pharmacy chain, gaining a new source of revenue).

Involuntary Interorganizational Transactions

Market transactions and voluntary interorganizational transactions are not sufficient to manage all organizational interdependencies found in the health care sector. Examples include relationships with regulatory agencies, fiscal intermediaries, and utilization-management companies. Regulated organizations have an interdependent relationship with the organizations that regulate them. Such interdependence cannot be legally managed through market transactions, which, by definition, involve economic exchanges. Furthermore, the nature of the interdependent relationship between a regulated health care organization and its regulator means that the relationship is not subject to the voluntary types of interorganizational transactions described above.

These involuntary relationships lead to unique ways of managing interdependence. Many ingenious strategies have evolved (Altman, Greene, & Sapolsky, 1981). While these strategies are specific

MANAGERIAL GUIDELINES

The development of effective coordination mechanisms is one of the most difficult tasks managers face. This activity is especially difficult in health care organizations owing to their high degree of internal differentiation. Managing interdependencies among health care organizations can be even more complicated. To assist such endeavors, we offer the following suggestions:

1. Within health care organizations, managers must be aware of the relationship between functional specialization and the need for coordination. The establishment of additional organizational units may improve the coordination *within* such units, but the added units may make it more difficult to coordinate activities *among* all units within the organization or the multiorganizational system.

2. In their efforts to manage interdependencies among organizational units, managers select coordination mechanisms that best match the situation at hand. Factors to consider include task uncertainty, degree of interdependencies among units, and size of the organization.

3. In relationships with other interdependent organizations, health care managers should choose from a variety of interorganizational mechanisms for coordination. In making their selection, managers should carefully consider the relative benefits and costs inherent in available mechanisms.

to an individual organization's interactions with regulatory bodies, but they can be modified for use in other involuntary interorganizational transactions as well. Perhaps the most common approach, and always available to organizations in dealing with their regulators, is litigation. Most regulatory decisions can be appealed in the courts, which are sensitive to procedural errors or infringement of due process rights. Regulators who overlook requirements for notice, public hearings, or the opportunity for full consideration of issues invite litigation. While distasteful to many, another strategy organizations use to deal with their regulators involves cultivating supportive relationships with the executive and legislative branches and with state and federal regulatory agencies. Such political intervention strategies can afford effective protection against overly enthusiastic or even dutiful regulators. It is no accident that hospitals routinely place prominent public officials and politically connected private citizens on their governing bodies, that physicians are among the most generous political campaign contributors, or that well-connected consultants flourish in and around Washington, D.C., and state capitals.

Other strategies, unethical and/or illegal though they may be, are sometimes used by regulated organizations to attempt to manage relationships with their regulators. For example, one advantage regulated organizations often have over their regulators is their technical expertise and the ability to assemble and manipulate large volumes of data. When challenged, regulated organizations may flood their regulators with technical data seeking to justify their position, or simply obscure the issues as part of a data overload strategy intended to foster ambiguity. Although it is clearly illegal and unethical, outright deception is possible in relationships between organizations and their regulatory stakeholders. The cost and scope of projects can be understated; pertinent data can be fabricated or falsified; projects or protocols can be altered after approval. The complexity of projects, long lead times, turnover of regulatory staff, and the difficulty government agencies have in coordinating their programs can prevent close scrutiny of regulated organizations and encourage cheating.

Managing Interorganizational Linkages

As with intraorganizational coordination, it is important for a manager to use a contingency approach when establishing and maintaining relationships with interdependent organizations. The manager must do this both when selecting the interdependent organizations with which linkages should be established and when determining the most appropriate forms of linkages from the available menu. Chapter 11 elaborates on this process.

It is important to note here that interorganizational coordination is not achieved without costs. The obvious costs are time, personnel, and money needed to support the various forms of linkages. The less obvious, but very important, costs include what Porter (1985) has termed the cost of compromise and the cost of inflexibility. The cost of compromise arises in the context that effectively coordinating across organizational boundaries may require that an activity be performed in a consistent way that may not be optimal for any of the participants in the interorganizational relationship. From the manager's perspective, the cost of compromise can be reduced if an activity is designed for sharing. For example, two merger participants may find that a new management information system that is designed to accommodate the needs of the new organization is better than applying—either separately or linked—the previously existing management information systems.

The cost of inflexibility is not an ongoing expense of interorganizational coordination mechanisms, but arises with the need for flexibility, usually in the form of responding to a competitor's move or to a new market opportunity. It is simply a matter that linkages developed to manage interorganizational interdependencies involve added complexity and often greater inflexibility.

COMMUNICATION*

As noted, both coordination and communication present significant challenges to managers as they seek to effectively manage interdependencies by establishing linkages within and outside their organizations. As with coordination, communication becomes more important as interdependence moves from pooled to sequential to reciprocal forms.

Following the paradigm established by March and Simon (1958) in which they identified two primary types of coordination—programming and feedback—this section discusses the role communication plays in both approaches. Remember, as was discussed earlier in the chapter, that programming approaches to coordination seek to clarify work responsibilities and activities in advance of the performance of work, as well as specify the outputs of the work process and the skills required. In essence, programming approaches seek to standardize work activities. By contrast, feedback approaches to coordination entail the exchange of information among staff while the work is being carried out, which permits staff to change or modify work activities in response to unexpected requirements. Both programming and feedback approaches to coordination rely extensively on effective communication.

Communication, which is *the creation or exchange of understanding between sender(s) and receiver(s),* plays a vital role in both programming and feedback coordination mechanisms. It also serves other purposes as well. When managers communicate effectively, one of four things or some combination of them is accomplished: information

---

*Some portions of this section are adapted with permission from Longest, B. B., Jr., Rakich, J. S., and Darr, K. (2000). *Managing health services organizations and systems* (4th ed.). Baltimore, MD: Health Professions Press, Chapter 17. Some portions of this section are adapted with permission from Longest, B. B., Jr. (2004). *Managing health programs and projects.* San Franciso: Jossey-Bass, Chapter 6.

transmission, motivation, control, and emotive expression (Scott, Mitchell, & Birnbaummore, 1981).

Information about operating activities, resources, alternatives, and the plans and activities of others in the organization—information people need if they are to make good decisions or take appropriate actions—is routinely transmitted within health care organizations. Managers also provide information to their organizations' external stakeholders such as its potential customers, health plans, and regulators. Information transmission is essential if organizations are to function effectively within their environments.

Although motivation is a process internal to the person experiencing it (see Chapter 3), managers have an effect on motivation in others by informing them about rewards that will result from their performance, by giving them information that builds commitment to the organization and its objectives, and by using communication skills to help people understand and learn how to fulfill their personal needs. Managers also communicate with external stakeholders to influence and motivate them to act in ways that benefit the health care organization, such as selecting the organization as a provider of medical services, offering favorable reimbursement levels for services, or establishing favorable regulatory policies.

Many kinds of communications help control the performance of health care organizations and those who work in them: activity reports, policies to establish standard operating procedures, budgets, and face-to-face directives are examples. Such communications enhance control when they clarify duties, authorities, and responsibilities. These communications play a central part in coordination.

A final function of communication results from the fact that it permits people to express their emotions and feelings, such as satisfaction, happiness, sadness, and anger. Emotive communication permits necessary venting of feelings to occur among people within organizations. It also permits the health care organization to increase acceptance of the organization and its actions, both internally and with external stakeholders. Whether the purpose of communica-

tion is transmitting information, motivating, controlling, or emoting, and whether it pertains to programming or feedback approaches to coordinating, it is accomplished through a specific process.

The Communication Process

All effective communication, whether intraorganizational or communication with external stakeholders, involves the creation or exchange of understanding between sender(s) and receiver(s) through a process diagramed in Figure 8.3. In this model, **sender**—which can be one or more individuals, departments, or units of an organization, or a system of organizations—have ideas, intentions, and information that they wish to convey. A sender uses words and symbols to **encode** ideas and information into a **message** for the intended **receiver.**

Because words may have different meanings for different people, or people may not understand certain words, it is often useful to augment the words in a message with other symbols to make communication more effective. In health care organizations, many kinds of symbols, which may be physical things, pictures, or actions, play a role in communication. Consider how many words would be needed to explain a hospital's complex organization design in lieu of information displayed in an organization chart. Or, imagine the difficulty of trying to communicate all the information in a sophisticated image of a heart using only words. Finally, action is a symbol that communicates. A smile or a congratulatory handshake has meaning. A promotion or pay increase conveys a great deal to the recipient, as well as to others. Lack of action can also have symbolic meaning. When managers fail to follow through on promises of new resources or promotions, or fail to acknowledge work that is done especially well, they are sending clear messages.

The **communication channels** or methods of communication are the means by which messages are transmitted. Channels include face-to-face or telephone conversations involving an individual and/or groups of senders and receivers, e-mail, fac-

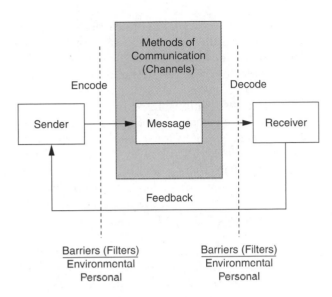

Figure 8.3. The Basic Mechanism of Communication

SOURCE: Longest, B. B. Jr., Rakich, J. S., and Darr, K. (2000). *Managing health services organizations and systems*, 4th ed. Baltimore, MD: Health Professions Press, p. 805.

simile messages, letters, memos, policy statements, operating room schedules, reports, electronic message boards, web pages, video teleconferences, newspapers, television and radio commercial spots, and newsletters for internal or external distribution.

The selection of channels is an important part of the communication process. Effective communication often involves using multiple channels to transmit a message. For example, a major change in an organization's human resources policy, such as changing the benefit package, might be announced in a letter from the vice president for human resources to all employees, graphically illustrated by posters in key locations, and then reinforced in group meetings where managers explain the policy and answer questions. A decision to lobby the state legislature for more generous Medicaid reimbursement might result in messages transmitted through channels such as letters to legislators, direct contact

between the organization's managers and trustees and legislators, and newspaper advertisements stating the organization's position. If other organizations would benefit from the legislation, they might participate, perhaps through an association, to produce and distribute television commercials or use other channels to increase support for their position.

Messages transmitted over any channel must be **decoded** by the receiver. Decoding means interpreting the words and symbols in the message. Because decoding is done by the receivers of messages, it is affected by their prior experiences and frames of reference. Decoding involves the receiver's perceptual assessment of both the content of the message *and* the sender, and the context in which the message is transmitted. The fact that messages must be decoded (interpreted) by the receiver raises the possibility that the message the sender intends is not the message the receiver gets. The closer the decoded message is to the one intended by the sender, the more effective the communication.

The most effective way to determine if messages are received as intended is through **feedback**. Without feedback, you have a one-way communication process. Feedback makes possible a two-way process, reversing the sender and receiver roles so that information can be shared, recycled, and fine-tuned to achieve an unambiguous mutual understanding (Dessler, 2004).

In intraorganizational communication, where interdependencies among individuals and units of an organization are significant, the feedback loop is very important in assuring that enough information is exchanged to effectively manage these interdependencies. Similarly, communication with external stake-holders is greatly improved if receivers provide feedback to senders, who can then adjust the message if it is not received as intended. Effective two-way communication occurs when a sender encodes and transmits a message to a receiver, who decodes the message and indicates understanding by giving feedback.

Feedback can be direct or indirect. Direct feedback is the receiver's response to the sender regarding a specific message. Indirect feedback is more subtle and involves consequences that result from a particular message. Internally, indirect feedback on a policy to change the organization's benefit package might include higher levels of employee satisfaction if the change is liked or increased turnover if the change is disliked. Externally, indirect feedback on attempts to change Medicaid reimbursement might include an increase in rates if the legislature agrees with the organization, no action if they disagree, or even hostile action if they disagree with the message or are upset by the methods used to communicate it.

Whether communication is within organizations or between them and external stakeholders, there are almost always barriers that must be overcome if communication is to be most effective. The environmental and personal barriers illustrated in Figure 8.3 are ubiquitous in the communication process, and can block, filter, or distort messages as they are encoded and sent and when they are decoded and received. **Environmental barriers to communication** are characteristics of an organization and its environmental context that block, filter, or distort communications. Such barriers can be nothing more than the fact that people have too little time to communicate carefully. Other environmental barriers include the organization's managerial philosophy, multiplicity of its hierarchical levels, and power/status relationships between senders and receivers.

Managerial philosophy can directly inhibit, as well as promote, effective communication. Requirements that all communication "flow through channels," inaccessibility, lack of interest in employees' frustrations, complaints, or feelings, and insufficient time allotted to receiving information are symptoms of a philosophy that retards communication. Managerial philosophy also has a significant impact on an organization's communications with its external stake-holders. This topic is addressed more fully in a later section.

Multiple levels in an organization's hierarchy, and other organizational complexities such as size or scope of activity, present barriers that tend to cause message distortion. For example, a message sent from the CEO to employees through several layers of an organization might be received in quite a different form than that originally sent. Or, a report prepared for the CEO that passes through the hierarchy may not reach its destination because it is lying on a desk and is, in essence, blocked.

Power/status relationships can also present barriers to effective communication by distorting or inhibiting transmission of messages. How often does the nurse with 20 years of experience tell a new medical resident that a procedure or treatment thought to be appropriate and about to be ordered is not efficacious? How is the nurse's message encoded—bluntly or obliquely?

Another environmental barrier stems from the fact that managers in health care organizations may use terminology that is very different from that used by those responsible for direct care. Both may use terminology unfamiliar to external stakeholders. This barrier is widespread in communication within health care organizations; it is almost universal in communications between them and many of their external stakeholders.

Another set of barriers—**personal barriers to communication**—are always potentially present when people communicate. These barriers arise from the nature of people, especially in their interaction with others and apply equally to communication within organizations and between them and their external stakeholders. Examples of personal barriers to effective communication include people distorting the encoding or decoding of their messages according to their frames of reference or their beliefs and values. People may also consciously or unconsciously engage in selective perception, or permit their emotions—such as fear or jealousy—to influence their communications.

Unless one has had the same experiences as others, it is difficult to completely understand messages from them or to construct messages that others completely understand. The wealthy may have difficulty understanding the concerns of people without health insurance. Because personalities and backgrounds differ, people have idiosyncratic opinions and prejudices in areas such as politics, ethics, religion, equity in the workplace, sex, race, and lifestyle. These biases, beliefs, and values filter and distort communication. Selective perception means that people tend to filter out the "bad" of a message and retain the "good," usually because it makes them feel better or helps them protect their status quo.

Awareness that environmental and personal barriers to effective communication exist is the first step in minimizing their impact, but positive actions are needed to overcome them. Although the specific steps necessary to overcome the barriers depend on circumstances, several general guidelines can be suggested.

Environmental barriers are reduced if receivers and senders ensure that attention is given to their messages and that adequate time is devoted to listening to what is being communicated. In addition, a management philosophy that encourages open and free flow of communications is constructive. Reducing the number of links (levels in the organizational hierarchy or steps between the organization as a sender and external stakeholders as receivers) through which messages pass reduces opportunities for distortion. The power/status barrier is more difficult to eliminate because it is affected by interpersonal and interprofessional relationships. However, consciously tailoring words and symbols so messages are understandable and reinforcing words with actions significantly improves communications among different power/status levels. Finally, using multiple channels to reinforce complex messages decreases the likelihood of misunderstanding.

Personal barriers to effective communication are reduced by conscious efforts of sender and receiver to understand each other's frame of reference and beliefs. Recognizing that people engage in selective perception and are prone to jealousy and fear is a first step toward eliminating or at least diminishing these barriers. Empathy with those to whom messages are directed may be the surest way to increase the likelihood that the messages will be received and understood as intended.

Effectively communicating among component organizations in a health system can be especially demanding. Barriers resulting from organizational complexity in systems can be quite formidable.

Adapting Porter's (1985) approach to achieving effective linkages among business units in a diversified corporation suggests ways for managers to overcome some of these barriers to effective communication within a system.

- Use devices or techniques that cross organizational lines, such as partial centralization and interorganization task forces or committees, to actively facilitate communication. At the governance level, systems can enhance communication through interlocking boards, which are defined as boards with overlapping membership.

- Use management processes that include cross-organizational dimensions in areas such as planning, control, incentives, capital budgeting, and management information systems to enhance communication.

- Use human resource practices that facilitate co-operation among the organizations in a system, such as cross-organizational job rotation, management forums, and training because these increase the likelihood that managers in one part of the system will understand their counterparts elsewhere in the system and that they will communicate more effectively.

- Use management processes that effectively and fairly resolve conflicts among organizations in a system to enhance communication. The key to such processes is that corporate management installs and operates a process that fairly settles disputes among component organizations in the system. Equitable settlement of disputes facilitates effective communication.

Making the Communication Process Effective

Managers use the process outlined in Figure 8.3 when they communicate. Their success in achieving understanding when they communicate depends upon a number of variables. Shortell (1991, pp. 70–92) identifies several key elements of effective communication in a model developed for physicians

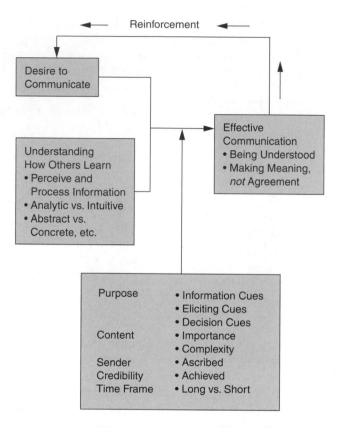

Figure 8.4. Elements of Effective Communication: A Guiding Framework

SOURCE: Shortell, S. M. *Effective Hospital-Physician Relationships.* Chicago: Health Administration Press, 1991; p. 87. Reprinted by permission.

and hospitals to improve their communications. The following summarizes these elements, and Figure 8.4 illustrates their interrelationships.

1. An effective communicator must have a *desire to communicate,* which is influenced both by one's personal values and the expectation that the communication will be received in a meaningful way.

2. An effective communicator must have an *understanding of how others learn,* which includes consideration of differences in how others perceive and process information. For example, is the receiver analytic or intuitive?

Does the receiver prefer abstract versus concrete information? Is the receiver better able to interpret verbal or written information?

3. The receiver of the message should be cued as to the *purpose* of the message. That is, whether the message is to provide information, elicit a response or reaction, or to arrive at a decision.

4. The *content, importance, and complexity* of the message should be considered in determining the channels through which the message is communicated.

5. The achieved or ascribed *credibility of the sender* affects how the message will be re-

ceived—"trust" (an achieved credibility) being most significant.

6. The *time frame* associated with the content of the message (long versus short) needs to be considered in choosing the channels through which and the manner in which the message is communicated. That is, faster channels and more precise cues are needed with shorter time frames.

The application of these elements of effective communication can improve a manager's communications, especially if they are considered in conjunction with the process model described in Figure 8.3. The elements of effective communication, and the process itself, apply whether communication is the intraorganizational communication that takes place within a health care organization or the communication between an organization and its external stakeholders.

Intraorganizational Communication

Intraorganizational communication flows downward, upward, horizontally, and diagonally within organizations, with each direction of flow having its appropriate uses and unique characteristics. Typically, downward flow is communication between superiors and subordinates in organizations; upward communication uses the same channels but in the opposite direction. Horizontal flow is manager to manager or worker to worker. Diagonal flow cuts across functions and levels. While this violates an organization's hierarchical chain of command, it may be permitted in situations where speed and efficiency of communication are particularly important.

Downward Flow

Downward communication flow primarily involves passing on information from superiors to subordinates in organizations. It commonly consists of information, verbal orders, or instructions from organizational superior to subordinate on a one-to-one basis. It may also include speeches to groups of employees or meetings. The myriad of written methods such as handbooks, procedure manuals, newsletters, bulletin boards, and the ubiquitous memorandum are also channels of downward communication. Computerized information systems contribute greatly to downward flow in many health care organizations.

Upward Flow

Upward communication flow serves to provide managers with decision-making information, reveal problem areas, provide data for performance evaluation, indicate the status of morale, and generally underscore the thinking of subordinates. Upward flow becomes more important with increased organizational complexity and scale. This is especially emphasized with the organizational growth of health care organizations and their participation in systems. Managers rely on effective upward communication, and they encourage it by creating a climate of trust and respect as integral parts of the organizational culture (Robbins & Coulter, 2005).

In addition to being directly useful to managers, upward communication flow helps employees satisfy personal needs. It permits those in positions of lesser organizational authority to express opinions and perceptions to those with higher authority; as a result, they feel a greater sense of participation. The hierarchical chain of command is the main channel for upward communication in health care organizations, but this may be supplemented by grievance procedures, open-door policies, counseling, employee questionnaires, exit interviews, participative decision-making techniques, and the use of ombudspeople (Luthans, 2003).

Horizontal and Diagonal Flows

Unhindered downward and upward communication are insufficient for effective organizational performance. In complex organizations, which are frequently subject to abrupt demands for action and reaction, horizontal flow must also occur. For example, the work of interdependent patient care units must be coordinated. Health care organizations using matrix designs, as described in Chapters 7 and 10, illustrate

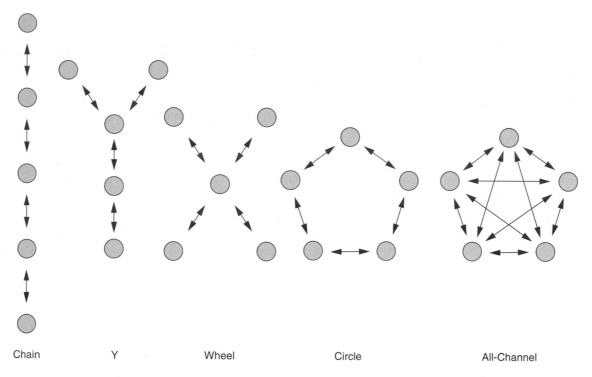

| Chain | Y | Wheel | Circle | All-Channel |

Figure 8.5. Common Communication Networks

SOURCE: Longest, B. B. Jr., Rakich, J. S., and Darr, K. (2000). *Managing Health Services Organizations and Systems*, 4th ed. Baltimore, MD: Health Professions Press, p. 813. Reprinted by permission.

the value of horizontal communication and coordination in these organizations. Committees, task forces, and cross-functional project teams are all useful mechanisms of horizontal communication.

The least common flows of communication in health care organizations are diagonal flows, although they are growing in importance. For example, diagonal communication occurs when the director of a hospital pharmacy alerts a nurse in medical intensive care about a potential adverse reaction between two medications ordered for a patient. Diagonal flows violate the usual pattern of upward and downward communication flows by cutting across departments, and they violate the usual pattern of horizontal communication because the communicators are at different levels in the organization. Yet, such communication is extremely important in health care organizations. Commit-

tees, task forces, quality circles, and cross-functional project teams made up of members from different levels of the organization or system can each serve as useful mechanisms of diagonal communication.

Communication Networks within Organizations

Downward, upward, horizontal, and diagonal communication flows within organizations can be combined into patterns called **communication networks**, which are communicators interconnected by communication channels. Figure 8.5 illustrates the five common networks: chain, Y, wheel, circle, and all-channel. The *chain network* is the standard format for communicating upward and downward and follows line authority relationships. An example is a staff nurse who reports to a nurse manager, who reports to a nursing supervisor, who reports to the vice president for nursing, who reports to the president.

The *Y pattern* (turned upside down) shows two people reporting to a superior who reports to two others. An example is two staff pharmacists who report to the pharmacy director, who reports to the vice president for professional affairs, who reports to the president. The *wheel pattern* shows a situation in which four subordinates report to one superior. There is no interaction among subordinates, and all communications are channeled through the manager at the center of the wheel. This pattern is rare in health care organizations, although elements of it can be found in the situation in which four vice presidents report to a president if the vice presidents have little interaction among themselves. Even though this network pattern is not used routinely, it may be used in circumstances in which urgency or secrecy is required. For example, the president with an emergency might communicate with vice presidents in a wheel pattern because time does not permit using other modes. Similarly, if secrecy is important, such as during an investigation of possible embezzlement, the president may require that all relevant communication with the vice presidents be kept confidential for a period of time.

The *circle pattern* allows communicators in the network to communicate directly only with two others, but since each communicates with another communicator in the network, the effect is that everyone communicates with everyone and there is no central authority or leader. The *all-channel network* is a circle pattern except that each communicator may interact with every other communicator in the network.

Communication networks vary along several dimensions. The most appropriate pattern depends upon the situation in which it is used. The wheel and all-channel networks tend to be fast and accurate compared with the chain or Y-pattern networks, but the chain or Y patterns promote clear-cut lines of authority and responsibility. The circle and all-channel networks enhance morale among those in the networks better than other patterns because everyone is equal in the communication activity, but these patterns result in relatively slow communica-

tion. This is a serious problem if an immediate decision or response is needed. Managers must construct communication networks to fit the various communication situations they face.

Informal Communication

Coexisting with formal communication flows and networks within organizations are **informal communication** flows, which have their own networks. Like informal organization structures, informal communication flows and networks result from the interpersonal relationships of people in organizations. The common name for informal communication flows is *grapevine*, a term that arose during the Civil War, when telegraph lines were strung between trees much like a grapevine (Newstrom & Davis, 1993, p. 441). Messages transmitted over those flimsy lines were often garbled. As a result, any rumor was said to come from the grapevine.

By definition, the grapevine, or informal flow of communication, consists of channels that result from the interpersonal relationships in organizations. Informal communication flows in an organization are as natural as the patterns of social interaction that develop in all organizational settings. Like the informal organization structure, informal communication flows coexist with the formal flows established by management. There is no doubt that informal communication channels can be and routinely are misused in health care organizations, especially in transmitting rumors. For example, in times of crisis, organizations are rife with rumors; frequently, the rumors are wrong. Yet, properly managed, informal communication flows can be useful. Downward flows move through the grapevine much faster than through formal channels. In a health care organization, much of the coordination among units occurs through informal give-and-take in informal horizontal and diagonal flows. In the case of upward flow, informal communication can be a rich source of information about performance, ideas, feelings, and attitudes. Because of their potential usefulness and pervasiveness, managers should try to understand informal communication flows and use them to advantage.

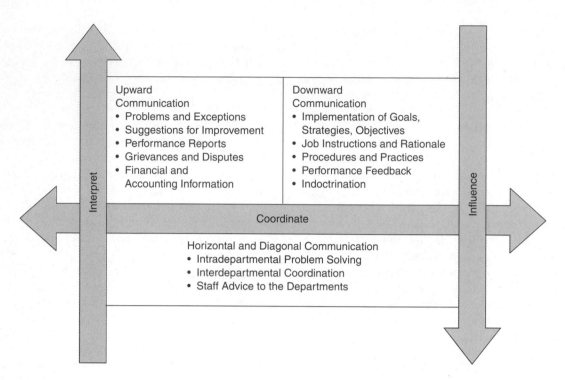

Upward
Communication
• Problems and Exceptions
• Suggestions for Improvement
• Performance Reports
• Grievances and Disputes
• Financial and
  Accounting Information

Downward
Communication
• Implementation of Goals,
  Strategies, Objectives
• Job Instructions and Rationale
• Procedures and Practices
• Performance Feedback
• Indoctrination

Interpret

Influence

Coordinate

Horizontal and Diagonal Communication
• Intradepartmental Problem Solving
• Interdepartmental Coordination
• Staff Advice to the Departments

Figure 8.6. **Communication Flows in Health Care Organizations**

SOURCE: Daft, R. L. & Steers, R. M. *Organizations: A Micro/Macro Approach*, 538. Reading, MA: Addison-Wesley Educational Publishers, Inc., 1986. Reprinted by permission.

The multidirectional communication flows and the networks they form within organizations each have a purpose, and each is an important tool for managers. To the extent these flows are planned and designed into the organization, they are part of its formal design, and they represent formal communication channels and networks. To the extent they are natural communication between and among people arising outside the formal design, they are informal communication channels and networks. Figure 8.6 summarizes the key uses of downward, upward, horizontal, and diagonal communication flows in health care organizations.

Communicating with External Stakeholders

Health care organizations typically maintain relationships with a large and diverse set of external stake-holders (Longest, 1990), which can be shown in a *stakeholder map,* such as the one for the Indiana State Health Department shown in Figure 8.7. Effective communication between a health care organization and its external stakeholders is necessary because these organizations are affected, sometimes quite dramatically, by what the external stakeholders think or do. A health care organization's external stakeholders include the individuals, groups, or

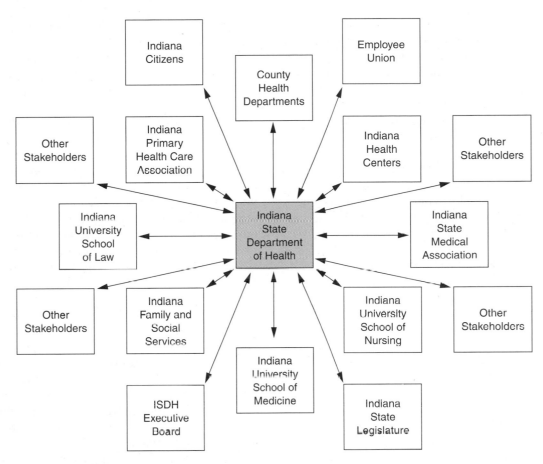

Figure 8.7. Indiana State Department of Health Stakeholder Map

SOURCE. Ginter, P. M., Swayne, L. M., and Duncan W. J. *Strategic Management of Health Care Organizations,* 3rd ed., 458. Malden, MA: Blackwell Publishers Inc., 1998. Reprinted by permission.

organizations outside the organization that have a stake in its decisions and actions and attempt to influence those decisions and actions (Blair & Fottler, 1998). The sheer number and variety of external stakeholders complicate communication with them. Communication is further complicated by the nature of the relationships. Positive relations with external stakeholders usually makes it easier to manage the relationships, and communication flows tend to be more effective than when relations are negative.

Boundary spanning is another name for the process through which organizations communicate with their external stakeholders, and *boundary spanners* are the people who carry out this process. On the one hand, boundary spanners obtain critical information from external stakeholders that can be useful to the organization. Strategic planning and marketing departments or functions are examples of such boundary spanning. On the other hand, boundary spanners also represent the organization to external stakeholders. This activity takes many forms, including marketing, public relations, guest or patient relations, government relations, or community relations. Because information is the object of these boundary-spanning activities, communication is critical to their success. An organization's ability to glean necessary or useful information from its external stakeholders or to be effectively represented to them depends upon effective communication.

While the communication process with all external stakeholders is essentially the creation of understanding between sender and receiver utilizing the process outlined in Figure 8.3, each stakeholder must be considered in terms of its unique dimensions if effective communication is to occur. This is illustrated in two examples of communicating with external stakeholders: the public sector with which the organization interacts and in health care organizations' commercial marketing activities.

Communicating with the Public Sector

Health care organizations, perhaps as much or more than any organizations in American society, are affected by public policies—the formal decisions made in the public sector. The fact that they are affected by so much public policy stems from the fundamental contributions health care organizations make to the physical and psychological condition of the American people, as well as the role these organizations play in the nation's economy. In view of these very important contributions, it should not surprise anyone that government, at all levels, is keenly interested in the performance of health care organizations. Nor should there be surprise that this intense interest results in numerous public policies—including policies affecting the provision and financing of health care services as well as the production of inputs (e.g., the education of health professionals and the development of health technology) to those services (Longest, 2002). The importance of public policies to health care organizations makes effective communication

with the public sector vital to the well-being of these organizations.

Managers have two important categories of communication responsibilities regarding the public sector environments of health care organizations (Longest, 1997). First, they are responsible for analyzing this environment. Done properly, this analysis permits them to acquire sufficient information and data to understand the strategic consequences of events and forces in their organization's public policy environment. Such analysis yields an accurate assessment of the impacts—both in terms of opportunities and threats—of public policies on the organization. Furthermore, such analysis permits managers to position their organizations to make strategic adjustments that reflect planned responses to these opportunities and threats.

Second, managers of health care organizations are responsible for influencing the formulation and implementation of public policies. This responsibility derives from the fact that effective managers seek to make their organization's external environment, including the public policy component of that environment, as favorable to the organization as possible. Inherent in this responsibility are requirements to identify public policy objectives that are consistent with their organization's values, mission, and objectives and to seek through appropriate and ethical means, such as advocacy and joining with associations, to help shape public policies accordingly.

Advocacy

Advocacy, which is defined as the effort to influence public policy through various forms of communicating persuasively, is a primary mechanism through which managers can influence public policy. It has been argued that every manager involved in health services is an advocate, and that success at advocacy depends directly on communicating effectively (Filerman & Persaud, 2003).

Figure 8.8 illustrates advocacy as a six-step process: analysis, strategy, mobilization, action, evaluation, and continuity. Each of the steps in the process de-

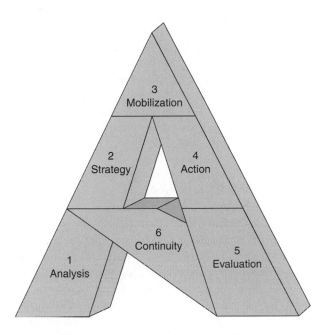

Figure 8.8. "A" Frame for Advocacy

Source: Adapted with permission of the Center for Communication Programs, Johns Hopkins University, Bloomberg School of Hygiene and Public Health. (See http://www.jhuccp.org/topics/advocacy.shtml.)

pends upon effective communication and is described in greater detail at http://www.jhuccp.org/topics/advocacy.shtml.

Analysis. Analysis is the first step to effective advocacy, just as it is the first step to any effective action. Activities or advocacy efforts designed to have an impact on public policy start with accurate information and in-depth understanding of the problem, the people involved, the policies, the implementation or nonimplementation of those policies, the organizations, and the channels of access to influential people and decision makers. The stronger the foundation of knowledge on these elements, the more persuasive the advocacy can be.

Strategy. Every advocacy effort needs a strategy. The strategy phase builds upon the analysis phase to direct, plan, and focus on specific goals and to position the advocacy effort with clear paths to achieve those goals and objectives.

Mobilization. Coalition-building strengthens advocacy. Events, activities, messages, and materials must be designed with your objectives, audiences, partnerships, and resources clearly in mind. They should have maximum positive impact on the policymakers and maximum participation by all coalition members, while minimizing responses from the opposition.

Action. Keeping all partners together and persisting in making the case are both essential in carrying out advocacy. Repeating the message and using the credible materials developed over and over helps to keep attention and concern on the issue.

Evaluation. Advocacy efforts must be evaluated as carefully as any other communication campaign. Since advocacy often provides partial results, an advocacy team needs to measure regularly and objectively what has been accomplished and what more remains to be done. Process evaluation may be more important and more difficult than impact evaluation.

Continuity. Advocacy like communication is an ongoing process rather than a single policy or piece of legislation. Planning for continuity means articulating long-term goals, keeping functional coalitions together, and keeping data and arguments in tune with changing situations.

Communicating in Marketing

The central purpose of marketing is to support the voluntary exchange of something of value between buyers and sellers (Kotler, 2002). Successful health care organizations produce services or products that are of value to certain people, groups, or organizations (e.g., individual patients/customers, health plans, or government) and make the services or products available to them. In turn, individuals, groups, or organizations seek out the services or products and choose them. Communication is vital to how this process occurs; indeed, communicating effectively is necessary for the exchanges to occur at all.

Marketing can assure that an organization has patients/customers for its services or products, that their needs are identified and met, and that the organization receives value in return (Berkowitz, 1996; American Organization of Nurse Executives, 1999). The major activities in commercial marketing include:

- Determining what groups of potential patients/customers (or markets) exist; determining their needs; and identifying which of these groups of potential patients/customers the organization wishes to serve. In essence, these activities determine an organization's target markets. If the organization has competitors, it is also necessary to determine what they are doing or may do in regard to the target markets.

- Assessing the organization's current service mix or product line relative to the identified target market's needs in order to determine what products or services the organization can provide in response, or can develop and then provide.

- Deciding how to facilitate exchanges between the organization and its target markets and implementing these decisions. Prerequisites to mutually satisfactory exchanges between a health care organization and its target markets include responding to how and where customers prefer to gain access to and use the products and services, as well as developing pricing structures that both attract patients/customers and provide the necessary financial resources to support the organization. Accomplishing both requires communicating information effectively to the target markets.

Carrying out all of the activities involved in commercial marketing depends on information being exchanged through effective communication.

Listening to External Stakeholders

When managers in health care organizations want to effectively listen to their external stakeholders, they approach the task in a systematic, analytical way called *stakeholder analysis*. By doing so, the chances increase of acquiring useful or necessary information from external stakeholders—whether they be the public sector, the community, or any of its other external stakeholders.

Although specific approaches for systematically listening to external stakeholders vary widely, these efforts generally include a set of interrelated activities akin to the environmental assessments organizations make in the context of their strategic management. In conducting environmental assessments, health care organization managers *scan* their environments to identify strategically important issues, *monitor* the issues, *forecast* trends in the issues, *assess* the importance of the issues for the organization, and *diffuse* information obtained to those in the organization or system who need it (Ginter, Duncan, & Swayne, 2002; Longest, 1997). In conducting stakeholder analyses, managers also *scan* to identify important stakeholders, *forecast* or project the trends in stakeholders' views or positions, *assess* the implications of the stakeholders' views and positions for the organization, and *diffuse* the results of the first four steps to those in the organization who need to know the views and positions of external stakeholders.

Scanning activities involve acquiring and organizing important information about who are the organization's external stakeholders. In most instances, this is rather straightforward to determine and can readily lead to the development of a stakeholder map, such as the one shown in Figure 8.9.

Considerations about who are an organization's external stakeholders are frequently judgmental. In order to ensure quality in these judgments, it is useful to use ad hoc task forces or committees of people from within the organization, perhaps with the aid of outside consultants. Any of several formal expert-based techniques of assistance help determine who are the stakeholders. The most useful among these are

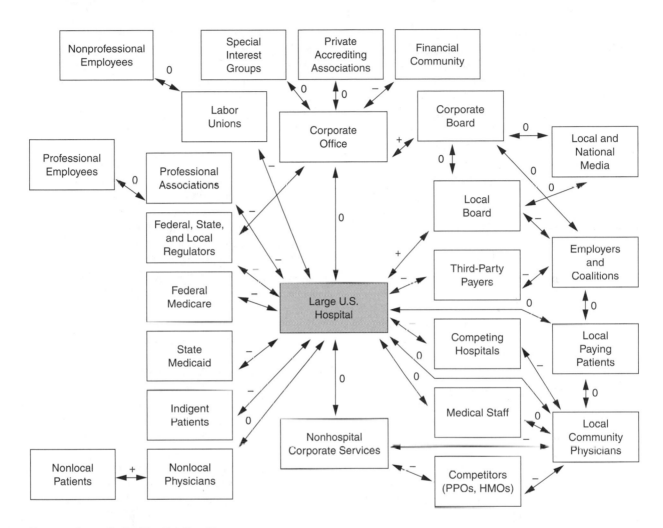

Key: + = Generally Positive Relationship
     0 = Generally Neutral Relationship
     − = Generally Negative Relationship

Figure 8.9. Stakeholders in a Large Hospital

SOURCE: Fottler, M. D., Blair, J. D., Whitehead, C. J., Laus, M. D., and Savage, G. T. "Assessing Key Stakeholders: Who Matters to Hospitals and Why?" *Hospital & Health Services Administration*, Vol. 34, No. 4 (Winter, 1989), p. 530. Copyright 1989, Foundation of the American College of Healthcare Executives.

the Delphi technique, the nominal group technique, brainstorming, focus groups, and dialectic inquiry (Ginter, Duncan, & Swayne, 2002, pp. 77–79).

Scanning to identify external stakeholders must be followed by the next step, monitoring the identified stakeholders by tracking or following closely their views and positions on matters of importance. Monitoring is especially important when the views and positions are dynamic, not well structured, or are ambiguous as to strategic importance. Monitoring stakeholder views and positions permits clarification of the degree to which they are strategically important. As with scanning, techniques that feature the acquisition of expert opinions can help managers determine which stakeholders should be monitored.

Effective scanning and monitoring cannot provide managers with all the information they need about the frequently quite dynamic views and positions of their organization's external stakeholders. Managers need forecasts of stakeholders' emerging views and perceptions. Such forecasts, if accurate, can give managers ample time to factor these views and preferences into their decisions and actions.

Scanning and comprehensively monitoring the views and positions of an organization's external stakeholders, and even accurately forecasting trends in their views and positions, are not enough to ensure good stakeholder analysis. Managers must also concern themselves about the specific and relative importance of the information they are receiving. That is, they must be concerned with an assessment or interpretation of the strategic importance and implications of this information.

Minimally, this involves characterizing stakeholders as negative, positive, or neutral, as in Figure 8.9. While the determination of these positions is relatively easy to make, based on past experience if nothing more, careful assessments of stakeholders' importance is far from an exact science. Intuition, common sense, and best guesses all play a role in this determination. Aside from the difficulties encountered in collecting and properly analyzing enough information to fully inform the assessment, there sometimes are problems derived from the influence of personal prejudices and biases of those making judgments. This can force assessments that fit some preconceived notions about which stakeholders are strategically important rather than the realities of a particular situation (Thomas & McDaniel, 1990).

The final step in the process of conducting useful stakeholder analyses involves diffusing or spreading the results of the effort to all those in the organization who need to have access to this information. This step is frequently undervalued as part of the process and, in extreme cases, even overlooked. Unless it is effectively carried out, however, it really does not matter how well the other steps in the stakeholder analysis are performed. Thus, attention must be given to the task of diffusing the results of these analyses if the analytical process is to have its desired useful effect.

There are two basic ways that those who have produced information about the external stakeholders of an organization can diffuse this information into the organization or system. They can rely upon the *power* of senior-level managers to dictate diffusion and use of the information, including using coercion or sanctions to see that the information is diffused, and even used, in the organization or system. Or they can use *reason* to persuade or educate those involved in the organization's decision making to utilize the information. Combinations of power or reason-based approaches to stimulation use of this information tend to work best.

Diffusion of strategically important information obtained from or about the organization's external stake-holders brings the process of stakeholder analysis to completion. The ability of any organization's managers to effectively listen to the organization's external stakeholders depends very heavily on the quality with which this process is conducted. In fact, today, given the vital linkage between health care organizations and their external stakeholders such as customers, payers, and regulators, it is unlikely that any organization can succeed in the absence of a reasonably effective process through which its managers effectively listen to the external stakeholders and respond to what is received in communication with them.

Communicating When Something Goes Wrong

Based on a large-scale study of medical errors (Brennan, Leape, Laird, et al., 1991), many things can go wrong in clinical settings. One of the verities of life for managers of health care organizations is that on occasion, even in well-managed organizations, something will go wrong (Kohn, Corrigan, & Donaldson, 2000). After all, health care organizations employ, under fallible human direction, dangerous drugs, devices, and procedures in their battles against disease and injury. This is complicated by the fact that these technologies are employed on behalf of people at vulnerable stages or moments in their lives, people who often have an inflated and unrealistic expectation of what can be done for them or their loved ones.

Clinical mishaps are not the only potential problems in health care organizations. These organizations are also important economic entities in their communities. They employ people, buy goods and services, and generate costs for others who pay for their services. The finances and operations of health care organizations provide another set of things that can possibly go wrong. Financial problems in health care organizations not only affect internal stakeholders, but also may have ramifications for external stakeholders. Indeed, health care organizations provide ripe conditions for things to go wrong, and for there to be serious consequences when they do.

There are direct and indirect consequences when something goes wrong in a health care organization. Clinical mistakes can cause pain and suffering directly, even death. Downsizing, laying off employees, or even terminating a program or department due to funding shortages is obviously felt directly by those who work in affected organizations, but may also ripple out into surrounding communities.

There are also important indirect consequences when things go wrong. Health care organizations

are integral components of habitable, stable communities. People want networks of supportive institutions in their communities. In addition to jobs and economic security, they also value good schools, comforting centers of religious life, responsive governments, effective public safety systems, *and* accessible, high-quality health services. Anything that diminishes these vital signs of stability and well-being also diminishes the quality of life. If something goes seriously wrong in a health care organization, this will invariably have a disturbing effect on its internal and external stakeholders, and intensify the need for effective communication.

The approaches managers can take to the fact that things can go wrong in their organizations are conceptually similar to what clinicians do regarding the safety of their patients. In both instances, clinicians and managers focus on *preventing* things from going wrong. However, when something does go wrong, the focus shifts to *containing and minimizing* the damage. Finally, the focus becomes one of *addressing* the consequences of negative occurrences.

In seeking to prevent mishaps, contain and minimize the resulting damage from them, and address the consequences of them, managers engage in different activities, although ideally the activities are integrated. Throughout, communicating plays a vital role. Each set of activities managers use to manage and communicate about things going wrong is considered below.

Preventing Things from Going Wrong

In attempting to prevent the occurrence of negative events, managers are increasingly turning to integrated sets of activities aimed at making certain that the right things are done, that they are done correctly, and that they are done correctly the first time (Deming 1986; Griffith & White, 2002; Juran, 1989). These sets of activities go by various names. A popular one is *continuous quality improvement* or CQI. By whatever name they are called, these substantial and organized efforts focus on continuous improvement in performance, including preventing negative occurrences, and provide a framework within which undesirable events, at least those under the control of managers, can be avoided or minimized. The framework works best in combination with activities designed to reduce risk and reap the benefits of organizational learning (Senge, 1990). Although there is no way to avoid all unwanted occurrences, concerted efforts can help reduce the frequency and severity in health care organizations.

Containing and Minimizing the Damage

No matter how hard managers work to prevent it, and no matter what means to this end they employ, things will go wrong in health care programs. The focus then becomes one of containing and minimizing the damage. In seeking to do this, managers engage in activities that are guided by concepts and models of assessing and controlling performance. In controlling, managers seek to assure that the processes used in their domains, as well as the outputs, outcomes, and impacts achieved in their domains, are continuously monitored, that the results are assessed, and, when necessary, that interventions are undertaken to contain the damage caused by something going wrong. In addition, the CQI and the risk management programs instituted to prevent problems also include elements intended to help contain the damage when such events occur.

In exerting control, managers seek to regulate activities and events in accordance with preestablished plans and standards. When control is exercised effectively, deviations from established standards are noticed quickly and corrective actions are taken to curb the damage that might otherwise be done. Both the detection of deviations and the corrective responses rely upon managers and other participants communicating effectively.

However, the reality is that when prevention fails, regardless of how effectively the resulting damage has been contained, some damage will have been

done. As noted above, damage done in health care organizations often has significant direct and indirect consequences for both internal and external stakeholders. When things go wrong, the manger's focus eventually shifts to addressing the consequences.

Addressing the Consequences

Before anything constructive can be done to address the consequences of something going wrong in a health care organization, those who suffer the consequences must be identified. Sometimes this is easily done. Patients/customers who are harmed, their families, employees who are injured on the job or who are laid off from their work, and their families endure obvious consequences. Less obviously perhaps, potential patients/customers and other employees who learn of such events and feel less positively about an organization are also experiencing consequences. Every storeowner who loses a customer feels the ripple effects of layoffs in a health care organization.

Indeed, when something goes wrong in a health care organization, there may be consequences for many individuals, groups, and organizations. Collectively, the people and organizations that might be harmed when things go wrong are the same as those who stand to benefit when things go right—the organization's internal and external stakeholders. The best way for managers to fully understand and appreciate the consequences of events for stakeholders is through communicating with them, or at least with representative samples of them.

Once those directly or indirectly affected have been identified, the ethically sound goal of fully addressing the consequences of a negative event requires restoring them as closely as possible to positions and conditions extant before the event. Achieving this goal across the board may not be possible (some wrongs can never be righted), but it is the appropriate goal and should guide decisions and actions, including how the manager communicates with the stakeholders.

Each instance of something going wrong requires its own unique set of decisions and actions

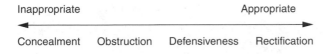

Figure 8.10. Management Approaches When Something Goes Wrong

to appropriately manage the event's consequences. There are few hard-and-fast rules to guide managers in developing these sets of decisions and actions, although their potential decisions and actions range along a rather clear-cut continuum of appropriateness, as illustrated in Figure 8.10.

At one end of the continuum, the most inappropriate responses are characterized by attempts to conceal the fact that something has gone wrong—in effect, to do and communicate as little as possible about what has happened or, in the extreme, to lie and mislead about what has happened. Somewhat less extreme is to respond by acknowledging that something has gone wrong, but denying wrongdoing, avoiding or minimizing responsibility, and taking no action to address the consequences. Guided by a preference for this type of response, a manager most likely will take an obstructionist approach regarding the event, and communicate about it only minimally.

A third type of response to something going wrong is labeled defensiveness. The manager (or another spokesperson if legal counsel has become involved, for example) acts and communicates about what has gone wrong in a way that complies with the letter of the law. This is a common response to serious negative events and reflects the intention to minimize legal liability. Decisions and actions based on this approach may be entirely legal, but they also can be far from the ethical high ground.

A defensive approach to dealing with the consequences of an untoward event partly reflects how costly taking responsibility can be. Serious problems involving human health and life can be very expensive. However, a defensive approach may be

taken even when the issues are layoffs, service reductions, downsizing, or closings, or other operational problems that affect internal or external stakeholders. Managers can find themselves conflicted over fully addressing the consequences of untoward events and their responsibilities to preserve their organization's financial assets as well as its good name and reputation. But the defensive position, so often occupied when something goes wrong, falls short of the most appropriate response.

At the most appropriate end of the continuum in Figure 8.10 is a type of response called rectification. Rectification is characterized by fully accepting warranted responsibility for what has gone wrong and undertaking aggressive actions to address the consequences for and rectify the harms to all those who have been affected, including communicating extensively with them.

Managers who pursue a rectification response take a positive and proactive stance toward addressing the negative consequences. Their decisions and resultant actions reflect this stance. Communications are characterized by openness and candor about what went wrong, its causes, and the actions being taken to deal with the consequences.

The pattern of response to things going wrong builds upon itself. Responses characterized by concealment, obstruction, and to a large extent, defensiveness, once detected by stakeholders, add mistrust to the concerns already in their minds, and invite intensified scrutiny of the immediate situation and of similar future situations. To the contrary, health care organizations with established histories of undertaking rectification responses when things go wrong build trust among their stakeholders. With such histories, little or no effort is wasted by stakeholders wondering whether they are being provided all relevant information about a negative event or about an organization's determination to fully address its consequences. The payoff for organizations whose managers behave in this way includes an easier and faster return to a suitable equilibrium with stakeholders after untoward events.

MANAGERIAL GUIDELINES

1. A key to assigning the proper managerial priority to coordination and communication efforts is the degree to which *interdependence* exists between or among people and units within an organization, and between the organization and its external environment. Assessing the degree and nature of interdependence is the first step toward effective coordination and communication strategies.

2. Managers should pay careful attention to selecting and implementing compatible and, whenever possible, mutually reinforcing mechanisms of coordination and communication if they are to successfully link together the people and units within their organizations and link their organizations to its external stakeholders.

3. The predominance of professionals in health care organizations both facilitates and complicates coordination and communication. Their presence facilitates because professional education prepares these people to link their efforts with those of others as part of the normal course of their work. But their presence also requires careful attention to maintaining collegial and consultative relationships, which, in turn, should guide managers' choices about coordination and communication.

4. Coordination and communication, while treated separately in this chapter for ease of presentation, are in fact highly interrelated and interactive phenomena. Managers should always consider the communication implications and opportunities when seeking to coordinate, and vice versa.

Obviously, the best way to manage negative events in health care organizations is to prevent their occurrence. Carefully orchestrated CQI efforts can be very beneficial in preventing or minimizing the occurrence of problems. When prevention fails, however, managers must turn their attention to containing the damage that flows from unwanted events and to addressing their consequences. In this, managers are best served by aggressive, positive, and proactive efforts to identify the harmed stakeholders and to make them whole again, and to communicate with them openly and extensively in doing so.

DISCUSSION QUESTIONS

1. Distinguish between intra- and interorganizational coordination in health care organizations. What are the key mechanisms available to managers to achieve each type of coordination?

2. Define *communication* and draw a model of the basic technical process. How can managers overcome the barriers to effective communication?

3. Discuss the various types of communication flows in organizations and the uses of each. Discuss the various types of communication networks and describe the advantages and disadvantages of each.

4. You have just been appointed manager of a joint venture between the hospital where you work and some members of its medical staff to operate an ambulatory surgery center. One of your initial concerns is the establishment of effective linkages to the hospital. Drawing upon the material in this chapter, develop your approach to this task and indicate the reasons for your plan.

5. Think of a situation in which a health care organization receives bad press. How might the organization respond? How should it respond?

REFERENCES

Altman, D., Greene, R., & Sapolsky, H. M. (1981). *Health planning and regulation: The decision-making process.* Ann Arbor, MI: Association of University Programs in Health Administration Press.

American Organization of Nurse Executives. (1999). *Market-driven nursing: Developing and marketing patient care services.* San Francisco: Jossey-Bass.

Andrews, L. B., Stocking, C. T., Krizek, T., Gottlieb, L., Krizek, C., Vargish, T., & Stegler, M. (1997, February). An alternative strategy for studying adverse events in medical care. *Lancet, 349,* 309–313.

Auerbach, A. D., Nelson, E. A., Lindenauer, P. K., Pantilat, S. Z., Katz, P. P., & Wachter, R. M. (2000). Physician attitudes toward and prevalence of the hospitalist model of care: Results of a national survey. *American Journal of Medicine, 109*(8), 648–653.

Baggs, J. G., Ryan, S. A., Phelps, C. E., Richeson, J. F., & Johnson, J. E. (1992). The association between interdisciplinary collaboration and patient outcomes in a medical intensive care unit. *Heart and Lung, 21*(1), 18–24.

Bazzoli, G. J., Chan, B., Shortell, S. M., & D'Aunno, T. (2000). The financial performance of hospitals belonging to health networks and systems. *Inquiry, 37*(3), 234–252.

Berkowitz, E. N. (1996). *Essentials of health care marketing.* Gaithersburg, MD: Aspen Publishers, Incorporated.

Blair, J. D., & Fottler, M. D. (1998). Effective stakeholder management: Challenges, opportunities and strategies. In W. J. Duncan, P. M. Ginter, & L. E. Swayne (Eds.), *Handbook of health care management* (pp. 19–48). Malden, MA: Blackwell.

Brennan, T. A., Leape, L. L., Laird, N. M., et al. (1991). Incidence of adverse events and negligence in hospitalized patients: Results of the Harvard Medical Practice Study. *New England Journal of Medicine, 324*(6), 370–376.

Byrne, M. M., Charns, M. P., Parker, V. A., Meterko, M. M., & Ray, N. P. (2004). The effects of organization on medical utilization: An analysis of service-line organization. *Medical Care, 42*(1), 28–37.

Charns, M. P., & Schaefer, M. J. (1983). *Health care organizations: A model for management.* Englewood Cliffs, NJ: Prentice-Hall.

Charns, M. P., & Tewksbury, L. J. (1993). *Collaborative management in health care.* San Francisco: Jossey Bass.

Cleland, D., & King, W. R. (1997). *Project management handbook.* New York: John Wiley & Sons.

Daft, R. L., & Steers, R. M. (1986). *Organizations: A micro/macro approach.* Reading, MA: Addison-Wesley Educational Publishers, Inc.

Deming, W. E. (1986). *Out of the crisis.* Cambridge, MA: Massachusetts Institute of Technology, Center for Advanced Engineering Study.

Dessler, G. (2004). *Management: Principles and practices for tomorrow's leaders.* Upper Saddle River, NJ: Prentice Hall.

Diamond, H. S., Goldberg, E., & Janosky, J. E. (1998). The effect of full-time faculty hospitalists on the efficiency of care at a community teaching hospital. *Annals of Internal Medicine, 129*(3), 197–203.

Filerman, G. and Persaud, D. (2003). Advocacy Defines the Health Care System. In Leatt, P. and Mapa J. (Eds.). Government Relations in Health Care: A Leadership Essential. Toronto, Quorum/Greenwood Publishing.

Flood, A. B. (1994). The impact of organizational and managerial factors on the quality of care in health care organizations. *Medical Care Review, 51*(4), 381–428.

Fottler, M. D., Blair, J. D., Whitehead, C. J., Laus, M. D., & Savage, G. T. (1989, Winter). Assessing key stakeholders: Who matters to hospitals and why? *Hospital and Health Services Administration, 34*(4), 525–546.

Ginter, P. M., Duncan, W. J., & Swayne, L. M. (2002). *Strategic management of health care organizations* (4th ed.). Malden, MA: Blackwell.

Ginter, P. M., Swayne, L. M., & Duncan, W. J. (1998). *Strategic management of health care organizations* (4th ed.). Malden, MA: Blackwell.

Gittell, J. H., Fairfield, K. M., Bierbaum, G., Head, W., Jackson, R., Kelly, M., Laskin, R., Lipson, S., Silisky, J., Thornhill, T., & Zuckerman, J. (2000). Impact of relational coordination of quality of care, postoperative pain and functioning, and length of stay: A nine-hospital study of surgical patients. *Medical Care, 38*(8), 807–819.

Greenberg, G. A., Rosenbeck, R. A., & Charns, M. P. (2004). From professional-based leadership to service line management in the Veterans Health Administration: Impact on mental health care. *Medical Care, 41*(9), 1013–1023.

Griffith, J. R., & White, K. R. (2002). *The well-managed healthcare organization* (5th ed.). Chicago: Health Administration Press.

Hage, J. (1980). *Theories of organizations: Forms, processes, and transformations.* New York: Wiley-Interscience.

Hoff, T. H., Whitcomb, W. F., Williams, K., Nelson, J. R., & Cheesman, R. A. (2001). Characteristics and work experiences of hospitalists in the United States. *Archives of Internal Medicine, 161*(6), 851–858.

Jaklevic, M. C. (2004). A deal that's hard to refuse. *Modern Healthcare, 31*(49) 4–5.

Joint Commission on Accreditation of Healthcare Organizations. (1997). *Accreditation manual for hospitals,* Continuum of Care (cc5). Chicago: Author.

Juran, J. M. (1989). *On leadership for quality: An executive handbook.* New York: Free Press.

Kanter, E. M. (1990). *When giants learn to dance.* New York: Simon and Schuster.

Kapp, M. B. (1990, March). Cookbook medicine: A legal perspective. *Archives of Internal Medicine, 150,* 496–500.

Knaus, W. A., Draper, E. A., Wagner, D. P., & Zimmerman, J. E. (1986). An evaluation of outcome from intensive care in major medical centers. *Annals of Internal Medicine, 104*(3), 410–418.

Kocher, C., Kumar, K., & Subramanian, R. (1998). Physician-hospital integration strategies: Impact of physician involvement in hospital governance. *Healthcare Management Review, 23,* 38–47.

Kohn, L. T., Corrigan, J. M., & Donaldson, M. S. (Ed.). (2000). *To err is human: Building a safer health system.* Washington, DC: National Academy Press.

Kotler, P. (2002). *Social marketing* (2nd ed.). Thousand Oaks, CA: Sage Publications.

Kraut, A. I., Pedigo, P. R., McKenna, D. D., & Dunnette, M. D. (1989, November). The role of manager: What's really important in different management jobs. *The Academy of Management EXECUTIVE, 3*(4), 286–293.

Lawrence, P. R., & Lorsch, J. W. (1967, June). Differentiation and integration in complex organizations. *Administrative Science Quarterly, 11*(3), 1–47.

Likert, R. (1967). *The human organization.* New York: McGraw-Hill.

Longest, B. B., Jr. (1990, Winter). Interorganizational linkages in the health sector. *Health Care Management Review, 15,* 17–28.

Longest, B. B., Jr. (1997). *Seeking strategic advantage through health policy analysis.* Chicago: Health Administration Press.

Longest, B. B., Jr. (1998, March/April). Managerial competence at senior levels of integrated delivery systems. *Journal of Healthcare Management, 43*(2), 115–135.

Longest, B. B., Jr. (2002). *Health policymaking in the United States* (3rd ed.). Chicago: Health Administration Press.

Longest, B. B., Jr., Rakich, J. S. & Darr, K. (2000). *Managing health services, organizations and systems* (4th ed.). Baltimore, MD: Health Professions Press.

Luke, R. D., Begun, J. W., & Pointer, D. D. (1989). Quasi firms: Strategic interorganizational forms in the health care industry. *The Academy of Management Review, 14*(1), 9–19.

Luthans, F. (2003). *Organizational behavior* (9th ed.). New York: The McGraw-Hill Companies.

March, J., & Simon, H. (1958). *Organizations.* New York: John Wiley & Sons.

Marshall, M. N., Shekell, P. G., Leatherman, S., & Brook, R. H. (2000). The public release of performance data, what do we expect to gain? A review of the experience. *Journal of the American Medical Association, 283*(414), 1866–1874.

Mintzberg, H. (1979). *The structuring of organizations.* Englewood Cliffs, NJ: Prentice-Hall.

Mintzberg, H. (1992). *Structure in fives: Designing effective organizations.* Englewood Cliffs, NJ: Prentice-Hall.

Newstrom, J. W., & Davis, K. (1993). *Organizational behavior: Human behavior at work* (9th ed.). New York: McGraw-Hill, pp. 102.

Parker, V. A., Charns, M. P., & Young, G. J. (2001). Clinical service lines in integrated delivery systems: An initial framework and exploration. *Journal of Healthcare Management, 46*(4), 261–275.

Pearson, S. D., Goulart-Fischer, R. N., & Lee, T. H. (1995). Critical pathways as a strategy for improving care: Problems and potential. *Annals of Internal Medicine, 123*(12), 941–948.

Pfeffer, J., & Salanick, G. R. (1978). *The external control of organizations: A resource dependence perspective.* New York: Harper & Row.

Pointer, D. D., Begun, J. W., & Luke, R. D. (1988, Summer). Managing interorganizational dependencies in the new health care marketplace. *Hospital and Health Service Administration, 33*(2), 167–177.

Porter, M. E. (1985). *Competitive advantage: Creating and sustaining superior performance.* New York: The Free Press.

Robbins, S. P., & Coulter, M. K. (2005). *Management* (8th ed.). Upper Saddle River, NJ: Prentice-Hall.

Satinsky, M. A. (1998). *The foundations of integrated care.* Chicago: American Hospital Publishing.

Scott, W. R. (1982, Fall). Managing professional work: Three models of control for health organizations. *Health Services Research, 17*(3), 213–240.

Scott, W. R., Mitchell, T. R., & Birnbaummore, P. H. (1981). *Organization theory: A structural and behavioral analysis* (4th ed.). Homewood, IL: Richard D. Irwin.

Senge, P. M. (1990). *The fifth discipline: The art and practice of the learning organization.* New York: Bantam Doubleday Dell Audio Publishing.

Shortell, S. M. (1991). *Effective hospital-physician relationships.* Chicago: Health Administration Press.

Shortell, S. M., Gillies, R. R., Anderson, D. A., Erickson-Morgan, K., & Mitchell, J. B. (1996). *Remaking healthcare in America: Building organized delivery systems.* San Francisco: Jossey-Bass.

Shortell, S. M., Zimmerman, J. E., Rousseau, D. M., Gillies, R. R., Wagner, D. P., Draper, E. A., Knaus, W. A., & Duffy, J. (1994). The performance of intensive care units: Does good management make a difference? *Medical Care, 32*(5), 508–525.

Starkweather, D. B. (1981). *Hospital mergers in the making.* Ann Arbor, MI: Health Administration Press.

Thomas, J. B., & McDaniel, R. R., Jr. (1990). Interpreting strategic issues: Effects of strategy and the information-processing structure of top management teams. *Academy of Management Journal, 33*(2), 288–298.

Thompson, J. D. (1967). *Organizations in action.* New York: McGraw Hill.

Van de Ven, A., Delbecq, A., & Koenig, R. (1976, April). Determinants of coordination modes within organizations. *American Sociological Review, 41,* 322–338.

Weick, K. (1976). Educational organizations as loosely coupled systems. *Administrative Science Quarterly, 21*(1), 1–19.

Young, G. J., Charns, M. P., Daley, J., Forbes, M. G., Henderson, W., & Khuri, S. F. (1997). Best practices for managing surgical services: The role of coordination. *Health Care Management Review, 22*(4), 72–81.

Young, G. J., Charns, M. P., Desai, K., Khuri, S. F., Forbes, M. G., Henderson, W., & Daley, J. (1998). Patterns of coordination and surgical outcomes: A study of surgical services. *Health Services Research, 33*(5).

Young, G. J., Charns, M. P., & Herren, T. (2004). Product-line management in professional organizations: An empirical test of competing theoretical perspectives. *Academy of Management Journal.*

Zuckerman, H. S., & Kaluzny, A. D. (1991, Spring). Strategic alliances in health care: The challenges of cooperation. *Frontiers of Health Services Management, 7*(3), 3–23.

CHAPTER 9

Power and Politics

Jeffrey A. Alexander, Ph.D., Thomas G. Rundall, Ph.D.,
Timothy J. Hoff, Ph.D., and Laura L. Morlock, Ph.D.

CHAPTER OUTLINE

LEARNING OBJECTIVES

After completing this chapter, the reader should be able to:

1. Distinguish between rational and political models of organization and their appropriateness to health services organizations.

2. Know the practical and managerial implications of the effective use of power in health services organizations.

3. Identify the conditions that promote the use of power, politics, and informal influence in health services organizations.

4. Understand the range of political strategies and tactics employed by members of health services organizations.

5. Understand the source of power in health services organizations.

6. Know the approaches for consolidating and developing power by managers, physicians, and other groups in health services organizations.

KEY TERMS

Alliances

Authority

Coalitions

Code of Ethics

Control of Information

Coping with Uncertainty

Dependency Relationships

Formal Authority System

Influence

Interdependency

Interests

Network Centrality

Nonsubstitutability

Organizational Decision-
    Making Processes

Political Games

Political Model of
    Organization

Politics

Power

Public Good

Rational Model of
    Organization

Sources of Power

❧ IN PRACTICE   Turf Battles Among the Medical Staff

Terry Johnson leaned back in her chair feeling overwhelmed by the stacks of memos and reports piled on the desk before her. As the new administrative resident at Suburban Healthcare System, she had been delighted when Sandy Shulman, the chief operating officer, suggested that Terry assist her and the finance director to prepare for a series of meetings with clinical chiefs that would help develop the next three-year capital budget.

Sandy had handed over a thick folder filled with budget requests and then explained that Terry's role would be to help track down any additional patient volume and market-area data that could help determine both the need for and the desirability of each of the major proposals for equipment or renovations. Delight had quickly faded to dismay, however, as Terry wondered what types of information could possibly be helpful to senior management and the governing board as they tried to evaluate the array of proposals with their competing priorities and sometimes contradictory assumptions.

A good example was the proposal from the Department of Surgery for renovation funds and equipment to create their own capability within the department for performing coronary angiographies. Currently this procedure was performed in laboratories within the Department of Radiology, but according to the Department of Surgery

proposal, the limited space and equipment available could no longer accommodate the growing demand. Terry noted that the budget request from the Department of Radiology included funds to purchase an additional image intensifier as well as other equipment needed to increase the capacity of radiology for performing angiographies and other interventional radiological procedures.

At Sandy's suggestion, Terry had met with the manager in Radiology responsible for scheduling these procedures. It appeared that afternoon time slots were almost always available without a long waiting period for an appointment. Competition was severe, however, among physicians trying to schedule patients in the early morning, particularly during the 7 A.M. to 9 A.M. periods. In addition, during the past few months, a number of complaints had resulted from emergency cases "bumping" patients undergoing elective procedures from the schedule. Perhaps additional capacity was needed, but in which department?

There also seemed to be several other duplicate proposals with requests for similar equipment purchases. It appeared, for example, that both the Department of Radiology and the Obstetrics and Gynecology Service were planning to double their capacity to perform pelvic ultrasounds and mammography. Terry was aware that a large freestanding diagnostic imaging center recently

(continues)

IN PRACTICE *(continued)*

had opened nearby and wondered whether the utilization projections of either proposal would be likely to materialize.

In a subsequent meeting with Sandy to go over detailed population projections by gender and age group for their market area, Terry voiced her confusion regarding the duplication in requests for new equipment. Could it be cost-effective for the same types of procedures to be performed by multiple specialties in different clinical services within the health system?

Sandy commented that this question was being pondered throughout the country as technological advances continued to create important new devices and techniques that are not clearly the domain of any one specialty. In some hospitals, for example, general surgeons and gastroenterologists argued over who should be credentialed to perform laparoscopic cholecystectomies—a surgical procedure that allows a patient's gallbladder to be removed through small incisions in the abdomen. In other medical centers, disputes waged whether obstetricians-gynecologists or radiologists were better trained to

perform and interpret pelvic ultrasounds and mammograms; and whether radiologists or gastroenterologists should perform gastrointestinal endoscopy. In some hospitals, heated discussions were occurring regarding whether general surgeons or otolaryngologists were more appropriately trained to conduct head and neck surgery; and whether carotid endarterectomies were more appropriately performed by vascular surgeons or neurosurgeons.

Sandy emphasized that such "turf disputes" were only likely to intensify as technological advances continued to outstrip the development of medical standards and guidelines for designating the credentials appropriate for performing specific procedures and utilizing specialized medical equipment. These uncertainties were often compounded by the difficulties in obtaining adequate data on patient outcomes and costs in order to compare alternatives. Terry realized that these controversies were likely to have important economic consequences as physicians attempted to retain and further expand their patient bases. But how, she wondered, could these types of conflicts be resolved?

CHAPTER PURPOSE

Whether at hospitals, health maintenance organizations (HMOs), group practices, or preferred provider organizations (PPOs), the conflicts presented at Suburban Healthcare System are not unique. Managers of health care organizations are continually required to balance the rational, or task-oriented, with the social reality of organizational life (Buck, 1966; Cyert & March, 1963; MacMillan, 1978; March & Olsen, 1976). This chapter will discuss the (1) importance of power and politics to organizational functioning; (2) the sources of power; (3) when power is likely to be used in organizations, and for what types of issues; (4) strategies and tactics for increasing power; (5) the conditions

that give rise to power abuse by managers in organizations; and (6) the various ways in which employees may respond to the use of power in organizations.

THE IMPORTANCE OF POWER AND POLITICS IN HEALTH SERVICES ORGANIZATIONS

Health managers continually strive to improve efficiencies and productivity in the delivery of clinical care as well as meeting established organizational goals. Yet the reality is that these goals are not easily defined or universally accepted by organizational members. As we see at Suburban Healthcare System, interests within a given organization vary widely across departments, occupational groups, and individuals; and the role of management is to achieve a sense of balance. Success requires that managers must be cognizant of the distribution of power in their organization, the circumstances under which power is utilized, and tactics and strategies associated with the effective use of such power (Pfeffer, 1981, 1992).

When asked, many health services managers would acknowledge the existence and importance of informal power and politics as central forces in their organizations. However, these same managers are often reluctant to legitimize power and politics as acceptable management processes (Pfeffer, 1992). Such power is viewed as illegitimate by many managers because it often operates outside the formal authority system of the organization (Kanter, 1979; Kotter, 1985). Yet, informed power and political activity are commonplace in most organizations (Parker, Dipboye, & Jackson, 1995). Any casual examination of the organization chart of a large tertiary hospital would reveal a complex system of reporting relationships and authority channels (see Chapter 10). This official system of accountabilities, control, and influence, however, does not fully represent what transpires between managers, physicians, and other groups of health care providers (Young & Saltman, 1985). What gets done, how it gets done, and even the establishment of organizational goals themselves may be determined largely through processes of coalition building and influence that operate outside of the formal authority structure expressed on the organizational chart (Perrow, 1961, 1963).

In early research on power in organizations, many researchers viewed the use of informal power as leading to subversion of organizational goals. Anything that occurred outside the formal authority structure of the organization was assumed to be potentially motivated by self-serving interests on the part of individuals or groups. Such behavior was often assumed to run counter to the attainment of officially sanctioned organizational goals (Pfeffer, 1992).

However, current views of the use of power in organizations are more positive. In many organizations faced with a turbulent, high-velocity environment the use of power may be helpful and necessary to effective performance. Because health care has been subject to a rapid pace of technological, financing, social, and market change, there has been a corresponding need for health care organizations of all types to make decisions rapidly, respond quickly to competitors' actions, develop new services, and enter new markets in a timely fashion. Under such time-related pressures, health care organizations can no longer depend on traditional, vertical channels of authority and reporting relationships to make decisions and implement them quickly. Less hierarchical methods of getting things done are becoming the norm, and those methods often rely on informal power and influence, negotiation, and network positioning rather than formal authority (Pfeffer, 1997).

The importance of informal power and politics is further increased by the ambiguity and uncertainty surrounding the establishment of organizational goals in health services organizations and the means to achieve them. Ambiguity and uncertainty in health services organizations is in large measure due to the existence of disagreements about what organizational goals should be, how they should be measured, how they should be prioritized, and the means by which they should be achieved creates situations where different perspectives and interests come into play (Kotter, 1977; Kouzes & Posner, 1988; Salancik & Pfeffer, 1977). The pervasiveness of ambiguity and uncertainty in health delivery organizations suggests that problems, particularly important problems, are typically not solved exclusively by logical analysis and sound reasoning. Managerial success in organizations is frequently a matter of working with and through other people, not simply using hierarchical position to achieve stated objectives (Pfeffer, 1992). Indeed, organizational success is often a function of how well individuals can coordinate their activities (Bennis & Nanus, 1985; Kotter, 1978). This coordination is often a direct outcome of the effective use of power (both formal and informal) by managers. Informal power, although frequently operating outside the boundaries of the formal authority system of health care organizations, is not necessarily antithetical to the achievement of organizational goals. To acknowledge power and its importance in organizations is simply to acknowledge the diversity of interests and goals within the organization, the existence and normalcy of conflict, and that organizational results may stem from the political behavior of participants with different preferences (Morgan, 1986). Power can be analyzed systematically, and politics employed selectively, so as to make management more effective.

Power, Influence, and Politics— Definitions

Power has been notoriously difficult to define and measure in organizations. This is primarily because power is an intangible force in organizations. It cannot be seen, and it is not wholly captured in formal organizational charts. Indeed, power, and related concepts such as **influence**, and politics have been used in a variety of ways in the literature on organizations and management. For example, while power is often defined as the potential ability of one person or group to influence other persons or groups to carry out orders (Dahl, 1957) or to do something they otherwise would not have done (Astley & Sachdeva, 1984; Kaplan, 1964), other definitions emphasize that power is the ability to achieve goals or outcomes that power holders desire (Salancik & Pfeffer, 1974).

For the purposes of this chapter, we incorporate elements of both of the above definitions and define **power** as the ability of one person or group in an organization to influence other people to bring about desired outcomes (Daft, 2001). Influence refers to actions that either directly or indirectly cause a change in the behavior and/or attitudes of another individual or group. Influence might be thought of as the explicit act of using power to change the behavior of others (Cialdini, 1984; Mintzberg, 1983). Finally, we define organizational **politics** as activities to acquire, develop, and use power and other resources to obtain a preferred outcome (Pfeffer,1981). In any complex organization uncertainty and conflict over decisions are natural and inevitable, and politics is the mechanism for reaching agreement. In this sense, politics does not inherently produce either good or bad outcomes for an organization.

Why Systems of Power and Politics Arise

Most writers agree that the use of informal power and politics in organizations occurs most frequently in situations where goals are in conflict, where formal power is decentralized or diffused throughout the organization, where information is ambiguous, and where cause-and-effect relationships between actions and outcomes are uncertain or unknown (Mintzberg, 1983; Morgan, 1986; Perrow, 1961, 1963; Pfeffer, 1981). Although health service organizations are far too varied to claim that they all meet these conditions, one could easily see how, for certain decisions and domains of activity, these characteristics might easily apply to organizations as diverse as hospitals, HMOs, nursing homes, and group practice organizations. It is often the case, for example, that governing boards and senior management have difficulty expressing clear, unconflicting goals and objectives capable of being operationalized by the formal structure and control systems of the organization (Crozier, 1964; Young & Saltman, 1985).

Many argue that political activity and informal influence systems arise because of inherent failings in the formal system of authority. This perspective is based on the notion that an important function of the formal control system is to articulate and operationalize organizational goals and to direct the behavior of organizational members toward the achievement of these goals (Mintzberg, 1983; O'-Donnell, 1952). In many organizations, particularly health care organizations, this is at best an imperfect process since many goals are operationalized quite imperfectly, and some, such as the quality of medical care and service, are difficult to operationalize at all. In addition, most health services organizations have multiple goals such as providing high-quality and accessible care and maintaining financial viability. However, organizational participants are rarely provided with the means to weigh the importance of different goals in order to direct their activities.

The ambiguity and uncertainty in how to operationalize and prioritize organizational objectives creates an arena for potential conflict among even the most dedicated, well-intentioned participants (Morgan, 1986). As illustrated by the turf battles at the Suburban Healthcare System (see In Practice, p. 277), this situation may be reinforced by the complex division of labor and differentiation that occurs in many health care organizations. This pattern may be due to the assignment of different tasks and sometimes different organizational goals to different units or occupational groups. The tendency is for each unit or subgroup to emphasize the importance of its own activities and to sometimes treat its own tasks as ends in themselves rather than focusing on large organizational goals (Lourenco & Glidewell, 1975; Perrow, 1970). Such differentiation creates group pressures that promote solidarity within the group and mistrust or misunderstanding of other groups—a we-they relationship (Morgan, 1986; Pfeffer, 1992). Table 9.1, for example, illustrates the differences in principal orientations of managers and physicians that often foster conflict between the two groups. Together, these types of organizational factors generate attempts to influence decisions and activities outside of the formal system of authority in organizations. Of primal importance here is that such systems of power and influence outside the formal authority system are naturally occurring phenomena in organizations and must be acknowledged and used by managers to effectively render some decisions and to implement those decisions in such a way as to benefit the organization as a whole.

Rational versus Political Perspectives on Management

The acknowledgment and effective use of power, influence, and politics in organizations requires a fundamentally different outlook on organizational life than that prescribed in many graduate programs of health administration. The key differences between the **rational** and **political models of organizations** are displayed in Table 9.2. Rational models imply that the managers of health care organizations are orchestrating the activities of a team whose members all subscribe to a common set of goals and objectives. Organizational members—whether physicians, nurses, ancillary care personnel, or others—are expected to perform the roles for which they have been appointed. Their behavior should be consistent with the achievement of commonly agreed upon organizational goals. Conflict in this context is seen as a source of trouble and an unwanted intrusion. Formal authority or professional expertise are the only legitimate sources of power, and all others are viewed as antithetical to the attainment of organizational goals.

By contrast, managers who acknowledge the existence of power and influence beyond that vested in the formal authority system or professional expertise have a fundamentally different view of organizational life. These managers recognize that individuals and groups have different **interests**, aims, and objectives and that organizational membership is often a platform for pursuing their own ends. The central task of management is to balance and coordinate the various interests of organizational members so that concerted effort can be achieved to work within the constraints set by the organization's former goals. Perhaps most importantly, the manager who explicitly acknowledges the importance of informal

Table 9.1. Cultural Differences between Health Care Executives and Physicians

Attribute	Health Care Executives	Physicians
Basis of knowledge	Primarily social and management sciences	Primarily biomedical sciences
Exposure to relevant others while in training	Relatively little exposure to physicians, nurses, other health care professionals, or patients	Great deal of exposure to nurses, other health care professionals, and patients; little exposure to broader business or economic world of health care
Patient focus	Broad: all patients in the organization and the larger community	Narrow: one's individual patients
Time frame of action	Middle to long run; emphasis on positioning the organization for the future	Generally short run; meet immediate needs of patients
View of resources	Always limited; challenge lies in allocating scarce resources efficiently and effectively	More limited view emphasizing resources needed for one's own patients; resources should be available to maximize the quality of care
Professional identity	Less cohesive; less well developed	More cohesive; highly developed

SOURCE: S. Shortell, *Effective Hospital-Physician Relationships.* Ann Arbor, MI: Health Administration Press, 1992. Reprinted with permission from the Hospital Research and Educational Trust.

organizational power often uses uncomfortable situations involving disagreements and conflicts and turns them into positive aspects of organizational life. Conflict, for example, can energize an organization and keep it from becoming lethargic, stale, and subject to inertia (Hannan & Freeman, 1984). Conflict can motivate employees to engage in self-evaluation (Tushman, Newman, & Romanelli, 1986). Indeed, organizations themselves are viewed from this perspective, not as unified systems, but as loosely coupled systems where semi-autonomous parts strive to maintain a degree of independence while working under the same name and framework provided by the organization. To be successful, managers must have the ability to read developing situations, analyze the interests that affect or are affected by these situations, understand conflicts, and explore power relations.

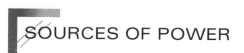

SOURCES OF POWER

Effective use of power assumes that one has the requisite amount of power to influence the outcomes of organizational decisions. Thus, understanding the **sources of power** is an important first step in acquiring or increasing such power. Some power is derived from personal attributes such as sensitivity, articulateness, and self-confidence. Employees may also increase their power by becoming knowledgeable or expert about certain activities important to the organization or by taking on difficult tasks.

Table 9.2. Rational versus Political Models of Organizations

Organizational Characteristic	Rational Model	Political Model
Goals, preferences	Consistent across members	Inconsistent, pluralistic within the organization
Power and control	Centralized	Diffuse, shifting coalitions and interest groups
Decision process	Logical, orderly, sequential	Disorderly, give and take of competing interests
Information	Extensive, systematic, accurate	Ambiguous, selectively available, used as a power resource
Cause-and-effect relationship	Predictable	Uncertain
Decisions	Based on outcome maximizing choice	More limited view emphasizing resources needed for one's own patients; resources should be available to maximize the quality of care
Ideology	Efficiency and effectiveness	Struggle, conflict, winners and losers

Generally, however, structural sources of power are more important (Brass, 1984; Hickson, Hinings, Lee, Schneck, & Penning, 1971; Mechanic, 1962; Pfeffer, 1992). From this perspective, power is derived from where individuals are situated in the division of labor and the communications system of the organization. One's placement in these structures imbues one to a lesser or greater extent with power from the institutionalized authority attached to one's position (formal power), as well as power one derives from one's control over resources, decision-making processes and information, and one's ability to manage the organization's strategic contingencies (often informal power). Below we describe these sources of power and discuss how they are typically related to an organization's hierarchical structure. We also discuss ways in which these sources of power can be used to increase power re-

gardless of one's location in the organization's formal structure.

Authority Linked to Formal Position

Perhaps the most obvious source of power in organizations is that which is vested by formal authority associated with the role or position of an individual in the organizational hierarchy (Tannenbaum, 1968; Weber, 1947). When observing an organizational chart, such as that depicted in Figure 9.1, it is relatively easy to discern what positions have **authority** over others and what positions are subordinate to higher ranked positions. The **formal authority system** of the organization is usually defined in terms of position-linked rights and obligations that are widely accepted in the

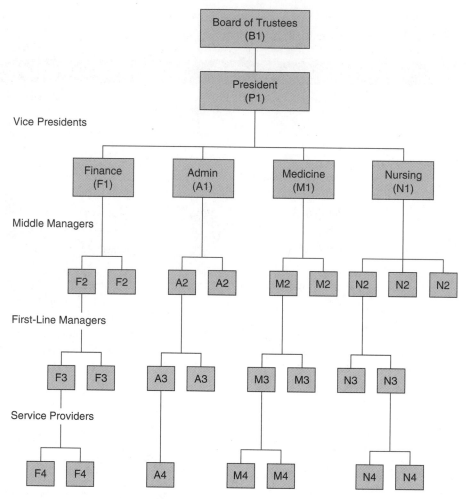

Figure 9.1. Formal Authority Structure: Acute Care General Hospital

organization. Hence, authority has three properties that distinguish it as a special type of power (Daft, 2001, p. 449). First, authority is vested in organizational positions. Employees have authority because of the positions they hold, not because of personal characteristics or control over important resources. Second, subordinates accept the authority of superiors because they believe that position holders higher up in the hierarchy have a legitimate right to exercise authority. Third, authority flows down the vertical hierarchy along a formal chain of command. Typically, those in higher positions are vested with the power to direct and influence those in lower positions. However, even power vested by the formal authority structure of the organization holds only so long as those who are subject to this kind of authority respect and accept the nature of that authority. Although formal authority is supported by strong beliefs and values within organizations, under certain circumstances it can erode or even be lost entirely. This sometimes occurs in situations where a tyrannical boss will so alienate the workers of an organization that they will refuse to further acknowledge his authority and his power by refusing to carry out his orders or by quitting the organization.

Control over Resources

Health services organizations such as hospitals require substantial resources to perform day-to-day operations and achieve long-term, strategic goals. Although control over resources is often linked to position in the organizational hierarchy, this is not always the case. Departments or individuals that generate income and other valued resources have greater power. These resources are used by the organization to construct buildings, pay salaries, purchase capital equipment and supplies, and pay for hundreds of other costs. In most cases, top managers control these resources through management of the organization's budgeting process. Each year, resources are allocated to departments in the form of budgets. Departmental budgets are typically proposed by department managers, modified through a negotiation with other department managers and organizational leaders, and ultimately are approved by top managers. These negotiations are often contentious, not only because managers differ in the way they prioritize organizational needs, but because control over a resource is itself a desired source of power in the organization. For example, the ability of a hospital's strategic planning department to offer physicians even modest compensation for participating in nonclinical planning committee work is a means of rewarding those physicians for their participation and increasing their loyalty to the department. Control over resources may have an even greater effect on the strength and breadth of one's influence by making it possible to establish **dependency relationships**—situations in which units or individuals depend on access to resources outside their immediate control to accomplish their goals. Research suggests that the amount

of dependency-related power linked to one's ability to control a resource depends on three attributes of the resource. The resource must be (1) essential to the functioning of the organization; (2) in short supply (or concentrated in terms of the number of people); and (3) nonsubstitutable. These three attributes make the resource critical for the organization and thus create organizational dependency on those individuals or groups who control its availability and use. The power of a given department is created in part by the dependence of others, and that dependence is a function of how much others need the resource the department controls, as well as how many alternative sources for that resource there are (Blau, 1964; Jacobs, 1974; Pfeffer & Davis-Blake, 1987). For example, many physicians in health services organizations will emphasize the revenue-generating capabilities of their clinical departments as the basis for influencing future capital acquisition or the purchase of new medical technology. One hospital physician noted, "Of course, our argument about our financial contribution to the hospital is primarily useful with the administration and the board. It should also have some meaning to other physicians, however, if our work conditions become so intolerable that we are unable to continue maintaining our quality of service, there will be financial ramifications for everyone associated with the hospital" (Young & Saltman, 1985).

It is important to note that access to and control over critical resources can occur at lower as well as higher levels in health services organizations (Mechanic, 1962). For instance, a purchasing agent often has considerable latitude regarding negotiating contracts for equipment and supplies. She can seriously inconvenience a surgical suite by dragging her feet on ordering replacement equipment or by refusing to expedite a request.

The acquisition of power through control over resources is often accomplished through the formation of **alliances** and **coalitions** (Gamson, 1961; McNeil, 1978). Alliances and coalitions are developed through several different mechanisms,

IN PRACTICE — Competing Goals and Conflicting Cultures

As head of this region's largest radiology group, George Watts had worked at Fairhope Medical Center for over 15 years. So when owner Medmark Corp., a large investor-owned system, sent in a new administrator, Mr. Wade Baron, last year, Dr. Watts paid what he expected to be a courtesy call. But as the doctor now recalls it, the visit was neither friendly nor courteous. "You don't want me for an enemy," he says the new hospital chief executive warned him.

The context of the exchange soon became clear. Dr. Watt's group has long provided radiology services to other hospitals in addition to Fairhope, including Medmark's archrival. Without warning, the new chief executive issued an ultimatum: Split away from your group and practice only at Medmark—or leave. While the same mandate was issued for other physicians in other specialties at Fairhope, Dr. Watts emerged as Mr. Baron's chief foe. He and other members of his group continue to practice at the group's outpatient facility, at several other hospitals, and, for the moment, at Fairhope.

"I'm offended that a businessman is trying to tell me when or with whom I can be a doctor," Watts states. Mr. Baron counters: "No one likes change and here's a new guy nobody knew wanting to institute change." Each boasts decades of health care experience. Each claims the moral high ground, saying that if his opponent wins, patient care will suffer.

---

including helping people to obtain positions of power through appointments and promotions and doing favors for those whose support is needed (Pfeffer, 1992). Although these strategies may seem manipulative, and even illegitimate, they are often necessary in complex, interdependent systems with many actors and points of view such as those demonstrated at the Fairhope Medical Center (see In Practice, above). In health services organizations, alliances often emerge among the chiefs of clinical services in their requests for capital improvements. For example, the chief of radiology and the chief of orthopedic surgery may support each other in their respective request for a portable fluoroscope and for renovations to department facilities. Their combined power increases the probability that their requests will be approved. Also, such alliances may be used to mount a campaign against capital requests by other service chiefs.

Control over Decision-Making Processes and Information

Another source of power among top managers is the control they have over **organizational decision-making processes**. The decisions top managers make about organization-wide goals and objectives, such as the organization's growth strategy, comprehensiveness of service offerings, and the emphases placed on quality improvement, cost control, and community service, constrain decisions made at lower levels in the health services organization. These types of decisions provide others in the organization with strategic and operational goals to which department-level goals, objectives, work plans, and budgets must be rationally linked. Other ways managers can control decision-making processes include setting the scope of authority for standing and ad hoc committees, prescribing the acceptable parameters of problem solutions being developed by committees or task forces, and appointing to such committees and task forces employees with whom close ties have been developed. In one health services organization, the chief executive officer (CEO) appointed a committee to recommend a new chief operations officer (COO). The CEO provided the committee with a detailed list of the qualifications the new COO should have. He also selected the people to serve on the committee. In this way, the CEO shaped the decision process within which the new COO would be chosen. Actions such as these by top managers place limits on the decisions of lower-level managers and thereby influence the outcomes of their decisions (Daft, 2001).

The **control of information** can also be a source of power. The primary basis for the power of a hospital's medical staff, for example, is usually perceived to be its control over a specialized body of knowledge and technical skills required to diagnose and treat patients (Burns, Andersen, & Shortell, 1989; Scott, 1982; Shortell, 1992). Because patients are vital to the hospital's continued viability, physicians' expertise gives them a strong power base within the organization. However, it has recently been recognized that the expertise required to deal effectively with financial system coordination and the legal complexities of health care organizations is also crucial to the viability of the organization. Expertise in these matters has increased the power of management in their relationships with physicians over the past two decades (Davies, Rundall, & Hodges, 2003; Moore & Wood, 1979; Rundall, 2004; Rundall, Davies, & Hodges, 2004; Shortell & Rundall, 2003). A related source of power is the control managers have over what business-related information is collected, how it is interpreted, and how it is shared (Davenport, Eccles, & Prusak,1992; Larson & King, 1996). Top managers generally have access to more information than do other employees, and this information can be released as needed to shape the preferences and decisions of other people. However, it is well known that middle managers and lower-level employees may manipulate the information they provide to top managers in order to influence decisions (Daft, 2001).

Network Centrality

One's physical and social location in the organization contributes to one's power. A central location lets one be visible to key people and become part of important interaction networks (Daft, 2001). However, **network centrality** can also be enhanced by being part of major communication pathways that link individuals within the organization. Power accrues as a function of one's position in the network of communications and social relations within the organization (Hackman, 1985; Izraeli, 1975; Pfeffer, 1992). In general, being centrally located puts one in contact with many others in the organization and provides access to information and people that are critical to the organization's success. Although typical of top managers, all organizational members, regardless of their place in the formal organizational hierarchy, may be embedded in multiple communication and social networks and are thus able to use the information and relationships derived from these networks to build alliances and influence organizational decisions. The advances made in computer technology, through extensive use of e-mail and instant messaging systems, allows managers to now be even more central in the organization's communication networks.

Nonsubstitutability

Power is also a function of an employee's or department's **nonsubstitutability**: the extent to which it is difficult for the employee's or department's function to be performed by other readily available resources (Daft, 2001). Nonsubstitutability in combination with importance of function increases power. For example, if an employee has specialized skills that cannot be easily replaced, such as a critical care nurse in a tight nursing job market, her power is greater. Or, if an organization has no alternative source of knowledge about computers and information systems, the power of the information technology department in a health system will be greater.

Management of Strategic Contingencies

Strategic contingencies are activities and events both inside and outside an organization that are essential for attaining organizational goals (Daft, 2001). Individuals and departments involved with managing strategic contingencies for an organization tend to have greater power, even if they do not possess great formal power as in the case of Emily Clayton (see In Practice, p. 289). Coordinating complex patient care processes; maintaining positive relationships with physicians; creating and maintaining administrative and clinical information systems; building a reliable, low-cost supply chain; and managing accreditation and licensing processes are examples of managing strategic contingencies in a hospital. Managers in health care organizations who are equipped to deal with these types of contingencies gain power because their work is critical to the viability of the organization (Alexander, Morrisey, & Shortell, 1986; Glandon & Morrisey, 1986; Roemer & Friedman, 1971). It should be noted that the power derived from an individual's or group's ability to deal with strategic contingencies is directly related to the centrality of their functions to the organization and inversely related to the degree to which their skills are substitutable. For example, a political analyst in a health care organization whose responsibility is to interface with state regulatory agencies may lose some of her power if such functions can be performed equally well by a member of the hospital's marketing department.

The management of strategic contingencies is closely linked to a related source of organizational power: **coping with uncertainty** (Brass, 1984;

Fligstein, 1987; Hickson et al., 1971; Pfeffer, 1992). Internal and external environments of health services organizations can change quickly and in complex and unpredictable ways. Such change generates uncertainty among managers about what are appropriate courses of action. Departments that cope with this uncertainty will have more power. However, as noted by Daft (2001, p. 457), the mere presence of uncertainty does not provide power, but reducing uncertainty on the behalf of other departments will. The uncertainty created by interdepartmental dynamics; demands by physicians, nurses, and other occupational groups; competitive market forces; volatile capital markets; governmental regulations; and many other factors provide opportunities for those with relevant knowledge and skills to explain, interpret, and mediate as necessary to reduce the uncertainty faced by the organization's managers.

Tactics for Increasing Power

The previous discussion argued that power in organizations is not primarily a characteristic of the individual. Rather, power is related to the individual's position in the organization, the resources commanded by the individual's department, the functions performed by the department, and the environmental contingencies with which the department copes. However, individuals can use a variety of tactics to increase the power of their position or department. This section briefly describes tactics for increasing organizational power.

Our discussion of the sources of power suggests the following tactics for increasing power.

- Provide resources to other departments and operating units. Since resources are always important to organizational survival, a department that generates resources and provides them to other organizational units in the form of money, information, or facilities will increase its power.

- Create dependencies. When the organization depends upon a department for information, knowledge, or skills, that department will increase its power relative to others.

✣ IN PRACTICE   Managing Strategic Contingencies

University Medical Center is scheduled to go through the Joint Commission on Accreditation of Healthcare Organizations (JCAHO: http://www.jcaho.org/) reaccreditation process in the next year. In recent years, JCAHO has revised existing standards and established many new standards, particularly in the area of assuring patient safety. Given these changes, everyone at University Medical Center knew that this reaccreditation process would be unlike any other they experienced. Emily Clayton, a project manager at the hospital with a history of working on temporary assignments assisting various departments during times of staff shortages or special project development, was asked to accept responsibility for preparing the physicians, nurses, and other clinical and nonclinical hospital staff for the JCAHO reaccreditation. Viewing this assignment as important to the hospital and as an opportunity to show senior management what she could do, Emily quickly accepted the job. Emily and her small team of assistants began the difficult process of revising the hospital's policies to conform to the new standards of care, and getting formal approval of those new policies from all affected clinical departments. The task required diligence, commitment to participatory decision making, frequent communication with key players up and down the administrative and medical hierarchies, negotiation and conflict resolution, and patience with those who resisted change. Emily consulted extensively with JCAHO to acquire expertise in the new standards, organized and ran innumerable meetings with clinicians to discuss the changes in clinician behavior required by the new standards, and sought input from clinicians about how to implement these policies in ways that made sense in their hospital. Most importantly, this work had to be done in a way that moved the educational

activities and policy decisions forward in a timely way without alienating the clinicians affected by the changes. As Emily's work progressed, she encountered a good deal of resistance from many quarters, but the most difficult person to work with was Dr. John Thomas, the vice president for clinical affairs, who consistently attempted to block or dilute the policy changes Emily believed were necessary to ensure reaccreditation. How should Emily deal with this problem? What power does Dr. Thomas have? What power does Emily have in this situation? What tactics can Emily use to overcome the resistance of this senior manager?

Here is what actually happened.

Emily knew that her power in this situation was based on the fact that she was known to be effectively managing a strategic contingency for the hospital, knew more about JCAHO accreditation standards and processes than anyone else in the hospital, and that the process she was using gave her access to an extensive network of senior administrative and clinical staff in the hospital. She was at the center of all communications about JCAHO reaccreditation, and knew the views and preferences of all the hospital's leaders. Emily's information-sharing and educational activities with key hospital leaders had been largely successful, establishing their support for the policy changes she believed were essential if the hospital was to be reaccredited. Many of the e-mail and other communications could be shared with the vice president of clinical affairs, and Emily made certain that the agenda she set for the planning and decision meetings she arranged gave senior managers and clinicians opportunities to express their support for the policy changes. In time, Dr. Thomas realized that other senior leaders, including all of the chiefs of the major departments were supportive of the changes, and he became

(continues)

IN PRACTICE *(continued)*

less resistant to the changes. In the end, developing expert knowledge about the JCAHO reaccreditation standards and processes, extensive and broad communication and educational activities, establishing coalitions, and demonstrating effectiveness at managing this strategic imperative enabled Emily to overcome the resistance of a powerful senior manager.

- Take responsibility for areas of high uncertainty. When department managers identify and remove uncertainties, the department's power will be increased.

- Satisfy strategic contingencies. When contingencies are not being satisfied or new contingencies arise, there is an opportunity for a department to take responsibility for managing those critical activities and events and increase its power.

- Build coalitions. Coalition building requires taking time to meet with other managers or external stakeholders one-on-one or in small groups to present views and negotiate agreements. In coalition building it is especially important to build good relationships through establishing mutual trust and respect. Top management often spends considerable time in external coalition building as illustrated by the activities of CEO John O'Connor (see In Practice, p. 291).

- Expand networks. Networks can be expanded by extending communication and personal contact to managers outside your existing network. Also, networks can be expanded by influencing personnel recruitment, transfer, and promotion decisions in order to place people in key positions, people who are supportive of your department's goals.

- Control decision processes. Decision processes can be controlled in a variety of ways. Selectively limiting or choosing the data and information available at the time an important decision is being made is one tactic. The most common version of this is to make certain that information about your department demonstrates meaningful contributions to important organizational goals and presents the department in the best possible light. Another tactic is to constrain the decision process by influencing who will make a decision and/or influencing the items placed on the agenda for an important meeting.

WHEN POWER IS LIKELY TO BE USED

To effectively use power, it is important to recognize the conditions under which it is most appropriately used. First, because power is a finite resource, organizational members are more apt to employ it for decisions they consider to be important such as those made at higher organizational levels and those that involve crucial issues like reorganization and budget allocations (Pfeffer & Salancik, 1974). Second, power is more likely to be a factor for those domains of activity in which performance is more difficult to assess (e.g., staff activity rather than line production) and in situations in which there are likely to be uncertainties and disagreement (e.g., goals, priorities, and the means to achieve them) (MacMillan, 1978; Salancik & Pfeffer, 1974).

It is interesting to note that all of these conditions are evident in the description of turf battles among medical staff members at Suburban Healthcare System (see In Practice, p. 277). The decisions to be made involve critical resource allocations across departments that will determine what major equipment purchases and renovations will be made during the next three years. These decisions are

Building External Coalitions Results in Internal Success

John O'Conner has been successful as CEO of Urbanwide Health Plan largely because of the external base of influence that he has developed. To ensure that his Atlanta-based company provides cutting-edge insurance products in his market, O'Conner realized that he must take specific steps to find out how other businesses are run, develop a broader knowledge of political behaviors within organizations, and establish coalitions of external stakeholders. He became involved with the Atlanta Chamber of Commerce, and as a result of informal ties to local executives, was asked to join a number of boards of directors. He was elected president of the local Trade Association of Health Insurance Executives and later served as an officer in the national association of the same organization. He testified frequently before Congress on matters of health insurance and writes guest columns in several widely read health and business periodicals. These and similar activities have enabled O'Conner to become a more effective manager by positioning him to scan the external environment for both opportunities and threats that might affect Urbanwide and provide him with tremendous informational authority and leverage among potential purchasers of his firm's products. Although some of his vice presidents joke that he is rarely around the office, they all acknowledge that his wide array of activities conducted outside the formal chain of command of Urbanwide are what maintains the firm's leadership position in its market.

likely to have important economic consequences for the departments involved as well as for individual physicians. Moreover, the major disagreements described are in new areas of activity in which performance is difficult to assess due to the lag time involved in developing medical standards, including appropriate certification and credentialing requirements for innovative diagnostic and therapeutic procedures. The situation is also characterized by disagreements regarding which specialties are more competent to perform specific procedures and who should have priority in scheduling patients and accessing equipment and support staff. In addition, there are uncertainties regarding future demand for the new technologies and the likely impact of increased competition in the market area. These circumstances in combination are highly likely to stimulate attempts to influence decisions and events through the exercise of political power.

The conditions described above are created by **interdependencies** among organizational members or units. Interdependence exists whenever one actor does not entirely control all the conditions necessary for the achievement of an action or for obtaining the outcomes desired from the action. When interdependence exists, our ability to get things done requires us to develop power and the capacity to influence those on whom we depend (Pfeffer, 1981, 1992). The development and use of power is particularly important when the people or groups with whom we are interdependent differ in their point of view from ours and thus cannot be relied upon to do what we would want. Even where there is clear agreement on these goals, different perspectives have a way of presenting problems.

Given the complex and interdependent nature of patient care activity, there is often a high need for interdepartmental coordination. Further, there tends to be higher degrees of interdependence at higher levels of the organization, where tasks are less likely to be either simple or self-contained (e.g., strategic planning, restructuring).

It is important to note, however, that *very* high degrees of interdependence do not promote political activity because failure to cooperate under such conditions would assuredly mean the demise of the organization or the organizational unit. For example, very little political maneuvering occurs in the operating room or in intensive care units where interdependence is extremely high and where strong incentives to work together and coordinate activities are tantamount to organizational success. Taking the opposite perspective, we would expect power and political activity to be relatively low in those organizational settings that are characterized by simple or self-contained tasks (Hinings, Hickson, Pennings, & Schneck, 1974). In the hospital setting, for example, housekeeping and security might be examples of functional units that reflect a low degree of interdependence and, thus, limited political activity.

The degree of interdependence in organizations is, in part, determined by the amount of resources available to the organization (Pfeffer & Salancik, 1978). Slack resources reduce interdependence, while scarcity increases it. When resources are plentiful, individual and departmental interests are more easily satisfied (Pfeffer, 1992). Organizational members and units tend to depend less on each other for the achievement of their personal or subunit interests, and thus interdependence is decreased. However, when resources are scarce, interdependencies are increased. The allocation of scarce resources means that some organizational units will benefit while others will lose.

These ideas are easy to illustrate with respect to medical staff turf battles. For example, conflict can be decreased and the resulting political activity dampened if resources are plentiful enough to decrease departmental interdependence by providing duplicate equipment, space, and support staff.

Bloom (1991) describes a hospital where an intense dispute arose between radiologists and cardiologists regarding the most effective size for the lens on an image intensifier—a piece of equipment used during catheterizations and angiographies. Although both groups of specialists performed the

same procedures and used the same type of equipment, the radiologists preferred a 14-inch lens, while the cardiologists had a strong preference for a 9-inch lens. To satisfy both groups, hospital management purchased image intensifiers with lenses of each size and established separate catheterization and angiography laboratories with their own distinct support staffs. If patient volumes and financial resources are not adequate to support such duplication, however, it is likely that conflicts of this type will be resolved through the political process.

Interdependence as a catalyst for the use of power and politics in organizations is only applicable if the players in the interdependent situation possess different points of view. If everyone has the same goals and shares the same assumptions about how to achieve those goals, there will be minimal conflict and thus little room for power and influence. Such differences in points of view are more likely to emerge where there is a higher degree of task specialization or differentiation in the organization (Hinings et al., 1974). Simply put, when work is divided into different backgrounds and training, which will cause workers to take different views of similar situations. Table 9.1, for example, illustrates some of the fundamental differences in orientations between managers and physicians that may promote different perspectives on organizational goals, "best practices," and legitimate authority. These are graphically illustrated in the different points of view expressed by Dr. Watts and Mr. Baron (see In Practice, p. 286).

It is important to note that, even if the above conditions are met, power and influence should not be used indiscriminately. Because power is a valuable and finite resource, it is typically conserved for important issues. Thus, power is more likely to be exerted in situations involving major capital outlays, budget allocations, or strategic change as opposed to decisions on dress codes or changes in reporting forms. However, even minor decisions can sometimes hold significant symbolic importance in their ability to convey the appearance of power. For example, decisions regarding the relative location of the offices or parking spaces of the vice president for planning and marketing and the vice president for finance may be bitterly disputed since locations are often symbolic of an individual's or department's power within the organization (Edelman, 1964).

ISSUES ON WHICH POWER IS LIKELY TO BE USED

There are four main domains of activity that tend to be linked most strongly with the use of power and politics in organizations. These are structural change, interdepartmental coordination, management succession, and resource allocation and budgeting. Structural change is important because it potentially reallocates formal authority on the organizational chart. If, for example, a hospital is considering shifting from a functional to a divisional design, change in responsibility and tasks attendant to such design changes will also affect the underlying power base of various departments and individuals within the organization. Because of the potential effect on increasing and decreasing power among certain groups or individuals, political activity is often needed to initiate and implement such a change (Eisenhardt & Bourgeois, 1988).

Because formal rules, policies, and procedures with respect to conducting tasks are often department-specific, there are a few rules to guide the way in which departments should coordinate with one another. Perhaps more important, coordination often has implications for the responsibility and prerogatives of departments involved in a particular task. Hence, it is often the case that political processes and influence help define respective authority and task boundaries (Morgan, 1986). For instance, in some institutions medical staff turf battles have resulted in the clear delineation of practice domains. To cite one example, it may be determined that radiology should have the authority to control cardiac catheterization laboratories with their associated technology, technicians, and policies, while other

specialists may request use of the facilities. In many health care organizations today, there is a great deal of instability in the ranks of mid-level and top-level management. Whether succession involves hiring new executives, promoting individuals from within, or transferring management to other units within a hospital or multi-institutional system, such changes may bring with them considerable change in the power structure of an organization. A new manager often brings a new set of alliances or values that can upset existing alliances and working relationships, as well as previous agreements among organizational personnel. From another perspective, managerial hiring or promotion can be used as a strategy to enhance one's political position if the new manager has allegiances or values consistent with those of particular coalitions in the organization (Pfeffer, 1981, 1992). Politically based promotions are often apparent when "unobvious" choices are picked for advancement. This means that the candidate may be chosen for promotion not based on her skills, expertise, or experience but on her loyalty or similarity to the dominant political coalition in the organization.

On the surface, resource allocation should be made on the basis of rational considerations such as allocating funds to those activities or units most central to the achievement of key organizational or strategic goals. However, the value of resources within organizations is so high that survival of various individuals and departments often depends on obtaining adequate resources. Resource allocation and budgeting become, in effect, the battlegrounds over which organizational priorities are debated (Davis, Dempster, & Wildavsky, 1966). The allocation of resources, the budgeting process, and political influence in setting the organization's agendas are inextricably interrelated. Such political action becomes particularly important in periods of resource decline. If resources are plentiful, all departments potentially receive an allocation that permits them to pursue their own goals and interests. However, as the pie gets smaller, a zero-sum game mentality sets in such that resources allocated to one department are viewed as resources denied another. As illustrated in the next section, this sets the stage for considerable political activity within organizations (Hills & Mahoney, 1978).

POWER STRATEGIES AND TACTICS: GAMES PEOPLE PLAY

Power may be converted into political influence within the organization. The exercise of such influence is often described as a set of "games," each with its own structure and rules that are played outside the legitimate system of authority (Allen, Madison, Porter, Renwick, & Mayes, 1979; Maccoby, 1976; Mintzberg, 1983). The most common **political games** and the reasons they are played are listed in Table 9.3.

The insurgency games are usually played to resist authority, or as a means to affect or prevent change in the organization. Frequently they are played at the point in the authority hierarchy where decisions are implemented. They may be played by lower-level participants who attempt to circumvent, sabotage, or manipulate elements of the authority system and are often played by managers who distort or limit the amount of information sent to superiors in the authority structure. They can be played subtly by individuals or small groups or aggressively by a large number of participants willing to take unified visible action.

The insurgency games are sometimes met by attempting to increase authority (i.e., by tightening personnel and bureaucratic controls and by administering sanctions). They may also be countered in a retrospective or perspective fashion by the counterinsurgency games. The most frequent are limiting the amount of information available to subordinates, fostering competition among subordinates to maintain control, and various forms of cooptation.

A variety of political games are played to build power bases. Sponsorship games have simple rules:

Table 9.3. Political Games

Games to resist authority	Insurance games
Games to counter the resistance to authority	Counterinsurgency games
Games to build power bases	Sponsorship games (with superiors)
	Alliance-building games (with peers)
	Empire-building games (with subordinates)
	Budgeting games (with resources)
	Expertise games (with knowledge and skills)
	Lording games (with authority)
Games to defeat rivals	Line vs. staff games Rival camp games
Games to effect organizational change	Strategic candidates games
	Whistle-blowing games Young Turks games

SOURCE: Adapted from Henry Mintzberg, *Power in and Around Organizations*, copyright © 1983, p. 188. Reprinted by permission of Prentice-Hall, Inc., Englewood Cliffs, New Jersey.

The individual attaches himself to a rising star—or already one in place—and professes loyalty in return for a piece of the action. The alliance-building game is played by individuals or groups who negotiate with their peers' implicit contracts of support for each other. The empire-building game is played by individuals to enlarge their power base by collecting subunits or loyal subordinates. In her study, *Men and Women of the Corporation*, Kanter (1977) found that individuals who wanted to have significant influence on the organization had to play at least one of these three games: "people without sponsors, without peer connections, or without promising subordinates remained in the situation of bureaucratic dependency."

Budgeting games are used to acquire more resources for the positions or units the individual already has under his or her control. They are the best known of the political games, probably because they are the most visible and have the most well-defined rules. With respect to operating budgets, a variety of strategies are used to gain the largest possible allocation (e.g., always requesting more than required in the knowledge that a given percentage will be cut in the final negotiations). In the case of capital budgets, methods are typically found to underestimate costs and overestimate benefits (Table 9.4).

Professionals may play a variety of games in which their expertise is exploited as a political means of influence. These games are played offensively by emphasizing the uniqueness and importance of their skills and knowledge and defensively by both limiting the access of others to their expertise and discouraging attempts on the part of managers and others to rationalize or routinize it (i.e., to disaggregate it into easily learned steps). The lording games involve the utilization of legitimate authority or certified expertise for illegitimate, usually personal reasons.

Games to defeat rivals, such as the line vs. staff or rival camp games, are zero-sum struggles for control over organizational resources, decisions, and/or activities by weakening or sometimes eliminating competitors.

The strategic candidates game is the most common of the games played to effect organizational change. An individual or group seeks a strategic change by promoting through the legitimate systems of influence its own project, proposal, or person as a "strategic candidate." The decision-making process involving strategic decisions often is relatively unstructured, thus encouraging political influence attempts. Furthermore, power within the organization is frequently redistributed during periods of strategic change, usually in favor of those who initially proposed and fought for it. Although strategic candidates in this game are promoted through the legitimate channels of influence, it is important to note that they are supported, at least

in part, for nonlegitimate reasons (e.g., in order to defeat rivals or to facilitate empire building).

The whistle-blowing game is usually played by an individual at a relatively low level in the hierarchy of authority who questions the legitimacy of actions by superiors and appeals to powerful individuals outside the organization for support. In the young Turks game, a small group, often with a significant power base, uses political means in attempts to affect fundamental changes in the organization's mission or in the systems of authority, expertise, or ideology. For example, in one religiously sponsored multi-institutional system, a group of newly hired MBA graduates working at the corporate level engaged in a campaign to shift the emphasis of the system toward a bottom-line orientation and away from a traditional, mission-driven orientation.

Most health care organizations must coordinate the activities of a diverse group of highly trained professionals. The traditional system of formal authority tends to be relatively weak in these organizations. Specifically, there is often ambiguity in how to operationalize or prioritize organizational goals, particularly with respect to the curing, caring, and rehabilitation functions of health services organizations. In addition, because of the difficulties involved in measuring outcomes of professional performance, when goals are imposed on professionals by a managerial hierarchy, they are often easy to deflect. Second, among highly trained professionals, identification with a discipline and professional society may well be stronger than with the organization. When many types of professionals are present, intergroup conflict is likely as factions develop along lines of varying professional interests, orientations to patient care, or status distinctions among such groups. Third, highly skilled professionals have a tendency to invert means and ends—to focus on maintenance and further development of their own skills rather than broader organizational objectives. Further, although the skills themselves may be well defined, the situations to which they may be most appropriately applied often are not. As the opening case illustrates, this situation may lead to territorial

Table 9.4. Budgeting Games

Strategy	Description
Games to Obtain Funding for New Programs or Equipment	
Foot in the Door	Initially request funding for a modest program. Conceal its actual magnitude until it has gotten underway and built a vocal constituency.
Keeping Up With the Joneses	Base the budget request for new program funding on the rationale the Joneses that the organization must stay abreast of the competition (whether or not there is a demonstrated need for the new program.)
Keeping Up to Date	The rationale is based on the argument that the organization must be a leader and therefore must adopt the latest technology. An actual "Jones" need not be found or cited.
Call It a Rose	Utilize appealing (but misleading) labels. A classic example is the strategy used to obtain additional space by the National Institutes of Health in the early 1960's. During this time period it was impossible to obtain budget approval for new building construction, but it was possible to get funding to build "annexes." It is probably not surprising that at least one "annex" is more than double the size of the original building.
Games to Maintain Programs at Their Current Levels and to Resist Budget Cuts	
Sprinkling	Increase budget estimates by only a few percent, either across-the-board or in areas difficult to detect. Frequently this is done in anticipation that arbitrary cuts will be made. The goal is to attain a final budget allocation that is at the level it would have been without "sprinkling" or arbitrary reductions.
Create a Public Outcry	When budget reductions are ordered, decrease or eliminate a popular program in an effort to elicit client support and divert attention away from less popular program areas where cuts might indeed be feasible. A common example is the reduction of firefighter and police force positions that big city mayors often make when asked to reduce their budgets. The action is often taken in an effort to elicit popular support for budget restorations.
Witches and Goblins	Make the assertion that, if the budget request is not approved, dire consequences will follow. Appeals are based on emotion, not evidence.
We Are the Experts	Assert that the proposed budget must be approved because it reflects expert knowledge that "mere managers" cannot hope to understand. This strategy is frequently used by professional types, including scientists, military officers, professors, and physicians.

SOURCE: Adapted from Robert Anthony and Regina Herzlinger, *Management Control in Nonprofit Organizations.* 3rd ed. (Irwin, 1980), pp. 344–353.

disputes over patients, clients, and activities among different disciplines and specialties within health services organizations. Finally, professionals traditionally have been expected to give the highest priority to the needs of their own individual patients or clients—an expectation likely to generate conflicts both with other professionals serving as patient or client advocates and with managers espousing organization-wide objectives. This combination of weak formal authority and highly developed systems of expertise creates strong catalysts for the use of politics as a means for achieving organizational goals or implementing major decisions.

The ambiguities and conflicts generated by strong expertise and weak authority systems are most likely to give rise to those political games in which peers compete with each other for the allocation of resources. Alliance and empire building, budgeting, rival camps, and strategic candidates games tend to be particularly important. It is also important for managers to note that they can often exercise considerable influence in health services organizations not by relying on the formal system of authority but by their centrality in the organization and a willingness to engage in the political process. When conflict resolution emerges as a critical organizational function, managers may attain influence commensurate with their skills in mediation and negotiation.

EMPLOYEE RESPONSES TO THE USE OF POWER

To this point, the chapter has outlined ways in which managers can acquire and use power and politics to advance legitimate organizational goals. However, it is also important to understand and anticipate the responses of employees to the use of power by managers. Power involves individuals exerting their will over others in the making and implementing of decisions. Employees may react negatively to the use of power. These reactions may include decreased trust in the organization, increased employee dissatisfaction, increased conflict within the organization, decreased morale and effort by line employees, and increased employee turnover.

By creating this negative fallout, power use may undermine future operations and decision making. In this way, the responses of employees to the use of power must be prioritized and addressed by managers.

Maintaining employee trust is an important goal for managers in limiting potential negative fallout within the organization from the use of power. High levels of trust serve as psychological buffers for employees, allowing them to accept that power must be used and yet believe that its use involves functional and ethical actions by managers. Low levels of trust within the organization make any instance of power use by managers risky. The presence of trust within an organization among employees towards management means that when power is used, employees have positive expectations about why it is being used, and the outcomes that will derive from it. When trust is not present, employees may perceive that the use of power has only negative or secretive aspects associated with it. Over time, these expectations can translate into overt responses such as decreased job satisfaction and morale.

Managers can build a work environment facilitating trust in several ways. First, rewards and incentive systems can be aligned for managers and employees, so that employees understand that any use of power affects both groups similarly (Whitener, Brodt, Korsgaard, & Werner, 1998). Formal training programs around how to build and maintain trust can be implemented within the organization (Caudron, 1996). Creating work processes that involve high levels of interdependency increases the degree to which individuals must rely upon each other in the organization. This mutual reliance fosters trusting relationships. Establishing reward systems for lower-level employee feedback around poor performance or quality improvement also enhances trust, making employees believe that their voice is valued by management (Hoff, 2003).

THE ABUSE OF POWER IN ORGANIZATIONS

It is important for managers to view the use of power as necessary at times for their organization in helping to achieve its goals in an efficient manner. Managers should, however, balance this functional view of power with a more critical perspective that views the use of power as potentially abusive to the organization's employees (Hardy & Clegg, 1996).

Power abuses occur within organizations for two main reasons: to achieve personal or organizational goals. An example of a power abuse used to pursue personal goals could involve a chief executive officer creating a board of directors consisting solely of friends or business partners, who yield to the CEO's insistence that they misrepresent financial and performance data to outside stakeholders, thereby enabling the CEO to earn incentive bonuses. Power can also be abused to advance organizational goals. This form of power abuse is not easy to discern, nor do all groups within the organization necessarily agree that abusing power to achieve organizational ends in a given situation has negative consequences. In fact, such abuse may be sanctioned by numerous stakeholders both within and external to the organization. An example of a power abuse motivated by the pursuit of organizational goals is laying off employees to reduce costs without attending to the fundamental organizational problems or bad management decisions causing poor performance.

Regardless of the ends pursued, the abuse of power by managers elevates the potential for negative fallout to occur in the organization. Perhaps most important is the crisis of trust that can occur when managers or executives abuse power. This trust crisis is expressed in two primary ways: (a) loss of faith by customers and external stakeholders (e.g., regulators, shareholders, funders) in the organization, and (b) loss of faith by employees

towards management. Both crises have recently gained center stage in light of corporate scandals in health care and other industries. Loss of faith by customers and other external stakeholders can meaningfully affect organizational performance and survival, in the form of lost business for the organization, reduced financial capital, stricter regulatory scrutiny, and the development of a negative reputation that allows other competitors to gain a long-term edge over the organization (Fukuyama, 1995; Miles & Snow 1992; Sitkin & Stickel, 1996).

Loss of trust by employees towards managers when power is abused reduces the potential for positive dynamics within the organization that enhance performance. Examples of positive dynamics negatively affected by power abuse include teamwork, cooperative behavior, communication quality, citizenship behavior, and job satisfaction (Axelrod, 1984; Blau, 1964; Hoff, 2003; Whitener et al., 1998). Other negative fallout that may occur includes increased organizational complacency, decreased work effort or "shirking" on the part of employees, slower organizational adaptation to change, and decreased quality of services or products (Burawoy, 1979). While not a certainty, the abuse of power can seriously impact organizational performance, lead to lost business, and in some cases facilitate collapse in the form of bankruptcy or dissolution.

Several conditions facilitate the abuse of power within organizations. These include high information ambiguity within the organization, high ends-means ambiguities, an overly centralized decision-making structure, the scarcity of rival coalitions both internal and external to the organization, low or one-sided interdependencies between key organizational stakeholders, an existing culture of organizational complacency, and short time horizons for decision making within the organization (Brass, Burkhardt, & Marlene, 1993; Crozier, 1964; Kotter, 1979; Mintzberg, 1983; Perrow, 1989; Weber, 1978). Ironically, the conditions that create the potential for power abuse derive in large part from the same general conditions that give rise to power use. This highlights the paradoxical nature of power within organizations, in that the factors that allow power to grow and be used effectively are also those that, when manipulated in certain ways or taken to extremes, provide fertile conditions for power to be abused. Given this reality, a key managerial task is to institutionalize a structural framework and culture within the organization, which limits the probability that power use conditions are manipulated.

For example, the ability to create dependencies in relationships is a potential source of organizational power within organizations. However, too much of an imbalance in terms of the extent to which a dependency relationship favors one group over another creates the potential for power abuse (Brass et al., 1993). As discussed, individuals who have access to resources create dependencies for others and the organization as a whole, both of which must rely on those controlling the resources to function properly (Blau, 1964). This situation is exacerbated when the resources in question are scarce, essential, and non-substitutable. Thus, for example, private practice surgeons who bring patients to a particular hospital to perform their surgeries, or who perform surgeries for hospital patients, create dependencies in the form of the hospital and its employee staff, relying upon both the surgeons' patient business and their skills for existing patients to generate revenue and preserve jobs. This is especially true if the amount of surgery business is a significant portion of hospital revenue, and the surgical services provided cannot be found with abundance in the community.

In this situation, there is high potential for power abuse on the part of the surgeons. For instance, facing their own business challenges or simply desiring to grow profit, these surgeons may leverage their resource control in such a way as to negotiate more favorable reimbursement terms for their services that negatively affect the hospital's ability to provide other services. They may be less willing to compromise their demands because of their greater bargaining power vis-à-vis the hospital. In addition, their desire to be autonomous may tempt them to use their resource control to apply greater pressure on the hospital to overlook instances of poorer

quality or efficiency in the provision of their services, for example, by threatening to move their business elsewhere. They may also refuse to subscribe to hospital norms and rules around outcomes like quality and patient satisfaction. This, in turn, could negatively affect the morale of other hospital employees, hinder teamwork and cooperation in the operating room environment, and cause other surgeons and physicians to question the validity of these norms and rules, making management more difficult.

Control over information is another legitimate source of organizational power that, when taken to extremes, often results in power abuse. Individuals who position themselves at the center of communication and information networks within the organization are in a position to exercise power. Information is a resource that allows individuals to set decision-making premises within the organization and control uncertainty (Crozier, 1964; Perrow, 1989). However, to the extent managers or others within the organization gain exclusive control over information (i.e., to the extent that specific individuals or groups can create gaps or ambiguities in understanding within the organization), a foundation for power abuse is created. This source of power abuse is evident with respect to recent scandals involving chief executive officers and their staff who were selective regarding the types of financial and performance data presented to employees, boards of directors, and auditors, mainly to cover up poor performance or pursue personal ends.

The building of coalitions and alliances is a source of organizational power. However, an organizational environment in which there is a single dominant coalition or alliance provides a foundation for power abuse. Any leader-centered coalition that does not adhere to a diversity of viewpoints and perspectives can create an autocratic situation in which the leader's will and preferences become those of the larger group (Mintzberg, 1983). This leads to negative outcomes such as groupthink (Janis, 1989). The absence of rival coalitions within the organization creates a situation for power abuse, mainly by lessening the capacity for creative tension and ideas to compete with each other on the basis of their informational, logical, and strategic merits. This decreased capacity encourages the dominant coalition to introduce mechanisms by which to minimize deviation from the preferred status quo (Salancik & Pfeffer, 1977). This may hurt the organization in terms of performance and ability to adapt to changing demands in the environment.

Nowhere is this dynamic seen more clearly than in the case where a chief executive officer builds a power base for her influence over time by creating a board of directors consisting of close friends, business partners, or individuals who share a similar viewpoint. Taken to the extreme, these types of boards become "rubber stamps" that often fail to carry out their fiduciary responsibility as counterbalances to executive control within the organization. They also reduce the quality of strategic decision making because they abdicate their role as the critiquers of management decisions. In the final analysis, this allows executives to make decisions that potentially benefit their own ends at the expense of customer, employee, or shareholder ends. The case of HealthSouth fits this profile, as the existing board under the leadership of the founder and CEO consisted in part of individuals who had either personal or business reasons for not questioning executive decisions. One director co-owned a venture capital fund in which the CEO invested hundreds of thousands of dollars ("Board Walks," 2003). Another director's company supplied millions of dollars of commercial glass to a Health-South hospital, despite being the high bidder for the contract ("Board Walks," 2003). And a third director personally invested in a company set up by HealthSouth ("Two HealthSouth Directors," 2003). Although HealthSouth is not the only example of compromised boards of directors, it did, in this case, lead to serious power abuses that went unchecked and undiscovered for some time.

Managers can take several steps to guard against the abuse of power within their organizations. These steps include structuring communication networks to create greater transparency in terms of or-

ganizational decision making, implementation, and evaluation, using boards of directors and advisory groups as counterbalances to managerial authority, creating a strong code of ethics within the organization, designing appropriate appraisal systems, and emphasizing personal integrity in the hiring function (Alford, 2001; Hoff, 2003; Kotter, 1979, Thibodeaux and Powell, 1985; Westheafer, 2000).

Creating transparency involves making information a "**public good**" within organizations. This means, for example, allowing access to performance data at all levels of the organization, so that everyone from line employees to the chief executive appreciates the logic by which specific decisions are made. In establishing greater internal transparency, managers end up becoming more accessible to employees. This enhances trust within the organization, and while it does not preclude the use of power as a necessary dynamic, it is likely to identify instances of abuse in a timely manner. External transparency also limits power abuse. Providing key constituents such as shareholders, regulators, and customers with complete, accurate, and timely performance data prevents executives and boards of directors from making decisions that are not rooted in strategic logic but instead derive more from the manipulation of circumstances on the part of individuals or groups in the organization.

Many recent corporate scandals that involved managerial abuse of power could have been prevented through the use of independent oversight mechanisms in the form of boards of directors and external auditors. Many boards are laden with members who are connected to the organization in some manner that makes them reluctant to enact their oversight role. Such characteristics make boards less useful for controlling power abuse in organizations. Organizations that staff boards of directors with individuals who: (a) have the time to fulfill the oversight role and (b) have no personal stake involved in the results of that oversight place themselves in the best position to allow the use but not abuse of power by managers.

Creating a strong code of ethics and institutionalizing it into the organization's culture also limits power abuse (Hatcher, 2002). Recent examples of power abuses within organizations have been found to result in part from the presence of work environments that tolerated and even promoted unethical (not necessarily illegal) behavior in relation to the use of power. Establishing a **code of ethics** gives managers and employees formal guidance about how to act across different situations where power may be exercised. This limits individual discretion in using power. It also conveys a sense that there are risks or potential sanctions to using power in an abusive way (Thibodeaux & Powell, 1985). Key to the success of a code of ethics is the overt dedication of top management to it.

Designing performance appraisal and hiring systems that emphasize and reward ethical behavior also limits the potential for power abuse within organizations. For example, power abuse by managers towards employees through the use of formal position in the hierarchy is minimized when appraisal systems exist that judge employee performance across a range of objective performance dimensions. Considering personal values and ethical behavior as important factors in the hiring and evaluation of managers and employees heightens the probability that the organizational workforce consists of individuals who are less likely to take advantage of any power at their disposal. Over time, it creates an organizational culture in which a negative view towards power abuse becomes a shared norm. The creation of such a culture is shown in the process of moving to a service line structure in a VA health facility (see In Practice, p. 302).

POWER, POLITICS, AND ORGANIZATIONAL PERFORMANCE

This chapter began with the claim that many managers view the use of power and politics in their organizations as dysfunctional for the attainment of organizational goals and positive organizational performance. Recent writings, in contrast, have maintained that the use of power and politics in organizational settings can serve to facilitate the implementation of important decisions in these organizations. In all likelihood, the truth probably lies somewhere between these two extremes. There is no doubt that influence attempts can be expensive and time-consuming. Engaging in political activity, for example, may dissipate the energies and focus of management in health care organizations, restrict the flow of important information to decision makers, and distort perceptions about the opinions of others in the decision-making process. Managers of successful health services organizations who desire to reduce inefficiencies stemming from political activity in their organizations might choose several approaches.

- If possible, increase the level of slack resources in their organizations to reduce conflict and to allow subunits to attain their own goals.
- Reduce differentiation and heterogeneity among organizational members and units so as to promote consensus in organizational goals, common views of means to achieve these goals, and a common culture to bind organizational members together.
- Divide organizational rewards more evenly so that nothing substantial is to be gained from attempts at political influence.

Such strategies for reducing the level of influence and politics in organizations are also appropriate for managers who simply do not feel comfortable or have the skills associated with using power in organizational settings.

However, in the current health care environment, few organizations can be successful without adapting, often in significant ways, to the changing demands imposed by stakeholders, regulators, or competitors. In situations where major changes in strategy, technology, approach to the market, and management of the workforce are required, power and influence processes may be useful and even necessary to achieve such transformations. Over time, power may become

IN PRACTICE

Managing to Succeed and Not Abuse Power in the Upstate New York Veterans Health System

In the late 1990s, the Veterans Health System faced a crisis that threatened its very existence. Calls to privatize the health care system for veterans in the United States, negative publicity in the media about the care received by veteran patients, stagnant funding, and increased congressional oversight were environmental factors that coalesced to threaten the organization's existence as a public sector agency. As one of 22 health care delivery networks in the country, the Upstate New York Veterans Health System (VHS) needed to improve quality of care, become more efficient, redefine its customer base, and shift its strategic focus to new forms of care in order to survive. The major decision Upstate New York VHS leadership made was to move to a service-line structure for care delivery. This structure organized services according to specific products or outputs (e.g., mental health, medicine, geriatrics) rather than by the functions or inputs that combined to produce those services (e.g., nurses, psychologists, physicians), and the geographic locations in which those services were delivered (i.e., hospitals in different parts of Upstate New York).

In particular, the rapid move to the service-line structure, the need for immediate change in organizational outcomes, a centralized decision-making hierarchy within the service line, high levels of complacency among a demoralized VA provider staff, and high uncertainty and ambiguity regarding how to achieve improved service outcomes within the new structure created the potential for power abuse by top management within each of the four clinical service lines established in the new structure. For one of the service lines focused on mental health, the Behavioral Health Service Line (BHSL), this abuse did not materialize. Instead,

BHSL leadership took specific actions to make sure the potential for managerial abuse of power was minimized.

To offset the negative effects of a centralized decision-making structure, service-line leadership created a parallel decision-making structure comprised of frontline providers and staff. This parallel structure, manifested in the form of "network groups," was given formal responsibility for examining strategic issues such as new program growth within the service line, as well as evaluating the implementation of management decisions across various programs. Their job was to help critique how major strategic decisions played out in the organization. In this way, the network groups provided one form of check on management discretion, while also getting individuals closest to the point of production involved in decision making. Service-line management also delegated a large amount of responsibility to frontline workers in mental health programs for implementing strategic initiatives. To facilitate this involvement, a formal "Goalsharing" incentive program was created within the Veterans Health System. This program allowed workers to develop their own performance goals and then be financially rewarded for meeting those goals. This program was intended to also get employees to feel more appreciated for having to respond to stakeholder demands quickly, without feeling that they were not being consulted.

By delegating much of the responsibility for program implementation down to the frontline workers, service-line management was ceding control over the operational details of new initiatives, thus minimizing their potential ability to abuse the power given to them in running the

BHSL. By doing this, service-line managers acknowledged ambiguity to employees around the program's means (ambiguity being a precondition for power abuse), but encouraged employees to be the ones to solve that ambiguity. For example, one new initiative involving the integration of mental health services into the network's primary care clinics was almost completely implemented using ideas generated by frontline mental health provider staff that volunteered to staff the primary care clinics. Service-line leadership took full responsibility over defining the types of outcomes each program and new initiative must achieve, but they stopped short of micromanaging the pursuit of those outcomes. They were also trying to raise the level of job satisfaction and morale, to create a more favorable work environment for employees.

Finally, service-line leadership involved all levels of the organization in performance monitoring. Mandated to meet a number of formal quality outcomes, the BHSL made those outcomes known to all, built evaluation systems that relied upon front-line input made performance data a "real-time" resource available to everyone in the organization simultaneously, and delegated responsibility for investigating and solving performance deficiencies to the programs themselves. In this way, service-line leadership sent a signal to frontline employees that they were to be privy to all the information management had in making their decisions. In this way, there would be no confusion or uncertainty (and thus, no potential for managers to abuse power) regarding where the service line was in successfully making the needed changes in service delivery. If success was achieved, then everyone would know about it at the same time, and frontline workers could take the credit for it as well as leadership.

The actions taken by service-line management to limit power abuse have not undermined success of the new service-line structure. The number of total patients served by the network as a whole increased over 40% between 1996 and 2000. Since the move to care lines in 1997, the network has led all other networks in terms of overall customer satisfaction. Cost per patient in the network decreased 40% between 1996 and 2000, and its $197 cost per outpatient in 2000 was the lowest nationally. As a subset of the network's overall performance in various quality arenas, the Behavioral Health Service Line's achievements are particularly noteworthy. It has been the national leader on several key performance measures, the overall level of employee satisfaction and the degree of efficiency in providing services. The network was the first to receive National Committee for Quality Assurance accreditation, and has recently received the Robert Carey Award for excellence in quality achievement. This award is given annually to only one organization within the Veterans Administration.

institutionalized in health services organizations (i.e., imbedded strongly in certain individuals, occupational groups, or departments). This is likely to result in a situation characterized by status quo orientation and inertia. Those in power will strive to keep that power by advocating positions that maintain the structures, strategies, and activities that brought them to power in the first place. As illustrated below, change and adaptation typically come only after great internal political struggle (see Debate Time 9.1). Thus, to effect change that will ultimately benefit the organization, managers must be prepared to utilize power in a fashion to overcome inertia, resolve turf battles, and channel the diverse interests of organizational members and stakeholders.

DEBATE TIME 9.1   What Do You Think?

Trauma services in Maryland are coordinated by the state's Institute of Emergency Medical Services, a broad network that included the State Shock-Trauma Center, other trauma centers strategically located in hospitals across the state, and the ambulance and helicopter personnel who transport patients. Since its founding a quarter of a century ago, the 130-bed shock-trauma facility has been reserved for the most critical trauma patients, many of whom are flown in from all regions of the state with life-threatening injuries due to auto accidents. The Shock-Trauma Center also performs medical triage for the statewide Emergency Medical Services (EMS) system.

For some years the Shock-Trauma Center shared facilities with the state's major University Hospital. Although they were both governed by the same not-for-profit corporation, the Shock-Trauma Center operated with considerable autonomy. In 1984 the state granted approval for a new $35 million separate facility for the Shock-Trauma Center. Part of the agreement included the decision to transfer all trauma care provided in the University Hospital Emergency Department, including patients with knife and gunshot wounds, to the Shock-Trauma Center, which would be located only a few blocks away. The rationale for this decision was to conserve resources by not duplicating trauma care personnel and equipment.

Although the move to the new building was completed in 1989, Shock-Trauma physicians resisted treating a category of patients that they perceived as diluting the center's main mission. In 1992 a new director for the Shock-Trauma Center was hired by the not-for-profit corporation that governed both that facility and the University Hospital. The Shock-Trauma Center was ordered by top managers of the corporation to begin treating

all trauma injuries that would in the past have been seen in the University Hospital Emergency Department. Three prominent Shock-Trauma physicians who resisted these changes were fired. At a well-attended news conference defending these changes, the new director, Dr. Bradley, explained that in an era of dwindling resources and soaring health care costs, it was important to end duplication and to move the Shock-Trauma Center into a closer collaboration with the adjacent university medical center.

Since the initial organization of the state's EMS system, the Shock-Trauma Center had assumed responsibility for medical triage, including directing the personnel transporting trauma victims to the most appropriate facility with available resources. The proposal to tighten the relationship between Shock-Trauma and University Hospital generated considerable concerns among other trauma system members regarding whether "patients would continue to be sent to where they could get the best treatment." Separate news conferences were called by a group of physicians representing other hospitals with trauma centers and by the state's volunteer firefighters responsible for the transport of trauma patients. The firefighters complained that they had not been consulted about recent changes in the EMS system. In addition, in separate statements to the press conflicting positions on these issues were adopted by the governor who supported the new Shock-Trauma director, and several key legislators who sided with the fired surgeons in their belief that broadening the center's focus would dilute its quality.

At this point in the conflict, the state's largest newspaper published an article comparing Dr. Bradley to the original founder of the Shock-Trauma Center, Dr. Gordon, who "was a one-man wrecking crew if someone got in his way." According to the newspaper, Dr. Gordon:

> . . . did not suffer fools or foes for very long. As he told colleagues, "Only a dog needs to be loved." The results, not his popularity, were all that mattered.
>
> And he succeeded brilliantly. Over the vehement opposition of other hospitals, jealous physicians, possessive bureaucrats and busy-body legislators, he carved out a new field of medicine— emergency medical services.
>
> Employing innovative techniques, he declared war on behalf of critically injured accident victims. By getting patients into the operating rooms in that first "golden hour," and by throwing teams of surgeons into the battle, he performed miracles. More often that not, he won the war. Thousands of lives were saved.
>
> Along the way, he collected enemies. It didn't faze him. He was smart enough to win the loyalty of a governor, key legislators, firefighters, and paramedics. Only when he was slowing down, when his own Shock-Trauma doctors turned against him in 1989 for creating "general chaos," did he step down. He died last fall.
>
> Now some of the same doctors are seeking another scalp: Dr. Bradley's. Their complaint is ironic: they don't want Shock-Trauma to change. Yet this is an institution created out of change—a dramatic rethinking of how to treat critically injured accident victims. Dr. Gordon's whole life at the Shock-Trauma Center was about change. He kept the place in constant turmoil.
>
> Time, especially in today's high-tech medical world, does not stand still. This is an era of severe government deficits, a time when the public is demanding accountability. Yet Shock-Trauma had been notorious for its lack of accountability and its free-spending ways. It insisted on total independence. That is now changing. Interdependence is the key word. And there is a strong effort to depoliticize what are essentially medical matters.
>
> Dr. Gordon was superb at getting what he wanted from the politicians and winning public acclaim. At this stage, Dr. Bradley lacks the political skills that served Dr. Gordon so well. The circus at Shock-Trauma is likely to continue. Dr. Bradley's foes will see to that. But, what the heck. As Dr. Gordon used to say, "You can tell the pioneers by the arrows in their backs."

Fortunately, most political conflict in organizations does not reach the level of intensity displayed in this example. It does provide a vivid illustration, however, of the types of conflicts that may be encountered in determining organizational goals, as well as the fragility of the balance of influence in many multi-institutional arrangements.

SOURCE: Adapted by permission from Barry Rascovar, "Shock and Trauma at the Shock-Trauma Center," *The Baltimore Sun,* August 9, 1992.

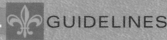

MANAGERIAL GUIDELINES

1. Recognize different sources of power. In the majority of health care organizations, power is derived from multiple sources—formal authority, control over critical resources, expertise, and to a lesser extent, individual charisma. Effective health care managers must be able to distinguish among different types of power, be sensitive to the source of their own power, and be careful to keep their actions consistent with others' expectations.

2. Use power selectively. Effective health care managers must understand the costs, risks, and benefits of using each type of power and must be able to recognize which to draw on in different situations and with different people.

3. Power and influence are not inexhaustible. Influence in health services organizations should be considered a finite rather than an unlimited resource. Managers should direct their influence attempts toward those issues of highest priority or where the greatest benefits are likely to result and be willing to defer in other areas.

4. Position yourself centrally in communications networks. The highly complex and professional nature of most health service organizations usually results in multiple power centers. Managers can often exercise considerable influence not by relying on the formal system of authority but rather by establishing themselves in a central position vis-à-vis other power holders and being willing to engage in the political process.

5. Use negotiation and mediation skills to control conflict. The diffuse power arrange-ments and multiple goals of health services organizations may lead to recurring conflicts among individuals and groups.

6. Develop power by controlling strategic contingencies and resources. Be aware of less visible but important power relations that occur outside the formal system of authority in organizations. Increase individual and departmental power by effectively dealing with strategic contingencies that face the organization.

7. Political behavior and conflict are normal aspects of organizational change. Regard political behavior and conflict as expected, normal aspects of organizational life. To be an effective agent for change, use power through building coalitions, cooperation of influential members of the organization or external stakeholder groups, and the control of decision-making premises.

8. Use politics under conditions of ambiguity and uncertainty. Employ principles of the rational model of organizations when goals are well defined and easily measured, when alternatives are clear, and when the relationship is unambiguous. When these conditions are not present, consider using the political process to achieve desired ends.

9. Power abuse can be avoided through organizational strategies. Managers can avoid situations of power abuse through development and maintenance of trust, mutual dependencies, information sharing, a code of ethics, and reward systems that emphasize ethical behavior. Managers should also establish multiple, diverse groups in the organization with authority to provide input into organizational strategy

DISCUSSION QUESTIONS

1. Using concepts from the chapter, can you identify the various political strategies used by Dr. Gordon and Dr. Bradley in Debate Time 9.1?

2. As illustrated in Debate Time 9.1, what are some of the functions and possible dysfunctions of using political strategies to effect change in organizations?

3. Do you agree that a strong effort should be made to "depoliticize what are essentially medical matters"?

4. Do you agree with Dr. Gordon's statement, "You can tell the pioneers by the arrows in their backs"? Is this type of outcome inevitable for change agents? (You may want to base your reasoning on concepts from this chapter and Chapter 12.)

REFERENCES

Alexander, J. A., Morrisey, M. A., & Shortell, S. M. (1986). The effects of competition, regulation and corporatization on hospital-physician relationships. *Journal Health and Social Behavior, 27,* 220–235.

Alford, C. F. (2001). *Broken lives and organizational power.* Ithaca, NY: Cornell University Press.

Allen, R. W., Madison, D. L., Porter, L. W., Renwick, P. A., & Mayes, B. T. (1979). Organizational politics: Tactics and characteristics of its actors. *California Management Review, 22,* 66–83.

Astley, W. G., & Sachdeva, P. S. (1984). Structural sources of intraorganizational power: A theoretical synthesis. *Academy of Management Review, 9,* 104–113.

Axelrod, R. (1984). *The evolution of cooperation.* New York: Basic Books.

Bennis, W., & Nanus, B. (1985). *Leaders: The strategies for taking charge.* New York: Harper and Row.

Blau, P. M. (1964). *Exchange and power in social life.* New York: John Wiley.

Bloom, S. L. (1991, Winter). Hospital turf battles: The manager's role. *Hospital and Health Services Administrations, 36*(4), 590–599.

Board walks: Five conflicted HealthSouth directors will resign. (2003, December 4). *The Birmingham News.*

Retrieved June 28, 2004, from LexisNexis Academic.

Brass, D. J. (1984). Being in the right place: A structural analysis of individual influence in an organization. *Administrative Science Quarterly, 29,* 518–539.

Brass, D. J., Burkhardt, M. E., & Marlene, E. (1993). Potential power and power use: An investigation of structure and behavior. *Academy of Management Journal, 36*(3), 441–471.

Buck, V. E. (1966). A model for viewing an organization as a system of constraints. In J. D. Thompson (Ed.), *Approaches to organizational design.* Pittsburgh, PA: University of Pittsburgh Press.

Burawoy, M. (1979). *Manufacturing consent.* Chicago: University of Chicago Press.

Burns, L. R., Andersen, R. M., & Shortell, S. M. (1989). The impact of corporate structures on physician inclusion and participation. *Medical Care, 27*(10), 967–982.

Caudron, S. (1996). Rebuilding employee trust. *Training and Development Journal, 50*(8), 19–21.

Cialdini, R. B. (1984). *Influence: Science and practice* (2nd ed.). Glenview, IL: Scott, Foresman.

Crozier, M. (1964). *The bureaucratic phenomenon.* Chicago: University of Chicago Press.

Cyert, R. M., & March, J. G. (1963). *A behavioral theory of the firm.* Englewood Cliffs, NJ: Prentice-Hall.

Daft, R. L. (2001). *Organization theory and design* (7th ed.) (pp. 440–462). Cincinnati, OH: South-Western College Publishing.

Dahl, R. (1957). The Concept of Power. *Behavioral Science,* July, 1957, 202–3.

Davenport, T. H., Eccles, R. G., & Prusak, L. (Fall, 1992). Information politics. *Sloan Management Review,* 53–65.

Davies, T. O., Hodges, C. L., & Rundall, T. G. (2003, March). Views of doctors and managers on the doctor-manager relationship in the NHS. *British Journal of Health Care Management, 326,* 626–628.

Davis, O. A., Dempster, M. A. H., & Wildavsky, A. (1966). A theory of the budgeting process. *American Political Science Review, 60,* 529–547.

Edelman, M. (1964). *The symbolic use of politics.* Urbana, IL: University of Illinois Press.

Eisenhardt, M., & Bourgeois, L. J. (1988). Politics of strategic decision making in high-velocity environments: Toward a midrange theory. *Academy of Management Journal, 31,* 737–770.

Fligstein, N. (1987). The intraorganizational power struggle: Rise of finance personnel to top leadership in large corporations, 1919–1979. *American Sociological Review, 52,* 44–58.

Fukuyama, F. (1995). *Trust: The social virtues and the creation of prosperity.* New York: Free Press.

Gamson, W. A. (1961). A theory of coalition formation. *American Sociological Review, 26*(3), 373–382.

Glandon, G. L., & Morrisey, M. A. (1986). Redefining the hospital-physician relationship under prospective payment. *Inquiry, 23,* 175–186.

Hackman, J. D. (1985). Power and centrality in the allocation of resources in colleges and universities. *Administrative Science Quarterly, 30,* 61–77.

Hannan, M. T., & Freeman, J. (1984). Structural inertia and organizational change. *American Sociological Review, 49,* 149–164.

Hardy, C., & Clegg, S. R. (1996). Some dare call it power. In S. Clegg, C. Hardy, & W. Nord (Eds.), *Handbook of organizational studies* (pp. 622–640). Thousand Oaks, CA: Sage Publications.

Hatcher, T. (2002). Ethics and HRD: A new approach to leading responsible organizations. Cambridge, MA: Persuns Publishing.

Hickson, D. J., Hinings, C. R., Lee, C. A., Schneck, R. E., & Penning J. M. (1971). A strategic contingencies theory of intraorganizational power. *Administrative Science Quarterly, 16,* 216–229.

Hills, F. S., & Mahoney, T. A. (1978). University budgets and organizational decision making. *Administrative Science Quarterly, 23,* 454–465.

Hinings, C. R., Hickson, D. J., Pennings, J. M., & Scheck, R. E. (1974). Structural conditions of intraorganizational power. *Administrative Science Quarterly, 19,* 22–44.

Hoff, T. J. (2003). *The power of frontline workers in transforming government: The Upstate New York Veterans Healthcare Network.* Washington, DC: IBM Endowment for the Business of Government.

Izraeli, D. N. (1975). The middle manager and the tactics of power expansion: A case study. *Sloan Management Review,* 57–70.

Jacobs, D. (1974). Dependency and vulnerability: An exchange approach to the control of organizations. *Administrative Science Quarterly, 19*(1), 45–59.

Janis, I. L. (1989). Groupthink. In W. E. Natemeyer & J. S. Gilberg (Eds.), *Classics of organizational*

behavior (2nd ed.) (pp. 179–187). Danville, IL: The Interstate Printers and Publishers, Inc.

Kanter, R. M. (1977). *Men and women of the corporation.* New York: Basic Books.

Kanter, R. M. (1979). Power failure in management circuits. *Harvard Business Review, 57*(4), 65–75.

Kaplan, A. (1964) Power in perspective. In R. L. Kahn & E. Boulding (Eds.), *Power and conflict in organizations* (pp. 11–32). London: Tavistock.

Kotter, J. P. (1977). Power, dependence and effective management. *Harvard Business Review, 55*(4), 135–136.

Kotter, J. P. (1978). Power, success, and organizational effectiveness. *Organizational Dynamics, 6*(3), 27–40.

Kotter, J. P. (1979). *Power in management.* New York: Amacom Publishing.

Kotter, J. P. (1985). *Power and influence: Beyond formal authority.* New York: Free Press.

Kouzes, J. M., & Posner, B. Z. (1988). *The leadership challenge: How to get extraordinary things done in organizations.* San Francisco: Jossey-Bass.

Larson, E. W., & King, J. B. (1996). The systematic distortion of information: An ongoing challenge to management. *Organizational Dynamics, 24*(3), 49–61.

Lourenco, S. V., & Glidewell, J. C. (1975). A dialectical analysis of organizational conflict. *Administrative Science Quarterly, 20*(4), 489–508.

Maccoby, M. (1976). *The gamesman.* New York: Simon & Schuster.

MacMillan, I. C. (1978). *Strategy formulation: Political concept.* St. Paul, MN: West Publishing.

March, J., & Simon, H. (1958). *Organizations.* New York: John Wiley and Sons.

March, J. G., & Olsen, J. P. (1976). *Ambiguity and choice in organizations.* Bergen, Norway: Universitetsforlaget.

McNeil, K. (1978). Understanding organizational power: Building on the Weberian legacy. *Administrative Science Quarterly, 23*(1), 65–90.

Mechanic, D. (1962). Sources of power of lower participants in complex organizations. *Administrative Science Quarterly, 7,* 349–364.

Miles, R. E., & Snow, C. C. (1982, Summer). Causes of failure in network organizations. *California Management Review,* 93–72.

Mintzberg, H. (1983). *Power in and around organizations.* Englewood Cliffs, NJ: Prentice-Hall.

Moore, T., & Wood, D. (1979). Power and the hospital executive. *Hospital and Health Services Administration, 24,* 30–41.

Morgan, G. (1986). *Images of organization.* Beverly Hills, CA: Sage.

O'Donnell, C. (1952). The source of managerial authority. *Political Science Quarterly, 67,* 573–588.

Parker, C. P., Dipboye, R. L., & Jackson, S. L. (1995). Perceptions of organizational politics: An investigation of antecedents and consequences. *Journal of Management, 21*(5), 891–912.

Perrow, C. (1961). The analysis of goals in complex organizations. *American Sociological Review,* 854–866.

Perrow, C. (1963). Goals and power structures: A historical case study. In E. Friedson (Ed.), *The hospital in modern society.* New York: Macmillan.

Perrow, C. (1970). Departmental power and perspectives in industrial firms. In M. N. Zald (Ed.), *Power in organizations* (pp. 58–59). Nashville, TN: Vanderbilt University Press.

Perrow, C. (1989). *Complex organizations: A critical essay.* New York: McGraw-Hill, Inc.

Pfeffer, J. (1981). *Power in organizations.* Marshfield, MA: Pitman Publishing.

Pfeffer J. (1992). *Managing with power: Politics and influence in organizations.* Boston: Harvard Business School Press.

Pfeffer, J. (1997). *New directions for organization theory.* New York: Oxford University Press.

Pfeffer, J., & Davis-Blake, A. (1987). Understanding organizational wage structures: A resource dependence approach. *Academy of Management Journal, 30,* 437–455.

Pfeffer, J., & Salancik, G. R. (1974). Organizational decision making as a political process: The case of a university budget. *Administrative Science Quarterly, 19,* 135–151.

Pfeffer, J., & Salancik, G. R. (1978). *The external control of organizations: A resource dependence perspective.* New York: Harper and Row.

Roemer, M. I., & Friedman, J. W. (1971). *Doctors in hospitals.* Baltimore: Johns Hopkins University Press.

Rousseau, D. M., & Parks, J. M. (1983). The contracts of individuals and organizations. In B. M. Staw & L. L.

Cummings (Eds.), *Research in organizational behavior,* vol. 15 (pp. 1–43). Greenwich, CT: JAI Press.

Rundall, T. G. (2004). Hospital-physician relationships: Comparing administrators' and physicians' perceptions. In H. T. O. Davies & M. Tavakoli (Eds.) *Policy, finance, and performance in health care* (pp. 47–79). Alderstot, U.K.: Ashgate Publishers.

Rundall, T. G., Davies, H. T. O., & Hodges, C. L. (2004). Doctor-manager relationships in the United States and the United Kingdom. *Journal of Healthcare Management.*

Salancik, G. R., & Pfeffer, J. (1974). The bases and use of power in organizational decision making: The case of a university. *Administrative Science Quarterly, 19,* 453–473.

Salancik, G. R., & Pfeffer, J. (1977). Who gets power—and how they hold on to it: A strategic contingency model of power. *Organizational Dynamics,* 3–21.

Scott, W. R. (1982). Managing professional work: three models of control for health organizations. *Health Services Research, 17,* 213–240.

Shortell, S. M. (1992). *Effective hospital-physician relationships.* Ann Arbor, MI: Health Administration Press.

Shortell, S. M., & Rundall, T. G. (2003). Understanding physician-organization relationships: Social networks and strategic intent. In S. S. Mick & M. Wyttenbach (Eds.), *Advances in health care organization theory* (pp. 141–173). San Francisco: Jossey-Bass Publishers.

Sitkin, S. B., & Stickel, D. (1996). The road to hell: The dynamics of distrust in an era of quality. In R. M. Kramer & T. R. Tyler (Eds.), *Trust in organizations* (pp. 196–215). Thousand Oaks: CA: Sage.

Tannenbaum, A. S. (1968). *Control in organizations.* Englewood Cliffs, NJ: Prentice-Hall.

Thibodeaux, M. S., & Powell, J. D. (Spring, 1985). Exploitation: Ethical problems of organizational power. *SAM Advanced Management Journal,* 42–44.

Tushman, M. L., Newman, W. H., & Romanelli, E. (1986). Convergence and upheaval: Managing the unsteady pace of organization evolution. *California Management Review, 29,* 29–44.

Two HealthSouth directors step down. 2003, December 16. *The Birmingham News.* Retrieved June 28, 2004, from LexisNexis Academic.

Weber, M. (1947). *The theory of social and economic organization*. New York: Free Press.

Weber, M. (1978). *Economy and society: An outline of interpretive sociology* (2 vols.) (G. Roth & C. Wittich, Eds.). Berkeley, CA: University of California Press.

Westheafer, C. (2000). Integrating perspectives within a framework: Taming the dark side. *Organizational Development Journal, 18*(3), 63–74.

Whitener, E. M., Brodt, S. E., Korsgaard, M. A., & Werner, J. M. (1998). Managers as initiators of trust: An exchange relationship framework for understanding managerial trustworthy behavior. *Academy of Management Review, 23*(3), 513–530.

Young, D. W., & Saltman, R. B. (1985). *The hospital power equilibrium: Physician behavior and cost control.* Baltimore: The Johns Hopkins University Press.

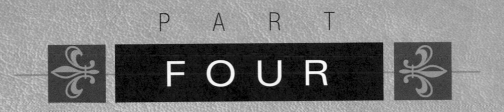

Positioning the Organization for Success

THE NATURE OF ORGANIZATIONS: FRAMEWORK FOR THE TEXT

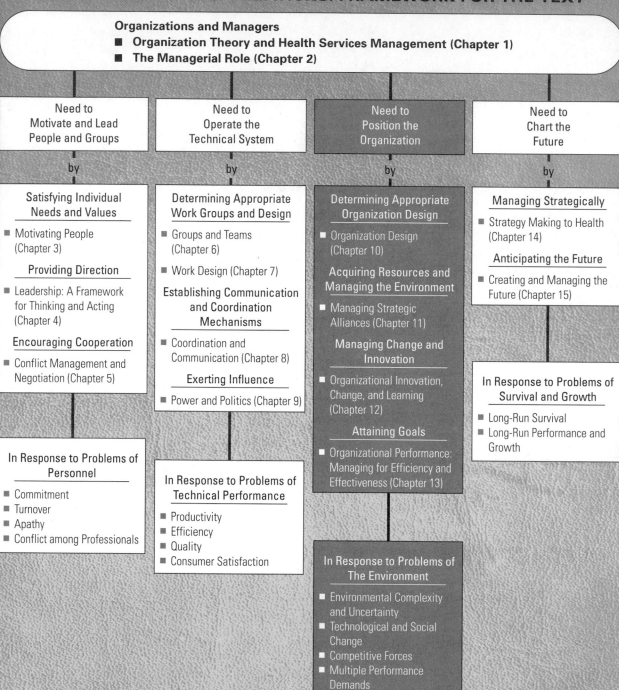

Organizations and Managers
- **Organization Theory and Health Services Management (Chapter 1)**
- **The Managerial Role (Chapter 2)**

Need to Motivate and Lead People and Groups

Need to Operate the Technical System

Need to Position the Organization

Need to Chart the Future

by

by

by

by

Satisfying Individual Needs and Values
- Motivating People (Chapter 3)

Providing Direction
- Leadership: A Framework for Thinking and Acting (Chapter 4)

Encouraging Cooperation
- Conflict Management and Negotiation (Chapter 5)

Determining Appropriate Work Groups and Design
- Groups and Teams (Chapter 6)
- Work Design (Chapter 7)

Establishing Communication and Coordination Mechanisms
- Coordination and Communication (Chapter 8)

Exerting Influence
- Power and Politics (Chapter 9)

Determining Appropriate Organization Design
- Organization Design (Chapter 10)

Acquiring Resources and Managing the Environment
- Managing Strategic Alliances (Chapter 11)

Managing Change and Innovation
- Organizational Innovation, Change, and Learning (Chapter 12)

Attaining Goals
- Organizational Performance: Managing for Efficiency and Effectiveness (Chapter 13)

Managing Strategically
- Strategy Making to Health (Chapter 14)

Anticipating the Future
- Creating and Managing the Future (Chapter 15)

In Response to Problems of Survival and Growth
- Long-Run Survival
- Long-Run Performance and Growth

In Response to Problems of Personnel
- Commitment
- Turnover
- Apathy
- Conflict among Professionals

In Response to Problems of Technical Performance
- Productivity
- Efficiency
- Quality
- Consumer Satisfaction

In Response to Problems of The Environment
- Environmental Complexity and Uncertainty
- Technological and Social Change
- Competitive Forces
- Multiple Performance Demands

Organizations operate within a complex and dynamic environment. Health care executives thus manage the environment as well as the operations within their own organization. The four chapters in this section highlight the nature of the managerial role in terms of understanding and developing strategies for effective intervention.

Chapter 10, "Organization Design," focuses on fundamental principles, evolution, and alternative designs in terms of their strengths and limitations. The chapter addresses the following questions:

- What is organization design? What is the role of management in the design and redesign of organizations?

- What are the components and characteristics of design?

- What designs are available, and what are their strengths and weaknesses relative to different environments?

Chapter 11, "Managing Strategic Alliances," deals with the emergence and operations of such alliances. The chapter focuses on the following questions:

- What are the types and forms of alliance structures?

- What are the processes and dimensions that distinguish these structures?

- What are the stages or processes involved in the development of an alliance?

Chapter 12, "Organizational Learning, Innovation, and Change," presents an analysis of the change process and the various types of changes involved in health services organizations. Among the questions it addresses are the following:

- What are the stages of the change process, and what factors facilitate or inhibit that process?

- What are the different types of changes that may occur, and what strategies are appropriate to ensure successful implementation and institutionalization?

Chapter 13, "Organizational Performance: Managing for Efficiency and Effectiveness," provides an overview of the various dimensions of performance and the issues that face health care managers and their organizations. Among the questions addressed are the following:

- What is organizational performance?

- What criteria are appropriate to differential performance?

- What can managers do to improve quality and increase value?

Upon completing these four chapters, readers should understand the fundamental design of organizations, their relationship to other organizations, and how this relationship affects organizational performance and change.

CHAPTER 10

Organization Design

Peggy Leatt, Ph.D.,G. Ross Baker, Ph.D., and John R. Kimberly, Ph.D.

CHAPTER OUTLINE

- The Meaning of Organization Design
- Levels of Organization Design
- Systematic Assessment before Design
- Designs for a Variety of Health Services Organizations
- Influences on Future Organization Designs
- Organizations in Transition

LEARNING OBJECTIVES

After completing this chapter, the reader should be able to:

1. Understand the principles of organization design.
2. Have an awareness of the evolution of organization design.
3. Use a framework for understanding organization design considerations.
4. Analyze common organization designs in terms of their applicability, strengths, and limitations.
5. Consider guidelines for changing organizations designs.

KEY TERMS

Assessment for Design	Design Process	Matrix or Mixed Design
Bureaucratic Organization	Divisional Design	Organizational Assessment
Centralization and	Environmental Assessment	Parallel Design
Decentralization	Functional Design	Political Process Assessment
Collectivist-Democratic	Human Resources	Product-Line or Program
Organization	Assessment	Design
Cultural Assessment	Levels of Organization Design	

❧ IN PRACTICE   Patient Safety at Children's Hospitals and Clinics[1]

Julie Morath joined Children's Hospitals and Clinics as chief operating officer and vice president for care delivery in May 1999. Children's Hospital provides pediatric health services in six facilities in the greater Minneapolis–St. Paul area. In her new role, Julie saw an opportunity to create an environment and structure focusing on improving quality of care and patient safety. The importance of this issue was highlighted later that year when the Institute of Medicine (IOM) released a study, "To Err is Human," that made patient safety a critical priority for American hospitals. Using data from research studies, the IOM Committee estimated that from 44,000 to 98,000 Americans die each year from preventable adverse events. Moreover, while health care organizations had traditionally held physicians and other professionals accountable for such incidents, the IOM made it clear that health care managers and boards were also responsible for creating an environment where improved patient safety was possible. But how can hospitals help to identify errors and reduce their impact?

Morath set out by collecting information within the hospital and from elsewhere about patient safety. She talked to staff, including the vice president of medical and other key clinical leaders, and she held focus groups with frontline staff to identify experiences in Children's Hospital where patients had been injured during their care. By the end of 1999 the Board of Children's Hospitals and Clinics had agreed to add patient safety to the organization's key goals and to start an agenda to implement patient safety efforts. The plan had three key elements: (1) transforming the organizational culture to encourage reporting of adverse events and errors, (2) redesigning the medication administration system to reduce adverse drug events, and (3) developing a structure that enabled staff to identify and work on these issues.

Morath created a Patient Safety Steering Committee (PSSC) to oversee the safety efforts. The committee had 19 members from different areas of the organization. This group set the goals for the safety initiative, identified changes needed in policies and procedures, and reviewed the work of "safety action" teams—cross-functional groups that were created to work on specific issues such as medication safety within different clinical areas. Each safety action team reviewed the patient safety needs in their area, including reports of "near misses" and incidents that might indicate the need to improve systems of care. These teams of frontline staff worked to identify local solutions to patient safety issues.

As the work of the Patient Safety Steering Committee expanded, Morath realized that

(continues)

> ## ❧ IN PRACTICE *(continued)*
>
> dedicated leadership was needed to take on this effort. In January 2001, the PSSC hired Dr. Eric Knox to take on the role of director of patient safety.
>
> To enable leaders to identify the progress made in these patient safety efforts, the PSSC helped to identify a series of patient safety performance measures including the number of patient safety reports, the percentage of patient safety work plan ideas implemented, and the number of medication best practices implemented in each site. These performance measures, together with other measures of hospital and clinic performance, allowed both the PSSC and the senior leadership to monitor the progress toward safer care.

[1]Based on Morath (2002), A. Edmondson, M. A. Roberto, and A. Tucker,

CHAPTER PURPOSE

As experienced by Julie Morath when she joined Children's Hospitals and Clinics, health services organizations are constantly challenged to explore ways in which organizations, especially health services, make decisions about designing and redesigning organizational structures. Given the complex nature of the external environment in which organizations must operate in order to survive, managers must actively decide who has responsibility for making which decisions at various levels. In other words, who will have power in the organization and for what purposes? The focus of this chapter is on exploring a variety of organization designs that are typical of health services organizations and analyzing where the designs seem to work best. Given the changing environment of health care, designs that will help organizations maintain high performance, including quality and patient safety, during times of transition are highlighted.

THE MEANING OF ORGANIZATION DESIGN

Design Is Dynamic

Organization design refers to the way in which the building blocks of organization—authority, responsibility, accountability, information, and rewards— are arranged or rearranged to improve effectiveness and adaptive capacity. Organization design and redesign are dynamic, being simultaneously both an outcome and a process. As an outcome, organization design can be represented by the boxes and lines on an organization chart. These represent how the building blocks are arranged. As many organizations face increasingly uncertain and rapidly changing environments, new ways of representing organization are emerging, replacing boxes and lines. Intersecting circles, inverted triangles, and lattices are alternative ways of describing the outcomes of design and redesign.

Design outcomes, however, are generally transitory. Top management of most organizations is always searching for more effective ways to carry out its mission, and as external circumstances change, redesign may well be indicated. In effect, then, design and redesign constitute a process whereby current arrangements are evaluated and new ones are introduced, in some cases almost continuously.

Although we might like to think of organizational design as a rational, deliberate, and planned series of activities in which men and women of vision create organizational arrangements supportive of mission and strategy and are performance-enhancing, in reality—particularly in a sector as volatile as health care—the **design process** often reflects underlying political dynamics. Changes in leadership, goals, and strategies, and pure accident are all reasons why a change in design may not occur on a perfectly "rational" basis (Kimberly, 1984).

Management's Role in Organization Design

Management's primary task is to maintain and improve performance. In fact, management texts refer to organization design as one of management's most critical functions (Daft, 1998; Morgan, 1997; Nadler, Gerstein, Shaw, & associates, 1992). Usually, the activities of design are seen as the responsibilities of senior management. However, many of the most successful designs appear to be those that have been built with input from a broad range of organizational members, including key external and internal stakeholders and persons at all levels within the organization. Outside consultants are sometimes brought in to provide technical advice on the range of designs that might be considered.

Do not make the mistake of thinking of organization design as a "once and for all event" parallel to an architect or engineer designing and constructing a new building. When a new organization is formed, a new design will be created; however, the redesign of the organization is an ongoing process in which the design needs will change as the organization's needs change. This idea is most important for managers who may not only have responsibility for redesigning their organizations but also for ensuring that the design is implemented.

The design process is not carried out in isolation from other management activities. In fact, ideas about the type of design that might be appropriate should be derived from the organization's mission and strategic planning process (Pearce, 1982). For example, if a pharmaceutical company decides to expand its product lines, it may be necessary to reorganize its research and development division. If the Department of Public Health decides to close down its immunization program, it may be necessary to regroup ongoing services within the organization.

The way in which an organization is designed also has considerable importance for the nature and content of the information system needed by the organization. Since an organization design specifies who has power to make which decisions, it also indicates which positions need what types of informa-

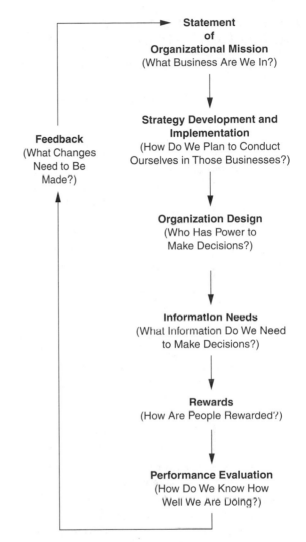

Figure 10.1. Organizational Design in Relation to Other Management Activities

tion and at what times. Organization design also has implications for how performance will be evaluated and rewarded. Finally, the knowledge gathered from performance indicators will be fed back to subsequently influence the organization's mission. The relationships of organization design to these other management activities can be seen in Figure 10.1.

When Should an Organization's Design Be Re-thought?

A number of circumstances would suggest that a manager should be reconsidering the appropriateness of an organization's design. Some examples of triggers or indicators that the best design may not be in place include:

- *The organization is experiencing severe performance problems.* Indicators of inadequate performance may be presented to the manager from external reviews such as accreditation processes and customer satisfaction surveys or from internal reviews such as financial statements, medication error reports, and clinical audits. These problems may be identified at varying levels within the organization, for a particular position, a work group or team, a department, or a total organization.

- *There is a change in the environment that directly influences internal policies.* In some circumstances, there may be major changes in the environment, such as capitation payment for all health services received by a given population or new policies regulating pharmaceutical manufacturing or sales. These changes may require a redesign and refocusing of key organizational groups.

- *New programs or product lines are developed.* When an organization recognizes certain markets or product lines as high priority, an organization design change may be necessary to infuse resources into the new areas. Conversely, when old programs are to be dropped, new structural arrangements may be necessary.

- *There is a change in top leadership.* New leadership may provide considerable opportunity to rethink the way in which the organization has been designed. New leadership tends to view the organization from a different perspective and may bring innovative ideas to the reorganization.

In summary, health services organizations are redesigned to adapt to an environment where prevention of disease and promotion of healthy lifestyles are encouraged, where incentives exist to redirect patients to utilize more cost-effective ambulatory care services, and where there is a market pressure to provide high-quality and safe care at a competitive price while improving patient satisfaction (Gillies, Shortell, & Young, 1997; Shortell, Gillies, Anderson, Mitchell, & Morgan, 1993).

LEVELS OF ORGANIZATION DESIGN

Several aspects of an organization can be redesigned or changed. For example, decisions can be made to change the overall size of the organization, the number and types of units or departments within, and how these units may be grouped. We can also decide to change the span of control of individual managers, reorganize tasks, specify rules and procedures in a formalized or standardized way, reallocate decision-making authority, alter communication channels, change mechanisms of control and reward, create new roles or positions, and determine how coordination will be achieved.

We typically think of design being achieved for a whole organization, such as a nursing home, a hospital, or a public health unit; however, design may take place for a particular group of departments, for an individual unit or department, or for a specific position (also see Chapter 7). Mintzberg (1983) has pointed out that the design of individual positions forms the basic building blocks on which the design of a whole organization is developed. On a wider scale than a single organization, we may also create a design for a network of organizations in a given community or for a system of organizations (also see Chapter 11). These interlocking **levels of organization design** are illustrated in Table 10.1.

Designing a Position

In terms of designing individual positions in the organization, there may be hundreds from which to

Table 10.1. **Levels of Design in Health Services Organizations**

Renewing the Organization	
Levels	**Some Illustrations**
Individual positions	Managers
	Staff positions
	Health professionals
	Other workers
Work groups	Task forces and committees
	Teams
	Units and departments
Clusters of work groups	Division of two or more units
	Medical staff organization
Total organizations	Hospitals
	Primary care centers
	Public health units
	Long-term care facilities
	Health maintenance organizations (HMOs)
	Multispecialty group practices
Network of organizations	Strategic alliances between physicians and health systems
	Organizations providing services for oncology patients
	Preferred provider organizations (PPOs)
	Affiliated groups of hospitals
Systems	A group of hospitals under single ownership
	All home health services in a state
	A national system of health services
	An integrated health system

choose, depending upon the organization's size and complexity. For example, a new manager might be hired into a health services organization as an executive assistant to the president. If you were in this position, you would likely be excited about the possibilities and ask the president for a copy of your job description. The president, being amused, might inform you that your first task is to prepare a draft of your own position description for management's approval.

In designing an individual job or position for any level within an organization, it is necessary to identify the breadth and scope of tasks that can be performed and the extent to which the work can be standardized. Both of these factors have implications for the skills and training that will be necessary for the persons filling the job. Some of the basic parameters that should be identified include the major responsibilities and roles inherent in the position, to whom the position is accountable, for whose work the position is accountable, and the relationship of other peer positions to it. See for example Table 10.2, which illustrates a position for a patient safety officer.

Designing a Work Group

Increasingly the use of teams in health services organizations is required by the complexity of health care work (Katzenach & Smith, 1993; Mohrman, Cohen, & Mohrman, 1995). Quality improvement teams are often cross-functional, and can examine work processes that cut across organizational units (Gaucher & Coffey, 1993; McLaughlin & Kaluzny, 2006; Melum & Sinioris, 1992). Managers often need to create a task force or quality improvement team to solve a complex problem in a short time frame. For example, a health services manager may be interested in improving the speed with which the results of blood tests are reported. A quality improvement team could be formed for this task and the manager should clarify the specific purpose of the team, the time frame for completion of the problem solving, and the boundaries of the group's authority. The manager should also make decisions about the skills and knowledge necessary to complete the task. In this case, to investigate the issue with the results of blood tests, it may be appropriate to use a multidisciplinary approach that includes a

Table 10.2. Patient Safety Officer*

Position Summary:

The designated safety officer will have primary oversight of the facility-wide patient safety program. This leadership role will direct others within the facility towards process improvements that will support the reduction of medical/health care errors and other factors that contribute to unintended adverse patient outcomes. This practitioner provides leadership for safety assessments, coordinates the activities of the Patient Safety Committee, educates other practitioners on the system-based causes for medical error, consults with management and staff, and communicates literature-based ideas regarding effective patient safety strategies to others within the organization.

Essential Functions: The Patient Safety Officer will . . .

1. Oversee the creation, review, and refinement of the scope of the Patient Safety Program within the facility on an annual basis.
2. Coordinate the activities of the Patient Safety Committee.
3. Serve as liaison between the CEO, the Board of Trustees, and the Safety committee.
4. Oversee the management and use of medical error information. Review internal error reports and utilize information from external reporting programs (e.g., ISMP Medication Safety Alert™ and ECRI Health Device Alerts).
5. Investigate (along with risk management if a separate position) patient safety issues within the facility. Participate in Root Cause Analysis of internal error reports.
6. Recommend and facilitate change within the organization to improve patient safety, based on identified risks.
7. Collaborate the development of policy and procedures effecting organizational safety.
8. Develop a mechanism for internal communication of patient-safety related information.
9. Design and implement educational presentations that facilitate the understanding and implementation of patient safety standards within the organization.
10. Serve as a resource for clinical departments on issues of patient safety.
11. Support and encourage error reporting throughout the organization through a nonpunitive error reporting system.
12. Support the development of a recognition program aimed at improving patient safety.
13. Report to the governing body on the occurrence of known medical and health care errors and identified near misses and dangerous conditions within the facility, as well as actions taken, either proactively, or based on occurrences. Barriers to the implementation of safety programs should be addressed.

Qualifications:

1. An advanced degree in a health care related field is desirable. A bachelor's degree with appropriate prerequisite knowledge, experience, and skills should also be considered.
2. Experience with the organization's identified quality improvement model/program.
3. Knowledge of risk management principles and issues regarding patient safety.
4. Superior interpersonal skills.
5. Strong leadership qualities (task completion, motivation).
6. Effective change agent.

*The content herein was developed under a project supported by the Delaware Valley Healthcare Council and is subject to the copyright of ECRI, ISMP, and DVHERF.

SOURCE: From Pathways for Medication Safety.® 2002, the American Hospital Association, the Health Research and Educational Trust, and the Institute for Safe Medication Practices. Available at www.medpathways.info.

nurse, physician, laboratory manager, laboratory technician, hematologist, orderly, or other health workers. A similar design approach may be used for deciding upon more permanent work groups, such as clinical units or "microsystems" responsible for the provision of clinical care, strategic business units, departments, or other groups. These issues are further discussed in Chapters 6, 7, and 15.

Designing a Cluster of Work Groups

In some circumstances it may be necessary to redesign a cluster of departments or units within an organization or a system. One of the most important design decisions to be made in clustering work groups is determining the most appropriate grouping of units to achieve integration. Grouping of units implies that the units will share a common manager, common resources, and common performance measures. To illustrate the various ways in which units may be grouped, we use the example of the physician organization arrangements (POAs). POAs are structural mechanisms (joint ventures) to facilitate integration of physicians into a network of integrated health systems (Alexander et al., 1996; Zuckerman et al., 1998). Shortell, Gillies, Anderson, Erickson, and Mitchell (1996) found that greater physician integration was significantly related to higher inpatient productivity and higher levels of integration. POAs may be designed in a number of ways. For example, physician groups may be grouped by knowledge and skill or by specialty and subspecialty (such as all medical specialties and all surgical specialties). Physicians may also be grouped by work process, for instance, by placing the operating rooms, intensive care units, and parts of radiology under the same management, because they have a common patient flow. Ambulatory care clinic physicians may be grouped by time if they tend to hold clinics in the same time frame. Physicians may be grouped by commonality of clients or patients, for example, cardiology and cardiovascular surgery. Finally, physicians may be grouped because they are geographically located in

the same hospital or facility. Chapters 6 through 9 provide further discussion of these issues.

Designing and Redesigning a Total Organization

The challenge of designing or redesigning a total organization is enormous, and the amount of investment necessary to manage the redesign process is extensive. Perhaps most important, the process has to unfold in such a way that behaviors, not just formal structures, change (James, 2003) and the organization that is in place becomes a learning organization (see Chapter 12).

Designing a Network

A network of organizations comprises those organizations that exist in a particular community or environment, which may be loosely or closely connected to achieve a common purpose or serve a common clientele (Kaluzny, Morissey, & McKinney, 1990). An example is the network of health and social services that may exist in a community to provide services to individuals with dementia and their families. Types of organizations within the network may include an acute hospital, psychiatric hospital, nursing home, home health services, day care services, Meals on Wheels, housing and transport services, social services, and so on. The objective in the design of the network is to ensure coordination of services and smoothness of client flow between organizations to maximize effectiveness. One of the key tasks in designing a network is identifying the target population, such as individuals with dementia, to be served by the network. The main demographic and health characteristics of the specific target population such as age, sex, cultural group, language, and morbidity and mortality rates by specific diseases must be identified. At the network level, the design process is relatively complex because it involves examining the nature of the relationships among the organizations in the network (Gittell & Weiss, 1997). Design decisions may include deciding which organizations should have the most power, which resource transactions may take place, and how innovations will be diffused. These issues are also considered in Chapter 11.

Designing a Health System

A health system is a network of organizations that provides or arranges to provide a coordinated continuum of services to a defined population and is willing to be held clinically and fiscally accountable for the outcomes and the health status of a population served (Gillies et al., 1997). At the system level, design decisions are even more complex, depending upon the purpose(s) of the system and the heterogeneity of the programs provided. One of the most important factors to be analyzed at the system level is the degree of **centralization and decentralization** of decision making. For example, given a system that may include as many as 80 acute health care organizations or groups, it is essential to clarify which decisions will be made at the corporate level and which decisions will be made at the regional or individual organization level. Such decisions can be further categorized as those involving the setting of policy (e.g., wage and salary guidelines), initiating activities (e.g., hiring new staff), and granting final approval (e.g., capital budgets). When the majority of decisions are centered at the corporate office, the organization is said to be vertically centralized. In high-technology industries such as health care, greater vertical decentralization is expected because of the expertise at lower levels in the organization. As a general rule, decisions should be made at the lowest possible levels, especially when the majority of workers are professionals. Horizontal decentralization refers to the extent to which influence and decision making is shared laterally. In the design of a health system, for example, an important design factor may be deciding upon the extent to which individual operating units can develop their own strategic plans separately from those developed by the corporate office. A major part of the activities at the de-

centralized level are concerned with the implementation of policies and ensuring quality.

Table 10.3 shows health system design for two organizations: PennCARE and the Henry Ford Health System. In describing the two cases, Dubbs (2002) illustrates the importance of being consistent in the creation of organizational designs. While these health systems have different design configurations—PennCARE uses a virtually integrated, loose contract-based model and Henry Ford employs a vertically integrated tight ownership model—their overall designs reflect the similarities in principles and values within each organization. The comparison of the cases illustrates how each organization has been able to effectively manage relationships by synchronizing each organization's governance structure, organizational culture, strategic planning, and management processes.

SYSTEMATIC ASSESSMENT BEFORE DESIGN

Earlier in this chapter, we emphasized the need to match a design with the organization's mission and strategies as well as obtaining participation from major stakeholders. An organizational model or conceptual framework is an essential tool to guide this analysis and action. Most people who have been exposed to organizations have an implicit experience-based model; however, organizational theorists and researchers have now developed general models for thinking about organizations as total systems. The major factors that are essential to consider in an organizational **assessment for design** are shown in Figure 10.2. These factors reflect the need to consider organization design decisions in the context of a broad managerial framework where several key factors are assessed simultaneously. The factors are the mission, **environmental assessment**, **organizational assessment**, **cultural assessment**, **human resources assessment**, and political process assessment.

Table 10.3. Organizational Design Consistency

Characteristics	PennCARE	Henry Ford Health System
Governance Structure	■ Virtual arrangement of connecting organizations ■ Contract-based ■ Not ownership-based	■ Vertically integrated system with tight arrangements ■ Centralized control at the system level ■ Governance by ownership
Organizational Culture	■ No overarching organizational culture ■ Eleven cultures at the local level ■ Preservation of local cultures encouraged	■ Strong organizational culture ■ Common organizational vision ■ A history of strong ties between hospitals and physicians
Strategic Planning Process	■ There is a designated planning group that assists in identifying new opportunities ■ No written formal strategic plan	■ Responsibility for strategic planning rests with a senior vice president ■ Written strategic plans are updated annually for each region/operating unit and then integrated into a central plan
Decision-Making Procedures	■ Initiatives for strategic decision making occur at local levels ■ Decentralized structure	■ Key decisions are approved centrally ■ Responsibility for implementing decisions is decentralized ■ Standardized rules and operating procedures
The Value of Organizational Design Consistency	■ Organizational design is characterized by "loose" consistency across the key characteristics	■ Organizational design is characterized by "tight" consistency across the key characteristics

SOURCE: Adapted from Dubbs, N. L. (2002). Organizational design consistency: The PennCARE and Henry Ford Health System experience. *Journal of Healthcare Management, 47*(5), 307–318.

The Mission

One of the first and most important considerations in beginning an organization design strategy is to identify the mission of the organization. The mission may have been established through a strategic planning process in which a wide range of stakeholders worked together to provide a clear statement of the vision for the organization. Usually a mission statement identifies "what business the organization is in." It may also include statements about the values and ideology of the organization in terms of client services and management. A mission statement usually outlines some more specific formal goals for the organization. Gellerman quotes the American architect Louis Sullivan, who in 1890 wrote, "Form follows function." Gellerman (1990) reaffirms that this principle also applies when designing organizations. They should be designed for a specific purpose or function, hence the impor-

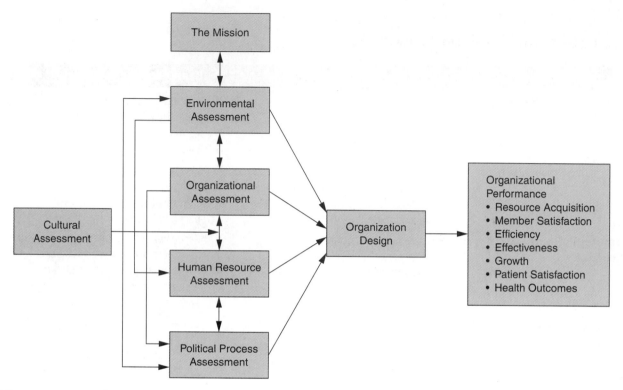

Figure 10.2. Overall Framework for Organizational Design Considerations

tance of the mission statement.

Environmental Assessment

Assessing the environment of an organization is important to ensure that the organization will achieve desired levels of effectiveness. Complex environments create instability and uncertainty, which can be countered by developing different organizational designs. Environmental uncertainty affects the degree of formality of structure, the nature of interpersonal relationships, and the time orientation (short versus long run of employees). As uncertainty increases—that is, as environmental conditions become less stable—organizations may divide into specialized operating units. These units may develop varying priorities and have different time hori-

zons. To ensure expected levels of effectiveness, managers must design a variety of mechanisms to achieve integration across operating units. The absence of such mechanisms may lead to conflict and diminished performance.

What design options are available to the manager faced with the consequences of increasing environmental uncertainty? In their classic work, Lawrence and Lorsch (1967) advocate the creation of lateral relations such as direct managerial contact across functions, cross-functional teams (either permanent or temporary), liaison roles, and integrating departments. Such design strategies have the ultimate effect of improving coordination and decentralizing decision making so that it takes place at the level of the organization where the necessary information exists. Discussion on the parallel organizational design that Stein and Kanter (1980) suggest as one mechanism for integrating persons from all levels in the organization in the decision-making process will be covered later in this chapter.

Organization design may also be contingent upon the technology of the organization. Rapidly changing diagnostic procedures, treatment, and drug therapies as well as changing information technologies in the environment of health services organizations demand more complex, flexible, and nimble designs that can adapt quickly to innovations.

Organizational Assessment

An important stage in preparing to redesign an organization is to identify the strengths and limitations of the organization. This process is frequently referred to as a SWOT analysis (strengths, weaknesses, opportunities, and threats). Since every organization is different, this assessment can be carried out in a number of ways. A frequently used approach is to conduct focus group discussions of the most important strengths and weaknesses of the organizations. This knowledge is useful for organizations to build on their strengths and address their weaknesses. Focus groups for this kind of task are usually multidisciplinary and are made up of key stakeholders of the organization.

Cultural Assessment

Greater attention is being given to the importance of organizational culture to organization success, especially in bringing about organizational change. Culture has been variously defined as the values and beliefs, norms or behaviors that characterize the work of the organization. Culture essentially addresses the question of "what is it like to work here?" Strong cultures may provide greater cohesion for organizational members and allow easier achievement of mission and goals. Different cultures may evolve or exist at different operating units in an organization. Most organizations are "multicultural." Different unit or different professions may vary in their

beliefs and behaviors. Measuring organizational culture is difficult and may require a combination of focus groups for brainstorming, assessment instruments, and observation. Indications of an organization's culture can include employees' favorite stories about heroes of the organization, the celebrations and traditions, the language used, and other indications of patterns of behavior that make the organization a good or bad place to work (Siehl & Martin, 1990; Zammutto & Krakower, 1991).

Human Resources Assessment

Organizations are made up of people who give life to the organizations. The availability of individuals with appropriate knowledge and skills to carry out the mission of the organization is critical. It may not be possible, under some circumstances, for an organization to obtain highly specialized expertise when it needs it. Accordingly, organization designs are influenced by the availability of critical human resources to match the organization's mission and goals.

Political Process Assessment

All organizations have an informal structure as well as a formal one. Managers need to understand the nature of this informal structure, for example, who the key leaders are, and how this network can influence changes in organization design. For instance, informal leaders can facilitate or create barriers to the implementation of a new organization design; therefore, it is essential for managers to be aware of the informal political processes underpinning the organization's life.

In the framework shown in Figure 10.2, we see the systematic assessment of mission, environment, organization, culture, human resources, and political processes necessary to tailor an organization design for the specific needs of the organization. With this systematic approach, it is more likely that the design will facilitate the organization to achieve high levels of performance.

IN PRACTICE

The Visiting Nurse Agency: A Changing Environment

The Visiting Nurse Agency (VNA) was founded over 100 years ago by Jennie Johnson. Johnson's mother and grandmother before her had been known in their local community as persons who had always been called by neighbors to help deliver babies or provide support when family members were sick. Johnson saw VNA as an opportunity to carry on the family tradition by providing expert nursing services to those in need of care when sick in their homes.

The VNA was located in a rapidly growing suburb of a large city. During the initial years, VNA concentrated on two goals: first, attracting enough families to provide services to mothers with new babies and elderly persons requiring personal care at home; second, developing a reputation for providing a high-quality, personal, and caring service. All patients and clients appeared content with the service, and the agency, a private nonprofit organization, was in a financially stable situation.

During the late 1990s, VNA's growth slowed. Although VNA was perceived to provide good care in the home, a number of new nursing services were being provided by private agencies. These agencies were providing more extensive home visits for postnatal care in the evenings and on weekends. Nurses were providing extensive nursing services in conjunction with a local nursing home and a home for the aged on an outreach basis. Their services were available 24 hours a day, seven days a week. The local community general hospital was also experimenting with health promotion clinics where services were being provided at a minimal charge to local residents. The VNA was seen as a very traditional "nursing" agency with rather

specialized nursing services in the home and insufficient flexibility to meet the new needs of the community.

The VNA's hours of operation were Monday to Friday, 8:30 A.M. to 4:30 P.M. In 1994, VNA employed 51 registered nurses and five nurse-managers. The agency prided itself on the fact that all the nurses were registered nurses, and about half of them had a university education. Johnson, however, was becoming increasingly concerned by the decreasing demand for their services. By 1995, Johnson had begun to replace some of her nurse managers, hoping to bring in new energy and fresh ideas. She still believed that the agency was respected because of its high-quality nursing services and the good relationships the agency enjoyed with established families in the community. Johnson called in the nurse-managers and stressed the importance of the quality philosophy to them. She emphasized the need for careful supervision of the nurses. She said all nurses must arrive at their house calls on time; punctuality was very important. She stressed the need for all nursing procedures conducted in the home to adhere to predefined standards. She pointed out the importance of the need for regular performance evaluations for the nurses so that they could be given immediate feedback on areas in which they were not following the exact protocol of the agency. As new nurse-managers gained experience in VNA, they began to propose changes. One nurse-manager suggested that they establish an advisory board to serve as a liaison between the VNA and the local community. The advisory board would be made up of Johnson and key people from the local area, such as business people, women, minority group members, and senior citizens group members. The nurse-manager who proposed the idea argued that advisory board members could counsel prospective clients about the nursing services and in general provide a public relations function for VNA.

Another new nurse-manager proposed that the VNA engage in more advertising and marketing strategies. She argued that the agency nurses should become more involved in community groups such as the community center's senior citizen events. She also argued that the VNA should be prepared to respond to proposals for contracts with Health Maintenance Organizations.

As Johnson considered these and other proposals, the government announced approval of funding for a major expansion of the Metropolitan Home Care Program. Home care programs had been successful in other metropolitan areas and had been shown in some cases to be an excellent alternative to in hospital care, especially because a range of community support services could be provided. The new funding seemed to favor the provision of a variety of professional services in the home including nursing, medical, rehabilitation, and several homemaker services. The new funding was to be available on a competitive basis to both for-profit and not-for-profit agencies. Jennie Johnson and the nurse-managers were very concerned about whether they could compete and the impact these developments could have on VNA.

In January 1998, Johnson felt overwhelmed and wondered whether she was up to managing the VNA. The agency had grown little over the past five years and was receiving fewer and fewer referrals from its long-standing clients. The impact of the expanded Home Care Program was difficult to anticipate, and she was not sure how VNA should respond. Two of the sharpest nurse-managers had been to see her about a change in strategy. They encouraged the creation of several internal committees to study the problems. They also suggested that VNA begin planning the formation of specialized teams, organized around clients' needs and more appropriately able to respond to special interest groups. "The home nursing service industry is becoming more complex and is very competitive," one nurse-manager argued, "and if we don't adapt to it, we will be left behind: we need to find partners!" Johnson thought the best thing might be to retire and get out of the provision of visiting nurse services—so dear to her family tradition.

The Visiting Nurse Agency (VNA) (see In Practice, p. 326) provides an example of a health services organization that is facing changing times and is thinking about changing its organization design. How should this organization reconsider its mission in relation to the changing environment? What strengths and weaknesses does the organization have? What is the prevalent culture? How might the work of the nurse-managers be propagated?

DESIGNS FOR A VARIETY OF HEALTH SERVICES ORGANIZATIONS

Figure 10.3 provides the overall framework for organizational design considerations. This framework stresses that the design must be tailored to the

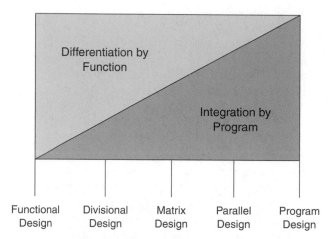

Figure 10.3. Continuum of Organizational Design

SOURCE: Adapted from Charnes & Tewksbury, (1993). *Collaborative management in health care* (p. 28, Figure 2.1). San Francisco: Jossey-Bass. This material is used by permission of John Wiley & Sons, Inc.

individual needs of the organization. Two main requirements of contingency theory are that organizations must cope simultaneously with needs to differentiate work and needs to integrate work (Charnes & Smith-Tewksbury, 1993). Differentiation is the requirement to divide work into specialized parts or functions; integration is the requirement to coordinate the work across different operating units or functions. All organizations must do both; but the common forms of organizational designs may be described along a continuum, as shown in Figure 10.3. The designs arranged along the continuum emphasize differentiated designs at one end (the left side of Figure 10.3) and integration at the other end (the right side of Figure 10.3). All of these designs may be found at the different levels of organization design shown in Figure 10.1. Most organizations' designs are less neat and tidy than these illustrations.

Specific design options available for health services managers depend on environmental demands, the organization's strategies, how activities can be grouped, and how decisions will be made.

Functional Design

A **functional design** exists when labor is divided into departments specialized by functional area. An example is shown in Figure 10.4. This kind of design is typical of a nursing home, chronic-care facility, or small (less than 100 beds) community general hospital. The basic hotel services are separated from the clinical services. The actual number of functional departments (and departmental manager positions) depends upon the size of the organization. From the management's viewpoint, the functional design enables decisions to be made on a centralized, hierarchical basis. Departmental managers are usually promoted from within the organization and have a depth of technical knowledge in the functional area.

The functional design is most appropriate when an organization is in a relatively simple, stable environment in which there are few changes taking place and there are a limited number of other organizations with which the organization has contact. A functional design becomes unsuitable when an organization grows and begins to diversify its services because interdepartmental coordination tends to be poor and decisions pile up at the top. If the environment becomes unstable, the functional design cannot cope because it does not have the facility to handle rapid information input or output and the response time is generally too slow. This type of design was most commonly seen in health care organizations 20 years ago. It is less common today because of increasing environmental uncertainty.

Divisional Design

The **divisional design** is often found in large academic medical centers (AMCs) that operate under conditions of high environmental uncertainty exacerbated by relationships with the medical school and high technological complexity because of intensive research activities (Heyssel, Gaintner, Kues, Jones, & Lipstein, 1984). It is also frequently found in pharmaceutical companies and health supplier organizations where a large variety of products and

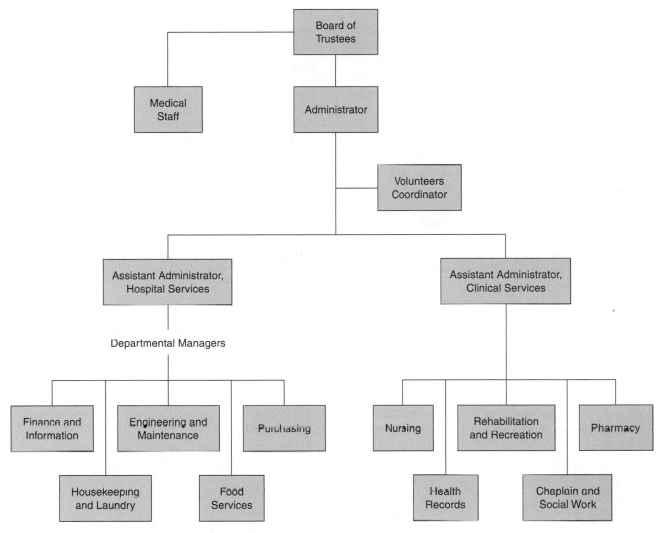

Figure 10.4. A Functional Design: Nursing Home or Chronic-Care Facility

markets are involved. It is most appropriate for situations where clear divisions can be made within the organization and semiautonomous units can be created. Traditionally, in teaching hospitals the way of grouping units has been relatively clear-cut. Units have been grouped according to the traditional medical specialties, such as medicine, surgery, pediatrics, psychiatry, radiology, and pathology. More recently, AMCs are beginning to question the ap-

propriateness of these traditional groupings and are moving toward defining product lines that cross traditional boundaries. Examples of product lines are those organized around health promotion; disease prevention programs; or diagnostic, therapeutic, and rehabilitation services; or those grouped around services to specific populations, such as the elderly or persons with cancer or cardiac problems. Similarly, in pharmaceutical companies, divisions are being created among related drugs. Divisionalization decentralizes decision making to the lowest level in the organization where the key expertise is available. Individual divisions have considerable autonomy for the clinical and financial operations. Each division has its own internal management structure, as illustrated in Figure 10.5.

The model illustrated in Figure 10.5 shows the physician in charge of each clinical service as the person with direct authority over all divisional operations. Each division has a manager of nursing or patient services, a manager of administrative services, and a finance officer. These managers work as a team to direct the division's operations. The managers are also accountable to the vice presidents of their disciplines. In some academic medical centers, a collaborative model is used to provide leadership of the team at the divisional level—that is, physicians, nurses, and administrators combine their skills to ensure knowledge of both the clinical and financial operations.

This operating unit structure enables the specialized units to handle relevant elements of the environment directly, enhancing the organization's capacity to exchange information with the environment and to develop strategies tailored to the product lines. In many instances, the divisions purchase central services from within the hospital and are provided incentives to operate their units cost-effectively. At the same time, the central service units are driven to operate efficiently; otherwise, the divisions may choose to purchase services outside the hospital at a better rate.

Difficulties with the divisional design tend to occur in times of resource constraints, when priorities must be set at higher organizational levels. For example, an academic health science center may have difficulty arriving at a consensus about which patient programs should be given priority if divisional managers cannot see the perspective of the whole organization. In times of resource constraints, greater sharing of resources between divisions is required, and more effective horizontal integrating mechanisms need to be established (Smith, Leatt, Ellis, & Fried, 1989). Divisons may also compete for resources or power, creating friction within the organization.

Matrix Design

To overcome some of the problems of the functional and divisional designs and allow competing bases of authority to jointly govern the workflow, **matrix or mixed designs** have evolved to improve mechanisms of lateral coordination and information flow across the organization (Scott, 2003). An example of a matrix organization for a psychiatric center is provided in Figure 10.6.

The matrix organization, originally developed in the aerospace industry, is characterized by a dual-authority system. There are usually functional and programs or product-line managers, both reporting to a common superior and both exercising authority over workers within the matrix. Typically, a matrix organization is particularly useful in highly specialized technological areas that focus on innovation. The matrix design allows program managers to interact directly with the environment vis-à-vis technological developments. Usually each program requires a multidisciplinary team approach; the matrix structure facilitates the coordination of the team and allows team members to contribute their special expertise.

The matrix design has some disadvantages that stem from the dual-authority lines. Individual workers may find having two bosses to be untenable since it creates conflicting expectations and ambiguity. The matrix design may also be expensive in that both functional and program managers may spend a considerable amount of time in meetings attempting to keep everyone informed of program activities. Additional costs may also be incurred because of the frequent requirement for dual accounting, budget, control, performance evaluation, and reward systems.

The use of the matrix design in health services organizations is becoming more common, particularly in organizations in which multidisciplinary approaches and patient-focused care are being encouraged. To some degree, most health services organizations have many characteristics of a matrix organization, al-

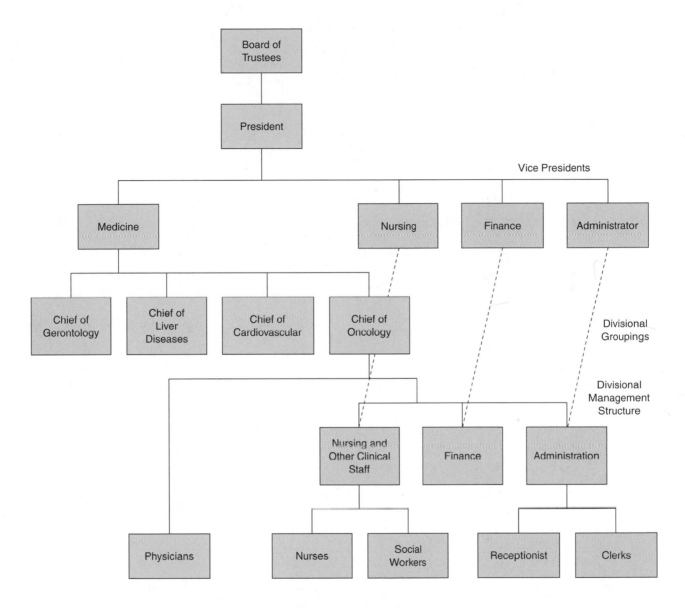

Figure 10.5. A Divisional Design: An Academic Health Science Center

though their design may not be formally named as such. For example, multiple authorities over patient care are clearly apparent in most hospitals. Most health professionals—such as nurses, psychologists, physiotherapists, pharmacists, occupational therapists, and social workers—have formal reporting re-

lationships to their functional departments but are also accountable to physicians for the quality of care provided. Multidisciplinary teams, which facilitate lateral communication and coordination of work, are an essential feature of almost all health services organizations, including community health, long-term care,

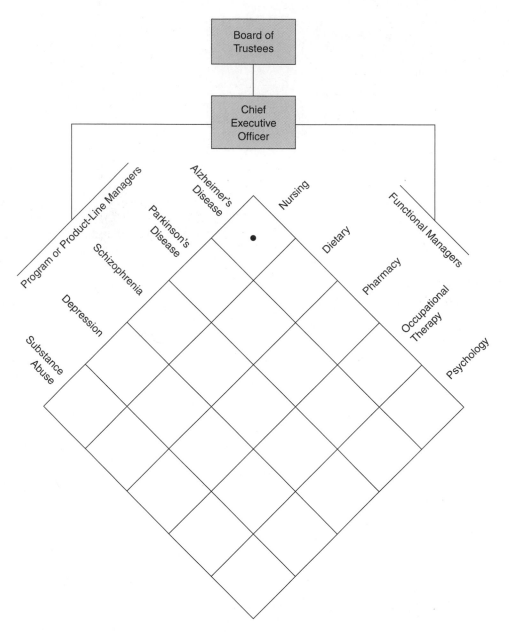

Figure 10.6. A Matrix Design: A Psychiatric Center

home care, and hospitals. As a result, learning to manage in matrix structures is particularly important for health services managers.

Parallel Design

The parallel structure was originally developed as a mechanism for promoting quality of working life in organizations (Stein & Kanter, 1980). The **bureaucratic** or functional **organization** retains responsibility for routine activities in the organization, while the parallel side is responsible for complex problem solving requiring participatory mechanisms. The parallel structure is a means of managing and responding to changing internal and external conditions. It also provides an opportunity for persons occupying positions at various hierarchical levels in the bureaucratic structure, and across functional areas, to participate in organizational designs.

The **parallel design** is one we commonly see being used by organizations implementing CQI/TQM (continuous quality improvement/total quality management) approaches. CQI/TQM places the clients or patients and their concerns at the center of the organization. The parallel side of the organization is often headed by a quality council made up of members of the bureaucratic side of the organization. The quality council then identifies areas where CQI/TQM teams may be established to investigate work processes where improvements in client services can be made. Representation on the teams is drawn from all levels in the hierarchy and from all departments that are involved in the work process under investigation. An example of a parallel structure for an acute general hospital is shown in Figure 10.7.

Advantages of the parallel structure to individual staff members are perceived to include expansion of their power, opportunities to affect the organization's decisions, the feeling of being involved in organizational issues, and the potential for individual growth through broadening of the range of work activities. Advantages to the organization are potentially those of increased performance and quality. Some possible disadvantages of the parallel structure are: (1) organization members may spend too much time in meetings, thus increasing costs of operations; (2) the parallel structure may begin to assume responsibilities for routine decisions, consequently overriding the bureaucratic structure; and (3) conflicts over perceived priorities and resource allocation may occur between the bureaucratic and parallel structures.

Product/Service Line or Program Design

Product-line management is defined as the placement of a person in charge of all aspects of a given product or group of products. An organization form that is well accepted among manufacturing, pharmaceutical, and health care supply organization, this type of structure has gained popularity among hospitals. The product line is a revenue and cost center, and the person in charge is responsible for all budgetary and financial responsibilities associated with the product. The person is also responsible for coordinating all the functional resources (e.g., planning, marketing, human resources) required to successfully manage the product line. Product-line management can provide important advantages by increasing operational efficiencies and enhancing market share. Operational efficiencies can be gained by analyzing cost and revenues across related product lines so that redundancies will be eliminated and synergies captured. Market share can be enhanced by targeting marketing strategies to the group of products and being able to promote these to different segments of the market as appropriate (e.g., the elderly, women, and children).

The major challenges health services organizations face in implementing product-line management include educating the relevant groups to the change, choosing criteria for grouping the products, and selecting and training the product-line managers. These changes require board and top management support and appropriate involvement and support of key leaders throughout the organization. People must

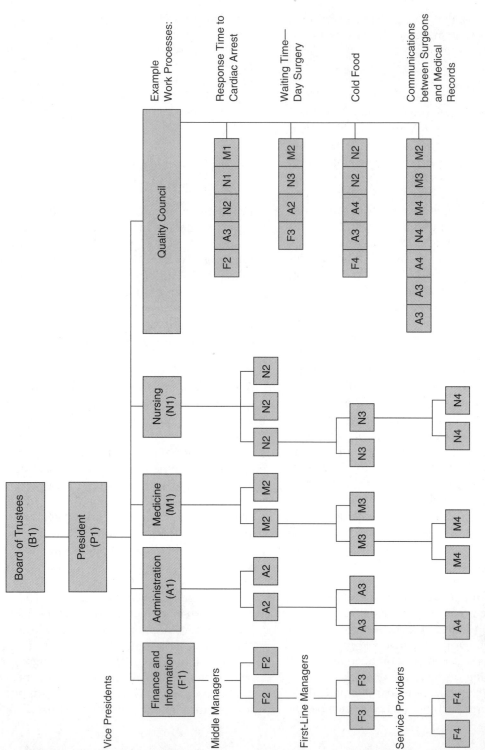

Figure 10.7. A Parallel Design: An Acute General Hospital

see it as a better way to manage resources, maintain or enhance quality, and increase overall value.

While many criteria can be used for grouping products, the most common are similarity of technology, markets, production process, distribution process, and use of human resources. By grouping products with these kinds of similarities, economies of scale and synergies (2 + 1 = 5 solutions) can be generated. Based on these criteria, for example, a hospital can consider the following product-line candidates: women's health, oncology, cardiology, rehabilitation, substance abuse, long-term care, and health promotion.

The selection and training of the product-line managers is particularly important. Individuals must be identified who have good technical knowledge of the product line and good analytical and interpersonal skills. In particular, they must be innovative, feel comfortable with ambiguity and complexity, and be able to work with more than one manager. The latter is reflected in Figure 10.8. This chart shows a matrix-type organization in which the product-line

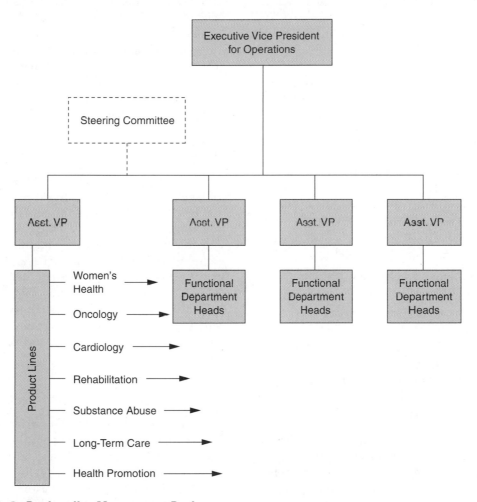

Figure 10.8. Product-line Management Design

managers work with both the functional department heads and the product-line assistant vice president. Recognizing that many problems and issues cut across the product lines, hospitals may establish a committee to deal with these issues. This committee can be composed of both product-line managers and functional department heads charged with reviewing the overall performance of the product lines and recommending addition, deletion, or modification of existing product lines.

Key success factors for this **product-line or program design** include (Leatt, Lemieux-Charles, & Aird, 1994):

- A strong management information system that links clinical, financial, and volume data by product
- A strong budgeting financial system that can disaggregate costs and revenues so that accountability can be appropriately assigned
- Reward systems to encourage innovation and risk taking
- Relevant clinical involvement of physicians, nurses, and other health professionals to deal with new technology, diagnosis and treatment patterns, quality, and patient convenience issues
- A strong support staff, particularly in the areas of marketing, finance, and planning
- The need to align authority and responsibility
- The need for integrative mechanisms that cut across product lines; hence, the development of the steering committee
- The need for a concerted management development program that emphasizes the ability to work with more than one manager, communication skills, conflict management skills, computer literacy, and creativity

Whether the product-line structure has an impact in actual operation within a hospital setting remains to be determined. A recent study of 11 general hospitals (Young, Charns & Heeren, 2004) suggests that a product-line structure was not associated with service quality or innovation and was negatively associated with human resource outcome such as professional development and job satisfaction.

INFLUENCES ON FUTURE ORGANIZATION DESIGNS

Based on the previous sections, a number of suggestions can be made about particular factors, somewhat unique to health services organizations, which may influence design decisions. These factors are generic and are likely to vary in importance through time and in various geographic locations. These influences may be classified according to whether they originate from the mission, environment, organization, culture, human resources, or the political process (see Figure 10.2).

The Mission

The most important factor relating to the mission of health services organizations is concerned with the level of specificity of the mission in determining what will be an appropriate design. As noted previously, health services organizations are beginning to narrow their focus and identify key market-driven areas in which they will operate. The move to identify specific target populations where inputs and health outcomes can be measured is a trend toward increasing the accountability of organizations for a social contract with the community.

The Future Environment

The future environment for most health services organizations is predicted to be both complex and dynamic (see Chapters 1, 2, and 15). A variety of pressures will be exerted externally that will, by necessity, influence design decisions. Some of the most important pressures will be as follows:

- Changing demographic characteristics of the population being served with an increase in the proportion of elderly persons needing services

- Greater sophistication of the general public and consumers of health services in terms of their demands on the system

- Increasing range of services being provided outside of traditional hospitals including ambulatory care programs, home care, long-term care, community health centers, and so on

- Growing involvement with the community to address underlying health issues, such as teenage pregnancy, substance abuse, and violence

- Increasing competition among health services organizations providing similar services in the same geographic location to maximize their market share

- Increasing attempts by governments at all levels to regulate the quantity and quality of services provided

- Changing systems of reimbursement to health services organizations to control costs

- Expanding private-sector involvement in health services organizations to augment services and control costs

- Increasing involvement of trustees, physicians, and other health professionals in the strategic planning and management of health services organizations

- Increasing attempts by external professional associations and accrediting bodies to set standards for professional conduct in health services organizations

- Increasing demand for outcome accountability and greater value

- Increasing focus on patient safety and quality of care by insurers and employer groups

- Rapidly developing medical technologies and proliferation of increasing specialized services

- Increased information demands, development of real-time information-processing systems to re-

late to the external environment, and growth of artificial intelligence systems

The Organization

Internal to most health services organizations are a series of structural and operating processes that provide opportunities or constraints on design decisions. For example:

- Greater emphasis on teamwork

- Greater accountability for the governance of the organization in terms of a social contract

- Increasing corporatization of the structure of health services organizations

- Demands to improve the quality of care

- Demands to control costs, operate efficiently, and increase productivity and overall value

- Increasing need for comprehensive and integrated clinical and financial information systems

- Constrained financial resources

- Changing working relationships to create more situations with two or more supervisor systems

- Increasing use of information technology in the workplace

- Increasing need to coordinate activities internally and to manage conflict creatively

- Increasing recognition of the need for interorganizational collaboration among public and private organizations to more effectively deal with preventable diseases such as SARS, influenza, and AIDS and the challenges of community disasters

Culture

As radical reform takes place in health services organizations, the culture of organizations will also change. The values that are held in high esteem will be modified. For example:

- Increasing emphasis on the "customer" with implementation of processes for patient-centered care

- Increasing use of patient-client satisfaction surveys to modify care processes
- Greater emphasis on the development of broad sets of indicators (such as the balanced scorecard) to monitor performance
- Increasing understanding of the value of community-based care
- Increasing use of evidence, such as health outcome measures to modify care processes
- Increasing emphasis on challenging traditional ways of doing things and the willingness to experiment
- Value of employees who are committed to the organization
- Value of employees who are adaptable and able to embrace change
- Increasing value will be placed on nonhierarchical leaders who can lead change processes
- Increasing emphasis on cultures that facilitate teamwork and collaboration with nontraditional partners
- Increasing value of the need to integrate functions and clinical processes
- Increasing importance of physicians and other health professions to collaborate in developing trust in health services organizations
- Increasing attention to creating a culture for patient safety and ethical issues

Human Resources

The particular characteristics of employees and other service providers available now or in the future may strongly affect the types of design decisions that may be made. For example:

- Acute shortage of nursing personnel in most specialties
- Greater emphasis on cross-skill training versus traditional professional training
- Greater emphasis on horizontal teams and collaborative practices

- Greater pressure to substitute less costly health care workers for more expensive health professionals
- Greater numbers of women in managerial positions requiring flexibility such as accessibility of day care and job sharing
- Greater ethnic and cultural diversity of the workforce
- Greater need to experiment with new work arrangements such as self-managed work teams and CQI/TQM strategies
- Many physicians who historically have had considerable autonomy becoming employees
- Shortages of key health services professionals; for example, pharmacists, physical therapists, and occupational therapists
- Increasing need for managers with professional training
- Increasing unionization of workers in health services organizations
- Closer scrutiny by unions as some health services organizations undergo retrenchment
- Increasing need to educate all levels in strategic management and in adopting a marketing orientation
- The need for succession planning, career planning, and management development programs linked more closely to the organization's strategic plan
- Escalating pressures to provide continuing education programs to health professionals, especially clinical managers

The Political Process

Because of the uncertainty and ambiguities that may exist in health services organizations and the variety of professional groups involved, the informal network within organizations may be particularly active. Informal leaders may be especially helpful to managers in identifying how a change in organization design might be received. Informal leaders may be useful in communicating ideas about change to the grassroots level in the organization or in repressing incorrect rumors that could damage the implementation process. Through the informal network, managers can identify which units or departments might be most or least receptive and attempt to involve key players in the redesign process. Additional suggestions are discussed in Chapter 9.

Although these factors are perhaps not applicable in all circumstances, they are potentially important when considering a new organization design. Most importantly, they emphasize the need for designs that are flexible and that can breathe and grow with the organization.

ORGANIZATIONS IN TRANSITION

Life Cycles

Until now, our discussion has focused on the importance of designing organizations in keeping with their mission, environment, information needs, culture, human resources, and politics; however, these factors all change. To a certain extent, organizations go through relatively predictable cycles that have different design implications. For example, Starkweather and Kisch (1971) suggested four phases through which health services organizations pass. The first is the search phase, which is characterized by newness, innovation, and a sense of ascendancy as the organization procures resources and seeks to establish its identity. The design of an organization in this phase is typically open and informal. The success phase is characterized by achievement in procuring patients, staff, and financial resources. The design of the organization during this phase becomes somewhat more formalized to manage the usually larger scale of operation. The bureaucratic phase is characterized by a relatively rigid conformity to rules and procedures; the organization is isolated from its clients in that it receives little feedback from them. During this phase

the organization may begin to decline because of its inability to respond to changes in the environment or to alter the environment to fit its needs. The succession phase is characterized by the development of new ways of providing services, often through the development of new units within the organization.

Kimberly and Miles (1980) raise important questions about organization design issues associated with each stages of the life cycle. Given that managers wish to design organizations for optimal performance, it makes sense that different designs are more appropriate at different stages of an organization's development. For example, a functional structure might be appropriate for a new organization during its search phase. As the organization grows, achieves success, and perhaps diversifies, a different design such as a product-line or program design may be appropriate. During periods of temporary or permanent decline, the organization may need to consider the appropriateness of a parallel design to help generate new ideas and maintain quality of services. These issues are critically important for organizational viability as demonstrated in the challenges facing the Oriole Women's Shelter (see Debate Time 10.1).

Designs for Quality Improvement

Given the highly competitive environment of health services organizations in the United States, Canada, and worldwide, quality of care has become an increasingly important differentiator. Quality has always been a focus of discussion, debate, and concern within the medical profession; however, its prominence in discussions and debates recently and more generally reflects both concern that quality may slip in the face of efforts to "manage care" and a search on the part of payers for value in what they purchase. The former is fueled by a number of recent, highly publicized cases of alleged abuse by managed care organizations, while the latter is influenced by the development of capabilities—still primitive—permitting measurement and comparison

DEBATE TIME 10.1   What Do You Think?

The Oriole Women's Shelter is a not-for-profit corporation and registered charity that began its operation in 1984 as a crisis-care facility for physically and emotionally abused women and their children. The staff is organized as a feminist collective and works in conjunction with a volunteer board of directors. The collective was founded by a group of women and frontline social agency workers concerned about this unmet need within their community. Some had been victims of domestic violence; others came to the group because of feminist social philosophy and commitment to effect change at a grassroots level. The total annual budget for the facility is approximately $1.4 million. The mission statement of the shelter states:

The Oriole Women's Shelter is committed to reducing the incidence of violence and oppression against women and children. It is an emergency crisis facility for abused women and the children, which provides safety counseling, information, advocacy, and other assistance in a supportive environment, in times of personal or family crisis. Community outreach and political action are significant components of the collective's work.

The population served by the shelter is extremely diverse ethnically, and significant proportions are refugees and new immigrants to the country. Issues that have arisen include the need for increased funding for translation services, ethnic foods, and more staff to accompany residents to legal, immigration, and other interviews. Residents and staff addressed serious issues surrounding racism in addition to the emotional, mental, and physical stresses of working with clients who have been victims of abuse.

The problem of physical and emotional abuse of women and children by men has become more widely publicized in the years that the shelter has

been in operation. This publicity has led to increased success with in-house fundraising, as well as greater ease in obtaining government funding for the work of the shelter. Nevertheless, the slumping economy of the past year has taken a toll on all publicly funded programs, with the shelter being no exception.

From its inception, the shelter has rejected the concept of a traditional hierarchical structure, which is believed by the founders and staff to reflect a male-dominated social structure that has contributed to power imbalances in society. These imbalances are felt to allow segments of the population to be oppressed and abused. Instead, the staff is structured as a collective, with decisions made on the basis of consensus. The key characteristics of a **collectivist-democratic organization** are described in Table 10.4 (Rothchild & Allen, 1989). All staff (11 full-time equivalents) receives the same salary, regardless of prior education, experience, or seniority within the organization. There is no identified manager, no model of supervision; performance reviews are controversial and conducted by the collective in the context of staff meetings. Weekly staff meetings are facilitated in turn by collective members. The meetings tend to be long, emotionally charged, and perceived by some to be inefficient in conducting the business of the collective. Decision making is laborious and in many cases inconsequential.

Staff interactions have become exhausting and time-consuming. Staff meetings therefore evoke negative emotional reactions from the collective members. Fears of isolation or appearing to be out of tune with the culture of the organization are regularly expressed, and there is a tendency to see fault as lying elsewhere.

Anyone who assumes a leadership role, proffers skills or competence in certain areas, or expresses a political viewpoint that counters the prevailing attitude is seen as attempting to take control. Having power is seen as negative and abusive and a source of anxiety or fear on the part of those who perceive themselves as not having power. Although there is a strong commitment in principle to the collective process, many staff members believe that an informal hierarchy does exist. This has its basis along lines of seniority, race, personal characteristics, and depth of commitment to the political beliefs of feminism and collectivism.

The board consists of eight professional and businesswomen who could be described as successful in their respective professions. (Men are not accepted as board or staff, and a release regarding this policy has been obtained from the Human Rights Commission.) The personal and corporate culture of members of the board is typically hierarchical, and they are often in conflict with the organizational culture of the shelter. All agree with and support the concepts of feminism and collectivism but have difficulty reconciling the legal and practical requirements for structure with the collective's wish for its values to be supported and honored. Lack of accountability, responsibility, and commitment to task completion are problems identified by the board, which relate to the collective structure as it now stands.

During the past three years, there have been increasing difficulties with intrastaff and staff-board communication, perceived staff stress, and anger in the workplace. Serious problems have arisen in the areas of administrative activity and accountability. No single individual willingly accepts responsibility for specific tasks or assignments. Although attempts have been made to address individual issues, no long-term or comprehensive solutions have been achieved.

1. What is the nature of decision making in this organization? What are its strengths and weaknesses?
2. Is designated leadership essential to the operation of an organization? Can power and accountability be shared?
3. What might be the impact of a formal organization design on this organization?
4. What mechanisms might preserve the values or culture of the organization while facilitating decision making?

Adapted from Zahn, C. and B. Quinn (July, 1991). The Oriole Women's Shelter, Unpublished Paper, University of Toronto, Toronto, Canada.

---

of the clinical performance of both individual and institutional providers. Health care organizations of all types are under pressure to improve the quality of the products and services they provide—and to be able to demonstrate the quality of what they do.

Managers need to recognize that quality is an organizational problem; that is, variation in quality is as much due to the way in which care is organized and coordinated as it is to the competence of individual caregivers. In order to improve quality, new organization designs need to be developed, designs that emphasize the importance of organizing work around the patient and of reframing the role of the hospital in the context of a system of health services provided in multiple settings.

To accomplish this, managers need to understand that while the strategic issue of medical intervention is important, as important as the issue of how the medical intervention is carried out—the logistical component of care. The latter is not simply a matter of logistics but is a complex systemic problem requiring cooperation among all

Table 10.4. Comparisons of Two Ideal Types of Organization

Dimension	Bureaucratic Organization	Collectivist-Democratic Organization
1. Authority	1. Authority resides in individuals by virtue of incumbency in office or expertise; hierarchical organization of offices. Compliance is to universal fixed rules as these are implemented by office incumbents.	1. Authority resides in the collectivity as a whole; delegated, if at all, only temporarily and subject to recall. Compliance is to the consensus of the collective, which is always fluid and open to negotiation.
2. Rules	2. Formalization of fixed and universalistic rules; calculability and appeal of decisions on the basis of correspondence to the formal, written law.	2. Minimal stipulated rules; primacy of ad hoc, individuated decisions; some calculability possible on the basis of knowing the substantive ethics involved in the situation.
3. Social control	3. Organizational behavior is subject to social control, primarily through direct supervision or standardized rules and sanctions, tertiarily through the selection of homogeneous personnel, especially at top levels.	3. Social controls are primarily based on personalistic or moralistic appeals and the selection of homogeneous personnel.
4. Social relations	4. Ideal of impersonality, relations are to be role-based, segmental, and instrumental.	4. Ideal of community; relations are to be wholistic; personal, of value in themselves.
5. Recruitment and advancement	5a. Employment based on specialized training and formal certification.	5a. Employment based on friends, social-political values, personality attributes, and informally assessed knowledge and skills.
	5b. Employment constitutes a career, advancement based on seniority or achievement.	5b. Concept of career advancement not meaningful; no hierarchy of positions.
6. Incentive structure	6. Remunerative incentives are primary.	6. Normative and solidarity incentives are primary; material incentives are secondary.
7. Social stratification	7. Isomorphic distribution of prestige, privilege, and power (i.e., differential rewards by office); hierarchy justifies inequality.	7. Egalitarian; reward differentials, if any, are strictly limited by the collectivity.
8. Differentiation	8a. Maximal division of labor: dichotomy between intellectual work and manual work and between administrative tasks and performance tasks.	8a. Minimal division of labor; administration combined with performance tasks; division between intellectual and manual work reduced.
	8b. Maximal specialization of jobs and functions; segmental roles. Technical expertise is exclusively held; ideal of the specialist-expert.	8b. Generalization of jobs and functions; wholistic roles. Demystification of expertise: ideal of the amateur generalist.

SOURCE: Rothchild, J., & Allen, W. J. (1989). *The cooperative workplace. Potentials and dilemmas of organizational democracy and participation.* Cambridge University Press. Reprinted with the permission of Cambridge University Press.

parties. The role of the physician is to conceptualize the care required, while other health care personnel—rather than being simply followers of physicians' orders—become problem-solvers who are necessarily closely linked in their work to physicians.

If the patient trajectory is to become the focus, interfaces between and among hospital services and between these services and logistical services must be a primary concern. If the patient trajectory is the focus, intermediate levels of structure may be required to coordinate relations among work units or with other parts of the hospital structure. Similarly, since management of the patient trajectory is everyone's responsibility, an increasing amount of cross-functional interaction is required. All of this implies changing existing patterns, formal and informal—in other words, changing design.

Effective designs for quality improvement take into account the system's rigidity and partition-ing, the central position given to patients and their treatments, and the flows of information within the system. It is the integration of *all* these elements within a single framework that is the challenge for managers. Developments within the Veterans Healthcare System illustrates the dramatic effect changes in organizational design can have on both efficiency and effectiveness (see In Practice, below).

Organizational designs evolve and change over time. As illustrated by the evolving events at Intermountain Health Care (see In Practice, below), managers need to continuously examine accountability relationships within their organizations to ensure that it is clear who is responsible for which aspects of organizational functioning. An appropriate organizational design and a compatible culture are two ways in which senior managers can promote organizational efficiency and effectiveness.

IN PRACTICE   The Veterans Healthcare System

The Veterans Healthcare System (VHA), the largest fully integrated system in the United States, began a redesign effort in 1995 (Kizer, 1999; Young, 2000). The overall goal in redesigning was to systematize quality management (QM) to ensure the provision of consistent and predictable high-quality access by patients to the entire system. The VHA has four well-articulated missions: (1) improving the health and functioning of America's veterans and reducing the burden of illness, injury, and disability of those conditions related to their service in the armed forces of the United States (especially those conditions resulting from combat); (2) conducting education and training programs that enhance the quality of care provided to veterans; (3) conducting research that will enhance the care of veterans;

and (4) providing contingent backup to the Department of Defense medical system during times of war and providing assistance to public health services and the national disaster medical system in providing medical assistance in times of disasters.

It is estimated that about 10 percent of the U.S. population are veterans, totaling approximately 25.6 million people. The decision to reengineer the system of health care for this large population came about for a number of reasons including pressures from the external environment such as the market-based restructuring of health care in general, growth of scientific and biomedical knowledge, general dissatisfaction with health care (especially VHA), consumer expectations for

(continues)

IN PRACTICE *(continued)*

quality, and many managerial and operational problems. Examples of these problems are shown in Table 10.5.

Because of these factors the VHA embarked on an ambitious process to redesign the health system in order to improve effectiveness and efficiency in day-to-day operations and bring about a quality transformation. During 1994 and 1995 various planning efforts and consensus-building activities were carried out to design and begin to implement a new operating structure. The structure changed the basic operating unit within the system from individual hospitals and medical centers to 22 regional networks called Veterans Integrated Service Networks (VISNs). Funding of operations was then allocated on the basis of populations, and care patterns began to shift away from acute hospitals. The VHA system also began to increase collaboration with the private sector and other government-funded health care providers. These changes were a fundamental shift from the VAs former disease-oriented, hospital-based, and professional discipline-based paradigms to ones that are patient-centered, prevention-oriented, community-based, and premised on universal primary care. In the new system multidisciplinary teams had shared responsibility and accountability for patient care.

Results

The new organizational design was implemented in several stages. As noted previously, an extensive strategic planning process was carried out that included assessment of the external and internal environment, the organization's mission, vision, values, and culture. In the second stage, the new integrated service was operationalized, a network management structure was implemented, decision

making was decentralized, funding was allocated on a capitation basis, and new service models were introduced.

Although the VHA's transformation was an evolving process, early results have suggested a remarkable level of achievement. Between 1994 and 1998 (approximately), some of the successes were:

- Fifty-two percent (27,319 of 52,315) of all VHA acute care hospital beds were closed.
- VHA's bed-days of care per 1,000 patients decreased 62 percent. The current VHA rate is now about 5 percent lower than the projected Medicare rate for the same time period.
- Universal primary care has been implemented, and by March 1998, 80 percent of patients could identify their primary caregiver.
- Annual inpatient admissions were 32 percent (284,596), while ambulatory care visits per year increased 43 percent (from 25.0 to 35.8 million per year).
- The management and operation of 50 hospitals have been merged into 24 locally integrated health care systems.
- There were 216 new community-based outpatient clinics established to improve access to care. The clinics were funded from redirected savings—that is, there have been no "new" funds provided for these clinics.
- Surgeries performed on an outpatient basis increased from 35 percent to 75 percent of all surgeries. This change was accompanied by increased surgical productivity and reduced mortality.
- Systemwide staffing was decreased by 11 percent (23,112 of 206,578 full-time employee equivalents), whereas the number of

patients treated per year increased by 18 percent. This included 8 percent more psychiatric/substance abuse treatment patients, 19 percent more homeless patients, and 53 percent more blind rehabilitation patients.

■ Telephone-linked care ("call centers") has been implemented at all VA medical centers, as well as temporary lodging ("hotel") beds.

■ Over 2700 (67 percent) VHA forms were eliminated, and all remaining forms and directives were put on CD-ROM or other electronic means.

■ A pharmacy benefits management program has produced an estimated cumulative savings of $347 million.

The third and continuing stage of implementation has focused on issues of quality of care and patient safety. VHA has implemented a patient

safety improvement process with some of the elements shown in Table 10.6.

In conclusion, in 2003, Jha, Perlin, Kizer, and Dudley reported on an assessment of changes in quality of care indicators at VHA from 1994 through 2000 and compared these results for the VHA with the quality of care afforded by the Medicare fee for service system using the same quality indicators. Results showed VA patients were receiving appropriate care at 90 percent or greater for 9 of 17 quality indicators. These findings suggest that changing an organizational design that matches the characteristics of the external and internal environments and is in keeping with the vision and missions of the organization can increase the outcomes of the organization in terms of quality of services. (For additional information see http://www. va.gov.)

Table 10.5. Critical Problems of the "Old" Veterans Health Care System

■ Hospital-focused and specialist-based, resulting in uncoordinated and episodic treatment of illness

■ Independent, competing medical centers not functioning as or realizing the benefits of being a system

■ Substantial and unexplainable inter-facility and inter-provider variability in the provision of care

■ Difficult to access

■ Centralized and hierarchical management structure that suppressed innovation and was too slow in making decisions

■ An inefficient bureaucracy governed by volumes of rigid policies and procedures

■ Too inwardly focused

■ A very complex resource allocation system that perpetuated unnecessary inpatient care and other inefficiencies

■ Inconsistent leadership

■ Management, capital asset, and resource use decisions too often based on political considerations

Table 10.6. Elements of the VHA's Patient Safety Improvement Initiative

Establishment of high-level Office of Patient Safety

Development of a Patient Safety Reporting Analysis and Feedback System that includes:

     Revision and expansion of former Patient Incident Reporting System

     Establishment of a Patient Safety Expert Advisory Committee

     Implementation of pilot projects using Patient Safety Reports

Implementation of a National Patient Safety Improvement Oversight Committee at VHA headquarters

Initiation of a Patient Safety Awards Program

Establishment of a Center for Lessons Learned

Imposition of a continuing education requirement in quality improvement and patient safety

Development and/or implementation of specific interventions such as

     A nationwide policy on the presence of concentrated KCl for injection in patient care areas

     Blood transfusion bar coding

     National medication administration system (bar coding for medication administration)

     Computerized drug interaction system

     Computerized physician order entry

     Year 2000 compliance project

     Reengineering the VHA's internal safety alert process

Patient Safety Improvement Research Projects and Centers of Inquiry

Convening of the National Patient Safety Partnership

Provision of support for other programs

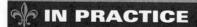 **IN PRACTICE**   Sustaining Quality Improvement Efforts Through Evolving Organizational Designs: The Case of Intermountain Health Care

History of Clinical Care Management at IHC

Intermountain Health Care (IHC) is lauded as a leader in clinical quality improvement among delivery systems. IHC's approach to clinical-care management changed course in 1995 when then IHC executive vice president Bill Nelson (now CEO) challenged Brent James (executive director of IHC's Institute for Health Care Delivery research) to fuse his "science projects"—Nelson's pet term for the proliferation of clinical and managerial quality improvement projects across IHC over the past nine years—into a comprehensive clinical management model. James explained, "There was a sentinel moment when we realized that our business was clinical medicine." He continued, "A big hindrance to quality improvement in health care centers around deployment . . . you tend to get these silo projects that just don't spread." Clinical process management would replace the previous piecemeal approach to improvement in health care delivery.

Interest in Quality Improvement

Reflecting on his tenure at IHC, James noted that IHC had begun to tinker with the concept of clinical-care management in 1986, with a series of investigations called QUE (quality, utilization, and efficiency) studies, which was classic health services research examining variation in clinical practice. While conducting the QUE studies, James attended a lecture by Dr. W. Edward Deming, known as the father of TQM, who introduced a "crazy" idea: Deming argued that higher quality could lead to lower cost. James returned to Salt Lake City and tested Deming's cost-quality hypothesis in preexisting IHC clinical trials: "We just started to add cost outcomes to our traditional clinical trials and proved it true within a few months." James realized that it was due to a "Godsend" that he was able to collect cost outcomes: In the early 1980s Steven Busboom in finance and Poulsen in business strategic planning had decided that they needed to measure the cost of clinical care. Busboom and Poulsen built an activity-based cost accounting system and implemented it across all facilities in the IHC system. James was able to attach costs to individual clinical activities and then build a cost profile of different strategies for managing a particular clinical condition.

Senior management within IHC felt they could realize Deming's maxim by allowing their physician population to self-manage. In 1986, Dr. Steve Lewis, a pulmonary intensivist and IHC's senior vice president for medical affairs, led the formation of The Great Basin Physician Corporation, similar to a Preferred Provider Organization (PPO) structure for community physicians within IHC. According to James, the model's emphasis on self-governance and protocols for care "helped pull the physicians together, but it never really materialized. It sort of died quietly on its own."

In 1998, IHC began to use outcomes data to hold IHC-associated employed and nonemployed professionals accountable for their clinical performance and to enable IHC to set and achieve clinical improvement goals. In 1999, the strategic task was to align financial incentives. To avoid passing on all the savings generated by clinical improvement to the payers, Burton and James found it necessary to build and test strategies to harvest part of those savings back to IHC Health Services and IHC's associated independent physicians, thereby making clinical management financially stable. Finally, in 2000, the board of trustees instructed IHC's senior management to roll Clinical Integration out across all operational functions.

Change Infrastructure

To facilitate the transition from a traditional management structure focused on managing the facilities where clinical care took place, to one oriented around clinical quality and clinical processes, Burton and James built a clinical administrative structure to be the clinical

(continues)

IN PRACTICE (continued)

counterpart of the administrative structure at each level in the organization.

Guidance Councils

The Guidance Councils were built around physician-nurse leadership dyads based in IHC's three urban regions. In each region, a Clinical Program physician leader was selected from practicing physicians. IHC bought one-quarter of their time for Clinical Program leadership activities, and provided additional training in quality management, leadership, and financial skills. A full-time nurse manager dealt with routine administrative matters and provided a direct link to clinical staff. The physician-nurse dyads within each region had two major responsibilities: meeting with clinical-care delivery groups that executed any of the key clinical processes in their Clinical Program and meeting with line administrative management structures in the region. See Figure 10.9.

Development Teams

Within each of the Guidance Councils were one or more permanent Development Teams that focused on select clinical processes. Guidelines, or protocols for specific procedures, were created by Development Teams; sent to the front lines for implementation, data collection, and review; and updated as results traveled back up the pyramid. Each Development Team comprised a physician leader, nurse, and physician team members drawn from frontline care deliverers who would actually implement any protocols the team developed, and a "core work group" of three or four expert physicians dedicated to following research around that specific key clinical process.

Integrated Management Structure

Having built a new clinical management structure parallel to the existing line management, James planned to merge the two over time. His strategy for merging the two structures was to encourage interdependence so the groups would realize "they have to be joined at the hip." Both branches of the parallel structure reviewed clinical goals and assessed outcome data according to their level of focus (i.e., individual physician, practice group, or region). Figure 10.10 provides more detail.

James continued, "We build it up parallel, give the medical management structure tight links and shared goals with the traditional administration, and then let the two management structures collapse together, into a single structure. We hope that over time they will experience and see the redundancy and ask themselves, 'Why are we holding two meetings?' and merge of their own accord."

James realized that it would take at least ten years to fully consolidate the clinical management structure and get all components of Clinical Integration running; however, that period was negligible compared to how long it would take to get IHC's physicians to subscribe to the concept. He commented, "Dr. W. Edwards Demming once said, 'If you want to convert the culture of an organization, and that organization contains *n* people, you first need to convert the square root of *n*.' Well, he should have added, 'You specifically need the early adopters.' It's not just any square root of *n*. I've got about 1,200 core physicians, so the square root is somewhere between 30 and 40. There was a palpable change in the medical staff when we crossed that number. It wasn't just Brent James, partially tainted by being over in the administration offices, saying that physicians as a profession needed to do this. It was a long list of respected physicians who could say, 'Guys, I've done this in my practice and it really makes *sense*. It's better care for our patients, a better

lifestyle for me, and more productive.' " For more information about IHC, visit *http://www.ihc.com*.

SOURCE: From Bohmer, R. M. J., & Edmondson, A. C. (2003). Intermountain Health Care (Case No. 9-603-066, p. 21). Harvard Business School.

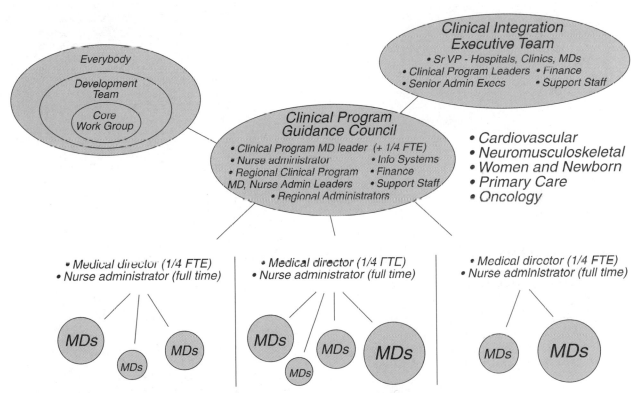

Figure 10.9. Guidance Council Structure: Intermountain Health Care

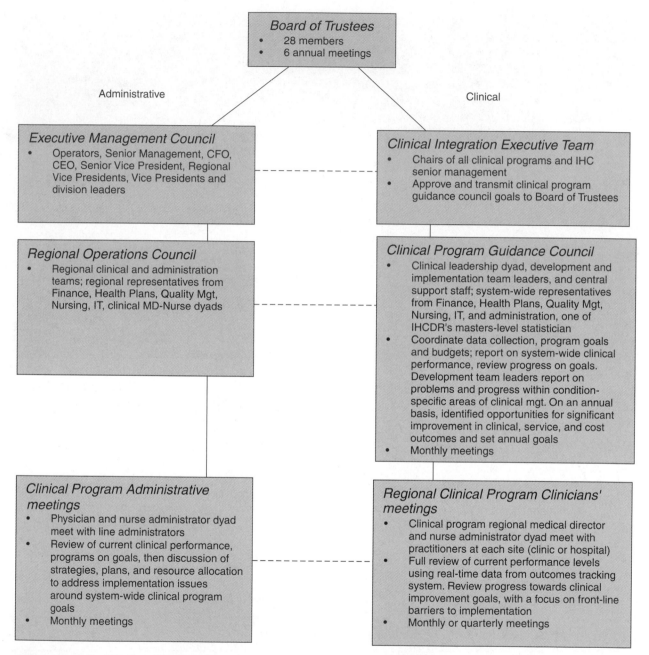

Figure 10.10. Parallel Administrative Structure: Intermountain Health Care

MANAGERIAL GUIDELINES

Design Preparation

- The organization must have a clear understanding of its mission (i.e., it should be clear to everyone what business the organization is in and what it is not).

- The external environment of the organization must be assessed in terms of its uncertainty. The social, technological, political, economic, legal, cultural, and ecological characteristics of the environment could have important consequences for the choice of organization design.

- It is important to understand the strengths and weaknesses of the organization so that the design strategy leverages the organization's competitive advantages.

- It is essential that managers understand the culture(s) of the organization and have a vision for creating a culture for the future that will facilitate organizational change.

- Assessment of the human resources available in the organization is essential to the task of organization design. There must be systematic understanding of the human resource capability, especially at the senior management level. It may be necessary to consider both short- and long-term succession planning as part of the preparation for redesign.

- The informal network inside the organization should be assessed so that key informal leaders can participate in the design process and, therefore, contribute to its success.

Design Process

- Key organizational leaders must anticipate that the process of organization design may take several weeks, months, or years depending upon the individual circumstances of the organization.

- Some organizations may find it useful to establish a task force or a team to consider alternative organization designs. Key members of senior management and major stakeholders may be members of this team, recognizing that the task force is advisory to the CEO. It is often helpful to expand the membership of the task force to selected individuals at other levels of the organization. For example, it may be useful to have representation from middle managers, unions, and client groups.

- An external consultant can also be useful in outlining the design options for the organization. Ultimately the decision on the actual acceptability of the design for the organization rests with the organization.

- It is important to recognize that the building blocks for future organizational designs will likely evolve from the "bottom-up" with individuals designing roles and work groups designing teams.

- During the design process, it is important to identify the ramifications of any new design. Who will stand to gain or lose from the changes being made?

Design Outcome

- Once an appropriate organization design has been agreed upon, it is important that a plan be developed for the communication of the design, its implementation, and evaluation.

- The new design must be communicated to everyone inside and outside the organiza-

(continues)

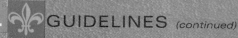

MANAGERIAL GUIDELINES *(continued)*

tion who is likely to be affected by the changes. Many organizations develop elaborate, staged plans to communicate the changes so that the individuals most affected by the design hear first.

■ Implementation of the new design will vary, depending upon how different the new design is from the old one. Implementation may evolve quickly or may be staged during three to five years in large complex organizations when the new design is radically different and when there is a need for extensive education of individuals to fill new roles. All the principles of

implementing change, outlined in Chapter 12, are applicable to implementing new designs.

■ Although not often carried out in the past, it is important to formally monitor the implementation of the design and assess the effect of the design on organizational performance. Recognizing that organization designs exist to help work get done and to achieve the mission of the organization, it is essential that an evaluation process be defined in order to assess the effects on clients, employees, and other relevant stakeholders.

DISCUSSION QUESTIONS

1. You have been hired as an assistant to a new CEO of an academic medical center. You have been asked to recommend a variety of organization designs for the 300-bed inpatient facility. The academic medical center is fully affiliated with the medical school, which is internationally renowned for its work in cardiovascular diseases, neurosciences, and transplant programs. The CEO's main objectives in the reorganization are to decentralize decision making to physicians and other clinicians, to pave the way for more effective information systems for monitoring quality and cost, and to break down traditional barriers between professional hierarchies and groups. What are your recommendations?

2. As administrator of a home care program in a city of 500,000 persons, you are planning

to expand your services. Your program has been in operation for about five years, and until now you have focused on clients with relatively short-term needs. Clients' average length of time in the program is 25 days. The expansion will consist of providing comprehensive services to persons who are chronically ill and who consequently require long-term home care. On the basis of a preliminary survey, you estimate that the size of your program will triple within a year. The chronic-care clients will most likely have problems of the circulatory system, neoplasms, or diseases of the musculoskeletal system. Most clients will need long-term nursing services, physiotherapy, occupational therapy, homemaking services, and a variety of supplies and equipment. Your organization is currently structured according to function (nursing, physiotherapy, homemaking, administration, finance). You have a staff of over 200, but with the new program you will probably need to double your staff. You are wondering about changing your organization design in preparation for the expansion. What would be the advantages and disadvantages of a program design for the home care program? On what basis might you group activities and personnel (e.g., by type of clients, by geographic area of the city, or by services)?

3. Pharmaceutical companies globally are faced by a set of similar strategic and organizational challenges: the cost of the research and development required to develop a new product, the amount of time it takes to get a new product to market, differential regulatory hurdles in different markets, changes in who the purchasers of their products are, and variably complex distribution arrangements from one country to the next. Pick any one of the above challenges and discuss how organization design principles might be used to meet it effectively.

4. You have just taken over the management of a rehabilitation center where the main clientele are those persons requiring rehabilitation services for post-hip and knee replacement surgery, postcardiac surgery, trauma accidents, and head and back injuries. These patients require a range of multidisciplinary services including medical, physical therapy, nursing, occupational therapy, psychology, and social work. How would you go about designing the teams to provide the necessary services?

5. The CEO of an Academic Medical Center has asked you to identify the key features of an organizational design that will facilitate quality services and maximize patient safety. Please prepare a presentation that the CEO can make to the hospital board.

6. Consider an organization you are familiar with (preferably one you have worked in). Reflecting on your experience in this organi-

zation, define at least one problem in its design. What were the symptoms of the problem? What might be (or should have been) done to solve the problem? Why do you think that nothing was done?

REFERENCES

Alexander, J. A., Vaughn, T., Burns, L. R., Zuckerman, H. S., Anderson, R. M., Torrens, P., & Hilberman, D. W. (1996, March). Organizational approaches to integrated health care delivery: A taxonomic analysis of physician-organization arrangements. *Medical Care Research and Review, 53*(1), 71–93.

Bohmer, R. M. J., & Edmondson, A. C. (2003). Intermountain Health Care (Case No. 9-603-066, p. 21). Harvard Business School.

Burns, L. R., Alexander, J. A., & Torrens, P. (1998, Spring). Physicians and organizations: Strange bedfellows or a marriage made in heaven? *Frontiers of Health Services Management, 14*(3), 3–34.

Charnes, M., & Smith-Tewksbury, L. J. (1993). *Collaborative management in health care.* San Francisco: Jossey-Bass.

Daft, R. L. (1998). *Organization theory and design* (6th ed). St. Paul: West Pub. Co.

Davis, J. (2003). Organizational downsizing: A review of literature for planning and research. *Journal of Healthcare Management, 48*(3), 181–199.

Dubbs, N. L. (2002). Organizational design consistency: The PennCARE and Henry Ford Health System experience. *Journal of Healthcare Management, 47*(5), 307–318.

Duncan, R. (1978, Winter). What is the right organization structure? Decision tree analysis provides the answer. *Organizational Dynamics, 7*(4), 59–80.

Edmondson, A., Roberto, M. A., & Tucker, A. (2002). Children's Hospital and Clinics (Case No. 9-302-050). Harvard Business School.

Gaucher, E. J., & Coffey, R. (1993). *Total quality in health care.* San Francisco: Jossey-Bass.

Gellerman, S. W. (1990). In organizations, as in architecture, form follows function. *Organizational Dynamics, 18*(3), 57–68.

Gillies, R. R., Shortell, S. M., & Young, G. L. (1997, Fall). Best practices in managing organized delivery systems. *Hospitals and Health Services Administration, 42*(3), 299–321.

Gittell, J. H., & Weiss, L. (1997, November). *How organization design shapes informal networks: The case of patient care coordination.* Working paper.

Harmon, J., Scotti, D. J., Behson, S., Farais, G., Petzel, R., Newman, J. H., & Keashly, L. (2003). Effects of high-involvement work systems on employee satisfaction and service costs. *Journal of Healthcare Management, 48*(6), 393–405.

Heyssel, R. M., Gaintner, J. R., Kues, I. W., Jones, A. A., & Lipstein, S. H. (1984). Decentralized management in a teaching hospital. *New England Journal of Medicine, 310*(22), 1477–1480.

James, C. R. (2003). Designing learning organizations. *Organizational Dynamics, 32*(1), 46–61

Jha, A. K., Perlin, J. B., Kizer, K., & Dudley, R. A. (2003). Effects of the transformation of the Veterans Affairs Health Care System on the quality of care. *The New England Journal of Medicine, 348*(2), 2218–2227.

Kaluzny, A., Morrissey, J., & McKinney, M. (1990). Emerging organizational networks: The case of the Community Clinical Oncology Program. In S. S. Mick & associates (Eds.), *Innovations in the organization of healthcare: New insights into organizational theory.* San Francisco, CA: Jossey-Bass.

Kaluzny, A. D. (1994). Centralization and decentralization in a vertically integrated system: The XYZ hospital corporation. In D. A. Conrad & G. A. Hoare (Eds.), *Strategic alignment: Managing integrated health systems* (pp. 125–131). Ann Arbor, MI: AUPHA Press/Health Administration Press.

Katzenbach, J. R., & Smith, D. K. (1993). *The wisdom of teams.* Boston: Harvard Business School Press.

Kimberly, J. R. (1984). The anatomy of organizational design. *Journal of Management, 10*(1), 109–126.

Kimberly, J. R., & Miles, R. H. (1980). *The organization life cycle: Issues in the creation transformation and decline of organizations.* San Francisco: Jossey-Bass.

Kimberly, J. R., & Minvielle, E. (2003). Quality as an organizational problem. In S. Mick & M. Wyttenbach (Eds.), *Advances in healthcare organization theory* (pp. 205–232). San Francisco: Jossey-Bass.

Kizer, K. W. (1999). The new VA: A national laboratory for health care quality management. *American Journal of Medical Quality, 14,* 3–20.

Lawrence, P., & Lorsch, J. (1967). *The organization and its environment.* Cambridge, MA: Harvard University Press.

Leatt, P., Baker, G. R., Halverson, P. K., & Aird, C. (1997, Summer). Downsizing, reengineering, and restructuring: Long term implications for health care organizations. *Frontiers in Health Service Management, 13*(4), 2–37.

Leatt, P., Lemieux-Charles, L., & Aird, C. (1994). *Program management and beyond: Management innovations in Ontario hospitals.* Ottawa, Canada: CCHSE.

Leatt, P., & Porter, J. (2003). Where are the healthcare leaders? The need for investment in leadership development. *Healthcare Papers, 4*(1), 14–33.

LeTourneau, B. (2004). Physicians and nurses: Friends or foes? *Journal of Healthcare Management, 49*(1), 12–15.

Longest, B. B. (2003). Strategic management and public policy. In P. Leatt & J. Mapa (Eds.), *Government relations in the health industry* (pp. 23–48). Westport: Greenwood Publishing Group, Inc.

McLaughlin, C. P., & Kaluzny, A. D. (2006). *Continuous quality improvement in health care: Theory, implications and applications,* Third Edition. Sudbury, Massachusetts: Jones and Bartlett.

Melum, M. M., & Sinioris, M. K. (1992). *Total quality management: The health care pioneers.* Chicago: American Hospital Publishing.

Mintzberg, H. (1983). *Structuring in fives: Designing effective organizations.* Englewood Cliffs, NJ: Prentice-Hall.

Mohrman, S. A., Cohen, S. G., & Mohrman, A. M., Jr. (1995). *Designing team based organizations: New form of knowledge work.* San Francisco: Jossey-Bass.

Morath, J. M., (2002). Individual Lifetime Achievement: Julianne M. Morath, RN, MS. Joint Commission Journal on Quality and Patient Safety, 28, (12), 637–645

Morgan, C. (1997). *Images of organization.* Thousand Oaks, CA: Sage Publications.

Nadler, D. A., Gerstein, M. S., Shaw, R. B., et al. (1992). *Organizational architecture: Designs for changing organizations.* San Francisco: Jossey-Bass.

Palmer, R. H., & Reilly, M. C. (1979). Individual and institutional variables which may serve as indicators of quality of medical care. *Medical Care, 17,* 693–717.

Pearce, J. A. (1982, Spring). The company mission as a strategic tool. *Sloan Management Review, 23*(3), 15–24.

Rothchild, J., & Allen, W. A. (1989). *The cooperative workplace: Potentials and dilemmas of organizational democracy and participation.* Cambridge, MA: Cambridge University Press.

Ruchlin, H. S., Dubbs, N. L., & Callahan, M. A. (2004). The role of leadership in instilling a culture of safety: Lessons from the literature. *Journal of Healthcare Management, 49*(1), 47–58.

Scott, W. R. (2003). *Organizations: Rational, natural and open systems,* (5th ed., p. 242). Upper Saddle, NJ: Prentice Hall.

Shortell, S. M., Gillies, R. R., Anderson, D., Erickson, K. M., & Mitchell, J. B. (1996). *Remaking health care in America: Building organized delivery systems.* San Francisco: Jossey-Bass.

Shortell, S. M., Gillies, R. R., Anderson, D., Mitchell, J., & Morgan, K. (1993). Creating organized delivery systems. The barriers and facilitators. *Hospital and Health Services Administration, 38*(4), 447–466.

Siehl, K., & Martin, J. (1990). Organizational culture: A key to financial performance? In B. Schneider (Ed.), *Organizational climate and culture.* San Francisco: Jossey-Bass.

Smith, T., Leatt, P., Effis, P., & Fried, B. (1989). Decentralized hospital management: Rationale, potential and two case examples. *Health Matrix, 7*(1), 11–17.

Starkweather, D., & Kisch, A. (1971). A model of the life cycle dynamics of health service organizations. In M. F. Arnold, L. V. Blankenship, & J. M. Hess (Eds.), *Administering health systems.* New York: Aldine Atherton Press.

Stein, B. A., & Kanter, R. M. (1980). Building the parallel organization: Creating mechanisms for permanent quality of work life. *Journal of Applied Behavioral Science, 16,* 371–386.

Trerise, B., & Lemieux-Charles, L. (1996). An assessment of the introduction of a multiskilled worker into an acute care setting. *Health Care Management Forum, 9*(3), 43–48.

Woolf, S. H. (2004). Patient safety is not enough: Targeting quality improvements to optimize the health of the population. *Annals of Internal Medicine, 140,* 33–36.

Young, G. J. (2000). *Transforming government: The revitalization of the Veterans Health Administration.* The Price Waterhouse Coopers Endowment of the Business of Government.

Young, G. L., Charns, M. P., & Heeren, T. K. (2004). Product-line management in professional organizations: An empirical test of competition theoretical perspectives. *Academy of Management Journal, 47*(5), 723–734.

Zahn, C., & Quinn, B. (1991). The Oriole Women's Shelter. Unpublished Paper, University of Toronto, Toronto Canada.

Zammutto, R. F., & Krakower, J. Y. (1991). *Quantitative and qualitative studies of organizational culture. Research in organizational change and development* (pp. 83–114). Greenwich, CT: JAI Press.

Zuckerman, H. S., Hilberman, D. W., Andersen, R. M., Burns, L. R., Alexander, J. A., & Toreens, P. (1998, Spring). Physicians and organizations: Strange bedfellows or a marriage made in heaven? *Frontiers of Health Services Management, 14*(3), 3–34.

CHAPTER 11

Managing Strategic Alliances

Edward J. Zajac, Ph.D., Thomas A. D'Aunno, Ph.D.,
Lawton R. Burns, Ph.D.

CHAPTER OUTLINE

- Alliances in Health Care
- Types and Forms of Alliances
- What Are Alliances Meant to Do?
- The Alliance Process: A Multistage Analysis
- Frameworks for Analyzing Alliance Problems

LEARNING OBJECTIVES

After completing this chapter, the reader should be able to:

1. Better understand why strategic alliances are increasing in use, particularly among health care organizations.

2. Distinguish between different types or forms of strategic alliances, using a number of dimensions.

3. Classify an alliance both in terms of what it looks like and what it is meant to do.

4. Understand how alliance motivation is often related to alliance structure and outcomes.

5. Identify whether your motivations for a strategic alliance are compatible with those of your alliance partner.

6. Think about strategic alliances in terms of the likely stages of development that alliances often experience and the critical issues that you may face at each stage.

7. Distinguish between an alliance problem and an alliance symptom and recognize the different implications for managerial intervention.

8. Understand both the pros and cons of alliances.

KEY TERMS

Alliance Problems versus
   Symptoms
Cost Reduction versus Rev-
   enue Enhancement
Ownership versus Control

Partner Orientation
Pooling
Strategic Alliance
Symbiotic versus Competitive
   Interdependence

Trading Alliances
Turbulent Environment
Uncertainty Reduction

✢ IN PRACTICE   The Yankee Alliance: Dealing with Adversity and Creating Growth

The Yankee Alliance began in 1984 with a few community hospitals in New England. By 2004, Yankee had grown to include 34 acute care facilities, 409 long-term care facilities, 23 community health centers, 345 home health sites, and 3,000 physicians.

It would be easy—and wrong—to think that Yankee's growth and success provide a simple blueprint for others to follow. Rather, Yankee's 20-year history reveals a great deal of complexity that has challenged its members and the management staff that has guided the Alliance from its inception. Indeed, the issues that Yankee has faced illustrate several key concepts and themes in this chapter.

To begin, though the Alliance had added several hospital members in the years after its founding, by 1995 growth in membership had not only stopped, but the size of the alliance actually decreased. One hospital left the Alliance when it joined a for-profit health system. Some members left due to mergers, and still others decided to join a competing national alliance (Voluntary Hospitals of America [VHA]). Further, some CEOs of member hospitals left their positions, and their replacements were not familiar with the Alliance. As Paul O'Neill, president of Yankee since its founding, put it: "One of the greatest challenges we faced was the changes within our own ranks."

At the same time, changes continued to occur in the environment of the Alliance and its members. Two of these changes figure prominently in Yankee's history. One is that hospital alliances, just like their member hospitals, merged to increase their size and market power. Specifically, in early 1996 there was a merger of three large, mainly hospital-based alliances: Premier, American Healthcare Systems (AmHS), and the Sun Health Alliance. This national alliance is called Premier and includes about one-third of all community hospitals in the nation (1,800 hospitals with 322,000 licensed beds), with $14 billion in annual supply purchases.

Yankee Alliance had been a member of AmHS for ten years. As a result, the merger that created Premier also created new opportunities—but also threats. One clear opportunity for Yankee was to take advantage of the size and market power of the new national alliance. To do this, however, Yankee members had to sign formal letters of commitment that obligated them to comply with contracts that Premier signs with various suppliers of goods and services. To benefit from the market power (lower costs) that comes from shared purchasing of materials, individual organizations must yield some autonomy. Otherwise, alliance size means relatively little.

The threat to Yankee stemmed from the fact that Premier's founding forced individual hospitals and health care systems to consider if they wanted to join Premier or its major competitor, VHA. Premier and Yankee fared well in this competition.

Premier's founding typifies the complexity of alliances in today's health care industry. Local

(continues)

CHAPTER PURPOSE

There is no doubt that the U.S. health care environment is undergoing major changes that could be characterized as turbulent. As illustrated by the challenges confronting the Yankee Alliance, turbulence characterizes rapidly changing environments where: (1) organizations are highly interconnected with one another, and (2) organizations are highly interdependent with the society in which organizations find themselves (Emery & Trist, 1965).

This emphasis on connectedness and interdependence is an important basis for viewing a specific organization's environment not as some amorphous external force but rather as the set of other organizations that are interconnected or interdependent with it. This organization, in turn, is part of the environment for the other organizations. In other words, when an organization looks out with concern or anticipation at its **turbulent environment**, what it sees is other organizations looking out at that organization (Shortell & Zajac, 1990).

This conceptualization of organizational environments suggests the need to focus more attention on how specific organizations interact with one another. This chapter emphasizes one such type of interaction—cooperative interorganiza-

tional relations. Longest (1990), in discussing what he terms "interorganizational linkages in health care," distinguishes between market transactions, voluntary relationships, and involuntary relationships. We focus most of our attention on those interorganizational relations that are noncoercive and entered into primarily for strategic purposes, that is, that are important to an organization's mission and expected to enhance organizational performance. We term such relationships **strategic alliances**, which are defined as any formal arrangements between two or more organizations for purposes of ongoing cooperation and mutual gain/risk sharing.

ALLIANCES IN HEALTH CARE

Alliances are often viewed as facing high failure rates; some claim 50% to 80%. For example, early research has argued that strategic alliances, by their very nature, are risky endeavors (Harrigan, 1985). The cooperative linkages between two or more organizations are viewed as somewhat fragile, exposing each party to the risk that the other party or parties may not continue to cooperate as expected. The business press has also had a penchant for describing, in detail, particular joint ventures or other alliances that failed. The failure of a cooperative alliance between two organizations often involves considerable drama, as interorganizational cooperation turns to conflict and sometimes litigation.

Although it is very important to recognize the pros and cons of alliances (see Debate Time 11.1), we believe that a fixation on the likely failure and inherent riskiness of alliances may be misguided. Specifically, we contend that any assessment of the *risk of strategic alliances* should be balanced with an assessment of the expected return or benefit of the alliance in terms of improved financial performance, innovation, and organizational learning, and the opportunity cost of not engaging in a strategic alliance. Regarding the first point, while financial performance is an obvious outcome to consider when analyzing the success or failure of a strategic alliance, it is not clear that it should be considered the most important, direct outcome. For example, innovation may be a driving force behind strategic alliances, and more generally, alliances may be viewed as a desirable way for organizations to learn about new markets, services, and ways of doing business (Zajac, Golden, & Shortell, 1991). These may actually be negatively correlated with financial performance, at least in the short run (Shortell & Zajac, 1988). This issue is discussed in greater detail in the section on how strategic intentions drive alliance activity.

In terms of opportunity cost, the relevant question is not, Is it risky?, but rather, Which is riskier: going it alone, doing nothing, or engaging in an alliance? Riskiness is not necessarily a problem. For example, the virtues of entrepreneurship are often extolled, despite the high risk and high failure rates involved. Strategic alliances may appear risky when the baseline comparison is not made explicit, but when compared with attempting a *de novo* entry into a new market or ignoring the market altogether, the alliance may actually seem like a relatively low-risk proposition (Shortell & Zajac, 1988). In fact, as subsequently discussed, the creation of a strategic alliance is often motivated by an organization's desire to reduce uncertainty.

The issues just raised are particularly relevant for health care organizations, which have seen an explosion of alliance building in the last few decades (Bazzoli, Chan, Shortell, & D'Aunno, 2000; Olden, Roggenkamp, & Luke, 2002). Alliance building is not limited to hospitals (Alter & Hage, 1993; Zuckerman & Kaluzny, 1991). There are alliances between hospitals and physician groups, between hospitals and health maintenance organizations (HMOs), and between hospitals, physicians, and agencies of the federal government (Kaluzny, Morrissey, & McKinney, 1990; Shortell, 1988). Nor are alliances limited to providers of care. Alliances known as business coalitions have emerged among buyers of care, that is, employers who band together to increase their effectiveness as purchasers of care for their employees. The variety of possible alliance partners is quite high, given the myriad of interdependencies between organizations in the health sector (see Table 11.1).

The causes for this outburst of activity are not difficult to identify. Perhaps the most important and obvious factor is that health care organizations are experiencing what Meyer (1982) has referred to as a series of "environmental jolts." These are relatively abrupt, major, and often qualitative changes in an environment that threaten organizational survival. The introduction of the Medicare Prospective Payment System, for example, qualifies as an environmental jolt and has led to massive changes in the strategies of hospitals in recent years (Shortell, Morrison, & Friedman, 1990; Zajac & Shortell, 1989). Further, a growing number of hospitals have closed. Other jolts include increased competition, a surplus of hospital beds, concern with cost containment, an increase in the number of uninsured patients, an aging population, and the AIDS epidemic.

These jolts create great uncertainty for health care managers. Alliances may reflect the reality that it is sometimes better to face life's uncertainties with partners than to go it alone (Kaluzny, Zuckerman, & Ricketts, 2002; Zuckerman, Kaluzny, & Ricketts,

DEBATE TIME 11.1 What Do You Think?

There are a few facts and many more unknowns about strategic alliances. One fact is that we are witnessing a substantial increase in strategic alliances in health care. An unknown, however, is whether this fact reflects a positive or negative development. An interesting example of an ongoing debate is found in Duncan, Ginter, and Swayne (1992). In this section, we consider some of the arguments swirling around the use of strategic alliances. Kaluzny and Zuckerman (1992) argue on the positive side for alliances, while Begun (1992) offers counterarguments on the negative side. The following list of issues summarizes their points of disagreement.

Positive

1. Alliances reflect a fundamental shift in how health service organizations do business; namely, a change from thinking in terms of control to thinking in terms of commitment, trust, shared risk, and common purpose.

2. Alliances provide organizations with a way to manage growing complexity and interdependence while maintaining a fair amount of individual organizational autonomy.

3. Alliances enable organizations to transcend the existing organizational inertia that is often created by complexity and vested interests seeking to maintain the status quo.

4. Alliances have been found to be effective in other sectors of our society, and failure to apply these concepts to health services would be a missed opportunity for meeting the challenges in the future.

Negative

1. Alliances distract organizations from their basic goal, which is to clobber your competitors or at least behave as if you have that need. Managers like the thrill of the competitive chase, and competition creates loyalty and team spirit in an organization.

2. Alliances are essentially a fad whose benefits have been exaggerated, similar to Theory Z, the pursuit of excellence, product-line management, and total quality management.

3. Alliances can lead to collusion between otherwise competing organizations, can lead to legal problems relating to antitrust challenges, and are attractive only to lazy organizations that are not interested in competition.

4. The process hassles of initiating and managing alliances are tremendous and costly, and these arrangements are quite fragile.

5. Governing an alliance means governing by committee, which we know to be an ineffective way to run a business. In particular, this problem reduces the speed and flexibility of an organization.

6. Cooperative strategy makes sense for large, multinational firms seeking to enter new and unknown markets or share expensive research and development projects, but not for health care organizations that face well-known local markets and do not need to finance much research and development.

Which of the above perspectives do you favor? How would you justify your position?

Table 11.1. Interdependencies Between Organizations in the Health Sector

In the health sector, focal organizations have potential inter-dependencies with organizations such as:

Accrediting agencies
Affiliated organizations
Alternative health systems
Competitors
Confederated organizations
Consortia members
Consumer representatives (public and private)
Employee representatives (unions)
Fiscal intermediaries
Financial organizations (bond rating)
Foundations
Government (all levels)
Health maintenance organizations (HMOs)
Independent practice associations (IPAs)
Insurance companies
Joint venture partners
Media
Physician-hospital organizations (PHOs)
Multi-institutional systems
Other partners
Owners
Political groups
Preferred provider organizations (PPOs)
Suppliers (including capital, consumables, equipment, and human resources)
Third-party association (TPAs)
Trade associations
Utilization management companies

SOURCE: Adapted from Longest B. Interorganizational linkages in the Health Sector. In *Health Care Management Review*, 1990; 15:17–28, with permission of Aspen Publishers, Inc., © 1990.

1995). Of course, alliances are but one response to the environmental changes described above. There has also been a marked increase in other types of multiorganizational arrangements, particularly multihospital systems (Shortell, 1988).

Further, other strategic adaptive responses to environmental change have emerged, including vertical integration and diversification (Clement, 1987). In short, as Starr (1982) argued over twenty years ago, the landscape of the health care field is itself changing: Where there were once many small and independent organizations there are now clusters of organizations, including alliances and other types of multiorganizational arrangements.

TYPES AND FORMS OF ALLIANCES

Alliances vary in regard to ownership, control, size, governance, and nature of participation.

Ownership versus Control

DeVries (1978) and others (e.g., Starkweather, 1971) have arrayed multi-institutional systems on a continuum of more autonomy to more **control**. However, these rankings often really reflect the degree of **ownership**, with complete ownership being equated with the highest form of control. While it seems reasonable to view ownership as related to control, we argue that this can sometimes be misleading.

For example, it is well known that McDonald's Corp. is very interested in maintaining control over its raw materials to ensure that quality is highly consistent. In dealing with its exchange partners who supply these raw materials, one might therefore expect that McDonald's would prefer an interorganizational arrangement that would involve substantial ownership interest in suppliers in order to have greater control. This is not the case, however. Even with no ownership interests, McDonald's simply communicates its quality requirements to the supplier organizations, and the organizations are typically quick to oblige.

How can this be? Two factors seem to be relevant. The first is obvious. McDonald's, by virtue of its size, enjoys substantial relative power in its relationship with suppliers; McDonald's represents a very large portion of a food supplier's business. This obviates, at least in large part, the need for McDonald's to also own some or all of the suppliers' assets. Ownership and control are essentially separated in this case. The second reason has much less to do with the relative power of the organizations involved and more to do with the establishment of a tradition of mutual gain and cooperation. Specifically, McDonald's has made it a policy to be loyal to high-quality suppliers and to use its size to protect the supplier from dramatic swings in sales revenue. In this way, both parties have incentives to ensure a long-term cooperative relationship—with no ownership interests.

This simplified example is not intended to show that ownership and control are usually unrelated, of course. Rather, the example demonstrates that tight control can exist even in cases where there is no ownership interest. In fact, Bazzoli and her colleagues (Bazzoli, Shortell, Dubbs, Chan, & Kralovec, 1999) analyzed all U.S. hospital systems (i.e., two or more hospitals have a common owner) and alliances (i.e., two or more hospitals agree to work together without common ownership) for the years 1994 and 1995 and found that there were alliances that exercised centralized control over a variety of decisions and systems in which control was decentralized. The lesson here is twofold: There are many dimensions upon which one can categorize strategic alliances, and one must exercise caution in interpreting what the dimension really represents. The discussion to follow addresses several additional dimensions upon which one can distinguish one type or form of strategic alliance from another.

Number of Members

Alliances vary greatly in size. They can consist of two organizations, but they often consist of many more. For example, as noted above Premier is a national hospital alliance that now includes 1,800 hospitals. Size makes a substantial difference in several ways. Larger alliances are more difficult to govern because it is more difficult to represent all members on a single board of directors. Larger size may also entail greater diversity among members, which in turn

may make it more difficult to find common ground on important issues ranging from alliance strategy (i.e., what are the overall purpose and goals of the alliance) to the management of alliance programs. Further, even when agreements are reached on alliance strategy and operations, larger size makes it difficult to coordinate members' efforts.

On the other hand, size has virtues. It creates power, as noted earlier. Larger alliances typically have more purchasing power because they can buy in larger volume (assuming, of course, that all members can agree on a particular vendor, which is often difficult). For example, Premier makes $14 billion dollars' worth of purchases per year. Similarly, larger alliances have more clout in lobbying at various levels of government. Further, larger alliances can generate capital easier simply from having a larger number of members' fees to collect.

Nonetheless, the costs and benefits of alliance size are difficult to assess in the abstract. What often matters most in determining an effective size for an alliance is its strategic purpose and particular situation. For example, a local or regional hospital network will have a relatively small number of members compared to other hospital alliances. Yet, it may have exactly the number of members it needs for its purpose, which is to provide the local area with a comprehensive service system.

Governance Structure

In the case of an alliance with two members, it is often not necessary to be concerned about establishing a way to govern alliance activities so as to give them direction. But beyond the simple case of a two-party alliance, governance issues can be considerably complex.

The governing bodies of many alliances, especially hospital alliances, tend to include at least one member from each participating organization, often the director or CEO of the member organization. This practice stems largely from important distinguishing features of alliances; that is, that they are a form of organization in which the members are equal and have a great deal of autonomy.

Further, the boards of health care organizations traditionally have been based on what Fennell and Alexander (1989) term a philanthropic model, which assumes that "bigger is better." In other words, boards were viewed as a key link to the local community and its resources; having more individuals on a board provided a hospital, for example, with greater community support and access to donors. Similarly, we have observed that alliance boards often are large so as to represent various interest groups.

Indeed, as Carman (1992) reports, alliance boards often have physician representatives, board members from participating organizations, and community members as well. Moreover, Carman argues persuasively that alliance boards should not consist entirely of CEOs. He points out that there is enough turnover among CEOs so as to create instability for an alliance if its governance rests only with them (Alexander, Fennell, & Halpern, 1993). In contrast, organizational commitment to the alliance is enhanced if it is represented in alliance governance by leaders other than CEOs.

As just noted, however, this means that larger alliances can have boards with dozens of members that, in turn, can make it difficult to achieve consensus and can slow decision making. Of course, large alliance boards can, and sometimes do, have executive committees that consist of a smaller subset of elected members who have the authority to make key decisions. Thus, an important choice for larger alliances is whether to represent all or some members on the alliance board and to determine what kinds of individuals (CEOs, physicians, trustees) should be alliance board members.

Mandated vs. Voluntary Participation

Another important dimension on which alliances vary is whether they are voluntary or mandated by an external group with legal or legitimate authority (Oliver, 1990). Most health care alliances are voluntary. These alliances reflect the efforts of individual organizations to strategically adapt to external changes by choosing to band together. But, it is important to recognize that even voluntary alliances may emerge in large part as a result of external pressure from powerful actors.

A central issue to note in comparing mandated and voluntary alliances is the extent to which the former are characterized more by style than substance and by instability than longevity. Scott (1987) argues that mandated forms of organization tend to be adopted only superficially and, as a result, also tend to be short-lived. Many international alliances (including the League of Nations and the United Nations) come to mind in this regard. Superficial compliance with a mandate to form an alliance is especially likely to occur when the participating organizations lack other motives for forming a relationship (Oliver, 1990). In general, managers and other organization members chafe under external constraints and regulation, even when such rules have some merit.

Discussion

Existing typologies have been useful in documenting and describing the common and different features of a wide range of interorganizational arrangements in health care. However, it is also important to ask what difference an organization should expect to see if it were to choose one form versus another.

In other words, what is the alliance intended to accomplish? For example, Zajac (1986), in an analysis of contract management arrangements, argues that organizations choosing to engage in a similar type of strategic alliance may have widely varying strategic intentions and that expected performance will vary correspondingly. In other words, the form of the alliance is not necessarily a good predictor of what the alliance can achieve.

WHAT ARE ALLIANCES MEANT TO DO?

Pooling versus Trading Alliances

Most broadly, one can distinguish between **pooling alliances** that bring together organizations seeking to contribute similar resources and **trading alliances** that bring together organizations seeking to contribute different resources (Doz & Hamel, 1998). This distinction is more precise than the often-made statement that organizations generally seek "complementarities" in alliances. The term *complementarity* suggests differences, but it is important to remember that similarities can often drive alliance activity as well. An example of a pooling or similarity-driven strategic intent for an alliance is one that seeks to gain purchasing power over a supplier or group of suppliers. Such alliances are often seen in health care, in the form of business coalitions (against hospitals) or hospital alliances (against health care supply organizations).

Examples of a trading or difference-driven alliance are a physician group–hospital joint venture, where each party contributes something distinct to the alliance, and a joint venture between two health care supply firms, such as Johnson & Johnson and Merck, where the former is known for its marketing expertise, the latter for its product development skills. These examples also highlight how strategic intent can often drive the form of a strategic alliance. Pooling strategies tend to involve more organizations and take the form of federations, consortia, or coalitions; and trading strategies tend to involve fewer (often only two) organizations and take the form of joint ventures, licensing agreements, and related arrangements. Of course, as mentioned, earlier alternative alliance forms can serve similar strategic intent in some cases. For example, a health plan can create a trading alliance with a pharmacy, benefits management firm, or it may seek to create a consortium of health plans that provides the same service.

Cost Reduction versus Revenue Enhancement

The strategic intent of alliances can also be examined in terms of their expected outcomes. An emphasis on expected alliance outcomes is relevant for several reasons: The success of an alliance will generally be defined by the degree to which the desired outcomes

are achieved; some performance outcomes may be largely incompatible with others; and one alliance partner's perception of the expected outcome may not be shared by that of other partners.

The first and most basic expected outcome refers to financial performance and addresses the issue of whether the alliance is primarily conceived for **cost reduction** or **revenue enhancement**. While this is not to say that the two outcomes are mutually exclusive, there are differences in the challenges for success for alliances, in how one gauges success, and in how cost-reducing versus revenue-enhancing alliances might be organized.

For example, consider a local alliance of four hospitals with historically complementary specialties (or distinctive competencies) that is seeking to increase the volume of patients to be treated in these specialties. Compare this alliance with a similarly sized and similarly located hospital alliance seeking to share the costs of providing indigent care to the local community. One would not measure success the same way, nor would the interaction between partners be the same in the two alliances. One might expect that the alliance motivated by the desire to increase patient volume would require substantial coordination, given that there is a reciprocal interdependence between the partners. In the case of the cost-sharing alliance, one would likely observe a combining of similar resources requiring relatively less active coordination, given that there is a pooled interdependence among the partners (Thompson, 1967).

Quality, Innovation, and Learning

Another way of classifying the intent of an alliance is the degree to which the alliance seeks to enhance outcomes such as innovation, organizational learning, and quality (Doz & Hamel, 1998; Zajac et al., 1991). These outcomes are distinct from those discussed above in that, while they may lead to revenue enhancement or cost reduction, their relationship to such financial performance measures may be difficult to discern, or in a more extreme case, may be negatively related to financially oriented targets (Shortell & Zajac, 1990).

For example, Zuckerman and D'Aunno (1990) noted that hospitals can increase their reputation for quality by joining a strategic alliance that involves other prestigious organizations. Membership in such an alliance may require only a minor contribution of time, effort, or capital. An interesting feature of such an alliance is that one partner's actions can damage the reputation of another by not delivering the expected level of quality. This suggests the need for appropriate screening of partners in terms of their commitment to quality.

There may also be regional differences in the degree to which membership is prestige-enhancing. One of the authors was involved in a research project on multihospital systems in which a voluntary membership affiliation with a large national, for-profit hospital system was viewed by the local community as an asset to the hospital. The name of the hospital system was proudly displayed at the hospital entrance and on hospital stationery. However, another hospital affiliated with that same system—but located in a different part of the country—made every attempt to downplay that affiliation. No signs were posted with the system name, and no trace of the system could be found on hospital stationery. The reason for this very different treatment? In the first example, the region had many for-profit affiliations, and several of the major hospital chains had their headquarters in that region of the country. In the second example, for-profit hospitals were much less common in the region and were viewed somewhat suspiciously by many in that environment. The point to be made is that, before seeking membership in an alliance for purposes of increasing actual or perceived quality, an organization must be aware of the limits of that benefit.

Other motives driving alliance activity, such as innovation and learning, are also conceptually distinct from other more straightforward motives. The payoffs from alliances that are driven by innovation and learning motives are often slow to emerge. This requires a particularly high level of partner commitment and patience. An additional factor to consider is that many organizations underestimate the involvement necessary to realize benefits such as innovation and learning. In these alliances, a more substantial personnel flow between partners can often accelerate the learning and innovation process.

Power Enhancement, Uncertainty Reduction, and Risk-Sharing

Power enhancement and **uncertainty reduction** are grouped together because one often has implications for the other. Specifically, alliances can be motivated by an organization's desire to gain influence over (or reduce dependence on) an aspect of the organization's environment. This reduction in dependence may also represent a reduction in uncertainty, although the two are conceptually distinct. An organization might be dependent on another organization, but if the more powerful organization is reliable, then the dependent organization may face little uncertainty.

This perspective can be seen in much of the early literature on interorganizational relations in health care. Longest (1990), for example, views the growth of multi-institutional systems as the result of an "external dependency relationship" between the hospital and its environment. In doing so, Longest is applying the resource dependence perspective to the health care industry (Pfeffer & Salancik, 1978). Longest (1990) uses the term *stabilization strategy* to characterize multihospital arrangements, which he explains are "formulated by people for a hospital that exists in relation to an external environment upon which the hospital is highly dependent."

Uncertainty reduction as an alliance motive can also be compared with a similar, yet distinct, motive: risk-sharing. The difference between the two motives is that the former highlights one organization's attempts to reduce its own uncertainty, whereas the latter emphasizes the joint reduction of uncertainty for both (or more) partners. Not surprisingly, the former is equated more with gaining influence of an exchange partner, while the latter is used more in terms of pooling resources to reduce common risk.

Summary

It is important to note that the above-mentioned strategic intentions that can drive alliance activity arc not mutually exclusive. For example, a business coalition may be formed because it wants to gain influence over local area hospitals, but it also has as its major objective a reduction in the cost of health care that the coalition members have had to pay. Thus, power and cost-reduction motives are both driving alliance formation. Similarly, a joint venture between a hospital and a multispecialty physician group may have as its objective the creation of new innovative services, yet also have the intent of increasing revenues (Longest, 1990).

Understanding the strategic intent of an alliance can be a critical success factor for the alliance. The understanding has several components, including understanding your own motivation for considering an alliance, expressing this understanding to your alliance partner, eliciting and then listening carefully to your partners' expression of their strategic intentions, and examining the compatibility (which could be compatibly similar or compatibly different) of your intentions and those of your partners. The lack of an articulated mission statement is often cited as the root of many failures in organizational strategy. The same is equally if not more true for strategic alliances, particularly given the potential for incompatible intentions across partners.

Physician-Hospital Trading Alliances

Physician-hospital alliances have spread across the health care system in response to several environmental jolts. The Medicare Prospective Payment System (PPS) altered the financial incentives of hospitals by using fixed, per-case payments but left physician incentives untouched. Because physicians control (directly or indirectly) up to 80% of hospital expenditures, hospitals began to develop relationships with their physicians in order to influence their thinking and practice behavior. The rapid increase in managed care (e.g., penetration by HMOs) in the late 1980s and early 1990s provided an additional spur to alliance formation (Olden et al., 2002). As HMOs sought to reduce their inpatient costs (e.g., through lower payments), hospitals looked for ways to cut costs through partnerships with their physicians. Moreover, some HMOs looked to pass on to providers the financial risks for their enrollees. Physicians and hospitals sought to develop alliances to accept and manage this risk. Finally, by the mid-1990s, HMO consolidations served to increase managed care's bargaining power over providers in local markets. Providers have responded to this threat by forming vertical alliances to pose a countervailing force (Burns, Bazzoli, Dynan, & Wholey, 1998).

Physician-hospital alliances take many forms, which contribute to the growing list of acronyms managers must now understand. Physician-hospital organizations (PHOs) constitute joint ventures designed to develop new services (e.g., ambulatory care clinic) or, more commonly, attract managed care contracts. Management services organizations (MSOs) constitute vehicles for the transfer of managerial expertise and administrative systems to physicians in small practices, and sometimes capital for expansion. Integrated salary models (ISMs) constitute vertically integrated arrangements in which the hospital purchases the physician's practice, establishes an employment contract with the physician for a defined period, and negotiates a guaranteed base salary with a variable component based on office productivity, with some expectation (or anticipation) that the physician will refer or admit patients to the hospital.

These alliances serve many purposes. They are generally designed to reduce uncertainty for both parties in dealing with an increasingly competitive and threatening environment. One objective is revenue enhancement: to increase the trading partners' success in obtaining managed care contracts and capitated revenues. Providers have anticipated the widespread use of capitation by HMOs, but this has varied greatly across the country. A second objective is to provide a platform for future physician-hospital collaboration in such areas as quality improvement and cost containment. Alliances are thus a vehicle for physicians and hospitals to begin working together in a risk-based and pay-for-performance environment. Because every physician is different, hospitals typically offer physicians a menu of alliances from which to choose (Dynan, Bazzoli, & Burns, 1997).

How well have these alliances performed? If success is gauged by provider interest, alliances are doing quite well. Recent evidence highlights the diffusion of alliances across U.S. hospitals, with continued high growth particularly among MSOs (American Hospital Association, 1998; Burns, Bazzoli, Dynan, & Wholey, 1997; Morrisey, Alexander, Burns, & Johnson, 1996). Other evidence, however, suggests that alliances have failed to achieve their specific objectives. With regard to managed care contracting, for example, barely half of all PHOs have risk-based contracts with HMOs, and most of the PHOs' "covered lives" are in PPO contracts that entail no capitation and little or no financial risk (Ernst & Young, 1995). PHOs and MSOs alike typically have fewer than 12,000 at risk lives under contract. With regard to collaboration, hospitals have succeeded in enlisting their physicians to join these vehicles. PHOs, for example, typically include 80% to 90% of the medical staff. Such wide-open participation is actually detrimental to the PHO's purposes, however, since the hospital is seeking physician partners who can practice more cost-effective medicine than the medical staff as a whole. Additional evidence suggests that PHO participation does not significantly increase the physician's perceived alignment and identification with the hospital (Burns et al., 1996).

Why are the results so disappointing, especially given the prevalence of alliances and the attention received in the trade literature? One reason is the structural form used to implement the alliance. These alliances are typically organized, financed, and controlled by the hospital with little physician participation. Not surprisingly, physicians balk at partnerships' in which they have not participated. Another reason (stated above) is the sheer size of

the physician panel. Alliances that fail to carefully screen their members resemble the medical staff at large and thus represent "business as usual." A third explanation is the lack of infrastructure found in many alliances. Too often hospitals will develop the alliances as external contracting vehicles to approach the managed care market, but fail to develop the internal mechanisms that will help the alliance partners to manage risk. Such mechanisms include physician compensation and productivity systems, quality monitoring and measurement, and physician selection (Burns & Thorpe, 1997).

More generally, research shows that hospital alliances have not produced as many operating efficiencies as expected (Clement et al., 1997; McCue, Clement, & Luke, 1999). But, research also shows that how alliances are organized makes a difference: Hospitals involved in strategic alliances that had more centralized decision making were likely to have better financial performance than hospitals in more loosely aligned alliances (Bazzoli et al., 2000).

For example, one national study of integrated delivery systems (including PHOs) conducted by the Center for Health Management Research (CHMR) examined the prevalence of three integrative mechanisms to help manage risk: physician panel sizing, physician compensation and productivity mechanisms, and physician leadership development. The study found that the three mechanisms were weakly developed, and especially so among loosely integrated arrangements such as PHOs (Burns, Walston, Alexander et al., 2001).

Another national study conducted by the Prospective Payment Assessment Commission (ProPAC) examined a different set of mechanisms in PHOs: the integration of clinical data across hospital departments, integration of clinical and financial data, the use of clinical guidelines, and the use of product-line management. The researchers found that the presence of any of these mechanisms inside the hospital was unrelated to the hospital's managed care activity, a major predictor of the presence of PHOs in hospitals (Morrisey, Alexander, Burns, & Johnson, 1996, 1999).

A third national study conducted by the American Hospital Association (AHA) found that while 38% of all integrated delivery systems had at least one capitated contract, only 17% of loosely integrated systems (e.g., PHOs) had such contracts (Bazzoli, Dynan, & Burns, 1999–2000). Thus, integrated delivery systems that featured PHOs were less likely to have a capitated contract, to have fewer such contracts, and to have fewer covered lives than integrated delivery systems with more tightly integrated physicians (e.g., acquired, salaried primary care physicians).

These findings suggest that implementation of the alliance and careful attention to developing its infrastructure is critical for the success of any alliance that physicians and hospitals form. In the absence of the mechanisms discussed above, one would expect PHOs to exert little impact on hospital quality and cost of care. In fact, two recent studies have addressed this issue directly. Cuellar and Gertler (2005) and Madison (2004) report that PHOs do not lower the cost of care. Indeed, they may lead to higher prices paid for care (for either the hospital or its physicians) due to the combined bargaining leverage of the two parties in the IDS model. Moreover, there is no evidence that PHOs improve quality of care, and in fact may damage it.

THE ALLIANCE PROCESS: A MULTISTAGE ANALYSIS

Previous studies of alliances have focused primarily on why they emerge, how they are structured, and what they do. Less attention has been given to how alliances evolve and behave over time (D'Aunno & Zuckerman, 1987a; Luke, Begun, & Pointer, 1989; Provan, 1984; Sofaer & Myrtle, 1991; Zajac & Olsen, 1993). Thus, we develop models that managers can use to understand how alliances develop as they do and what can be done to improve their chances for success.

Alliances can be considered within the context of a life-cycle model (Table 11.2). This model suggests that organizations often move through predictable stages of growth, with one or more factors triggering such movement. Further, each stage brings distinctive tasks that alliance leaders and members need to address.

Emergence: Finding Partners

In the first stage, environmental threats, opportunities, and uncertainty lead organizations with similar ideologies and dependencies to seek out each other. Further, this dance often begins when the potential partners relate to each other **symbiotically** as well as **competitively** (Hawley, 1950; Pfeffer & Salancik, 1978). In other words, alliances may be more likely to emerge when one organization uses some services or products of the other as opposed to the case when two organizations are vying for the same resources. A common example of symbiosis is a rural community hospital that refers cases for tertiary care to an urban teaching hospital.

Interorganizational exchange processes involve distinct stages (Zajac & Olsen, 1993). For example, in the early stage each organization engages in the process of projecting exchange into the future and constructing net present valuations of alternative exchange relationships on a continuum ranging from markets (i.e., arm's-length transactions with another independent organization), through strategic alliances (i.e., a formal cooperative arrangement between organizations, preserving the independent identity of each partner), and finally to hierarchies (i.e., the merging of two or more organizations into one organization) (Macneil, 1983). Perceptions of what each exchange partner seeks also emerge more clearly, enabling the more precise identification of similarities and differences that can form the basis for mutually beneficial exchange.

Thus, in the early stage there is preliminary communication and negotiation concerning mutual and individual organizational interests. An organization's behavior in this stage can set a precedent for future exchange and provide information through

Table 11.2. A Life Cycle Model of Organizational Alliances in Health Care

Stages			
Emergence	**Transition**	**Maturity**	**Critical Crossroads**
Key factors in development at each stage			
Environment poses threat to and uncertainty about valued resources	Motivation to achieve purposes of the alliance	Willingness to put alliance interests first	Increased centralization and dependence on alliance motivates members to seek hierarchy or withdraw from alliance
Organizations share ideologies and similar dependencies	Increased dependence on alliance for valued resources	Members receive benefits from previous investments	
Examples of tasks at each stage			
Define purposes of the alliance	Hire or form a management group	Attain stated objectives	Manage decisions about future of the alliance
Develop membership criteria	Establish mechanisms for coordination and control	Sustain member commitment	

which a firm can learn about the expected behavior of its partner. During this phase, initial relational exchange norms are being forged and commitments tested in small but important ways to determine credibility (Macneil, 1983). To summarize, in this initial stage, the purposes and expectations of the partners are stated, membership criteria are established, and group norms begin to evolve.

Though it is important for expectations to be realistic, it turns out that many young alliances have broadly stated goals that do not necessarily coincide with their activities. This is because goal statements reflect compromises made among members who are, as of yet, not willing to subordinate their interests to those of the group as a whole. Further, broad goal statements may attract other partners, and early members want to have the advantages that popularity typically affords.

Thus, in many cases, the criteria for alliance membership are selective and designed to ensure homo-

geneity among members. This reduces some of the governance and management problems discussed above. Further, many alliances seek to limit overlap in market areas so as to minimize competition among members and avoid antitrust issues.

At this initial stage, most alliances are not likely to form or hire a management group to direct their activities (D'Aunno & Zuckerman, 1987a), because organizations must initially identify and agree on a set of purposes. Organizations are also reluctant to yield authority and commit resources to a management group. Nonetheless, this is typically what happens in the second stage of alliance development.

Transition

In this stage the alliance establishes mechanisms for coordination, control, and decision making. This often entails forming or hiring a management group, moving the alliance to a form that Provan (1983) and D'Aunno and Zuckerman (1987b) term a *federation*. The transition may be rocky because, as just noted, organizations are reluctant to grant authority to others or to sacrifice their own autonomy. It is thus critical that alliance managers ensure that their efforts and programs are responsive to members' needs. During this stage the governance structure also takes shape. This may also be threatening to members, especially if they are not directly represented on the governing board.

Alliances vary in the extent to which their members are willing to commit resources to initiate and sustain programs and activities. An important weakness of many alliances is their inability to gain adequate commitment of members' resources. For example, there may be free-rider problems in that some members make little commitment but yet can benefit from the investments of others. It is likely that such problems are directly proportional to the value that members perceive in committing resources to the alliance. The more value that members perceive from active participation, the more resources (including autonomy) they are willing to commit to the alliance.

Of course, this leads to a challenging "chicken and egg" dilemma. On the one hand, members increase their commitment in proportion to threats from their environment and the alliance's ability to reduce threats and uncertainty. On the other hand, for the alliance to be effective in meeting members' needs, it may require the investment of valued resources from members as well as their willingness to coordinate efforts with each other. At some point, alliances require an investment of resources that are risked by members who have no certainty of return equal to their investment. At this point, trust becomes particularly important.

Maturity

The third stage of an alliance's life cycle is that of maturity and growth. In this stage it is critical that the alliance begin to achieve its objectives and aid members in coping with external threats. Such success enables an alliance to continue and to grow. It is also central that members be willing to put the interests of the alliance, at least sometimes, ahead of their own interests. This is necessary because alliances cannot meet the needs of all of their members, at least not simultaneously. Members must recognize that they will not necessarily benefit equally from alliance activities; it is essential, however, that they benefit as equitably as possible.

As alliances seek to attain objectives and sustain member commitment, several issues may arise. For example, alliances that add many members may find it impossible to avoid having members with overlapping market areas. If such overlap does occur, what role, if any, should the alliance play in mediating disputes that may arise among members?

Relationships between the members and alliance managers (if there are any) also become more complex. For example, are new programs initiated through the alliance manager's office, individual members, or both? If through the alliance office, what happens to similar programs already developed by individual members? For instance, suppose that a hospital alliance wishes to develop an alliance-wide HMO, but some members already have HMOs. Further, are there or should there be incentives for members to produce innovative programs that can be shared by all alliance members? In the absence of such incentives, how will the alliance develop innovations in management or services?

Zajac and Olsen (1993), in their discussion of the development of interorganizational relationships, note that alliances in this stage of development face some particularly sensitive issues because value is not only created but also claimed and distributed. Surrounding the issue of claiming and distributing value is the question of interorganizational conflict. Explicit or implicit norms for managing the divergence of interest will often arise (Zajac & Olsen, 1993). To the extent that these norms—defined as "shared and reasoned expectations that may arise from agreement or past acts"—emphasize the importance of joint value maximization, this should lead to searches for mutually satisfactory resolutions of conflict situations (Kaufmann, 1987). On the other hand, if these evolving norms do not develop in this way, the pursuit of individual firm interests would lead to an escalation of conflict that could ultimately be destructive to the strategic alliance. As noted in Chapter 5, the accepted use of conflict-resolution systems can limit the potential damage of interorganizational conflict (Ury, Brett, & Goldberg, 1988).

The continued development of trust is a key issue in this stage of interorganizational exchange. Trust stems from a growing confidence in a firm's expectations of the future (Luhmann, 1979). Schelling (1960) also notes that "trust is often achieved simply by the continuity of the relation between parties and the recognition by each that what he might gain by cheating in a given instance is outweighed by the value of the tradition of trust that makes possible a long sequence of future agreement."

Trust and conflict-management systems are subsets of other relational norms underlying the process exchange over time. These norms include shared expectations of reciprocity between alliance partners and a growing sense of the value of preserving the relationship (Macneil, 1983, 1986). These norms set the tone for the continued execution of contracts.

Critical Crossroads

As they evolve into the fourth stage of development, alliances move to what may be a critical crossroads. Up to this point, members became increasingly dependent on each other for needed resources, and there was growing pressure for greater member commitment to the alliance and more centralized decision making. In many ways, however, these developments run counter to the reasons why many organizations join an alliance. That is, alliances are attractive because they provide a relatively low-cost vehicle to reduce resource dependence while maintaining organizational autonomy. Thus, this stage may be a critical crossroads at which some members conclude that the price of belonging to an alliance is too high and withdraw. Indeed, it appears

that at least one hospital alliance collapsed precisely on this point (Ury et al., 1988). In contrast, others may decide that it is necessary to move toward more hierarchical arrangements to gain the full benefits of collective action.

The underlying issue is whether there is sufficient commitment or "glue" to hold alliances together over time (Zuckerman & Kaluzny, 1991). Though there may be common goals, ideologies, values, and inducements that keep members together, alliances typically remain loose arrangements. Can the degree of commitment required of members be secured in the long run? Will members be willing to sacrifice autonomy to allow for greater discipline in decision making? What coordination mechanisms are most appropriate and under what circumstances (Alter & Hage, 1993; Kaluzny & Zuckerman, 1992)? To survive, alliances must balance the need for and benefits of collective action with the need for individual members to retain adequate autonomy.

This critical crossroads represents a reconfiguring stage in the developmental process of a strategic alliance (Zajac & Olsen, 1993). It is usually triggered by reaching the end of the expected duration of the relationship or by changes in the partners' perceived level of the relationship's value. Reconfiguring may imply that an exchange partner will choose to leave, or it may mean that partners will join more tightly together by widening the scope of interorganizational exchange processes. For example, a group of hospitals may move from a shared purchasing arrangement to developing a joint preferred provider network.

With respect to perceived changes in the value of the strategic alliance, such changes may emerge from a new and changing environment or a historical comparison of actual to expected value creation. While this performance gap can lead to a reevaluation (positive or negative) of the interorganizational relationship itself, it may simply lead to a reassessment of the developmental processes. In other words, the reconfiguring stage may not involve a change in the type of strategic alliance per se but only a change in the process of interaction within the existing strategic alliance. These change options suggest that this stage may loop back to either the emergence stage, where value forecasts are respecified and strategic motivations are clarified for a new forecast period, or the transition stage, where the forms of exchange are revised and updated based on the continued experiences of the partners. Thus, the process model of strategic alliance development outlined here does not propose a one-way, deterministic path for alliances; instead, it highlights a sequence of likely phases that many alliances may experience and emphasizes a set of critical issues that health care organizations may face at the various stages of alliance development.

FRAMEWORKS FOR ANALYZING ALLIANCE PROBLEMS

A major difficulty that organizations face in addressing alliance problems is actually their inability to identify the problem correctly. By that we mean that individuals within an organization often don't know or disagree strongly on what the problem is, and this is compounded by differences of opinion between partners in alliance problem identification and diagnosis. These disagreements, we contend, can often lead to false diagnoses and the treatment of **alliance symptoms** rather than the root **alliance problems** facing the alliance. These incorrect interventions subsequently lead to greater friction, gridlock, and ultimately an increased likelihood of alliance failure (see In Practice p. 373). The three simple frameworks offered below are intended to lessen the likelihood of such failure.

Locating the Problem

If one were to ask several involved individuals why a particular alliance was in trouble, it is possible that one would get a uniform response. In such cases, locating the problem is simple. We argue, however, that

such agreement is the exception rather than the norm. Typically there are a host of possible reasons why an alliance might be facing difficulties. Without some way of organizing these reasons, there may be little hope of remedying the situation. We propose that alliance problems can be viewed as generally falling into the following categories (Johnson, 1986):

- Environmental problems
- Strategy problems
- Structure problems
- Behavior problems

These categories follow a macro to micro continuum, but more important for purposes of this chapter, they also tend to follow an uncontrollable to controllable continuum.

Consider the problems in health care alliances that require collaboration among professional groups with different training, time horizons, and economic incentives. For example, trading alliances between physicians and hospitals are particularly vulnerable to these difficulties. A recent analysis of six integrated systems in Illinois suggests that physician-hospital alliances have polarities to be resolved rather than problems to be solved (Burns, 1999). These polarities consist of nine areas in which the integrated system must seek to manage in two directions simultaneously (i.e., pursue the physicians' interests simultaneously with the hospital's interests). For example, the hospital system seeks to expose its physicians to practicing in a risk-based environment; at the same time, it is purchasing primary care physicians who are then given guaranteed salaries for several years—in effect, exempting them from all risk. As another example, the hospital system wishes to become "an organization of physicians," and yet the system is developed and controlled almost exclusively by hospital executives and serves primarily hospital purposes in the short term. For such alliances to be credible to physicians and work effectively, they need to satisfy the interests of both parties simultaneously. In terms of our framework, the problems lie not in uncontrollable environmental issues, or in the basic strategy of

⚜ IN PRACTICE   Strategic Alliances in the Pharmaceutical and Biotechnology Industry

In the past two decades, strategic alliances have become an important tool for pharmaceutical and biotechnology firms as they face increased competition, increased public scrutiny of their business practices and profits, and difficulties discovering new products. In the year 2001–2002 alone, there were 923 new (publicly announced) strategic alliances in this industry.

It's interesting to observe that a high proportion of these new alliances (404 of 923) were between partners who already had an ongoing relationship. New agreements among established partners may signal that the relationship has matured, as indicated in the life-cycle model of alliances presented in Table 11.2.

Of various possible new alliances (e.g., pairing a pharmaceutical firm with another pharmaceutical firm or with a biotechnology firm), the highest percentage (one-third) occurred between biotechnology firms. This suggests that these relatively small firms found alliances to be an especially important strategy to build the scale and scope needed to compete and perform well. Biotechnology firms may be creating pooling alliances that can allow them to reduce uncertainty and enhance market power.

In contrast, the second highest number of new alliances (217) was between pharmaceutical and biotechnology firms, probably reflecting pharmaceutical firms' needs for access to new products that the smaller, but more research-intensive, biotechnology firms have been generating. These may be trading alliances that allow pharmaceutical firms to gain access to innovations, while enabling biotechnology firms to gain access to the marketing capabilities that pharmaceutical firms possess. Some support for the view that pharmaceutical firms are using alliances to gain access to technical innovations is found in the fact that almost one-third of the new alliances involved genomics, the path-breaking science that can be used to develop treatments tailored to individuals' genetic types, making them highly effective.

Finally, it appears that firms are using alliances to enhance their capabilities in key markets. Most new alliances that focused on a specific therapeutic area were focused in the area of oncology, where there is both high demand for new, more effective treatments and the willingness to pay high prices for them.

For Discussion

What do you think are the possible major tensions that exist when a pharmaceutical firm forms an alliance with a biotechnology firm? How would you try to address those tensions? Identify different challenges that exist for maintaining or strengthening an ongoing alliance versus beginning a new relationship.

SOURCE: Reuters Business Insight. Pharmaceutical strategic alliances: Benchmarking 21st century deal-making. Retrieved August 16, 2004 from *http://www.the-infoshop.com*

deepening physician-hospital relationships, but in the fundamental structural decisions made and the behavioral problems created or exacerbated by those structural decisions.

The framework can be particularly valuable in highlighting disagreement as to what fundamental problems are facing a strategic alliance. We use an interesting nonhealth care example of an alliance failure to further illustrate this point.

In 1990, a consortium called U.S. Memories was conceived to provide a secure supply of chips for U.S. computer makers who were unhappy with the occasional shortages and price fluctuations brought on by Japanese chip makers, who controlled almost 90% of the DRAM market. This alliance, made up of U.S. chip buyers and a few U.S. chip makers, never got off the ground, as initial players backed out and new players refused to commit resources. Analysts offered several reasons as to why the alliance failed. Some attributed the failure to the fact that, once the temporary chip shortage was over, the alliance had no purpose. Others said it was ill-conceived and that the United States could never have competed with the more efficient Japanese chip makers. Some said that not enough players were involved; some said *too many* players were involved; and others said that the deal was not well structured. Finally, some blamed the leader of the consortium, saying that he was not well suited for such a position.

What do we make out of this mess? Could this alliance have been salvaged? Basically, we can start by using the framework above to categorize the myriad of alliance problems into environmental ("the market changed"), strategic ("it was a bad idea from the beginning"), structural ("it wasn't organized correctly"), and behavioral ("we had the wrong person at the top") problems. The point here is that, from a managerial perspective, a person responsible for gathering information about the alliance, processing that information, and making a decision on whether or how to intervene, can begin to piece together problems into useful clusters or categories.

Second, the categories themselves are useful in assessing the degree to which intervention can be effective. For example, after analyzing the categorized

reasons, a manager may believe that the primary problem is environmental—that is, the market conditions no longer support the alliance. This is largely an uncontrollable factor and, therefore, suggests that the alliance is not likely to succeed. On the other hand, the manager may believe the primary problem is structural—that the number or composition of the alliance is not right or that the incentives for participation are inadequate. This is more of a controllable factor and suggests that the alliance can be modified and thus face improved odds for success. In this way, the Environment→Strategy→Structure→Behavior framework can be a useful tool in identifying and diagnosing alliance problems.

Separating the Root Cause from the Symptom

If you had a rash and were to go to a physician, what would be the first thing the physician would do? Treat the rash or first ask a set of questions to discern why you have the rash? Hopefully, the latter approach is the more common. Unfortunately, many organizations involved in strategic alliances take the former approach. There's a problem; let's fix it. This "can do" attitude is laudable in one sense, but potentially reckless (even rash?) in another sense. Specifically, when one observes friction in strategic alliances, we argue that the most important response is to first delve more deeply to understand the source of that friction before attempting to treat the problem.

This advice regarding diagnosis before treatment may seem obvious, but it often is not done in alliances. The reason it is often not done stems from alliance partners' unwillingness or inability to put themselves in their partners' shoes. By this we mean that signs of noncooperative behavior from a partner are often viewed with hostility on the part of other partners. The other partners then devise their own response strategy before an analysis or diagnosis is done as to why the partner may appear to be acting noncooperatively. Quite simply, we are stating that the noncooperative behavior is only a symptom of a deeper problem.

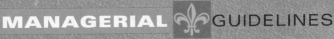

MANAGERIAL GUIDELINES

1. In assessing the risk of forming or entering an alliance, managers should compare the potential costs and benefits of alliances to doing nothing or to alternative strategies that involve going it alone; alliances may well be less risky than other strategies.

2. The form or structure of alliance should follow from its function—that is, what it is intended to do.

3. Managers should consider their options with respect to several important aspects of alliance structure, including ownership and control, number of members, governance structure, and mandated versus voluntary participation.

4. Many of the benefits of control in interorganizational relationships can be achieved without ownership; trust, commitment, and even power may be important substitutes for control based on ownership.

5. Increased size brings greater complexity and often more difficulty in coordinating efforts, but larger alliances tend to be more powerful for certain purposes (e.g., lobbying, purchasing in volume).

6. Large alliances often need more complex governance structures, and a key issue is who will be represented on an alliance board. It may be a mistake to have only CEOs or executive directors on alliance boards because the interests of other groups may be neglected; further, turnover among top managers is common and may disrupt the alliance if the board has no other types of members.

7. Mandated participation in an alliance is often less preferable to voluntary

participation. Alliances are not likely to succeed if members' only or most important motive for participation is to comply with external demands.

8. Recognize that alliances can be created to achieve one or more of the following objectives: to pool similar resources (e.g., as in joint purchasing arrangements); to trade dissimilar resources (e.g., as in a symbiotic relationship between a hospital and physician group); to reduce costs; to enhance revenues; to promote innovation, learning, or quality of services; or to enhance power, reduce uncertainty, or share risks among members.

9. From the above list, it is important to understand your own motives for seeking an alliance and to express these motives to potential or current partners.

10. Similarly, managers need to listen carefully to the intentions of potential or current partners in order to assess compatibility; failure to articulate a shared mission is an important reason for alliance failure.

11. Two kinds of problems are typical when it comes to alliance objectives. First, even though alliance objectives may be shared by members, the objectives may conflict with each other, especially over time. Second, there may be lack of consensus among members concerning alliance objectives. Both problems highlight the need for effective communication.

12. Recognize that alliances often develop in several stages that each bring distinctive threats and opportunities.

13. In the first stage (emergence), it is important to define the purposes of the

(continues)

MANAGERIAL GUIDELINES *(continued)*

alliance and select partners accordingly. Clear communication and acknowledgment of interests are critical.

14. After forming an alliance, managers must find ways to coordinate and control activities; this may entail hiring or forming a management group to focus specifically on alliance concerns.

15. As alliances mature, managers are likely to face complex issues about how much individual members must conform to and, indeed, place alliance interests ahead of their own. Further, there may be conflict about how to distribute the benefits (resources) that alliances have generated. Thus, managers need to focus on ways to sustain member commitment through trust, goal attainment, and the use of appropriate mechanisms to resolve conflict.

16. Mature alliances face the task of measuring up to members' original and changing expectations. Such alliances need to rethink their structure and objectives to make sure that they keep pace with members' needs.

17. More specifically, managers can diagnose alliance problems according to whether they are primarily environmental (i.e., stemming from external sources such as shift in market demands); strategic (i.e., concerning the overall purpose and direction of the alliance); structural (i.e., alliance form fits poorly with its purposes); or behavioral (i.e., skills are not adequate for carrying out alliance activities).

18. It is important to match alliance problems with appropriate means to deal with them, ranging from educating members to negotiating with them to coercing them.

19. Alliances can be just a management fad— be careful that you are forming one for the right reasons.

20. Recognize that alliances have their costs for managers in terms of time spent in understanding and negotiating with potential and current partners. In fact, alliances can slow decision making and make organizations less flexible—precisely what they are designed to avoid.

21. Select partners and develop ways of relating to them so as to avoid charges of collusion and antitrust problems.

22. Don't let alliance arrangements make your organization lazy and lose its interest in continuous improvement.

The obvious questions then become, What could the deeper problems be, and how do we treat them? We propose that there are at least four categories of problems:

- Parochial self-interest
- Misunderstanding and a lack of trust
- Different assessments
- Low tolerance for ambiguity

These categories, interestingly, match discussions of problems that exist in managing change (Kotter & Schlesinger, 1979). While the categories are not mutually exclusive, they are quite distinct from one another. For example, the first category represents rational, calculative, noncooperative behavior in which one partner knowingly acts in his own interest to the detriment of the other partner. The second type of problem is based less on selfishness than on the absence of accepted and well-developed norms;

that is, a trusting relationship between partners has yet to emerge. The third category differs from the first in that, while the first category (i.e., selfish, noncooperative behavior) reflects disagreement on ends and means, the third category reflects agreement on ends but not means. In other words, partners may share the same goal but diverge in their views on how to achieve that goal. Lastly, some alliance partners simply feel uncomfortable with the ambiguity and fluidity of alliances. The absence of full control, as is typical in strategic alliances, may not agree with some reluctant partners.

Identifying different categories of problems is in and of itself useful as a way to move beyond the symptom and toward the problem. Treating the problem is the next step, and we propose a simple principle: The treatment should match the problem. Again, while this seems obvious, we find that all too often in alliances the treatment is either insufficient or too harsh. Both of these situations are unfavorable. There are at least six ways of dealing with alliance problems:

- Education
- Participation
- Facilitation
- Negotiation
- Cooptation
- Coercion

Matching this set of treatments with the set of problems identified earlier represents a step toward effective alliance management (Kotter & Schlesinger, 1979). Consider the case where a partner faces a particularly calculative, self-interested partner. That partner is not lacking information; he knows what the situation is but does not want what his partner wants. In this case, an approach that emphasizes negotiation or cooptation is likely to be more effective than one that emphasizes participation or education. Contrast such a case with a partner whose actions are based on a misunderstanding. Here, negotiation as a response does not address the root problem; education and participation are more appropriate. We invite the reader to draw further matches between problem and treatment.

Know Thy Partner

A third framework that can be useful in addressing potential and ongoing alliance problems focuses more directly at understanding your partner's "type." Specifically, we suggest that it is a mistake to assume that your partner thinks about your alliance the same way that you do. Ideally, you will know what type of alliance partner you are dealing with at the earliest stages of the alliance. Unfortunately, it is our experience that many times a partner fails to take into adequate account the variety of partner types or **partner orientations** that exist. In our experience, there are five types of partners, ranging from the most desirable to the least desirable; each is discussed briefly below.

The Cooperative Partner

This partner is primarily interested in maximizing the joint gains in the alliance relationship, and recognizes that such maximization requires attention to what you need to achieve in the alliance. Thus, this partner will work with you in helping you achieve your goals, as well as his own. This is what you hope you have in an alliance partner, but it may be more rare than one thinks. This partner sees the alliance as win/win, and is interested in seeing that both sides win. A major pharmaceutical firm embodies this philosophy with the goal of being "the partner of choice" for biotech firms. This pharma company employs numerous alliance managers who see their role as "omsbudspersons" for the alliance.

The Quasi-Cooperative Partner

This partner is interested in making sure that you receive just enough value from the alliance so that you will not exit. By providing you with the minimally acceptable amount of value, you still prefer the alliance above other alternatives, but not by much. This relationship is unbalanced in terms of power and dependence, but can be stable, albeit not as rewarding for the weaker party. This partner sees the alliance in terms of keeping you interested, but barely.

The Indifferent Partner

This partner—for better or worse—is not particularly interested in your strategic aspirations at all. The partner sees the alliance primarily as a vehicle for the achievement of his/her strategic goals, and you are simply along for the ride. The partner has no objections to your expending effort for your purposes, as long as (1) he does not need to help you do this, and (2) the attainment of his objectives are not impeded as a result. This partner sees the alliance in terms of "I'll get mine, you find yours."

The Competitive Partner

This partner is worse than indifferent, insofar as he perceives your gains as implying a loss for him, even when really there is no such trade-off. This person is oblivious to the positive-sum possibilities of the alliance, and very sensitive to the zero-sum aspects. This partner cannot abide any asymmetry in alliance success that might favor you, even if such variation is a natural or short-term occurrence. This partner is so fixated on the relative comparison aspects of the relationship that he sees the alliance in terms of "your gain must mean my loss." Another major pharmaceutical firm had this philosophy, in that managers in this firm viewed a win/win alliance situation as one in which they felt they had "left money on the table." They would often seek to renegotiate win/win alliances.

The Vengeful Partner

This partner is even worse than a win/lose partner, because he is primarily focused on ensuring that you lose, even if he loses, as well. You might not think that such partners exist, and it is unlikely that you would knowingly ally with such a partner, but a partner can develop this orientation when problems in the alliance become personalized and negative emotion plays a larger role. Note that we readily accept the notion of positive emotion in alliances when we claim that trust between partners is a beneficial aspect of an alliance relationship. However, we suggest that when one partner feels that the other has somehow violated that trust, a sense of betrayal emerges that can lead a partner to act irrationally. This partner sees the alliance in terms of "I may lose, but you'll lose more." While this is admittedly rare, several alliances have had protracted legal battles when one party feels that the other party did not act "in good faith."

As you can see, there are multiple partner types, and most of them are not particularly attractive. So, how can you "know thy partner" in advance? First and foremost, you must pay careful attention during the alliance emergence process for cues from your alliance partner that suggest one type versus another. For example, we have observed in working with health care organizations that some alliance partners have little idea what their partners' strategic goals are. A cooperative partner would know this, and a lack of interest in the partner's goals is an early indication that your partner is indifferent, or worse. Similarly, explore with your partner alternative scenarios for the alliance, including some in which you do better initially, and gauge your partner's reaction. If your partner objects to the slightest asymmetries in alliance outcomes, this suggests a problem that will likely emerge again and again.

Finally, assuming you are comfortable with your partner's orientation at the inception of the alliance, you must still be vigilant to changes in that orientation that may arise due to changes in the context of the alliance, whether it be changes in environmental conditions or in personnel. Ideally, this type of "early warning system" will serve you well as the alliance relationship evolves. However, we also encourage you to utilize another valuable feature of strategic alliances: Be sure to have a clear written statement of exit provisions, by which you and your partner can extricate yourselves from an alliance that may no longer be serving its intended valued purpose.

DISCUSSION QUESTIONS

1. Under what circumstances would you agree with someone who said that alliances are very risky?
2. What dimensions would you use to classify the various types of strategic alliances? Why those dimensions?

3. Which alliance motivations do you think are the most compatible with each other?

4. What do you consider to be the likely stages of strategic alliance development? Does every alliance have to go through each stage?

5. What is the difference between an alliance problem and an alliance symptom, and what does this difference mean in terms of managerial intervention?

6. When can you tell if your partner is not likely to have a cooperative orientation?

REFERENCES

Alexander, T. A., Fennell, M. L., & Halpern, M. T. (1993, March). Leadership instability in hospitals: The influence of board-CEO relations and organizational growth and decline. *Administrative Science Quarterly*, 74–99.

Alter, C., & Hage, J. (1993). *Organizations working together*. Beverly Hills, CA: Sage.

American Hospital Association. (1998). *Hospital statistics*. Chicago: American Hospital Association Publishing.

Bazzoli, G. J., Chan, B., Shortell, S. M. & D'Aunno, T. (2000). The financial performance of hospitals belonging to health networks and systems. *Inquiry, 37*, 234–252.

Bazzoli, G. J., Dynan, L., & Burns, L. (1999–2000). Capitated contracting of integrated health provider organizations. *Inquiry, 36*(4), 426–444.

Bazzoli, G. J., Shortell, S. M., Dubbs, N., Chan, B., & Kralovec, P. (1999). A taxonomy of health networks and systems: Bringing order out of chaos. *Health Services Research, 33*(6),1683–1717.

Begun, J. W. (1992). Cooperative Strategies Weaken the Competitive Capabilities of Health Care Organizations. In W. Jack Duncan, Peter M. Ginter and Linda E. Swayne (Eds.) Strategic Issues in Health Care Management: Point and Counterpoint. Boston: PWS-KENT (44–50).

Burns, L. R. (1999). Polarity management: The key challenge for integrated delivery systems. *Journal of Healthcare Management, 44*(1), 14–33.

Burns, L. R., Alexander, J. A., Zuckerman, H. S., Andersen, R. A., Torrens, P., & Hilberman, D.

(1996, June). *The impact of economic integration on physician-organization alignment*. Paper presented at annual meeting of Association of Health Services Research, Chicago, IL.

Burns, L. R., Bazzoli, G. J., Dynan, L., & Wholey, D. R. (1997). Managed care, market stages, and integrated delivery systems: Is there a relationship? *Health Affairs, 16*, 204–218.

Burns, L. R., Bazzoli, G. J., Dynan, L., & Wholey, D. R. (1998, June). *HMO impact on integrated provider networks*. Paper presented at annual meeting of Association of Health Services Research, Washington, D.C.

Burns, L. R., & Thorpe, D. P. (1997). Physician-hospital organizations: Strategy, structure, and conduct. In R. Conners (Ed.), *Integrating the practice of medicine* (pp. 351–371). Chicago: American Hospital Association Publishing.

Burns, L. R., Walston, S., Alexander, J., Zuckerman, H., Anderson, R. and Torrens, P. (2001). Just how integrated are integrated delivery systems? Results from a National Survey. *Health Care Management Review 26*(1), 22–41.

Carman, J. M. (1992). *Strategic alliances among rural hospitals*. Berkeley, CA: Institute of Business and Economic Research, University of California, pp. 92–103.

Clement, J. P. (1987). Does hospital diversification improve financial outcomes? *Medical Care, 25*, 988–1001.

Clement, J. P., McCue, M. J., Luke, R. D., Bramble, J. D., Rossiter, L. F., Ozcan, Y. A., & Pai, C. W. (1997). Strategic hospital alliances: Impact on financial performance. *Health Affairs,16*(6), 193–203.

Cuellar, A., & Gertler, P. (2005, January). How the expansion of hospital systems has affected consumers. *Health Affairs, 24*(1), 213–219.

D'Aunno, T. A., & Zuckerman, H. S. (1987a). The emergence of hospital federations: An integration of perspectives from organizational theory. *Medical Care Review, 44*(2), 323–343.

D'Aunno, T. A., & Zuckerman, H. S. (1987b). A life cycle model of organizational federations: The case of hospitals. *Academy of Management Review, 12*, 534–545.

DeVries, R. A. (1978). Strength in numbers. *Hospitals: Journal of the American Hospital Association, 55*, 81–84.

Doz, Y. L., & Hamel, G. (1998). *Alliance advantage: The art of creating value through partnering.* Boston: Harvard Business School Press.

Duncan, W. J., Ginter, P. M., & Swayne, L. E. (1992). *Strategic issues in health care management: Point and counterpoint.* Boston: Kent Publishers.

Dynan, L., Bazzoli, G. J., & Burns, L. R. (1997). Assessing the extent of integration achieved through physician-hospital arrangements. *Journal of Healthcare Management, 43,* 242–262.

Emery, F., & Trist, E. (1965). The casual texture of organizational environments. *Human Relations, 18,* 21–32.

Ernst and Young. (1995). *Physician-hospital organizations: Profile 1995.* Washington, DC: Author.

Fennell, M. L., & Alexander, T. A. (1989). Hospital governance and profound organizational change. *Medical Care Review, 46*(2), 157–187.

Harrigan, K. R. (1985). *Managing for joint venture success.* Lexington, MA: Lexington Books.

Hawley, A. H. (1950). *Human ecology: A theory of community structure.* New York: Ronald Press.

Johnson, D. E. L. (1986). American healthcare systems. *Modern Healthcare, 16,* 78–82.

Kaluzny, A., Morrissey, J., & McKinney, M. (1990). Emerging organizational networks: The case of the community clinical oncology program. In S. Mick & associates (Eds.), *Innovation in health care delivery.* San Francisco, CA: Jossey-Bass.

Kaluzny, A., & Zuckerman, H. (1992, Winter). Strategic alliances: Two perspectives for understanding their effects on health services. *Hospital and Health Services Management, 37,* 477–490.

Kaluzny, A. D., Zuckerman, H. S., & Ricketts, T. C. (2002). *Partners: Forming strategic alliances in health care.* Beard Books, Washington, D.C.

Kaufmann, P. J. (1987). Commercial exchange relationships and the "negotiator's dilemma." *Negotiation Journal, 3,* 73–80.

Kotter, J. P., & Schlesinger, L. A. (1979). Choosing strategies for change. *Harvard Business Review, 57,* 106–114.

Longest, B. B. (1990). Interorganizational linkages in the health sector. *Health Care Management Review, 15,* 17–28.

Luhmann, N. (1979). *Trust and power.* New York: John Wiley and Sons.

Luke, R. D., Begun, J. W., & Pointer, D. D. (1989). Quasi firms: Strategic interorganizational forms in the health care industry. *Academy of Management Review, 14*(9), 19.

Macneil, I. R. (1983). Values in contract: Internal and external. *Northwestern University Law Review, 78,* 340–418.

Macneil, I. R. (1986). Exchange revisited: Individual utility and social solidarity. *Ethics, 96,* 567–593.

Madison, K. (2004). Hospital-physician affiliations and patient treatments, expenditures, and outcomes. *Health Services Research, 39* (2).

McCue, M. J., Clement, J. P., & Luke, R. D. (1999). Strategic hospital alliances: Do the type and market structure of strategic hospital alliances matter? *Medical Care, 37,* 1013–1022.

Meyer, A. (1982). Adapting to environmental jolts. *Administrative Science Quarterly, 27,* 515–537.

Morrisey, M., Alexander, J., Burns, L., & Johnson, V. (1999). The effects of managed care on physician and clinical integration in hospitals. *Medical Care, 37*(4), 350–361.

Morrisey, M. A., Alexander, J. A., Burns, L. R., & Johnson, V. (1996). Managed care and physician-hospital integration. *Health Affairs, 15,* 62–73.

Olden, P. C., Roggenkamp, S. D., & Luke, R. D. (2002). A post-1990s assessment of strategic hospital alliances and their marketplace orientations: Time to refocus. *Health Care Management Review, 27*(2), 33–49.

Oliver, C. (1990). Determinants of interorganizational relationships: Integration and future directions. *Academy of Management Review, 15*(2), 241–265.

Pfeffer, J., & Salancik, G. R. (1978). *The external control of organizations: A resource dependence perspective.* New York: Harper & Row.

Provan, K. G. (1983). The federation as an interorganizational linkage network. *Academy of Management Review, 8*(1), 79–89.

Provan, K. G. (1984). Interorganizational cooperation and decision making autonomy in a consortium multihospital system. *Academy of Management Review, 9,* 494–504. Reuters Business Insight, (August 16, 2004) "Pharmaceutical strategic alliance: Benchmarking 21st century deal-making" http//www.the-infoshop.com

Schelling, T. C. (1960). *The strategy of conflict.* Cambridge, MA: Harvard University.

Scott, W. R. (1987). The adolescence of institutional theory. *Administrative Science Quarterly, 32,* 493–511.

Shortell, S. M. (1988). The evolution of hospital systems: Unfulfilled promises and self-fulfilling prophecies. *Medical Care Review, 45*(2), 177–214.

Shortell, S. M., Morrison, E. M., & Friedman, B. (1990). *Strategic choices for America's hospitals: Managing change in turbulent times.* San Francisco: Jossey-Bass.

Shortell, S. M., & Zajac, E. J. (1988). Internal corporate joint ventures: Development processes and performance outcomes. *Strategic Management Journal, 9,* 527–542.

Shortell, S. M., & Zajac, E. J. (1990). Health care organizations and the development of the strategic management perspective. In S. Mick & associates (Eds), *Innovations in health care delivery: New insights into organization theory* (pp. 141–180). San Francisco: Jossey-Bass.

Sofaer, S., & Myrtle, R. C. (1991). Interorganizational theory and research: Implications for health care management, policy, and research. *Medical Care Review, 48,* 371–409.

Starkweather, D. B. (1971). Health facility mergers: Some conceptualizations. *Medical Care, 9,* 468–478.

Starr, P. (1982). *The social transformation of American medicine.* New York: Basic Books.

Thompson, J. T. (1967). *Organizations in action.* New York: McGraw Hill.

Ury, W. L., Brett, J. M., & Goldberg, S. B. (1988). *Getting disputes resolved.* San Francisco: Jossey-Bass.

Zajac, E. J. (1986). *Organizations, environments, and performance: A study of contract management in hospitals.* Unpublished dissertation, University of Philadelphia, Pennsylvania.

Zajac, E. J., Golden, B. R., & Shortell, S. M. (1991). New organizational forms for enhancing innovation: The case of internal corporate joint ventures. *Management Science, 37,* 70–84.

Zajac, E. J., & Olsen, C. P. (1993). From transaction costs to transactional value analysis: Implications for the study of interorganizational strategies. *Journal of Management Studies, 30,* 131–146.

Zajac, E. J., & Shortell, S. M. (1989). Changing generic strategies: Likelihood, direction, and performance implications. *Strategic Management Journal, 10,* 413–430.

Zuckerman, H. S., & D'Aunno, T. A. (1990). Hospital alliances: Cooperative strategy in a competitive environment. *Health Care Management Review, 15*(2), 21–30.

Zuckerman, H. S., & Kaluzny, A. (1991, Spring). The management of strategic alliances in health services. *Frontiers of Health Services Management, 7*(5), 3–23.

Zuckerman, H. S., Kaluzny, A. D., & Ricketts, T. C. (1995). Alliances in health care: What we know, what we think we know, and what we should know. *Health Care Management Review, 20*(1), 54–64.

CHAPTER 12

Organizational Learning, Innovation, and Change

Bryan J. Weiner, Ph.D., Christian D. Helfrich, Ph.D., and S. Robert Hernandez, Dr.PH

CHAPTER OUTLINE

LEARNING OBJECTIVES

After completing this chapter, the reader should be able to:

1. Identify the characteristics that make health care organizations complex systems.

2. Describe the five disciplines that promote organizational learning.

3. Explain why organizational learning often proves difficult in practice.

4. Describe the nature of the innovation process and the factors involved in that process.

5. Identify managerial actions that facilitate learning, innovation, and change.

KEY TERMS

Adaptive Learning

Adoption

Balancing Feedback Loops

Compatibility

Complexity

Change

Collective Innovations

Combinatorial Complexity

Dissemination

Diffusion

Double-Loop Learning

Generative Learning

Homophily

Implementation

Implementation Policies and
    Practices

Innovation

Innovation Effectiveness

Learning Organization

Mental Models

Moving

Network Externalities

Network Structures

Observability

Opinion Leaders

Performance Gaps

Personal Mastery

Policy Resistance

Refreezing

Reinforcing Feedback Loops

Relative Advantage

Restructuring

Shared Vision

Single-Loop Learning

Systems Thinking

Team Learning

Trialability

Unfreezing

❧ IN PRACTICE — How Will Your Drug Be Affected by Negative Study Results?

In March 2004, results were released from the Prove-It study, in which two cholesterol-lowering drugs (statins) were evaluated for their effectiveness in reducing LDL cholesterol to levels well below those recommended at the time (Cannon, Braunwald et al., 2004). The study immediately and dramatically affected sales of two widely prescribed statins: Pfizer's Lipitor and AstraZeneca's Crestor. The remarkable thing wasn't that Lipitor sales increased to 40% of all new statin prescriptions, versus 27% just days before the study results were released, but that sales dropped equally precipitously for Crestor, from 28% to 17% of all new statin prescriptions, even though Crestor was not one of the drugs studied. The study actually compared Lipitor with Pravachol, a statin manufactured by the study's sponsor, Bristol-Meyers Squibb. Pravachol sales remained steady at 7% of all new statin prescriptions. So why did Crestor, which was not even evaluated, get punished rather than Pravachol, which did poorly?

Just days before the release of study results, Public Citizen, an advocacy group, called upon the Food and Drug Administration (FDA) to recall Crestor because of severe side effects. While Crestor's sales dipped only modestly following Public Citizen's demand, the action may have made the drug particularly vulnerable to its primary competitor when strong evidence emerged for Lipitor's efficacy. But why did Pravachol sales not suffer as well, or even more, than sales of Crestor, given that Crestor actually lost to Lipitor in the head-to-head study? Possibly because sales of Pravachol were already much lower than for the other two drugs and were concentrated among niche patients with certain conditions. Physicians are reluctant to switch drugs for patients in stable condition. Thus, it probably would take more negative news to make physicians change their prescribing behavior (Winslow, 2004).

CHAPTER PURPOSE

The reaction of physicians and patients to the Prove It study illustrates the difficulty of predicting how events, even seemingly unrelated ones, will affect an organization's business performance, strategic plans, and innovation efforts. Indeed, health care leaders often find themselves puzzled by the "counterintuitive behavior" of health care organizations. Health maintenance organizations (HMOs) begin requiring physicians to choose less-expensive generic drugs, only to find that pharmaceutical costs rise rather than fall due to unintended changes in physician prescribing behavior. Hospitals implement quality management tools and practices that have been proven effective in manufacturing settings, only to find that quality of care worsens rather than improves. A physician group practice introduces electronic medical records and medical errors decrease, but only for a few months, after which they rise to levels even higher than before. A department manager introduces a flexible work schedule to improve job satisfaction and job retention, only to see morale plummet and turnover increase as nurses find themselves working longer hours with less predictability in assignments.

Social systems rarely behave the way we want them to, or even the way that we predict they will. Due to unanticipated consequences, yesterday's solutions become today's problems. Our efforts to introduce change provoke opposition by those who seek to maintain the status quo. We apply solutions that worked well before, only to find that they do not work again. So, we try harder, applying them with even greater fervor, but the problem only gets worse. Or the solution works, but introduces such deleterious side effects that the cure seems worse than the disease. In health care organizations, and all organizations for that matter, these unexpected dynamics produce **policy resistance**: the tendency for interventions to be delayed, diluted, or defeated by the response of the system to the intervention itself (Sterman, 2000).

Many believe that, to understand and mitigate policy resistance, health care leaders need to rethink their views of how organizations work and how they can be improved and changed. This chapter introduces a perspective of health care organizations that borrows from quantum theory and chaos theory. As described in Chapter 1, health care organizations are complex adaptive systems whose future states are unpredictable and unknowable. Moreover, we see innovation and change not as rational, controllable processes, but instead as complex, uncertain, nonlinear sequences of events and activities. Bridging these perspectives and integrating them is the notion of the **learning organization**, where innovation and change are seen as everyday activities and inputs for further learning (McGill & Slocum, 1993). The chapter concludes with managerial guidelines for generating learning, stimulating innovation, and implementing change.

CHANGE IN AN UNPREDICTABLE, UNKNOWABLE WORLD

Management theories reflect the "governing ideas" of their time. As noted in Chapter 1, scientific management and other closed-system theories reflected a mechanistic view of social and physical systems inspired by Newtonian physics. Structural contingency theory, population ecology theory, and other open-systems theories reflected an organic view of social and physical systems inspired by developments in the 1960s and 1970s in the fields of biology and ecology. Since the 1990s, new management concepts and theories have emerged as management scholars and practitioners absorb and apply recent developments in quantum theory and chaos theory (Begun, 1994; Plsek, 2001; Stacey, 1995; Zimmerman, 1999).

Quantum theory tells us that the world is not only unpredictable, but also fundamentally unknowable.

Classical theory in physics suggests that if we have enough information about the current state of a physical system, and enough processing capacity to analyze that information, we can accurately predict the future state of a physical system (Capra, 1982; Wheatley, 1992). Quantum theory denies this possibility, noting that the very act of measurement (i.e., collecting the information) alters the physical systems we hope to understand. Known as the Heisenberg principle, this seemingly counterintuitive finding appears even in social interactions. The simple act of taking a blood pressure measurement, for instance, may induce higher blood pressure if the patient feels anxious about the procedure or the situation. Likewise, administering a patient satisfaction survey may subtly influence a patient's feeling of satisfaction by calling her attention (through the survey questions) to some aspects of her visit, but not others. A key insight from quantum theory, therefore, is that continuous change, activity, and interconnectedness add an element of unpredictability to any system. As such, planned, controlled, orderly approaches to innovation or change are unlikely to perfectly achieve their intended outcomes.

Chaos theory also tells us that the future state of the world is unknowable because physical systems are highly sensitive to initial conditions. Chaos theorists semi-humorously illustrate such sensitivity with the notion that the flapping of a butterfly's wings in Brazil can initiate an atmospheric disturbance sufficient to create a tornado in Texas. "Butterfly effects" occur not only due to the sensitivity of systems to initial conditions, but also because most social systems—even very simple ones—exhibit interconnectedness and nonlinear dynamics. "Butterfly effects" occur in health care systems when seemingly simple, local changes rapidly lead to unanticipated, significant problems elsewhere in the system. For instance, small changes in personnel scheduling and hours of operation in a community health center can seriously disrupt a smoothly functioning emergency department at the local hospital. Likewise, small changes in information systems to address patient registration problems can lead to hundreds of thousands of dollars in lost

billing. Given the sensitivity of systems to initial conditions, chaos theory warns that programs, processes, or practices that work well in one health care organization may work poorly (or not at all) even when faithfully implemented (Wheatley, 1992). Even among health care organizations that look very much alike, small differences in initial conditions can lead to radically different outcomes.

So, where does this leave the health care executive? How does one manage and lead in a world that is unpredictable and fundamentally unknowable? No new management theory has emerged in response to quantum theory or chaos theory, but scholars and practitioners see two implications (Mintzberg, 1993; Senge, 1990; Stacey, 1995; Wheatley, 1992). First, we need to change the way we think about organizations. Organizations are more than simply open systems; they are complex adaptive systems. To grasp how complex adaptive systems work, we need new concepts and perhaps new ways of thinking that sensitize us to interrelationships, nonlinearity, and sensitivity to initial conditions (see In Practice, p. 386). Second, we need to rethink the roles of leadership and management. The classical management tasks of planning, organizing, deciding, and controlling are not sufficient to navigate complex adaptive systems such as health care organizations through an unpredictable, unknowable world. Rather the leader's new work consists of nurturing the development of organizations capable of learning in real-time and improvising in the face of frequent, unplanned changes (Senge, 1990).

HEALTH CARE ORGANIZATIONS AS COMPLEX ADAPTIVE SYSTEMS

Health care organizations are complex adaptive systems (Begun, Zimmerman, et al., 2003). What makes them complex adaptive systems is: (1) the individual

---

IN PRACTICE

New Concepts for Leading Health Care Organizations

For James Roberts, MD, senior vice president of VHA, Inc., the concepts of self-organization, coevolution, and emergence proved useful for understanding and guiding the creation of the VHA's Physician Leadership Network. The concept of coevolution, for instance, sensitized him to the interdependence that existed within VHA. As the organization developed a comparative database of physician practices, the relationships among the VHA's Dallas headquarters, the regional offices, and the physicians began to change. When relationships are coevolving rather than being dominated by one partner, ideas for new products, services, and processes emerge that no participant alone could have created or anticipated. "This idea of coevolving with our customers is one of the most powerful ideas around today. It's really forced me to think about the barriers to us really working together, coevolving. How do we blur the distinctions between providers, customers, and suppliers? After all, we are all in this together"(Zimmerman, 1999).

---

agents who work in them have the freedom to act in ways that are not always predictable, and (2) the actions of these agents are interconnected such that one agent's actions change the context for other agents (Plesk, 2001). Like other complex adaptive systems, health care organizations exhibit two forms of complexity. **Combinatorial complexity** (or "detail" complexity) arises from the number of constituent elements of a system or the number of interrelationships that might exist among them (Senge, 1990). For instance, the problem of optimally scheduling a suite of operating rooms in a hospital is highly complex. However, the problem's complexity lies in finding the best solution out of an astronomical number of possibilities. Dynamic complexity, on the other hand, arises from the operation of feedback loops (Sterman, 2000). There are two basic types of feedback loops. **Reinforcing feedback loops** amplify or intensify whatever is happening in a system. In everyday language, we refer to reinforcing feedback loops as self-fulfilling prophecies or the *Pygmalion Effect*. For instance, a physician group practice that delivers high-quality care develops a positive reputation, which, through positive word of mouth, generates more referrals. More referrals, in turn, generate

more resources that could be invested to further increase quality of care. **Balancing feedback loops** counteract or oppose whatever is happening in a system. For example, when the physicians in a group practice see more patients than they can realistically manage, patient satisfaction and possibly quality of care begin to suffer. Over time, negative word of mouth leads to fewer referrals and lighter schedules. Whereas reinforcing feedback loops drive a system toward disequilibrium and constitute the engines of accelerating growth or accelerating decline, balancing feedback loops drive a system toward equilibrium and constitute the engines of steady states or goal-oriented behavior. It is important to emphasize that reinforcing feedback loops can produce desirable or undesirable consequences. So, too, can balancing feedback loops.

Although combinatorial or detail complexity is important, dynamic complexity is critical to understanding the behavior of complex adaptive systems. When dynamic complexity exists (i.e., when feedback loops operate), the same action can have different effects in the short term and the long term. Likewise, actions can have one consequence locally and a different consequence elsewhere in the system. Policy resistance itself signals the presence of

DEBATE 12.1   What Do You Think?

Is there still a role for planning, organizing, deciding, and controlling in complex adaptive systems? Some management scholars and practitioners argue that organizational survival depends on managers giving up their "obsession with control, knowing what is going on, and seeking stability" (Berquist, 1992; McDaniel, 1997; Vaill, 1989; Wheatley, 1992). Others contend that classical management tasks still have a place in complex adaptive systems. For instance, Stacey (1996) proposes that, in complex adaptive systems, selecting the appropriate management or leadership approaches depends on two factors: the amount of certainty about cause-effect linkages (e.g., "If we do X, then Y occurs.") and the amount of agreement about an issue or decision (e.g., "What should we do?"). When high certainty and high agreement exist, classical management tasks work well. Plsek (2001) observes, for instance, that a surgical team doing a routine gallbladder surgery exhibits high certainty about the surgical procedures that lead to successful outcomes and high agreement about how to work together. Managing such situations calls for using data from the past to predict the future, planning paths of action to achieve outcomes, and then monitoring actual versus expected outcomes in order to reduce variation. When uncertainty is high and disagreement reigns, chaos and anarchy often result. In such situations, few management or leadership approaches work. When only modest levels of certainty and agreement exist, organizations enter the "zone of complexity" or the "edge of chaos," where high levels of creativity and innovation become possible. In this zone, managers cannot hope to understand what a complex adaptive system will do or how to optimize it. Hence, traditional management approaches lose their effectiveness. Instead, managers should lead by setting a few simple roles, establishing a "good enough vision," and creating a wide space for innovation.

dynamic complexity. What makes dynamic complexity "complex" is that feedback loops often contain delays—or interruptions between actions and consequences—that are poorly understood and often ignored. People have difficulty grasping system dynamics when cause and effect are distant from one another in space or time. In addition, most complex adaptive systems possess dozens or even hundreds of interlocking feedback loops. People can sometimes infer correctly the dynamics of systems possessing isolated loops; however, people's ability to predict the behavior of systems possessing multiple, interlocking loops is significantly challenged by their perceptual and cognitive limitations as individuals (Sterman, 2000).

Some management scholars and practitioners argue that, when we view organizations as complex adaptive systems, we see a need for leaders to play different roles and exercise different skills than those called for in classical organization and management theory (Senge, 1990; Stacey, 1995; Wheatley, 1992). In all of these prescriptions, learning takes center stage. As McDaniel (1997, p. 27) observes:

Both quantum theory and chaos theory led to the conclusion that future states of an organization are unknowable. Because the future is unknowable, success for health care organizations comes through organizational learning. Learning replaces control as complex adaptive systems anticipate the future (Gleick, 1987; Stacey, 1995; Zimmerman, 1993). Strategic leaders, therefore, should help organizations focus on learning rather than knowing. It is through this process that leaders and organizations can successfully cope with the turbulent unfolding of the health care world (see Debate Time 12.1).

ORGANIZATIONAL LEARNING

Learning itself is a feedback process. A person takes action, gathers information about the effects of her action, and then revises her understanding of the world and herself. In its simplest form, learning resembles a balancing feedback loop in which you compare your desired (or anticipated) state of affairs with the actual results of your conduct and then act in ways that you believe or hope will close the gap. Argyris and Schon (1978) refer to this type of learning as **single-loop learning**, a relatively simple error-and-correction process where problem-solvers look for solutions within an organization's policies, plans, values, and rules (Argyris & Schon, 1978). A more complex form of learning, which Argyris and Schon refer to as **double-loop learning**, occurs when problem-solvers attempt to close the gap between desired and actual states of affairs by questioning and modifying those organization's policies, plans, values, and rules that frame organizational problems and guide organizational action. Changes in underlying values and assumptions, in turn, prompt changes in action strategies (see Figure 12.1).

Both single-loop and double-loop learning are necessary and useful for health care organizations. Single-loop learning promotes **adaptive learning**, in which problem-solvers adjust their behavior and work processes in response to changing events or trends. For instance, a quality improvement team might invoke the Plan-Do-Study-Act (PDSA) cycle (Berwick, 1998)—a form of single-loop learning—in order to test the effectiveness of using posted

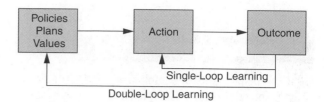

Figure 12.1. Single-Loop versus Double-Loop Learning

hand-washing reminders to reduce nosocomial (i.e., hospital-acquired) infections and thereby shorten lengths of stay. Double-loop learning promotes **generative learning**, in which problem-solvers attempt to eliminate problems by changing the underlying structure of the system. This underlying structure includes the operating policies of the decision-makers and actors in the system (e.g., their values and assumptions). For instance, a quality improvement team seeking to reduce handoffs among clinical professionals and thereby increase quality and safety might begin questioning deeply held assumptions about the value of staff specialization. On the basis of such questioning, they may redesign the care delivery system to employ multiskilled employees working in small, empowered work teams (Leander, 1996; Wermers, Dagnillo, et al., 1996). Organizational learning embraces both adaptive and generative learning.

Learning Organizations

While scholars and theorists have discussed organizational learning for some time, Peter Senge's 1990 book, *The Fifth Discipline,* popularized the term learning organization. In rather romantic terms, he described learning organizations as places where "people continually expand their capacity to create the results they truly desire, where new and expansive patterns of thinking are nurtured, where collective aspiration is set free, and where people are continually learning to learn together" (Senge, 1990, p. 1). In more prosaic language, Garvin (1993, p. 80) defined a learning organization as "an organization skilled at creating, acquiring, and transferring knowledge, and at modifying its behavior to reflect new knowledge and insights."

Although individual learning and organizational learning are inextricably intertwined, the latter involves collectively working together to gain experience, glean insights, build competence, and engage in new behavior (DiBella & Nevis, 1998). The knowledge and capabilities generated by organizational learning remain properties of the collective unit, reflected in its structures, processes, and culture. Thus, new knowledge and capabilities remain even if individual organizational participants leave.

Learning Disciplines

Senge (1990) describes five disciplines that, when combined, produce an organization capable of "expanding its capacity to create its future." He refers to these component technologies as disciplines because each involves a body of theory and techniques that must be practiced in order for mastery to develop. The disciplines are systems thinking, personal mastery, mental models, shared vision, and team learning.

- **Systems thinking** refers to the discipline of seeing wholes, perceiving the structures that underlie dynamically complex systems, and identifying high-leverage change opportunities. Systems thinking involves not only the recognition of the properties of complex systems, but also the skilled application of systems archetypes to illuminate the deeper structures that shape everyday organizational behavior and performance (see Figure 12.2). Through training and practice, organizational members can see where actions and changes in structures can lead to significant, enduring improvements (Senge, 1990, p. 114).

- **Personal mastery** is the discipline of individual learning, without which organizational learning cannot occur. Personal mastery involves continuously clarifying our individual sense of purpose and vision, and continuously learning how to see the world as it is without distortion. The tension created by the gap between vision and reality, if tapped creatively, generates energy for exploration and growth. Organizational members who demonstrate personal mastery are apt to exhibit greater commitment, take more initiative, learn faster, and feel greater responsibility. Fostering personal mastery requires, at a minimum, adopting Theory Y assumptions about human behavior and instituting organizational policies and practices that promote employee growth and development (see Chapter 3).

- **Mental models** refers to the discipline of constantly surfacing, testing, and improving our assumptions about how the world works. Mental models actively shape what we see and, therefore, how we act. By training and encouraging organizational members in the dual skills of reflection and inquiry (e.g., recognizing leaps of abstraction and uncovering censored thoughts and feelings), managers can promote organizational learning by loosening the grip of tacit, often faulty mental models (e.g., higher quality always costs more).

- **Shared vision** is the discipline of generating a common answer to the question, What do we want to create? Shared vision connects people through common aspiration and derives its motivational power by tapping people's personal visions. From shared vision comes the focus and energy for learning, the willingness to take risks and experiment, the mutual alignment of individual effort, and the commitment to the long-term view. Creating shared vision requires encouraging organizational members to develop and communicate personal visions, inquiring into the deeper vision that unites the diversity of expressed views, and staying the course through difficult times.

- **Team learning** refers to the discipline of creating alignment such that team members think insightfully about complex problems, synergize their knowledge and skills, and produce coordinated action. Team learning requires an organizational climate that promotes trust and respect—where it is safe for individuals to share both strengths and weaknesses. Such an environment diminishes individuals' inclination toward defensiveness as a protection from embarrassment or vulnerability to threat they may perceive in exposing such weaknesses to their colleagues. This can be achieved by promoting a mastery of open-minded dialogue where each individual learns from the others, the net result being a collective, organizational search for alternative meanings and new perspectives.

Senge emphasizes that all five disciplines matter because each builds upon and reinforces the others. Personal mastery, for instance, facilitates the integration of reason and intuition, which, in turn, enhances one's ability to see interrelationships among seemingly discrete events. Similarly, working with mental models loosens the grip of deeply held, often tacit assumptions that hinder systems thinking, shared vision, and team learning.

Limits of Organizational Learning

Although the promise of learning organizations is exciting, managers' enthusiasm for learning organizations needs to be tempered not only by the significant challenges involved in building such organizations, but also the seemingly intractable limits of organizational learning. First, organizational members usually possess only limited information, much of which is ambiguous or inaccurate. As Sterman (2000, p. 23) observes: "No one knows the current sales rate of their company, the current rate of production, or the true value of the order backlog at any given time. Instead, we receive estimates of these data based on sampled, averaged, and delayed measurements. The act of measurement introduces distortions, delays, biases, errors, and other imperfections, some known, others unknown and unknowable." In addition, expectancy gives rise to selective perception. In other words, we see or hear what we expect to see or hear, rather than what actually occurs (Bowditch & Buono, 2001). For instance, our mental models about what

is meaningful and important inform what we choose to define, measure, and monitor with our information systems; in turn, our information systems shape the perceptions that we form (Sterman, 2000). In this sense, we *enact* the environment in which we live (Weick, 1979).

Second, even with perfect and complete information, organizational members routinely engage in unscientific reasoning due to judgment errors and biases (Hammond, Keeney, & Raiffa, 1998). The human mind relies upon unconscious routines, called heuristics, to cope with complexity and uncertainty (Kahneman, Slovic, & Tversky, 1982). These heuristics, while efficient, often distort reasoning and judgment. Although the five learning disciplines can dampen the effects of recall bias, overconfidence, and other decision traps they cannot eliminate them or the poor learning that they produce.

Finally, organizational learning often bumps up against practical problems and competing priorities. For instance, many decisions and programs experience implementation delays or alterations as they encounter technical obstacles, resource constraints, or political resistance. Imperfect implementation hinders learning, especially when long time spans are involved. In addition, as Sterman (2000, p. 33) observes, "In the real world of irreversible actions and high stakes, the need to maintain performance often overrides the need to learn by suppressing new strategies for fear that they would cause present harm even though they might yield great insight and prevent future harm."

MANAGING ORGANIZATIONAL INNOVATION

Learning lies at the heart of both innovation and change. Learning, by definition, occurs when practice or experience lead to a relatively lasting change in knowledge or skill. Neither innovation nor change occurs without learning. **Innovation**

Using Systems Archetypes to Understand Organizational Behavior

System archetypes—or patterns of structure that occur again and again—represent the key tools of systems thinking. System archetypes enable people to *see* how interlocking reinforcing and balancing feedback loops influence the behavior of social systems; by seeing these structures at play, it becomes possible to identify those *high-leverage* actions that can produce lasting change. Senge (1990) describes several system archetypes, including one he calls "Limits to Growth." As illustrated in Figure 12.2, in Limits to Growth, a reinforcing feedback loop generates a spiral of success, but also triggers a balancing feedback loop that, after a delay, slows down the success. Limits to Growth structures explain why many efforts to improve quality and productivity (e.g., introducing quality circles) initially make progress, but later fail (Senge, 1990) as shown in Figure 12.3.

At first, these efforts promote more open communication between managers and employees, which, in turn, improves collective problem-solving ability. However, as the effort becomes more successful, it also becomes more threatening to the traditional distribution of power within the organization. Fearing a loss of power, union leaders begin undermining the effort by playing on workers' fears of being manipulated by management. Fearing that greater worker participation in decision making could undermine their power, managers begin to act defensively by only going through the motions of taking worker's input seriously. After an initial spurt of activity and some measure of success, the quality improvement initiative sputters and perhaps even dies. The key to *escaping* the limits to growth archetype is not to push harder (e.g., exhort, reward, and punish), but rather to address the limiting factor (e.g., adversarial union-management relationships). Senge contends that a small number of system archetypes account for a significant proportion of the behavior of complex adaptive systems and that understanding these archetypes enables managers to act intelligently and skillfully to change organizational behavior (Senge, 1990).

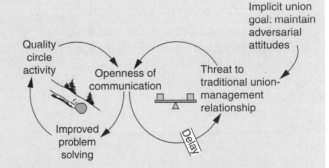

Figure 12.2. Reinforcing Feedback Loop

Figure 12.3. Balancing Feedback Loop

refers to the process by which an organization puts a technology or practice to use for the first time, regardless of whether other organizations have previously used the technology or practice (Emmons, 2000; Klein & Sorra, 1996; Nord & Tucker, 1987; Rogers, 1995, 2003). **Change** is a broader concept that deals with any modification in organizational composition, structure, or behavior—new or not new to the organization.

Managing organizational innovation is something like playing Blackjack against the house with a single deck of cards. Your skill usually has frustratingly little to do with the outcome of any single hand, but you can greatly improve your chances of winning overall by shrewdly estimating probabilities and playing strategically. And, like any gamble, pursuing organizational innovation inherently means taking on some risk.

How does one play strategically? Although innovation is perhaps the best-studied phenomena in management research, one of the most consistent findings is how unpredictable and complex the process is (Meyer & Goes, 1988), and this finding could ultimately be the most important lesson for managers to understand (Van de Ven, Polley, et al. 1999). However, as the saying goes, "chance favors the prepared mind." The best preparation may simply be to know the basic stages that *most* organizations go through when they try to innovate.

Before proceeding to describe these stages, however, two caveats merit discussion. First, innovation adoption and implementation processes may differ significantly for different types of innovations. For instance, innovation researchers often distinguish technical innovations from administrative innovations. In health care, technical innovations include ideas for new technologies (e.g., magnetic resonance imaging, or MRI), new products (e.g., new drugs), new services (e.g., telemedicine), and new clinical processes (e.g., administering aspirin immediately following a heart attack). Administrative innovations include new ideas or practices in the areas of personnel selection, resource allocation, task design, and organizational structure. Recent

examples of administrative innovations include total quality management (Kimberly & Minvielle, 2003), business process reengineering (Hammer & Champy, 1993), patient-focused care (Lathrop, 1993), clinical service lines (Charns & Tewksbury, 1993), and the balanced scorecard (Kaplan & Norton, 1996).

Second, a strong pro-innovation bias exists in management thinking and research and, perhaps, U.S. culture generally (Kimberly, 1981). As Downs and Mohr (1979) put it, "The act of innovating is still heavily laden with positive value. . . . Innovation, especially when seen as more than purely technological change, is still associated with improvement." However, not all innovations merit adoption or diffusion: Some cause more harm than good, while others seem appropriate only in limited circumstances. For instance, in the 1980s and 1990s, many hospitals developed cardiac surgery programs as an innovative, and lucrative, service; however, research subsequently showed that a large proportion of hospitals performing coronary artery bypass surgery (CABG) did not achieve sufficiently high volumes of surgery to maintain high-quality programs (Grumbach, Anderson, et al., 1995). Studies show that patients undergoing CABG at low-volume hospitals face a much higher risk of mortality than those undergoing the procedure at high-volume hospitals (Damberg, Chung, et al., 2001; New York State Department of Health, 2001), a finding that has prompted some state agencies to close some low-volume cardiac surgery programs and restrict the opening of new programs (Chassin, 2002).

The Innovation Model

Making sense of the voluminous management literature on organizational innovation is difficult without a framework for sorting the varied, and sometimes inconsistent, research findings and prescriptions found there. Everett Rogers (2003) offers a helpful, simple five-stage model of the organizational innovation process: agenda setting,

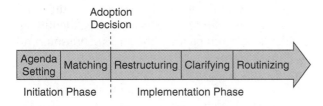

Figure 12.4. The Innovation Process
in an Organization

SOURCE: Adapted from Rogers, E. M. (2003). *The Diffusion of Innovations* (5th ed., p. 421). New York: Free Press.

matching, restructuring, clarifying, and routinizing (Rogers, 2003). (See Figure 12.4.) Although innovation in complex adaptive systems rarely occurs through the linear process described by the model, the model nonetheless offers a useful vehicle for discussing what we know, and do not know, about innovation.

Agenda Setting

Agenda setting often initiates the decision to adopt an innovation. Agenda setting refers to the ongoing process within organizations through which organizational members identify important problems and search for innovations to address these problems. **Performance gaps**—perceived discrepancies between expected and actual organizational performance—often trigger the innovation processes as organizational members look for new ideas or technologies to bridge the gap (Rogers, 2003). In some cases, organizational members begin with a perceived need and then search for innovations. In other cases, they first learn of an innovation and then find a need for it. Although this might seem illogical, it occurs because organizational members often face many pressing problems for which few solutions exist. In such cases, innovation results when organizational members opportunistically scan the internal and external environment for new ideas that might benefit the organization, and then find problems to solve (March, 1981).

Regardless of whether the problem or the solution comes first, the innovation process itself is largely driven by how organizational members perceive and prioritize needs. Two factors play a key role: who participates in the agenda-setting process, and how those participants perceive information. Given the hierarchical structure of most health care organizations, senior managers wield considerable influence over both the course and the outcomes of agenda setting. Indeed, research shows that senior managers' views of organizational priorities, attitudes towards change, and levels of technical training are strong predictors of whether or not organizations choose to adopt a given innovation, particularly those innovations that are new to a specific industry (Young, Charns, et al., 2001).

Although senior managers typically dominate agenda-setting processes, middle managers can contribute in significant ways by synthesizing and interpreting information from the external environment for the organization (Pappas, Flaherty, et al., 2004), discovering new opportunities, and accumulating and managing resources for strategic change (Floyd & Wooldridge, 1994). They can do so because of their unique experience on the front line and the social and professional networks they develop over time (Floyd & Wooldridge, 1994). Similarly, physicians, nurses, and other clinical professionals possess valuable information and unique perspectives on clinical workloads, patient care issues, intraorganizational coordination, and new technologies (Blumenthal & Edwards, 1995; Kirkley, 2004; McDaniel & Ashmos, 1986). Viewing organizations as complex adaptive systems calls attention to the value of greater involvement by middle managers and clinical professionals in agenda setting. The participation of these two groups increases not only the amount of information available but also the diversity of perspectives brought to bear on that information—permitting new insights and alternative meanings to emerge (Ashmos, Huonker, et al., 1998). Yet, despite these potential advantages, research suggests that strategic planning and other agenda-setting activities remain the almost exclusive province of senior managers (Mintzberg, 1997).

How agenda-setting participants perceive information also shapes the innovation process. Performance gaps often occur when organizational members perceive shocks in the regulatory, demographic, technological, social, and market environment (Drucker, 1998). However, people experience difficulty objectively appraising such events and trends partly due to the limits on organizational learning, mentioned earlier, and partly due to the propensity to view change in a negative light. Research shows that managers tend to view strategic issues as threats rather than opportunities (Jackson & Dutton, 1988), and, further, that perceived threat causes people to restrict the amount of information they attend to and the solutions that they consider (Billings, Milburn, et al., 1980; Staw, Sandelands, et al., 1981). Rather than triggering innovation, shocks might instead prompt managers to engage in wishful thinking, rely on faith, or resign their futures to fate (McCrae, 1984). Managers who perceive situations as opportunities rather than threats engage in more open-minded search for information searching and more explicitly weigh advantages and disadvantages of particular actions (Nutt, 1984). Even then, however, research shows that people generally value loss prevention over gain (Kahneman & Tversky, 1979); hence, they are more inclined to focus on mitigating perceived threats than identifying and exploiting opportunities. Health care managers can moderate people's tendency to bury their heads in the sand or otherwise pass on potentially valuable innovation opportunities by formally structuring the agenda-setting processes through the use of such tools as situational analysis, STEP analysis, and other decision-making and group process management techniques (see Chapters 6 and 14).

Matching

During the matching stage, the organization's needs and capacities are matched to the innovation and the decision to adopt or not adopt is made (Rogers, 2003). In the matching stage, organizational mem-

bers learn about the feasibility of adopting the innovation by anticipating benefits and costs, identifying problems that might arise in implementation, and outlining strategies for dealing with them. Matching is often not a formal, explicit process; moreover, matching may continue even after the innovation has been nominally adopted. Matching involves the interplay of two sets of factors: (1) innovation characteristics, and (2) social system characteristics.

Innovation Characteristics. Perceptions of the innovation predict between 49 percent and 87 percent of the variance in the diffusion, or rate of spread, of an innovation (Rogers, 2003). Five attributes of innovations affect the matching process and, ultimately, the adoption decision:

- **Relative advantage** refers to the degree to which the innovation is perceived as superior to current practice. Innovations perceived as superior are more readily adopted (Dirksen, Ament, et al., 1996; Meyer, Johnson, et al., 1997). Relative advantage is typically viewed in terms of benefits weighed against costs—though not necessarily in dollar terms. Advantages may accrue from prestige or social acceptance, for instance. Although seemingly straightforward, relative advantage is a matter of perception and therefore subject to the adopter's tolerance for uncertainty and propensity for risk.

- **Compatibility** refers to the degree to which the innovation is consistent with the values, beliefs, history, and current practices the potential users. Innovations that fit adopters' needs, values, and norms are more readily adopted (Aubert & Hamel, 2001; Denis, Hebert, et al., 2002; Foy, MacLennan, et al., 2002). Poor perceived compatibility might explain why physicians do not use formal, scientific protocols or clinical guidelines in their practice (Berwick, 2003). Some view guidelines as "cookbook" medicine, and hence, contrary to the value they place on professional autonomy. Others see merit in guidelines, but do not use them because they perceive a poor fit with their patient population or office workflow.

- **Complexity** refers to the degree to which organizational members perceive the innovation as difficult to understand or use. Other things being equal, simpler innovations spread faster than complicated ones (Denis, Hebert, et al., 2002; Meyer & Goes, 1988; Meyer, Johnson, et al., 1997). For example, it's easy for most employees to understand what it means to adopt new appointment-scheduling software; but how about adopting patient-focused care (Lathrop 1993)? Which would be easier to outline in a one-page memo?

- **Trialability** refers to the degree to which organizational members can experiment with the innovation on a limited basis. The ability to try an innovation without significant investment or irreversible commitment reduces uncertainty about expected consequences (Grilli & Lomas, 1994; Yetton, Sharma, et al., 1999). Some innovations, such as electronic medical records, require significant financial investment and widespread use before they generate benefits. Given such low trialability, it is not surprising that electronic medical records have been slow to spread among health care organizations.

- **Observability** refers to the degree to which the results of an innovation are visible to others. Innovations that generate benefits visible to intended adopters get adopted more readily (Denis, Hebert, et al., 2002; Grilli & Lomas, 1994; Meyer & Goes, 1988). Some innovations, such as total quality management, spread slowly because they generate benefits for the organization as a whole, but not necessarily for the adopting departments. Overall cost per case might decline, for example, even though nursing costs increase. By comparison, physicians might quickly adopt personal digital assistants containing patient data and drug formularies because such devices provide immediate, visible benefit.

It is important to emphasize that these attributes are perceptions, not objective features, of innova-

tions. Thus, health care managers can increase an innovation's attractiveness by influencing organizational members' perceptions of innovation attributes. For instance, managers can heighten the relative advantage of an innovation by stressing the potential benefits of adoption or lowering the costs or barriers to adoption (e.g., offering a trial period or free technical support). Likewise, managers can reduce the complexity of an innovation by allowing organizational members to simplify or experiment with the innovation (Markides, 1998).

Social System Characteristics. Innovation attributes are not the only factors that influence the matching process. Social system characteristics also influence organizational members' perceptions of an innovation as well as their assessments of the feasibility of adoption and implementation. Examples of broader contextual factors include:

- **Network structure**. Studies of technology diffusion among hospitals show that almost all of the geographic variation in technology adoption occurred *between* local communities of medical professionals, not *within* individual communities. In other words, medical professionals were keen to adopt innovations that their local colleagues had adopted (Greer, 1988). Doctors tend to operate in informal, horizontal networks, and nurses more often have formal, vertical networks (West, Barron, et al., 1999). In horizontal networks, peer influence and consensus tend to influence adoption decisions. In vertical networks, codified information (e.g., policy statements and practice guidelines) from authoritative sources tends to influence adoption decisions (Rogers, 2003; West, Barron, et al., 1999).

- **Homophily** refers to the degree of similarity between individuals, groups, or organizations. Individuals are more likely to adopt innovations if they are homophilous—in terms of socioeconomic, cultural, or professional backgrounds—with current users of the innovation (Fennell & Warnecke, 1988; West, Barron, et al., 1999;

Fitzgerald, Ferlie, et al., 2002). Similarly, organizations are more likely to adopt an innovation if other organizations in the same network—particularly those perceived as more prestigious—have already adopted the innovation (Burns & Wholey, 1993).

- **Opinion leaders** serve as hubs in social and professional networks and strongly influence how innovations are perceived, both within their organizations as well as in others (Becker, 1970; Coleman, Katz, et al., 1966). Opinion leaders can help both raise awareness about innovations and lend them credibility (Rogers, 2003). This may be particularly true of the health care sector where professional ties are strong and where the practice of medicine itself has a tradition of independence (Starr, 1982). Shrewd managers often try to recruit opinion leaders (e.g., respected physicians) to act as their lieutenants in efforts to raise or lower organizational members' enthusiasm for adopting an innovation. However, opinion leaders are often reluctant to sponsor innovations that deviate too much from group values and existing structures (Greer, 1988). Moreover, opinion leaders can "wear out" their credibility if they are perceived by their peers as too strongly identified with those who seek to promote or inhibit innovation adoption (Rogers, 2003).

Finally, some features of organizations have been shown to influence the adoption of innovations. Examples include the following:

- Boundary spanners refer to employees who have significant social ties both inside and outside the organization. Boundary spanners play a pivotal role in capturing ideas that become innovations (Kimberly & Evanisko, 1981; Rogers, 2003). Organizations that encourage employees to stay attuned to outside sources of ideas and opportunities are more likely to become aware of and adopt innovations (Barnsley, Lemieux-Charles, et al., 1998).

- Absorptive capacity refers to an organization's ability to acquire, assimilate, and apply new knowledge. Organizations with greater absorptive capacity more readily identify and adopt innovations (Barnsley, Lemieux-Charles, et al., 1998; Cohen & Levinthal, 1990; Zahra & George, 2002). Absorptive capacity is predicated on the organization's existing knowledge base, the deployment of the learning disciplines noted earlier, and the presence of leadership committed to sharing knowledge (Barnsley, Lemieux-Charles, et al., 1998).

- Organizational readiness for change also plays an important role in shaping organizational members' assessments of adoption desirability and implementation feasibility (Lehman, Greener, et al., 2002). Many elements contribute to organizational readiness for change, including motivational readiness (e.g., perceived need for improvement and pressure for change), institutional resources (e.g., physical space, staff availability, and training resources), and organizational climate (e.g., communication openness and stress levels).

In his study of the organizational dynamics or early-stage implementation of a behavioral health service line in the Upper New York VA, Hoff (2004) credited much of the success of the initiative to the organization's high level of readiness for change. For instance, the behavioral health service line director, who functioned as the "prime mover" for the innovation, generated significant motivational readiness in middle managers and frontline employees by establishing urgency, creating a guiding vision, and using every opportunity to communicate his message about the importance of the service line innovation to the organization's performance and survival. Equally important, the top management team exhibited strong social cohesion by (a) defending each other to criticism by outsiders, (b) viewing each other as integral to their own success in the job, (c) seeing the group as having meaningful input into decisions before they are made, and (d) expressing interest in cooperating and helping each other (Hoff, 2004; Shaw, 1981; Smith, Smith, et al., 1994). Finally, the implementation of the behavioral health service line benefited from a positive organizational climate characterized by rapid, open, and frequent communication about performance levels.

The matching stage concludes with the decision to adopt or not adopt an innovation. Conceptually, **adoption** is a discrete event that occurs at a single point in time. In reality, organizations revisit adoption decisions many times, provisionally adopting an innovation and then reassessing the decision as organizational members learn more about the innovation itself and the feasibility of implementation. For example, health care organizations sometimes "beta test" new information technology in order to find the optimal balance of performance, reliability, flexibility, and user-friendliness. The lessons learned from "beta testing" may prompt alterations in the technology's design, changes in the implementation plan, or even reconsideration of the adoption decision (Weiner, Savitz, et al., 2004).

Restructuring

Restructuring marks the beginning of the implementation phase of the innovation process. **Implementation** refers to the transition period during which targeted organizational members ideally become increasingly skillful, consistent, and committed in their use of an innovation (Klein & Sorra, 1996). Implementation begins with restructuring because implementation almost always involves the mutual adaptation of the innovation and the organization (Yin, 1979; Goodman & Steckler, 1989; Rogers, 1995, 2003). To illustrate, Weiner and his colleagues (2004) observed that innovative strategies for managing diabetes undergo considerable adaptation when implemented in physician group practices. In two of the group practices they studied, multidisciplinary committees first created and then modified several times both the content and the format of diabetes flow sheets (i.e. checklists that guide clinicians through a diabetes visit to ensure that essential diagnostic and treatment activities occur at the appropriate time). Similarly, at another practice, the nurse family practitioner responsible for diabetes management adapted instructional materials obtained from external sources as she designed the diabetes self-management course. Even seemingly

fixed innovations, such as a machine permitting in-office testing of hemoglobin A1c levels, underwent adaptation as physicians, pharmacists, and laboratory technicians tinkered to find what they considered the appropriate frequency of testing and the optimal range of values for diabetes management. Few innovations get implemented without undergoing some reinvention (Rogers, 2003). Permitting organizational members to adapt or modify the innovation can facilitate implementation by reducing the complexity of the innovation and increasing its compatibility with existing structures and practices. However, care must be taken to ensure the reinvention does not diminish the innovation's efficacy.

Organizational adaptation generally takes the form of **implementation policies and practices**, a shorthand phrase for the formal strategies that an organization employs in order to put the innovation into use, and the actions that follow from those strategies (Klein & Sorra, 1996). Implementation policies and practices vary from innovation to innovation but generally include training, technical support, recognition and reward, reorganization, job reclassification, workflow changes, and workload changes. Even seemingly simple innovations require changes in organizational policies and practices to support implementation. For instance, the physician group practice that purchased and installed the machine for in-office testing of hemoglobin A1c levels had to make significant changes in appointment scheduling, patient flow, patient charts, and staff responsibilities (Weiner, Savitz, et al., 2004). Like innovation adaptation, organizational adaptation facilitates implementation by reducing complexity and enhancing compatibility. Hoff (2004) found, for example, that organizational creativity played a significant role in Upstate New York VHA Network's effort to integrate mental health services and primary care services. Frontline management took a "trial-and-error" approach to staffing mental health providers in the Network's community-based outpatient clinics, allowing "real-time" information about patient flow and provider workload to guide decisions about the number and mix of mental health providers needed to implement this aspect of the behavioral health service line. Although some implementation policies and practices represent short-term, temporary measures, others, as illustrated by the implementation of the National Cancer Institute's (NCI) Community Clinical Oncology Program, become permanent organizational changes that require ongoing investment and support (see In Practice, below).

Clarifying

A brief window of time exists for restructuring to occur before the innovation enters the clarifying stage. In this stage, the innovation either diffuses within the organization or stalls (Rogers, 2003) as organizational members gain experience with an innovation, learn about its implications for them and for the organization, and begin comparing the actual versus expected benefits and costs of innovative

---

❧ IN PRACTICE   Improving Community Cancer Care

In 1983, the National Cancer Institute (NCI) introduced a radical concept—the idea of providing direct peer-reviewed funding to community oncologists for participating in NCI-sponsored clinical trials (Kaluzny & Warnecke, 2000). The Community Clinical Oncology Program funds consortia of community hospitals and physicians (CCOPs) to enroll patients in clinical trials developed by cancer centers and clinical cooperative groups that NCI has designated as "CCOP research bases." [Cooperative groups are consortia of research and provider institutions charged with identifying important questions in cancer research and designing clinical trials to address them.] Initially, the program focused on making therapeutic clinical trials available to community oncologists and their patients. In 1987, NCI expanded the program's scope by requiring CCOP research bases to design and conduct cancer prevention and control clinical trials and requiring CCOPs to meet annual cancer prevention and control accrual targets. *Prevention trials* evaluate new methods of detecting cancer risk and preventing primary and secondary cancers. *Cancer control trials* evaluate symptom management, rehabilitation, and continuing care interventions designed to minimize the burden of cancer and improve quality of life.

When the NCI added cancer prevention and control research as a CCOP requirement in 1987, many questioned whether a clinical research network accustomed to evaluating cancer therapies could move into this new investigative realm (McKinney, Barnsley, et al., 1992; McKinney, Morrissey, et al., 1993). Over the last decade, however, CCOP research bases have proven their collective capability to design and conduct cancer prevention and control trials, including large trials involving tens of thousands of study participants. Many cancer prevention and control trials have garnered national attention and, in some cases, changed the standard of care for at-risk populations and cancer patients (Minasian, McCaskill-Stevens, et al., 2004).

In a study of four CCOP research bases, Weiner and his colleagues found that those with productive cancer prevention and control research programs had tailored the innovation (i.e., cancer prevention and control research) to fit the interests, skills, and practice settings of group members (Weiner, McKinney, et al., 2004). At the North Central Cancer Treatment Group, for example, symptom management studies have become a mainstay, reflecting the resources and interests of its community investigators. The National Surgical Adjuvant Breast and Bowel Project (NSABP) moved into chemoprevention trials (i.e., studies involving drugs as preventive agents) as a "natural extension" of its research program on the effectiveness of adjuvant chemotherapies in reducing breast cancer recurrence among patients with early-stage disease. In addition, CCOP research bases with productive cancer prevention and control research programs had adapted their own organizational structures and processes to better fit the innovation. For example, they added new scientific committees that focused exclusively on cancer prevention and control research, allocated administrative staff to assist investigators in developing cancer prevention and control trials, hired new staff with the statistical skills needed to conduct cancer prevention and control research, invested in new information systems capable of handling the unique data demands of cancer prevention and control research, and allocated a small percentage of the research base's total budget to support pilot and developmental studies in cancer prevention and control. Many of these implementation policies and practices remain in effect to this day—thirteen years after the CCOP research bases adopted the innovation.

use. An important distinction exists between implementation effectiveness and innovation effectiveness (Klein & Sorra, 1996). Implementation effectiveness concerns the overall consistency and quality of organizational members' use of an innovation (e.g., do providers regularly update and use information in the clinic's diabetes registry?). **Innovation effectiveness** refers to the benefits the organization realizes from innovation use (e.g., does the diabetes registry improve patient outcomes?). Benefits may include increased organizational profitability, productivity, customer service, patient outcomes, or employee satisfaction. Implementation effectiveness is a necessary, but not sufficient condition for innovation effectiveness. That is to say, an innovation must be effectively implemented for the innovation to deliver the expected outcomes, but effective implementation does not guarantee that the innovation will be effective. Evidence-based clinical guidelines may represent a classical case of poor implementation effectiveness. Despite considerable evidence that clinical guidelines improve quality of care (Grimshaw & Russell, 1993), results from widespread adoption of clinical guidelines have been disappointing (Solberg, 2000). Perhaps the main reason is that guidelines have not been effec-

tively implemented. That is, the targeted users of guidelines—generally physicians—do not consistently and faithfully follow guidelines.

Organizations often struggle with a key activity of the clarifying stage: disseminating innovations from one part of the organization to other parts. Indeed, a chief concern in the business management literature over the past decade has been the problem of how to best make use of the knowledge and effective practices that already exist in different locales within an organization (Brown & Duguid, 2000; Carr, 1999; Gray, 2003; Hamel & Prahalad, 1994; Ulrich & Smallwood, 2004). Health care organizations are not immune to this problem. As Berwick (2003, p. 1971) notes, "even when an evidence-based innovation is implemented successfully in one part of a hospital or clinic, it may spread slowly or not at all to other parts of the organization." To illustrate, he reports that a large health maintenance organization (HMO) supported in one medical center an innovative asthma program that reduced hospitalization rates by two-thirds and brought prescribing practices into line with the best national recommendations. Unfortunately, the rest of the medical centers in the HMO did not embrace the innovation (Weiss, Mendoza, et al., 1997). He also notes that, despite evidence from randomized controlled trials that inexpensive antibiotics work best in treating first ear infections in children, nearly 30 percent of children with first ear infections enrolled in the Colorado Medicaid program received unnecessary, expensive, and hazardous antibiotics (Berman, Byrns, et al., 1997).

In part, the slow spread of innovations within organizations results from an overreliance on diffusion as opposed to dissemination. **Diffusion** is a *passive* process in which a growing body of information about an intervention, product, or technology is initially absorbed and acted upon by a small body of highly motivated recipients (Bero, Grilli, et al., 1998; Lomas, 1993). **Dissemination**, by comparison, is an *active* process whereby special efforts are made to ensure that intended users become aware of, receive, accept, and use an innovation (Lomas, 1993). Managers often seek to encourage the spread of innovations within their organizations by distributing information through written reports, newsletters, intranets, presentations, and various forms of continuing education. Yet research consistently demonstrates that informational strategies only raise awareness and knowledge; they do not alter behavior (Bero, Grilli, et al., 1998; Davis, Thomson, et al., 1995). Other approaches that enable intended users to experience the innovation firsthand or interact with "experts" who know the innovation well have been shown to promote greater acceptance and use of innovations (Davis, O'Brien, et al., 1999; Davis, Thomson, et al., 1995; Grimshaw, Shirran, et al., 2001; Oxman, Thomson, et al., 1995). Hence, managers seeking to transfer innovative knowledge, technology, or practice from one part of an organization to another would fare better using dissemination strategies such as cross-training, staff rotation, opinion leaders, and academic detailing (i.e., offering brief, one-on-one education and feedback).

Routinization

Routinization is the final stage in the innovation process where the innovation becomes incorporated into the regular activities of an organization and loses its distinct identity (Rogers, 2003). Routinization depends in part on the extent to which organizational members perceive the innovation as a legitimate and valued practice (Kanter, 1983). It is important to recognize that routinization does not necessarily depend on either implementation effectiveness or innovation effectiveness. An innovation can exhibit consistent, high-quality use by targeted organizational members and even deliver significant organizational benefits, yet still become discontinued because key supporters of the innovation leave or funding for the innovation disappears. Conversely, an innovation can exhibit inconsistent use, ritualistic use, or even nonuse, yet persist for years due to institutional inertia or political pressures.

Routinization depends on the continued allocation of five types of resources: budgetary resources, personnel resources, training programs, organizational policies and procedures, and supply and maintenance operations (Goodman & Bazerman, 1980; Yin, 1979). Ongoing monitoring of innovation use also supports routinization by signaling to targeted users the importance of continued innovation use and by providing performance feedback to enable users to make adjustments in their practice patterns (Weiner, Savitz, et al., 2004). While not all resource types are relevant to all innovations, the more resource types committed to sustaining an innovation, and the longer the duration of that commitment, the more routinized the innovation becomes (Yin, 1979).

Beyond committing resources and monitoring on an ongoing basis, organizational leaders can employ two interrelated strategies to improve the chances that an innovation will become routinized. First, research consistently shows that participation by end-users in decision-making processes tends to reduce resistance to change, build ownership of the change, and motivate people to make the change work (Ash, Lyman, et al., 2001; Gunasekaran, Marri, et al., 2001). With respect to innovation, participation may involve work on diagnosing and prioritizing needs (agenda setting); identifying, designing, and discussing innovations (matching); planning and implementation (restructuring and clarifying); or any combination of the above. Participation may promote greater acceptance of the innovation by facilitating the flow of information about what the innovation will be (i.e., reducing complexity) and why the organization is adopting it (i.e., clarifying relative advantage). Participation may also increase the quality of adoption decisions and the effectiveness of implementation efforts by shedding light on the requirements, opportunities, and constraints that exist at the local operating level. Finally, to the extent that end users feel invested in the innovation, participation may sustain innovation use even in the face of departure or reassignment of the initial individual or group that championed the innovation (Rogers, 2003).

Second, leadership can increase the prospects of routinization by providing organizational members latitude to reinvent or adapt the innovation. As with participation, organizational members feel a greater sense of ownership and commitment to the innovation if they have the opportunity to selectively implement or modify the innovation to better fit local needs, workflow, and resources. Berwick (2003) reports that Intermountain Health Care's Latter Day Saints Hospital reduced the rate of pressure sores in vulnerable patients by 80 percent by adopting a nationally disseminated clinical guideline. However, hospital staff did not implement the entire 30-page guideline; instead, they focused on two recommendations within the guideline that seemed to have significant potential—to calculate a decubitis ulcer (or pressure sore) risk score using an established scale, and then turn high-risk patients every two hours. By reinventing the guideline, hospital staff reduced the complexity of the innovation, making it much easier to implement and routinize as standard practice.

For certain kinds of innovations, routinization occurs only when the innovation achieves a "critical mass" of users (Frambach & Schillewaert, 2002). The term *critical mass* comes from nuclear physics and refers to the amount of radioactive material necessary to create a chain reaction where nuclear fission becomes self-sustaining. In innovation diffusion, critical mass is that point where "enough individuals in a system have adopted an innovation so that the innovation's further rate of adoption becomes self-sustaining" (Rogers, 2003). The idea of a critical mass holds true for all kinds of innovations, but is particularly powerful for innovations with **network externalities**, that is, innovations whose utility largely or entirely depends on others also using the innovation. A great example is e-mail: If you're the only person to adopt e-mail, it's totally useless because you have no one else to e-mail. As more people adopt e-mail, it becomes more valuable to each adopter; hence, the value depends on externalities related to the network of users. Cell phones, although they depended on the creation of a new infrastructure of transmitters and receivers, were still compatible with existing telephones, and so possessed more limited network externalities than e-mail did. Some health care innovations, such as electronic medical records and disease registries, also exhibit network externalities. Klein and Sorra (1996) refer to these types of innovations as **collective innovations** because they require the active, coordinated use of multiple members of the organization or social network in order to return benefits.

IMPLEMENTING LARGE-SCALE ORGANIZATIONAL CHANGE

Organizational learning and innovation often trigger large-scale organizational change efforts. Much of what we know about managing large-scale organizational change comes not from empirical research, but from managers and consultants who have led or facilitated such efforts. Most discussions of large-scale organizational change focus on the role of top management in designing and leading change. However, a growing number of management scholars and practitioners have questioned whether successful large-scale change efforts can be implemented in a top-down, linear, planned manner. Although senior managers can provide the leadership necessary to "set the wheels in motion" and support the change effort, two other groups play a critical role in shaping both the process and the outcome of large-scale change. These groups include the *implementers,* who translate broad change goals into specific action steps and champion the day-to-day execution of the change, and the *recipients,* who must adopt, adapt, and adjust to the change (Kanter, Stein, et al., 1992). Moreover, although plans provide useful roadmaps, successful large-scale organizational change often occurs through emergent, incremental steps as both problems and solutions arise through repeated interactions among leaders, organizational members, work processes, and environmental factors (Mintzberg, 1993). Accordingly, organizational learning and innovation not only trigger large-scale organizational change, but also permeate the change process itself.

As with innovation, linear stage models dominate much of the discussion of large-scale organizational change. For example, Kurt Lewin's (1951) classic three-step change framework of unfreezing, moving, and refreezing is perhaps the most well-known and influential model of organizational change. **Unfreezing** involves creating an awareness of the need for change and removing any resistance to change. **Moving** involves putting into place new strategies, structures, or practices; this stage often requires organizational members to accept of new ideas, attitudes, and behaviors—a process that managers or other change agents can facilitate with role modeling and training. **Refreezing** involves stabilizing the change by integrating the newly adopted strategies, structures, and practices into existing operating procedures and work routines and by reinforcing changes in the attitudes and behaviors of organizational members through, for example, altering recognition and reward systems.

A more recent change model, while still linear in form, more closely reflects the view of organizations as complex adaptive systems. Weick and Quinn

(1999) contend that change is an every day reality of today's workplace. Large-scale organizational change, therefore, represents a redirection of an ongoing process of change rather than an infrequent episode with a definite beginning and end. Turning Lewin's model on its head, they propose that organizational change occurs through freezing, rebalancing, and unfreezing. Specifically, they argue that organizations are locked in relative flux by an increasingly unpredictable environment. To sustain meaningful change, the organization first has to freeze itself to create stability. Only then can the organization assess where it is and orient itself vis-à-vis its values, attitudes, and behavior. Managers facilitate freezing by developing conceptual maps of the organization's strategies and relating stories that illustrate ideals or core assumptions. Once frozen, the organization reinterprets its disparate activities and events in its environment to rally around a coherent vision of where the organization wants to go. Managers can facilitate *rebalancing* by communicating core organizational values and linking them to strategic alternatives. Once equipped with a unifying vision, the organization *unfreezes* and its constituent parts resume their semiautonomous activities. Even though they engage with an ever-changing environment and no executive authority actively coordinates activities, constituents navigate by the core vision and maintain unity of mission. Managers facilitate unfreezing by communicating vision over the long term and being accepting of creativity.

Managing Change

These models, while useful for describing the change process, offer little guidance for managing large-scale organizational change. Kotter's (1996) organizational transformation model, on the other hand, proposes eight action steps for creating and sustaining large-scale change.

1. *Establishing urgency*—Examine market and competitive realities and create a sense of dissatisfaction with the status quo by identifying

and communicating crises, potential crises, and opportunities. It is not enough to identify performance gaps. The urgency level must be high enough to combat organizational complacency.

2. *Creating a guiding coalition*—Develop a team to lead the change effort. The key is to have a team that works well together and possesses the power, expertise, and credibility to make the change happen. A guiding coalition comprised solely of managers is bound to fail.

3. *Developing a vision*—Similar to Plsek's notion of "good enough vision" (2001), large-scale change requires a vision that is focused, flexible, and easy to communicate. Good visions provide a sense of direction, a touchstone for decision making, and a yardstick for gauging progress.

4. *Communicating the change vision*—Change does not sell itself. The vision must be communicated in a simple, jargon-free way in multiple forums. Change agents should use every possible opportunity to communicate the vision and should lead by example.

5. *Empowering broad-based action*—Barriers to change for employees always exist, and always so on multiple levels. Change agents need to provide training, change reward systems, revise reporting structures, alter standard operating procedures, and deal with difficult or resistant supervisors, managers, and executives.

6. *Creating short-term wins*—Major changes take time. Commitment and momentum will flag if the change effort does not produce visible, unambiguous short-term wins. Intentionally creating and celebrating short-term wins reenergizes members, generates confidence, and justifies sacrifices and hard work.

7. *Consolidating gains*—Resistance is always waiting to reassert itself. So is complacency. Change agents need to keep up momentum by building on short-term wins to campaign for the next, more difficult changes in interdependent systems, structures, and processes.

8. *Anchoring new approaches in the culture*—Change does not last if not fully integrated into the culture of the organization. This may require turnover among key personnel and changes in recruitment, selection, training, reward, and promotion processes.

Closer examination reveals that Kotter's model reflects a managerial elaboration of Lewin's three-stage model. The first four steps unfreeze the organization, the next three introduce change, and the last refreezes the organization by making the change permanent. Kotter argues that all successful large-scale change efforts go through all eight steps, although not necessarily in a linear fashion. Organizations can operate in multiple stages at once, but skipping a step or getting too far ahead generates only the illusion of progress. Sooner or later, the organization must return to the missed or hurried step. Kotter acknowledges that, "Those who attempt to create change with simple, linear, analytical processes almost always fail." At the same time, he observes that change efforts that do not generally follow the sequence he describes do not build and develop in a natural way, nor do they generate the momentum necessary to overcome the enormously powerful sources of inertia that confront any large-scale change effort.

The Art of Change

Guiding large-scale organizational change is more art than science. Although many business and management books offer ready-made answers and step-by-step instructions, it seems unlikely that large-scale organizational change can be implemented successfully in a programmed fashion, especially when one views organizations as complex adaptive systems. As the president and CEO of Group Health Northwest discovered, understanding and managing change is a learning process (see

IN PRACTICE   The Chief Mourner at the Funeral

Dr. Henry Berman, who was president and CEO of Group Health Northwest, an HMO in Spokane, Washington, for 15 years, learned a lot about the change process the hard way. When he first came to Spokane, the health plan was the stepchild of a developing national HMO. Although the clinical facilities were adequate, the administrative offices were housed in substandard space (e.g., some employees worked in a basement side-by-side with a water tank). When Group Health Cooperative, the large Seattle-based HMO, bought the organization, immediate plans were made to find new space for the administrative staff.

Dr. Berman describes what happened next: "We located good space on the second floor of an office building in a convenient location. Employees were being moved from cramped space with no windows to roomy quarters, many of which had windows and a lot of natural light. Every employee ended up with a better situation. Much to my surprise, everyone seemed unhappy, and grumbled about something or other that was a problem in the new space. I was dumbfounded—what did they want?

"Fortunately, the next year I attended an excellent conference on Leadership in Changing Times. One phrase from the many presentations has always stuck in my mind: 'Leaders have to be the chief mourners at the funeral.' Rather than being a cheerleader, telling everyone how good change will be, the role of the leader—from supervisors, to managers, to executives, to CEOs—is to commiserate with employees about how difficult change will be, and how you wish it could have been avoided, but it was necessary because of . . . (you supply the rest of the sentence). When the leader takes this role, it frees up the employee to look for the positive aspects of the change, and in future situations I often found myself being reassured by employees that everything would work out, and that they appreciated how concerned I was about them."

In Practice, above). The following questions illustrate the "art" of managing change (Bowditch & Buono, 2001; Jick, 1993). Careful consideration of these questions over the course of a change effort can provide useful diagnostic information.

- *Pace*—How long should the organization plan and design the change? How quickly can the change process advance? Should the pace of change be accelerated or slowed along the way?

- *Scope*—How much of the organization will be involved in the change process? Should the change "start small and grow" or should the change be implemented organization wide? If

the former, how will the change be diffused to other organizational units?

- *Depth*—How much change in a given area will be attempted? How many change initiatives can the organization effectively handle? Are the changes too intense or not intense enough?

- *Publicity*—How will the change initiative be publicized: with lots of fanfare or through a quiet, understated campaign? When will publicity begin? How often will it occur? What is the best way to communicate with different stakeholders in the change effort?

- *Supporting structures*—What new management structures or processes are needed to support the change effort? Will these structures and practices be transitional or permanent? If transitional, how will they be phased out?

- *Driver*—Who will drive the change: top management, middle management, clinical professionals, or lower-level employees? Is there an identifiable champion? Does he or she have the experience, skills, and the credibility to lead the change effort?

Common Organizational Change Approaches

Health care managers can draw upon several approaches to implementing large-scale organizational change. For many health care organizations, these change strategies represent innovations because they involve adopting new ideas, values, and practices. Because health care organizations are complex adaptive systems exhibiting sensitivity to initial conditions and nonlinear dynamics, managers must exercise care in implementing these change strategies and should not simply follow the approaches taken by other organizations. Both implementation effectiveness and innovation effectiveness depend on mutually adapting the innovation and the organization.

- Total quality management (TQM) encompasses several approaches, each differing somewhat in philosophy, principles, and methods. However, all embrace a philosophy of meeting or exceeding customer expectations through the continuous improvement of the processes associated with providing a good or service (Berwick, Godfrey, et al., 1990; Blumenthal & Scheck, 1995). Operationally, TQM combines three elements: organization-wide participation in the planning and implementation of continuous improvement, systematic use of statistical tools (e.g., control charts) to monitor and analyze work processes, and employment of process management tools (e.g., flowcharts) to help organizational members use their collective knowledge effectively (Hackman & Wageman,

1995; McLaughlin & Kaluzny, 2005). Unlike traditional quality assurance (QA) methods, which focus on correcting individuals' mistakes after the fact, TQM focuses on understanding and improving the underlying work processes and systems in order to add value (Berwick, 1989, 1990; James, 1989).

- Business process reengineering, like TQM, seeks to improve work processes, or sets of activities that, taken together, produce a result that is of value to a customer (Hammer, 1996; Hammer and Champy, 1993). The goal is to organize work processes around customers' needs or wants by breaking down the barriers of excess bureaucracy that may have evolved over time (Leatt, Baker, et al., 1997). Instead of attempting to improve existing processes, reengineering seeks to transform the organization by designing core work processes from scratch (Bowditch and Buono, 2001; Kissler, 1996). Key strategies include combining multiple jobs into one, empowering workers to make decisions, eliminating unnecessary process steps, and using information technology to replace complex checks and controls (Hammer & Champy, 1993).

- Patient-focused care equally emphasizes the quality of clinical care and the quality of service the patient experiences (Lathrop, 1993). Also called family-oriented care, it considers nurturing and caring service central to the healing mission. One important way organizations develop patient focus is by involving patients and their families in evaluating and planning changes. Key activities include reorganizing floors and units in order to group patients with more homogenous service needs, reconfiguring the location of diagnostic services, redesigning organizational roles, and creating patient care teams (Leander, 1996).

- Retrenchment (also known as downsizing) encompasses a variety of management cost-reduction strategies (Leatt, Baker, et al., 1997). Retrenchment seeks to improve efficiency by reducing labor costs, principally through personnel reduction. Retrenchment strategies include across-the-board cuts, delayering (e.g., eliminating middle management positions), early retirement programs, outsourcing, and substituting temporary employees for permanent ones.

- **Restructuring** focuses on bringing organizational processes, products, and people into concert around a shared vision and occurs on a more strategic level than reengineering. Typically this means reevaluating which lines of business it should be in, leading the organization to drop some, and perhaps add others. Restructuring assumes the organization needs to change its strategic focus and place more emphasis on core competencies (Leatt, Baker, et al., 1997). For example, a health care system might decide, after evaluating its market opportunities, to sell or close its health plan in order to focus more exclusively on patient care delivery.

Responding to the challenges of improving quality and patient safety, increasing access for underserved populations, and making health care more affordable will require significant changes in how health care organizations deliver care. Health care managers need to recognize that the future is unpredictable and unknowable, and that the successes of the past will not ensure success in the future. Health care managers and leaders of the future must be able to suspend their need of control; to see connections between seemingly isolated issues and events; to be creative, active problem solvers; and to exhibit empathy. Most of all, managers and clinical providers must be creators of learning organizations—organizations that combine adaptive and generative learning—and must be skilled in the art of managing innovation and implementing large-scale organizational change.

MANAGERIAL GUIDELINES

1. Encourage constant scanning for information about conditions and practices outside their units. Scanning promotes alertness, surfaces discrepant information, and uncovers new ideas. Scanning methods include benchmarking; ongoing contact with purchasers, suppliers, and partners; and soliciting feedback from employees, physicians, and patients.

2. Generate "creative tension" by promoting both a shared vision of the future and a realistic appraisal of current reality. Promoting organization-wide awareness of a performance gap creates awareness that new knowledge is needed and stimulates the learning process.

3. Develop metrics and measurement systems that gauge the performance of key work processes and track the progress of organizational learning. Measurement not only directs attention, but also generates

information that supports realistic appraisal of current reality and perhaps empirical challenge to people's mental models.

4. Encourage curiosity by valuing the questioning of long-held assumptions and permitting controlled experimentation. Computer simulations, tabletop exercises, and virtual worlds (Lewin, Parker, et al., 1998) provide low-cost laboratories for learning by allowing participants to engage in controlled experimentation without real-world consequences—though doing so with no intention of acting on the results can provoke cynicism.

5. Foster a climate of openness in which information flows freely, people can express their views, and decision making takes advantage of multiple perspectives. Defensiveness, secrecy, and disenfranchisement foreclose opportunities for learning and innovation and generate resistance to change.

6. Foster "continuous education" by committing financial resources and management support to education and training programs, personnel rotation, cross-training, part-time study, mentoring, and informal learning opportunities. Exposing individuals to new ideas and increasing interconnections supports both idea generation and knowledge transfer.

7. Seek out and support champions of innovation and learning. Champions not only preach the message, but also serve as role models. Assemble a guiding coalition of people with strong position power, broad expertise, and high credibility. Ensure that coalition members possess both leadership and management skills.

8. Get senior managers personally involved in organizational learning, innovation, and change. Personal, visible leadership sends a powerful message, creates opportunities for senior managers to learn, and provides role models.

9. Inculcate the discipline of systems thinking by encouraging organizational members to learn and make use of systems archetypes to understand work processes and outcomes.

10. Encourage systematic problem solving by adopting total quality management (TQM). TQM is a systemic approach to planning and implementing continuous improvement in performance. TQM embraces the use of statistical tools to monitor and analyze work processes including control charts, Pareto charts, and cost-of-quality analyses. TQM also embraces process management tools to help teams use their collective knowledge effective (Hackman & Wageman, 1995). Such tools include flowcharts, cause-and-effect (or "fishbone") diagrams, brainstorming, and storyboarding (see Analytical Tools for Improving Work Processes see Figure 12.5 pp. 407–408).

Analytical Tools for Improving Work Processes

Total quality management offers several analytical tools for assessing, analyzing, and improving work processes. For example, a *flowchart* is a pictorial representation of the steps in a work process (see Figure 12.5a). Flowcharts, which use standardized symbols to represent types of activities in a process, help members to identify activities that are repetitive, that add no value, or that excessively delay completion of the work.

A *control chart* provides a pictorial representation of the outputs of an ongoing process. Control charts allow the user to determine whether a given process is in need of improvement, identify points outside of the control range so that the causes of uncontrolled variance can be sought, and reassess the process after experimental attempts to improve it are completed.

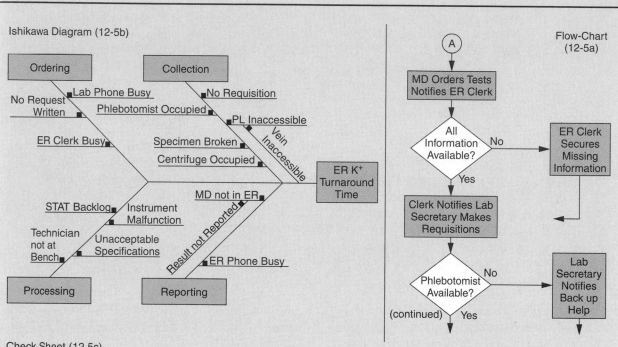

Check Sheet (12.5c)
Delays in production of Se K^+ results from 1/1/91 to 1/7/91

Code/Delay Type		Mon	Tue	Wed	Thur	Fri	Sat	Sun	Total
A	Request not Written by Physician	I	I				I		3
B	Lab Phone Busy > 2 minutes	I		I		II		I	5
C	Phlebotomists Unavailable	III	II	III	III	II	IIII	III	20
D	Requisition not Ready	II	I	I	I	I	III	II	11
E	Patient Inaccessible	I	I	II	I		II	I	8
F	Vein Inaccessible	I		II			II		6
G	Centrifuge Busy	II	I		I				4
H	Specimen Broken	II		I				I	4
I	STAT Backlog	III			I		II	I	7
J	Technician not at Bench	II		II		I	II	I	8
K	Unacceptable Specimen	I	I		II		I	II	7
L	Laboratory Secretary Unavailable to Report	III		I		I	I		6
M	ER Phone not Answered			I		I	II		4
N	MD not in ER	II		I		II		I	6
O	MD not Answer Page	I	I	II		II		II	8
P	Results not Reported by ER Secretary	II	I	II	I	III	II	II	13

Figure 12.5. Analytical Tools Used in FOCUS-PCDA

SOURCE: Adapted from Simpson, Kaluzny, & McLaughlin, 1994.

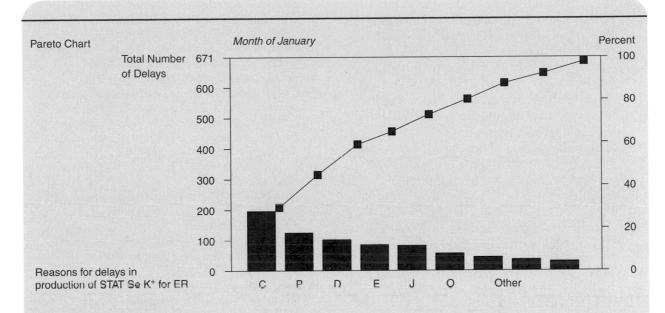

Figure 12.5. *(continued)*

A *cause-effect diagram* or "fishbone" graphically represents the relationship between a problem and its potential causes. Group members place the problem at the right-hand side of the page (the head of the fish). (See Figure 12.5b.) The "bones" of the fish are lines on which members list the potential causes by category; the generic categories of causes are people, tools, materials, and methods.

Finally, a *Pareto chart* highlights the major factors that contribute to a problem by arraying contributing factors in the order of their frequency of occurrence. (See Figure 12.5c.) This makes it visually apparent to the user which contributing factors represent high-leverage opportunities for change.

DISCUSSION QUESTIONS

1. As a manager, what does providing a "good enough" vision mean? Why are managers advised to develop a good enough vision of organizational change instead of an expansive, detailed vision?

2. How does "adaptive" learning differ from "generative" learning? How can managers promote and support generative learning?

3. What is the difference between technical innovation and administrative innovation? Provide an example of each not already provided in the text. For administrators, what is the problem with a pro-innovation bias?

4. When seeking to "routinize" an innovation, how long must monitoring continue? Is this the same for all innovations?

5. Within the context of organizational change, what does it mean to "unfreeze, move, and refreeze" an organization? Is this concept realistic?

6. Why should managers create "a climate of openness"? In what kinds of environments do you think it probably most difficult to reconcile "openness" and accountability?

REFERENCES

Argyris, C., & Schon, D. A. (1978). *Organizational learning.* Reading, MA: Addison-Wesley.

Ash, J. S., Lyman, J., et al. (2001). A diffusion of innovations model of physician order entry. *Journal of the American Medical Informatics Association, 8*(1) 22–26.

Ashmos, D. P., Huonker, J. W., et al. (1998). Participation as a complicating mechanism: The effect of clinical professional and middle manager participation on hospital performance. *Health Care Management Review, 23*(4), 7–20.

Aubert, B. A., & Hamel, G. (2001). Adoption of smart cards in the medical sector: The Canadian experience. *Social Science & Medicine, 53*(7), 879–894.

Barnsley, J., Lemieux-Charles, L., et al. (1998). Integrating learning into integrated delivery systems. *Health Care Management Review, 23*(1), 18–28.

Becker, M. H. (1970). Factors affecting the diffusion of innovation among health professionals. *American Journal of Public Health, 60,* 294–304.

Begun, J. W. (1994). Chaos and complexity: Frontiers of organization science. *Journal of Management Inquiry,* 329–335.

Begun, J. W., Zimmerman, B. J., et al. (2003). Health care organizations as complex adaptive systems. In M. E. Wyttenbach (Ed.), *Advances in health care organization theory.* San Francisco: Jossey-Bass.

Berman, S., Byrns, P. J., et al. (1997). Otitis media-related antibiotic prescribing patterns, outcomes, and expenditures in a pediatric medicaid population. *Pediatrics, 100*(4), 585–592.

Bero, L. A., Grilli, R., et al. (1998). Closing the gap between research and practice: An overview of systematic reviews of interventions to promote the implementation of research findings. The Cochrane Effective Practice and Organization of Care Review Group. *British Medical Journal, 317*(7156), 465–468.

Berquist, W. (1993). *The postmodern organization: Mastering the art of irreversible change.* San Francisco: Jossey-Bass.

Berwick, D. M. (1989). Continuous improvement as an ideal in health care. *New England Journal of Medicine, 320*(1), 53–56.

Berwick, D. M. (1990). Peer review and quality management: Are they compatible? *Quality Review Bulletin, 16*(7), 72–87.

Berwick, D. M. (1998). Developing and testing changes in delivery of care. *Annals of Internal Medicine, 128*(8), 651–656.

Berwick, D. M. (2003). Disseminating innovations in health care. *Journal of the American Medical Association, 289*(15), 1969–1975.

Berwick, D. M., Godfrey, A. B., et al. (1990). *Curing health care: New strategies for quality improvement.* San Francisco: Jossey-Bass.

Billings, R. S., Milburn, T. W., et al. (1980). Crisis perception: A theoretical and empirical analysis. *Administrative Science Quarterly 25,* 300–315.

Blumenthal, D., & Edwards, J. N. (1995). Involving physicians in total quality management: Results of a study. In A. C. Sheck (Ed.), *Improving clinical practice: Total quality management and the physician* (pp. 229–266). San Francisco: Jossey-Bass.

Blumenthal, D., & Scheck, A. C. (Eds.) (1995). *Improving clinical practice: Total quality management and the physician.* San Francisco: Jossey-Bass.

Bowditch, J. L., & Buono, A. F. (2001). *A primer on organizational behavior.* New York: John Wiley & Sons, Inc.

Brown, J. S., & Duguid, P. (2000). Balancing act: How to capture knowledge without killing it. *Harvard Business Review, 78*(3), 73–80.

Burns, L. R., & Wholey, D. R. (1993). Adoption and abandonment of matrix management programs— Effects of organizational characteristics and interorganizational networks. *Academy of Management Journal, 36*(1), 106–138.

Cannon, C. P., Braunwald, E., et al. (2004). Intensive versus moderate lipid lowering with statins after acute coronary syndromes. *New England Journal of Medicine, 350*(15), 1495–1504.

Capra, F. (1982). *The turning point.* London: Flamingo.

Carr, N. G., (1999). A new way to manage process knowledge. *Harvard Business Review, 77*(5), 24–25.

Charns, M. P., & Tewksbury, L. J. (1993). *Collaborative management in health care.* San Francisco: Jossey-Bass.

Chassin, M. R. (2002). Achieving and sustaining improved quality: Lessons from New York State and cardiac surgery. *Health Affairs, 21*(4), 40–51.

Cohen, W. M., & Levinthal, D. A. (1990). Absorptive capacity: A new perspective on learning and innovation. *Administrative Science Quarterly, 35*(1), 128–152.

Coleman, J. S., Katz, E., et al. (1966). *Medical innovations: A diffusion study.* New York: Bobbs-Merrill.

Damberg, C., Chung, L., et al. (2001). *The California report on coronary artery bypass graft surgery: 1997–1998 hospital data* (Technical Report). San Francisco, Pacific Business Group on Health and California Office of Statewide Health Planning and Development.

Davis, D., O'Brien, M. A., et al. (1999). Impact of formal continuing medical education: Do conferences, workshops, rounds, and other traditional continuing education activities change physician behavior or health care outcomes? *Journal of the American Medical Association, 282*(9), 867–874.

Davis, D. A., Thomson, M. A., et al. (1995). Changing physician performance. A systematic review of the effect of continuing medical education strategies. *Journal of the American Medical Association, 274*(9), 700–705.

Denis, J. L., Hebert, Y., et al. (2002). Explaining diffusion patterns for complex health care innovations. *Health Care Management Review, 27*(3), 60–73.

DiBella, A. J., & Nevis, E. C. (1998). *How organizations learn: An integrated strategy for building learning capability.* San Francisco: Jossey-Bass.

Dirksen, C. D., Ament, A. J., et al. (1996). Diffusion of six surgical endoscopic procedures in the Netherlands. Stimulating and restraining factors. *Health Policy, 37*(2), 91–104.

Downs, G. W., & Mohr, L. B. (1979) Toward a theory of innovation. *Administration & Society, 10*(4), 379–408.

Drucker, P. F. (1998). The discipline of innovation. *Harvard Business Review, 76*(6), 149–157.

Emmons, K. M. (2000). The relationships between organizational characteristics and the adoption of workplace smoking policies. *Health Education & Behavior, 27,* 483–501.

Fennell, M. L., & Warnecke, R. B. (1988). *The diffusion of medical innovations: An applied network analysis.* New York: Plenum.

Fitzgerald, L., Ferlie, E., et al. (2002). Interlocking interactions, the diffusion of innovations in health care. *Human Relations, 55*(12), 1429–1449.

Floyd, S. W., & Wooldridge, B. (1994). Dinosaurs or dynamos? Recognizing middle management's strategic role. *Academy of Management Executive, 8*(4), 47–57.

Foy, R., MacLennan, G., et al. (2002). Attributes of clinical recommendations that influence change in practice following audit and feedback. *Journal of Clinical Epidemiology, 55*(7), 717–722.

Frambach, R. T., & Schillewaert, N. (2002). Organizational innovation adoption—A multi-level framework of determinants and opportunities for future research. *Journal of Business Research, 55*(2), 163–176.

Garvin, D. A. (1993). Building a learning organization. *Harvard Business Review, 74*(1), 78–91.

Gleick, J. (1987). *Chaos: The making of a new science.* London: Heinemann.

Goodman, P. S., & Bazerman, M. (1980). *Institutionalization of planned organizational change. Research in organizational behavior* (pp. 215–246). Lexington, MA: JAI Press.

Goodman, R. M., & Steckler, A. (1989). A model for the institutionalization of health promotion programs. *Family & Community Health, 11*(4), 63–78.

Gray, D. (2003). Wanted: Chief ignorance officer. *Harvard Business Review, 81*(11), 22–24.

Greer, A. L. (1988). The state of the art versus the state of the science: The diffusion of new medical technologies into practice. *International Journal of Technology Assessment in Health Care, 4,* 5–26.

Grilli, R., & Lomas, J. (1994). Evaluating the message: The relationship between compliance rate and the subject of a practice guideline. *Medical Care, 32*(3), 202–213.

Grimshaw, J. M., & Russell, I. T. (1993). Effect of clinical guidelines on medical practice: A systematic review of rigorous evaluations. *Lancet, 342*(8856), 1317–1322.

Grimshaw, J. M., Shirran, L., et al. (2001). Changing provider behavior: An overview of systematic reviews of interventions. *Medical Care, 39*(8 Suppl 2), II2-45.

Grumbach, K., Anderson, G. M., et al. (1995). Regionalization of cardiac surgery in the United States and Canada. Geographic access, choice, and outcomes. *Journal of the American Medical Association, 274*(16), 1282–1288.

Gunasekaran, A., Marri, H. B., et al. (2001). Implications of organization and human behaviour on the implementation of CIM in SMEs: An empirical analysis. *International Journal of Computer Integrated Manufacturing, 14*(2), 175–185.

Hackman, J. R., & Wageman, R. (1995). Total quality management: Empirical, conceptual, and practical issues. *Administrative Science Quarterly, 40*(2), 309–342.

Hamel, G., & Prahalad, C. K. (1994). *Competing for the future.* Boston: Harvard Business School.

Hammer, H. (1996). *Beyond reengineering.* New York: HarperCollins Publishers, Inc.

Hammer, H., & Champy, J. (1993). *Reengineering the corporation: A manifesto for business revolution.* New York: HarperCollins Publishers, Inc.

Hammond, J. S., Keeney, R. L., & Raiffa, H. (1998). The hidden traps of decision making. *Harvard Business Review, 76*(5), 47–58.

Hoff, T. J. (2004). Early-stage success in service line implementation. *Health Care Management Review, 29*(1), 17–30.

Jackson, S. E., & Dutton, J. E. (1988). Discerning threats and opportunities. *Administrative Science Quarterly, 33*, 370–387.

James, B. C. (1989). *Quality management for health care delivery.* Chicago: Hospital Research and Educational Trust.

Jick, T. D. (1993). *Managing change: Concepts and cases.* Homewood, IL: Irwin.

Kahneman, D., Slovic, P., & Tversky, A. (1982). *Judgment under uncertainty: Heuristics and biases.* Cambridge: Cambridge University Press.

Kahneman, D., & Tversky, A. (1979). Prospect theory: An analysis of decisions under risk. *Econometrica, 47*, 263–291.

Kaluzny, A. D., & Warnecke, R. B. (Eds.). (2000). *Managing a health care alliance: Improving community cancer care.* Frederick, MD: Beard Books.

Kanter, R. M. (1983). *The change masters.* New York: Simon & Schuster.

Kanter, R. M., Stein, B. A., et al. (1992). *The challenge of organizational change: How companies experience it and how leaders guide it.* New York: Free Press.

Kaplan, R. S., & Norton, D. P. (1996). *The balanced scorecard.* Boston: Harvard Business School Press.

Kimberly, J. R. (1981). Managerial innovation. In W. H. Starbuck (Ed.), *Handbook of organizational design* (Vol. 1, pp. 84–104). Oxford: Oxford University Press.

Kimberly, J. R., & Evanisko, J. M. (1981). Organizational innovation: The influence of individual, organizational, and contextual factors on hospital adoption of technological and administrative innovation. *Academy of Management Journal, 24*(4), 689–713.

Kimberly, J. R., & Minvielle, E. (2003). Quality as an organizational problem. In M. E. Myttenbach (Ed.), *Advances in health care organization theory* (pp. 205–232). San Francisco: Jossey-Bass.

Kirkley, D. (2004). Not whether, but when: Gaining buy-in for computerized clinical processes. *Journal of Nursing Administration, 34*(2), 55–58.

Kissler, G. D. (1996). *Leading the health care revolution: A reengineering mandate.* Chicago: Health Administration Press.

Klein, K. J., & Sorra, J. S. (1996). The challenge of implementation. *Academy of Management Review, 21*(4), 1055–1080.

Kotter, J. P. (1996). *Leading change.* Boston: Harvard Business Press.

Lathrop, J. P. (1993). *Restructuring health care: The patient-focused paradigm.* San Francisco: Jossey-Bass.

Leander, W. J. (1996). *Patients first: Experiences of a patient-focused pioneer.* Chicago: Health Administration Press.

Leatt, P., Baker, G. R., et al. (1997). Downsizing, reengineering, and restructuring: Long-term implications for healthcare organizations. *Frontiers of Health Services Management, 13*(4), 3–37.

Lehman, W. E. K., Greener, J. M., et al. (2002). Assessing organizational readiness for change. *Journal of Substance Abuse Treatment, 22*, 197–209.

Lewin, K. (1951). *Field theory in social science.* New York: Harper & Row.

Lewin, R., Parker, T., et al. (1998). Complexity theory and the organization: Beyond the metaphor. *Complexity, 3*(4), 36–40.

Lomas, J. (1993). Diffusion, dissemination, and implementation: Who should do what? *Annals of the New York Academy of Science, 703*, 226–235; discussion 235–237.

March, J. G. (1981). Footnotes to organizational change. *Administrative Science Quarterly, 26*(4), 563–577.

Markides, C. (1998). Strategic innovation in established companies. *Sloan Management Review, 39*(3), 31–43.

McCrae, R. M. (1984). Situational determinants of coping responses: Loss, threat, and challenge. *Journal of Personality and Social Psychology, 46*, 919–928.

McDaniel, R. R. (1997). Strategic leadership: A view from quantum and chaos theories. *Health Care Management Review, 22*(1), 21–37.

McDaniel, R. R., Jr., & Ashmos, D. P. (1986). Strategic directions within health care institutions: The role of the physician. *Journal of the National Medical Association, 78*(7), 633–41.

McGill, M. E., & Slocum, J. W. (1993). Unlearning the organization. *Organizational Dynamics, 22*, 67–78.

McKinney, M. M., Barnsley, J. M., et al. (1992). Organizing for cancer control. The diffusion of a dynamic innovation in a community cancer network. *International Journal of Technology Assessment in Health Care, 8*(2), 268–288.

McKinney, M. M., Morrissey, J. P., et al. (1993). Interorganizational exchanges as performance markers in a community cancer network. *Health Services Research, 28*(4), 459–478.

McLaughlin, C. P., & Kaluzny, A. D. (2005). *Continuous quality improvement in health care: Theory, implementation, and applications* (3rd ed.) Boston: Jones and Bartlett.

Meyer, A. D., & Goes, J. B. (1988). Organizational assimilation of innovations: A multi-level contextual analysis. *Academy of Management Journal, 31*(4), 897–923.

Meyer, M., Johnson, D., et al. (1997). Contrasting attributes of prevention health innovations. *Journal of Communication, 47*, 112–131.

Minasian, L. M., McCaskill-Stevens, W. J., et al. (2004). *Implementing cancer prevention and control research.* The National Cancer Institute Perspective. Forthcoming.

Mintzberg, H. (1993). The rise and fall of strategic planning: Reconceiving roles for planning, plans, and planners. New York: Free Press.

Mintzberg, H. (1997). Toward healthier hospitals. *Health Care Management Review, 22*(4), 9–19.

New York State Department of Health. (2001). *Coronary artery bypass surgery in New York State: 1996–1998.* Albany, State Department of Health.

Nord, W. R., & Tucker, S. (1987). *Implementing routine and radical innovations.* Lexington, MA: Heath and Company.

Nutt, P. C. (1984). Types of organizational decision processes. *Administrative Science Quarterly, 29* 414–450.

Oxman, A. D., Thomson, M. A., et al. (1995). No magic bullets: A systematic review of 102 trials of interventions to improve professional practice. *Canadian Medical Association Journal, 153*(10), 1423–1431.

Pappas, J. M., Flaherty, K. E., et al. (2004). Tapping into hospital champions—Strategic middle managers. *Health Care Management Review, 29*(1), 8–17.

Plsek, P. (2001). Redesigning health care with insights from the science of complex adaptive systems. In *Crossing the quality chasm: A new health system for the 21st century* (pp. 309–322). Washington, DC: National Academy Press.

Rogers, E. M. (2003). *The diffusion of innovations.* New York: Free Press.

Senge, P. M. (1990). *The fifth discipline: The art & practice of the learning organization.* New York: Currency Doubleday.

Senge, P. M. (1990). The leader's new work: Building learning organizations. *Sloan Management Review, 32*(1).

Shaw, M. E. (1981). *Group dynamics: The psychology of small group behavior.* New York: McGraw-Hill.

Simpson, K., A., Kaluzng, C. McLaughlin, (1991) "Total Quality and the Management Laboratories," *Clinical*

Laboratory Management Review, 5:6, November/December.

Smith, K. G., Smith, K. A., et al. (1994). Top management team demography and process: The role of social integration and communication. *Administrative Science Quarterly, 39*(3), 412–438.

Solberg, L. I. (2000). Guideline implementation: What the literature doesn't tell us. *Joint Commission Journal on Quality Improvement, 26*(9), 525–527.

Stacey, R. D. (1995). The science of complexity: An alternative perspective for strategic change processes. *Strategic Management Journal, 16*, 477–495.

Stacey, R. D. (1996). *Complexity and creativity in organizations.* San Francisco: Barrett-Koehler.

Starr, P. (1982). *The social transformation of American medicine: The rise a sovereign profession and the making of a vast industry.* New York: Basic Books.

Staw, B. M., Sandelands, L. E., et al. (1981). Threat-rigidity effects in organizational behavior: A multi-level analysis. *Administrative Science Quarterly* (26), 501–524.

Sterman, J. D. (2000). *Business dynamics: Systems thinking and modeling for a complex world.* Boston: Irwin, McGraw-Hill.

Ulrich, D., & Smallwood, N. (2004). Capitalizing on capabilities. *Harvard Business Review, 82*(6), 119–128.

Vaill, P. B. (1989). *Managing as a performing art: New ideas for a world of chaotic change.* San Francisco: Jossey-Bass.

Van de Ven, A. H., Polley, D. E., et al. (1999). *The innovation journey.* New York: Oxford University Press.

Weick, K. (1979). *The social psychology of organizing.* Reading, MA: Addison-Wesley.

Weick, K., & Quinn, R. E. (1999). Organizational change and development. *Annual Review of Psychology, 50*, 361–386.

Weiner, B. J., McKinney, M. M., et al. (2004). *Implementing cancer prevention and control research: The cooperative group experience.* (Forthcoming).

Weiner, B. J., Savitz, L. A., et al. (2004). How do integrated delivery systems adopt and implement clinical information systems. *Health Care Management Review, 29*(1), 1–16.

Weiss, K. B., Mendoza, G., et al. (1997). *Improving asthma care in children and adults.* Boston: Institute for Healthcare Improvement.

Wermers, M. A., Dagnillo, R., et al. (1996). Planning and assessing a cross-training initiative with multiskilled employees. *The Joint Commission Journal on Quality Improvement, 22*(6), 412–426.

West, E., Barron, J. D. & Newton, J. N. (1999). Hierarchies and Cliques in the Social Networks of Health Care Professionals: Implications for the Design of Dissemination Strategies. *Social Science and Medicine,* (48), 633–646.

Wheatley, M. J. (1992). *Leadership and the new science: Learning about organization from an orderly universe.* San Francisco: Berrett-Koehler.

Winslow, R. (2004). Lipitor prescriptions surge in wake of big study: Gains of Pfizer drug come at expense of Crestor, latest statin contender. *Wall Street Journal,* p. 4.

Yetton, P., Sharma, R., et al. (1999). Successful IS innovation: The contingent contributions of innovation characteristics and implementation process. *Journal of Information Technology, 14*(1), 53–68.

Yin, R. K. (1979). *Changing urban bureaucracies.* Lexington, MA: DC Heath and Company.

Young, G. J., Charns, M. P., et al. (2001). Top manager and network effects on the adoption of innovative management practices: A study of TQM in a public hospital System. *Strategic Management Journal, 22*(10), 935–951.

Zahra, A. S., & George, G. (2002). Absorptive capacity: A review, reconceptualization, and extension. *Academy of Management Review, 27*(2), 185–203.

Zimmerman, B. J. (1992). The inherent drive toward chaos. In A. Van de Ven, P. Lorange, B. Chakravarthy, J. Roos (Eds.), *Implementing strategic processes: Change, learning, and co-operation.* Oxford, UK: Blackwell, 373–393.

Zimmerman, B. J. (1999). Complexity science: A route through hard times and uncertainty. *The Health Forum Journal, 42*(2), 42–46.

CHAPTER 13

Organizational Performance: Managing for Efficiency and Effectiveness

Ann B. Flood, Ph.D., Jacqueline S. Zinn, Ph.D., and W. Richard Scott, Ph.D.

CHAPTER OUTLINE

- ❧ The Challenge of Performance
- ❧ Issues in Assessing Effective Performance
- ❧ The Manager's Role in Creating High-Performance Health Care Organizations

LEARNING OBJECTIVES

After completing this chapter, the reader should be able to:

1. Understand the importance of assessing organizational performance.
2. Define performance measures for organizations.
3. Understand the important issues in defining, measuring, and using performance measures.
4. Evaluate professional work.
5. Compare management models based on quality assurance and quality improvement.
6. Manage for quality improvement in health care.
7. Understand management roles to create high-performance organizations.

KEY TERMS

Benchmarking

Cost-Effectiveness

Efficiency

Organizational Effectiveness

Outcome Measures of Quality

Process Measures of Quality

Productivity

Quality Assurance (QA)

Quality Improvement (QI)

Resource Acquisition

Structural Measures of
 Quality

Transformational Leadership

IN PRACTICE — Health Care Organizations and Medical Errors

In 2002, 16-month-old Delaney Lucille Gonzalez walked with her family into UCLA Medical Center for routine surgery to repair a cleft palate. Three days later, she was disconnected from life support and died in her mother's arms.

"To bring a healthy child in there for surgery so minor," her mother, Jodi, said recently, clutching a headband she had made for Delaney, "you just don't accept that she's going to die."

The simple explanation is that a breathing tube had been misplaced and had pumped air into the child's stomach rather than her lungs, according to Delaney's medical and autopsy records. Because her body was deprived of oxygen, Delaney's heart stopped. She suffered irreversible brain damage.

But the misplaced tube was just the first in a series of errors leading to the child's death, according to state health inspectors who reviewed the case in response to a complaint from Delaney's mother.

The operation was successful, according to medical records . . . but doctors told her parents that she would be able to go home the next day, the Gonzalezes said.

Jodi Gonzalez said that when she was allowed to see her daughter after 8 P.M., she saw a nurse pull the breathing tube out of Delaney's nose slightly as she turned to check a machine. The nurse immediately yelled for "Blake"—Dr. Blake

Alban—then a resident physician in the unit, Gonzalez said. The child's medical records do not refer to this incident—a lapse criticized later by state health inspectors.

The records indicate, however, that Alban ordered a chest X-ray at 8:50 P.M. and concluded that the breathing tube had not been moved. More than three hours later, he ordered another chest X-ray and made the same finding. On the basis of her own training as a nurse, Jodi Gonzalez questioned Alban's readings. Delaney's stomach was "hard as a rock," which she feared indicated that the breathing tube was pumping air into her stomach. "They kept doing more chest X-rays," she said, and they said "everything was fine."

But after being consulted by telephone three times during the night, supervising physician Irwin Weiss was concerned enough to come in around 3:15 A.M. Three minutes later, Delaney went into cardiac arrest.

In a report he signed the next day, Weiss concluded that two X-rays ordered by Alban had been misread. The hospital's radiology department, which typically reviews doctors' X-ray readings, didn't examine the records for more than 12 hours after the first one was taken, a delay criticized by the state health inspectors. Compounding the problem, Weiss noted, staff members also had disconnected a carbon dioxide monitor, which is designed to signal breathing problems, because they believed it wasn't working . . . the girl was not hooked up to another monitor until after her heart stopped.

Three days after the initial surgery, the doctors confirmed that the brain damage was permanent and that she had no chance of recovery. "I said, 'we can't keep her alive on life support. That's not fair to her,'" Jodi Gonzalez said. "They gave her morphine, put the baby in Jodi's arms and then turned everything off," Danny Gonzalez said. Delaney died less than an hour later.

Even in the most prestigious hospitals, medical errors sometimes kill patients. According to a landmark report in 1999, 44,000 to 98,000 people die annually in hospitals because of mistakes ranging from performing surgery on the wrong organ to prescribing the wrong type or dosage of medication.

Like Delaney, patients don't usually die from a single mistake. They die from a series of oversights, faulty assumptions, and missed opportunities— what some experts refer to as a systemic breakdown.

"One single problem is usually not sufficient. . . . It requires a chain reaction," said Dr. David G. Nichols, a professor of anesthesiology and critical care medicine and pediatrics at Johns Hopkins University School of Medicine.

With that in mind, leading hospitals and health networks, including UCLA, in recent years have designed ways to check and recheck medical decisions as they are made. They also have made a point of encouraging forthright discussion of mistakes with the aim of correcting faulty procedures.

Those who study medical errors say it is wrong to blame the individuals who commit the errors, when whole systems are probably at fault. "Even if you fired every person who you think you could attribute blame to, the systems wouldn't be any safer," said Maureen Bisognano, executive vice president and chief operating officer of the Institute for Healthcare Improvement in Boston.

In the last several years, many hospitals, consultants, and business groups have set out to design better systems to prevent—or at least to promptly catch—errors rather than to rely on astute doctors and nurses to correct them at the last moment.

Some hospitals, for example, have designed computer systems to process physician orders. Unlike the paper slips now used, the computer can flag potentially harmful drug interactions or dosage requests. Many hospitals also use bar-code systems to match medications in the right dosages to the right patients.

Source: Adapted from Ornstein, C. (2003, April 21). Series of errors led to girl's death, state says: The toddler entered UCLA Medical Center for routine surgery, but never recovered. *Los Angeles Times*.

CHAPTER PURPOSE

The demands for high performance in health care are unforgiving as demonstrated by the unfolding events experienced by Delaney Lucille Gonzalez at the UCLA Medical Center. This is reflected by an increasing demand for accountability, quality, efficiency, and safety. Insurers—including public insurance programs like Medicare and self-insuring businesses—seeking discounted prices or other forms of cost containment in return for their business. At the same time, decreases in utilization such as dramatically shortened average lengths of stay, alternative sites for care such as same-day surgery and home care programs, and growth in provider availability have led to increased competition among providers. While these trends have stimulated health services managers to focus on the business of health services—that is, on market share, pricing policies, marginal costs, and productivity—there are other managerial interests at work. Professional providers stress quality and adherence to high professional standards, clients and their families seek improved function and longer life, while public authorities retain an interest in access and equity and in promoting systems that serve the entire community.

Ultimately, if health care providers do not hold themselves accountable for performance, performance standards may be imposed on them (Their & Gelijns, 1998). For example, long-standing concerns about the quality of nursing home care prompted sweeping legislative changes, increasing the regulatory burden on facilities. Similarly, managed care organizations (MCOs) face an increasingly hostile public and regulatory environment prompting numerous bills and legislation at both the state and federal level, which are designed to protect patients' rights and constrain MCOs from attempts to implement cost-efficient strategies (Davies & Rundall, 2000; Mechanic, 1998; Pearson & Raeke, 2000; Shortell, Waters, Clarke, & Budetti, 1998). The objective of this chapter is to review the major issues related to assessing organizational performance, compare and contrast the approaches of quality assurance and quality improvement, and describe the strategies to achieve an effective health care organization.

THE CHALLENGE OF PERFORMANCE

Clearly, a major challenge to the health care executive is to put together an organization that maximizes productivity, quality, and market share while not losing sight of the organization's mission to serve the health needs of the community. Because they operate in an environment of constrained resources, balancing these pressures has meant having to trade off some programs, services, and markets for others. For example, nursing homes struggle to maintain a single standard of care for all residents in the face of inadequate Medicaid reimbursement. A hospital may agree to give up its maternity services in order to expand its medical-surgical services or may share high-technology resources with another hospital in order to concentrate more effort in expanding its ambulatory care programs. Alternatively, a hospital may agree to introduce a service critically needed in the community despite its being a net drain on its resources. Such trade-offs have meant that chief executive officers (CEOs) of today's health care organizations have to manage their organizations in relation to other organizations and the community's needs in addition to considering the performance of individual subunits.

Another set of internal pressures comes from the concerns of committed health professionals—managers, nurses, physicians, and others—to improve professional practice by using their knowledge, skills, and technology to the best of their abilities and to the improved capabilities permitted by advances in medicine. This force is often neglected when considering the other, perhaps more visible, concerns.

Finally, in addition to these reasons for managers to attend to performance issues, outcomes research and clinical guidelines have gained a new prominence as the federal government also seeks to evaluate health care in an effort to minimize use of ineffective services, contain costs, and yet hold providers accountable for fairly distributed and well-performed services.

More than anyone else, the manager is responsible for the performance of the organization, but in a professional organization, this responsibility is shared with providers. In a real sense, all of the preceding chapters are building blocks for assisting the manager to improve organizational performance. As outlined in Chapters 1 and 2, the manager's role includes attending to the performance of the internal environment (i.e., the various departments and activities within the organization that serve each other) as well as attending to external customers.

The successful manager needs to guide and oversee all of the subsystems of the organization, not just the maintenance or managerial subsystems, which have been traditionally emphasized in health administration. Thus, the manager can improve performance not only through attending to productivity and maintenance of the human and capital infrastructure but also to boundary spanning activities, adapting the organization to its ever-changing environment and advances in medicine, and governing, or holding the organization accountable for its actions. The performance of health care organizations in the future may increasingly depend on the ability of health care managers to truly lead, not just steer, through obstacles—that is, to mold and innovate within their environment rather than passively react to external changes (Nelson et al., 2002; Shortell, Gillies, Anderson, et al., 1996).

Organizational performance is generally depicted using four interrelated concepts. The first two terms center on evaluating an organization in terms of the goods or services it produces for external consumption. Both terms characterize the inputs needed, either using dollars or units of resources expended, to produce these goods or services. Note that these inputs can depict labor or capital or both components. **Productivity** is defined as the ratio of outputs to inputs. An example of hospital labor productivity is the total number of admissions divided by the total number of nursing staff hours. A comparable productivity measure in the home health setting is the number of registered nurse visits per day. **Efficiency** is defined as the cost per unit of output. An example is the average total labor costs per admission.

There are important and complex issues associated with assessing inputs. For example, should an efficiency measure include the costs of staff not directly involved in treating patients? Or, should productivity include physician hours when they are not paid by the hospital? In the nursing home, ancillary services are frequently provided by outside contractors. Should these services be included in assessing nursing home efficiency?

Despite the difficulty of addressing these issues, the biggest challenge is the problem of measuring outputs. For example, consider the output: hospital stays. Since most of the variation in resources or dollars used during specific hospital stays depends on the reasons for hospitalizing the patients and whether they received surgery, two measures of efficiency—one based on 100 normal births and the other on 100 patients with coronary artery bypass surgeries—are clearly not directly comparable. Even within discharge categories, differences in case mix intensity, such as the proportion of high-risk births, make direct comparison of outcomes problematic. The challenge is to create measures of efficiency or productivity that take into account such differences between patient stays that are due to patient-specific needs for care during an admission.

Given cost containment pressures, all health care organizations face the challenge of becoming more productive and efficient. Existing studies suggest that the factors associated with increased productivity and efficiency include use of the following:

- High standards and goals (Nauert, 1996; Shortell, 1985)
- Information and feedback (Nelson, Mohr, Batalden, & Plume, 1996; Nelson et al., 2002)
- Interdepartmental coordination and resource sharing
- Compensation systems oriented toward rewarding productivity or efficiency (Flood, Fremont, Jin, et al., 1998; Flood, Bott, & Goodrick, 2000)
- Physician involvement in decision making and governance (Shortell, 1983)
- Concentration of staff work and activity (Alexander & Rundall, 1985)
- Active governing boards that deal with environmental pressures (Choi, Allison, & Munson, 1986)
- Type of ownership (Aaronson, Zinn, & Rosko, 1994; Coyne, 1982; Institute of Medicine, 1986; Pauly, Hillman, & Kerstein, 1990; Rosko, Chilingerian, Zinn, & Aaronson, 1995)

- Chain ownership and contract management (Connor, Feldman, Dowd, & Radcliff, 1997; Menke, 1997; Miller & Luft, 1994; Zinn, 1994)
- Degree of system integration (Gillies et al., 1993)

Setting high standards for cost containment motivates organizational members, particularly when the compensation systems reinforce attainment of the productivity and efficiency standards. Productivity-based compensation incentives include sharing cost savings resulting from employee suggestions as well as year-end bonuses based on staying within budget or generating net profits beyond expectations. There is a downside to compensation packages, of course, when they inadvertently reward one behavior while hoping to encourage another (Kerr, 1975). While eliminating all financial conflicts of interest from compensation arrangements is not possible, attention to managing the magnitude of the effects from such conflicts is important (Ohsfeldt, 1993).

The second set of terms to evaluate organizational performance is consistent with a broader, open-system perspective of what the organization is trying to accomplish. **Organizational effectiveness** means the degree to which organizational goals and objectives are successfully met. An organization goal to be achieved could be a subobjective (e.g., recruiting a coordinator for the organization's quality assurance—improvement program), an intermediate level objective (e.g., reducing nursing staff turnover on the units), or an ultimate objective (e.g., reduction in risk-adjusted mortality for acute myocardial infarction cases). **Cost-effectiveness** is a composite measure that takes into account both cost and the degree of goal attainment. These measures can be sensitive to consumers' goals as well as organizational considerations (e.g., by incorporating quality-of-life outcomes or consumer satisfaction or by weighting the various outcomes by patients' preferences for them).

Assessing effectiveness is complicated because of the problems associated with defining and measuring organizational goals. As Scott (1977) notes, assessing organizational effectiveness largely depends on the kinds of goals organizations adopt and their reasons for doing so. Goals serve many purposes. They may:

- Motivate organization members to higher performance
- Act as criteria for evaluating performance
- Legitimize organizational activities
- Indicate to external agencies what the organization is about

So how should success in reaching a goal be measured? Different goals may be developed to serve these different purposes; alternatively, the same stated goals may be used differently in different situations to serve any or all of the above functions—with varying degrees of success.

The following section examines the major approaches to assessing organizational performance, particularly in regard to effectiveness. It is organized to highlight three types of problems and issues in evaluating performance: definitional (what is measured), technical (how to measure), and managerial (why it is being measured). These sections include a review of the factors that affect performance, focusing particularly on studies of quality in health care organizations. The managerial issues focus on internal strategies aimed to assure quality and to improve it. The chapter concludes with a discussion of high-performing health care organizations and associated managerial guidelines.

ISSUES IN ASSESSING EFFECTIVE PERFORMANCE

Evaluation systems are the principal devices managers have for attempting to influence and improve the performance of their organizations. It is important for managers to become aware of the limitations of any particular system. As Haberstroh (1965) noted, "First, performance reporting is omnipresent and necessarily so. Second, almost every instance of performance reporting has something wrong with it." These problems can be broadly classified into definitional, technical, and managerial issues of performance evaluation, although as Kanter (1981) remarks, "The most interesting questions in this area are not technical, they are conceptual: not *how* to measure effectiveness or productivity, but *what* to measure" [italics added].

Definitional Issues in Assessment

Fundamental Perspectives about Organizations

The most important definitional issue in measuring organizational performance is related to one's view of the fundamental purpose and nature of organizations because these views affect the most critical assessment questions: *what* will be measured and *why* it is being evaluated (Scott, 1977)? If organizations are conceived primarily as rationally designed instruments for the production of goods and services for external consumption, emphasis is placed on measures of productivity and efficiency. Alternatively, if organizations are viewed as collectivities capable of pursuing specific goals but primarily oriented toward their own survival—toward system maintenance—attention is diverted from output to support goals, such as members' satisfaction or morale or, more generally, the survival of the organization. If organizations are envisioned to be open systems that are highly interdependent with their environments, the key strategies leading to an effective organization involve acquisition of scarce resources (e.g., through the fundraising activities of volunteers and the choice of well-connected persons to serve on boards of trustees) and the capacity to adapt to a changing environment (e.g., through the creation of slack, or uncommitted resources). This view, by recognizing both an external and internal reality for organizations, underscores the importance of knowing why an evaluation is being performed: for internal consumption (e.g., to

take corrective action to solve a quality problem) or external (e.g., to demonstrate to an external group that accreditation standards were met).

Juxtaposing these different views of organizations not only exposes multiple ways to conceptualize effectiveness but also highlights the potentially conflicting features of performance in an organizational system. Two issues leading to discrepancies help illustrate this point.

First, the measures may not be mutually compatible. For example, efficiency in the attainment of specific goals may not be consistent with maximizing participants' satisfaction. More specifically, a teaching hospital, organized to maximize opportunities to train and take advantage of the availability of residents, can lead to greater dissatisfaction of patients as they experience a depersonalized and discontinuous array of providers and of nurses as they relinquish some valued aspects of their roles to inexperienced residents (Fleming, 1981). Similarly, while injuries may be reduced by the use of physical restraints in nursing homes as a safety measure, they may also negatively impact the quality of residential life and morale.

Second, different time frames for evaluating effectiveness can lead to discrepant evaluations. Particularly in a time of rapid environmental change, the organization that is well suited to deal with today's demands may by that very fact be ill-equipped to handle tomorrow's challenges. Weick (1977) notes that organizational features that preserve adaptability "look ugly and wasteful" in the present context but can prove invaluable when conditions change. Finally, the organization itself is seen as having a life cycle and all of its subunits are subject to changes that develop over time (Kimberly & Miles, 1980). Cameron and Whetten (1981) proposed that effectiveness varies according to the stage of organizational development. Effectiveness in earlier stages depends primarily on creativity and mobilizing resources; later stages emphasize commitment and cohesion among members; still later, formal processes of control and efficiency come to the fore; and finally, structural elaboration, decentralization, and flexibility receive emphasis.

Domain of Activity

Once a general framework or model has been selected to guide the investigation, it is necessary to determine which particular functions or activities will be evaluated (Dornbusch, Scott, & Busching, 1975). Most complex organizations serve a variety of aims and objectives. Modern hospitals, for example, not only provide a variety of types of patient care, including broad categories of services such as outpatient, inpatient, and emergency care, but many also pursue educational goals (e.g., residency training), research goals, and preventive and community service goals. Departmental and work group subdivisions often reflect—and protect—these differentiated purposes, with different subgroups and types of personnel performing quite divergent tasks and pursuing quite distinct objectives.

In some cases, these goals and the activities of the various groups are highly interdependent—in either negative or positive ways. Training objectives sometimes conflict with patient care as noted above, but they can also support and complement good care by making available advanced technology or encouraging providers to investigate unexpected results. In other cases, the goals and activities may be quite independent, the policies and practices of a labor and delivery center may be largely unaffected by those of the hospice program. In either situation—even if the same concept of effectiveness is being applied—the same organization may perform extremely well in one domain of activities but relatively poorly in another. For example, while long-term care settings provide both medical and social services for their residents, they may not provide both with equal effectiveness. The diversity of products in modern managed care organizations and integrated systems likewise exponentially increases the challenge to do all things well. Simply put, no organization can be equally effective with respect to all the objectives it pursues. Two implications are that there is no simple measure of overall effectiveness for a health care organization, but there is always room to continuously improve at least some aspect of performance.

Different Levels of Analysis

A third critical factor influencing conceptions of organizational performance is the level of analysis selected to guide the assessment. An important insight gained from open-systems theory is that all complex systems tend to be nested units, systems within systems. Thus, a hospital is composed of departments, and the departments are composed of work units, and the hospital as a whole is part of one or more larger systems, such as a multiunit hospital or regional health system. The boundaries that separate these levels are seldom clear and are often rather arbitrary. Further, many of these boundaries are not organized in neat concentric circles but frequently overlap and cross-cut one another. Individuals in modern societies are not completely contained within any single organization but instead are partially involved in several, and professional occupations and union organizations cross organizational boundaries in complex and unexpected ways.

Although there are obviously various possibilities, it is conventional to identify at least three system levels

- The organization itself, such as a health maintenance organization (HMO)
- A larger socially defined unit that contains the organization, such as a community, a health services region, or a system of hospitals
- Subunits contained within the organization, such as individual departments or practitioners.

Nerenz and Zajac (1991) propose yet another unit of analysis to assess performance in a variety of vertically integrated health systems. They propose that the basic unit of data collection should not be a service or a patient but an episode of care that embraces services provided across multiple sites and involving numerous actors. They challenge traditional measures of performance as containing inappropriate assumptions for today's complex systems, such as the presumed association between utilization and revenue or the assumption that the system's effectiveness can be maximized by maximizing the effectiveness of each component organization. They propose new ways to collect information that can aid future attempts to understand the relationship between system performance and system characteristics.

The unit of analysis selected can have a profound effect on the assessment of performance. For example, a strategy to measure efficiency of emergency services at the community level may differ considerably from an assessment focused on one hospital's emergency room. Most analyses of organizational performance focus on one or more of these three levels. The critical point, however, is that one should be as clear as possible about what level of analysis is selected.

It is also important to recognize that system performance at any given level may not be analyzable as a simple aggregation of system performance at lower levels. This is one of the principal features of any system: Its performance is determined as much, if not more, by the arrangements of its parts—their relations and interactions—as by the performance of the individual components. A number of highly qualified physicians do not necessarily add up to a high-quality medical staff. Rather, how the staff members are deployed by level of privileges and types of service, how their work is monitored and information fed back to allow improvement, the arrangements for continuing education, and other similar factors may be more decisive for many aspects of medical effectiveness (Flood & Scott, 1987).

One must be careful not to confuse level of analysis with the issue of whose interests are reflected in the determination of assessment criteria. For example, it is possible to focus on the performance of the hospital as a complex system but to assess this performance from the standpoint of the interest of the larger community. Whose interests are served in assessing effectiveness is best treated as a separate topic, a fourth factor that affects one's view of organizational performance.

Stakeholders

Early performance measures, based on small entrepreneurial organizations, focused primarily on profit for the owners or their agents (managers). For publicly traded health care organizations, like many nursing home, assisted living, and home health care providers, stockholder benefit remains a key measure of performance. It was not long before analysts noted that the interests of owners and their agents were far from being perfectly aligned and that other groups—such as professional workers, the public, and external clients—had interests in the organization's performance (Berle & Means, 1932; Burnham, 1941). Cyert and March (1966) described organizations in terms of shifting coalitions of interest groups—some internal, others external to the organization—that are constantly engaged in negotiating and renegotiating the conditions of their participation and thereby affecting the performance of organizations.

In any organization, both internal and external interested parties—stakeholders—have different desires and needs to be met by the organization. Certain views privilege the interests of shareholders, but many current observers of organizations insist that other interests including those of managers, staff, rank-and-file employees, clients, and the wider community—have equal standing (Ancona, Kochan, Scully, Van Maanen, & Westney, 1996; Harrison & Freeman, 1999). They want the organization to score points on different things. They have varying expectations and criteria for effectiveness. For example, internal stakeholders in hospitals include employees, physicians, and boards of directors. Most employees want meaningful work, opportunity for growth, and a reasonable degree of job security. Physicians want up-to-date technology, support services, and an environment in which they are free to practice medicine as they were trained. Physicians, while viewed primarily as internal stakeholders, can also be considered as external stakeholders, depending on the degree to which particular physicians identify with a given health care organization.

Health care organizations can also be external stake-holders for other health care organizations. For example, hospitals are a major source of referrals for home health agencies.

Other external stakeholders include suppliers, regulatory groups, competitors, third-party payers, and community groups. Third-party payers expect care to be provided in the most cost-effective manner possible. Patients have varying expectations depending on the severity of their illness, their education, and their financial resources. Regulators will be concerned with the organization's ability to maintain standards and contain costs. Suppliers of capital focus on the institution's bottom line. Given this disparate set of demands and expectations, it is not possible for a given organization to be seen as equally effective by all of its stakeholders or constituent groups at a given point in time.

Researchers have examined performance issues that involve multiple interested parties and coalition formation in health care organizations. Fennell and Alexander (1989) note that a board of trustees is supposed to represent the external stakeholders' interests and monitor and contain any self-interested actions on the part of hospital management and internal stakeholders. However, the stakeholders and customers in hospitals are often difficult to identify and sometimes hard to tell apart, resulting in continuous coalition formation among the interest groups.

This lack of clear-cut boundaries among the interests of various actors is further illustrated by proponents of quality improvement who argue that production of any service or product within the organization—such as filling a prescription or preparing a report for the government—involves a seemingly endless chain of suppliers, processors, and customers (Berwick, Godfrey, & Roessner, 1991). Rather than restrict the term *customers* to end users of an organization's product, this perspective emphasizes the complex web of parties with a stake in performance. This perspective is particularly useful in evaluating integrated delivery systems where complex supplier-customer relationships among system components abound.

Of course, not all interests are equally powerful. In most organizations, one can detect the presence of a dominant coalition whose interests carry more weight than others. But it is still important to note that in most organizations power is more widely dispersed today than in the past, and more diverse constituencies are perceived to be legitimate stakeholders in the enterprise.

One response to the disparate needs of multiple competing interests has been the development of a "community orientation" by health care organizations. Spurred by a variety of factors, there is a growing consensus among third-party payers, employers, community organizations, local governments, and other stakeholders that health services organizations like hospitals must reach beyond a narrow definition of their patients to enhance the health status of the entire population they serve (i.e., of their community). In this context, community includes all persons and organizations within a circumscribed geographical area in which there is a sense of interdependence and belonging. The degree of community orientation can be defined by the extent to which these organizations generate community intelligence, disseminate it internally and externally, and use it to develop community health interventions (Proenca, Rosko, & Zinn, 2000).

To summarize, a number of factors have been identified that have clear relevance to the evaluation of organizational performance. As illustrated by the challenges encountered by frontline personnel (see In Practice, Frontline Bureaucracy in Health Care and Access for the Uninsured, p. 425) the nature of organizations and the impact of time frames, the domains of the activities being evaluated, the level of analysis, and the perspective of interested parties are sufficiently complex that one may expect to find little consensus in the selection of criteria employed to evaluate organizational effectiveness (Campbell, 1977; Flood, 1994; Flood & Fennell, 1995; Steers, 1975).

Technical Issues in Assessment

Having described key definitional issues related to what should be measured, we now turn to problems

IN PRACTICE Frontline Bureaucracy in Health Care and Access for the Uninsured

"I feel that in the country we live in, everybody is entitled to health care, regardless of whether they can pay or not. But that's my personal opinion. And yes, sometimes it does influence me.
—Front desk clerk on processing uninsured patients

Each year, millions of uninsured individuals in the United States seek routine (nonemergency) health care services that they cannot afford, but most providers are not required to take care of them. Frontline bureaucrats—clerical staff who have direct contact with patients, including registration clerks, insurance verifiers, and patient representatives—in most health care organizations are charged not only with facilitating their employer's mission of caring for patients in need, but also with securing payment to cover the costs of that care. What do they do when these goals conflict, as is often the case when uninsured patients lack the resources to make required payments such as deposits at the time of care? How is it decided whether such patients will be seen or whether they will be turned away?

This study explored the role of frontline staff as gatekeepers of access to care, caught between administrative responsibility—which includes collecting revenue—and service to the client/patient—who sometimes cannot pay.

Many [managers and administrators] acknowledged that although they were eager to reduce the volume of self-pays, they were also concerned about the legal and political implications of denying services, public relations with their communities, and the costs of employing additional staff (e.g., financial counselors) to implement complex policies. A senior financial administrator . . . put it this way: "Of course we cannot specify that patients should be turned away. Those decisions are handled in each clinic differently, depending on the supervisors, the physicians involved, even on how busy the practice is on a particular day. When faced with such situations, the front desk staff will talk with their supervisors about what to do. Patients are generally called aside to prevent an unpleasant scene. The supervisor will generally understand when to consult the doctors about difficult situations." Several commented that the gaps and contradictions in policies reflected the need for considerable latitude in handling the politically charged issue of access, necessitating decision making on the front line.

Turning/Not Turning Patients Away

Seventy-one percent (39 of the 55) staff interviewed reported that they did not independently turn patients away. Although we found no written policies stating that patients are never to be turned away (not counting emergency room policies), a number of clerks believed otherwise, as reflected in statements such as the following: "One of the policies I'm pretty sure is that they don't turn away anybody, they don't turn away people."
—Representative

Others, although not referencing policy, stated the view as a matter of principle: "We just explain to them that they have to bring a deposit on their next visit. We don't turn away. I don't turn away patient care."
—Clerical

Finally, there was a third group that stated that they personally intervene to prevent patients from being turned away: "How they handle it with me—patients come in with no money and then dying and in need of health care and surgery, my department will tell you I am very voiceful about that. I don't feel

(continues)

IN PRACTICE (continued)

that it's right that you turn a person down that's dying. We used to hear, 'We are not about money, we are about health care and saving lives.' Not this hospital in some cases. They have their own picks and choices. . . ."

—Clerical

When asked, some of these individuals gave us examples of how they advocate for patients: "I had one patient . . . when she came in she only had, I think it was like $10 or something like that. And then I went over to a supervisor and I told her that she was in need of care and that she would be in next Friday when she got paid from her job, and she would come in and pay the remaining balance of the deposit. And they told me it's on your judgment if you think she . . . you know, if she looks like she will . . . And sure enough, she came back and she paid the remaining $40."

"(Recently) a mother brought a baby in. She didn't have insurance, but she applied—she had applied and so in that case I just went ahead and let her have the test done for the baby."

"We have a patient who is self-pay and she is on coumadin, and she needs to be checked ever so often . . . so she would be coming every week and that's too much for her to be paying. So we have actually—you know, let her go through without registering so we could help her out in a way."

Note three different approaches to advocacy: The first example involves "going out on a limb" for a patient; the second, categorizing a patient advantageously as "insurance pending" rather than as "self-pay"; the third instance illustrates a decision to act in contravention to policy.

In contrast, those who did report turning patients away expressed sentiments that might be described in the following examples as, respectively, *dispassionate, pragmatic, equivocal,*

and *regretful:* "I just do what the job tells me to do. As far as feeling sorry or anything, I don't get off into that part of it, I just do the job and if I have a problem or anything then I take it to the next in charge."

—Representative

"So in that way trying to work them through the system and keep the patient informed, but yet balance the needs of the hospital. I mean we can't give away everything, so in that way it gets tough."

—Utilization manager.

"We turn self-pay patients away from . . . for diagnostic testing. Okay. Those we do. We try to reschedule them. Not really turn them away, but we ask if we could reschedule."

—Utilization manager

The findings are consistent with studies of other human service bureaucracies. Prottas (1979) notes: "Numerous writers have noted that the political realities of public service programs require them to pursue several, sometimes incompatible, ends. The rules operationalizing those goals often operationalize those inconsistencies as well. . . . The result of these characteristics of bureaucratic rules is that the street-level bureaucrat achieves a wide latitude of discretion." It is therefore not surprising that a cadre of clerks, supervisors, and managers, in periodic consultation with nurses and physicians, could be left to grapple with the dilemma of rationing access to uncompensated care.

Source: Adapted from Weiner, S. J., Laport, M., Abrams, R. I., Moswin, A., & Warnecke, R. (2004). Rationing access to care to the medically uninsured: The role of bureaucratic front-line discretion at large healthcare institutions. *Med Care, 42* (4), 306–312.

of how to measure performance. The focus is on the generic problems and concerns that arise during the process of evaluating work performance.

Classes of Measures

Performance assessment requires that evidence be collected upon which evaluations can be based. More than 40 years ago, Donabedian (1966) noted that evaluators of the quality of health care answered the "how to" question by using one of three basic classes of measures: structural, process, and outcome measures. (See also, Donabedian, 1980.) Although he was referring to the evaluation of technical and psychosocial aspects of clinical care, these same categories are useful for evaluating nonclinical performance as well. Table 13.1 provides examples of each class of indicators applied to financial management, clinical care, and human resources management.

Structural Measures. Structural indicators are based on assessments of organizational features or participants' characteristics that are presumed to have an impact on organizational performance. As such, they can be thought of as input measures of an organization's capacity to permit or promote effective work. For example, in the opening scenario of UCLA Medical Center, **structural measures of quality** would portray the quality and number of staff in the operating room and the forms of coordination to carry out doctor's orders. Other indicators include the number and types of specialized equipment, such as carbon dioxide monitoring; the presence of an active peer review program; and the proportion of the medical staff that is board certified. Until recently, accreditation and certification reviews relied almost exclusively on either structural or process measures of performance; note too that accreditation itself can be used as a structural indicator of performance. For example, many managed care organizations require provider organizations to have accreditation by the Joint Commission on the Accreditation of Healthcare Organizations (JCAHO) as a prerequisite for contract participation.

Process Measures. **Process measures of quality** are based on evidence relating to the performer's activities in carrying out work. Examples include quality assurance activities such as reviews of physician decision making and orders provided to all patients dying in-hospital or reviewing nurse and physician conformance with standards for cleanliness on units with outbreaks of nosocomial infections. The proportion of residents physically restrained or catheterized are process "checkpoints" that may trigger more rigorous quality review in the federal nursing home certification process. Process measures can be directed at an organization or system of care as well—a review of the system for conducting and reporting the results of urgently requested laboratory tests. Process measures can also be used to assess the nonclinical aspects of performance. Examples in the financial area include liquidity ratios, such as the ratio of current assets to current liability, and activity ratios, such as the ratio of total operating revenue to total assets (Cleverly, 1981).

Outcome Measures. **Outcome measures of quality** are based on evidence gathered from the objects upon which the work is performed. Since assessments are made to determine whether changes have occurred in their characteristics that can be attributed to the work performed upon them, these can be thought of as measures of the output of work processes. Thus, for clinical care, changes in the patient's health status (to measure technical aspects of care) or satisfaction (to assess the interpersonal care) are assessed; for training institutions, changes in the student's knowledge, skills, or attitudes may be examined. In the financial area, outcome might be measured by the operating margin (ratio of operating income to operating revenue) or the return on assets (Cleverly, 1981).

These three classes of measures are not independent measures of performance, but linked in an underlying model. Structural measures of quality are valid to the extent that they motivate and encourage providers to choose efficacious, appropriate, or cost-effective actions. Process measures in

Table 13.1. **Examples of Performance Measures by Category**

	Domain of Activity		
	Clinical Care	**Financial Management**	**Human Resources Management**
Structure	*Effectiveness* ■ Percent of active physicians who are board certified ■ JCAHO accreditation ■ Number of residencies and filled positions ■ Presence of council for quality improvement planning	*Effectiveness* ■ Qualifications of administrators in finance department ■ Use of preadmission criteria ■ Presence of an integrated financial and clinical information system	*Effectiveness* ■ Ability to attract desired registered nurses and other health professionals ■ Size (or growth) of active physician staff ■ Salary and benefits compared with competitors ■ Quality of in-house staff education
Process	*Effectiveness* ■ Rate of medication error ■ Rate of nosocomial infection ■ Rate of postsurgical wound infection ■ Rate of normal tissue removed *Productivity* ■ Ratio of total patient days to total full-time equivalent (FTE) nurses ■ Ratio of total admissions to total FTE staff ■ Ratio of physician visits to total FTE physicians *Efficiency* ■ Average cost per patient ■ Average cost per admission	*Effectiveness* ■ Days in accounts receivable ■ Use of generic drugs and drug formulary ■ Market share ■ Size (or growth) of shared service arrangements *Productivity* ■ Ratio of collection to FTE financial staff ■ Ratio of total admissions to FTE in finance department ■ Ratio of new capital to fund-raising staff *Efficiency* ■ Cost per collection ■ Debt/equity ratio	*Effectiveness* ■ Grievances ■ Promotions ■ Organizational climate *Productivity* ■ Ratio of line staff to managers *Efficiency* ■ Cost of recruiting
Outcome	*Effectiveness* ■ Case-severity-adjusted mortality ■ Patient satisfaction ■ Patient functional health status	*Effectiveness* ■ Return on assets ■ Operating margins ■ Size (or growth) of federal, state, or local grants for teaching and research ■ Bond rating	*Effectiveness* ■ Turnover rate ■ Absenteeism ■ Staff satisfaction

turn are valid if they lead to improved products or better outcomes. This model overstates the simplicity of these relationships, which are loosely coupled at best and certainly should not be mistaken as substitutes for each other. It is important to recognize that each of these types of indicators is imperfect—subject to bias and misinterpretation. Process measures focus on energy and effort expended but neglect effects achieved. Moreover, measures based on process alone can only compare performance values with some specified standard; they cannot themselves assess the appropriateness of the standards employed. If process measures are once removed from effects, then structural indicators are twice removed, since they do not assess work performed or effort expended but only the organization's capacity for work. Presumed competencies may in practice turn out to be ineffectual, and existing capacities may on specific occasions be unemployed or underemployed. Outcome measures have the advantage of focusing attention on changes produced and results achieved. Their drawback is that they do not in themselves provide evidence that can connect observed outcomes to the effects of performance. Particularly in arenas such as medical care, it is common for poor outcomes to occur in spite of superior performance, and vice versa. Causal factors that are beyond the control of the caregiver are at work. And at a more general organizational level, a high proportion of good outcomes—patient recoveries, student achievements, profitability—may be more a function of selection procedures—admitting only the easiest patients or brightest students—than what the organization does. Finally, because full recovery is not the goal for much of health care, such as for chronic or mental illness and for care of the dying patient, a comparison of actual versus expected decline or comfort for such patients may be the most appropriate measure of outcome performance.

It is also important to distinguish objective measures of quality from people's perceptions. For example, a given home health agency may have the highest possible accreditation rating and best patient functional health status outcomes (objective mea-

sures) but be perceived by the community as having relatively low quality, perhaps owing to problems of convenience and access to services or an occasional war story of poor care. In the same vein, it is important to recognize that the public's perception of quality may differ from those of physicians and caregivers. For example, the public may give greater weight to access, convenience, comfort, and interpersonal relationships while the professional caregiver places greater emphasis on technical skill. In part, this is due to the public's relative inability to evaluate technical expertise. As a result, they use other criteria as proxy measures or assume technical quality as a given and then make choices based on the nontechnical criteria discussed above. Again, this points out the importance of deciding which stakeholder perspective(s) will be used to assess performance.

Preferences for Classes of Performance Measures

Associations are likely to exist between these classes of indicators and broadly defined categories of constituencies in organizations (Scott, 1977). Executives and managers typically prefer to employ structural measures of effectiveness since these are the types of indicators over which they have most control. Similarly, caregivers are likely to emphasize process measures because these activities are more under their control. By contrast, clients and representatives of the various external publics may prefer to focus attention on outcomes; never mind capacity or effort, what results were actually achieved? Patients, for example, are much more likely to be concerned about remission of symptoms and restoration of function than about the technical correctness of the procedures employed or the formal qualifications of personnel. Despite this preference, patients seldom can obtain good information about the average patient's experience with outcomes and must rely on the physician's judgment or structural indicators such as accreditation. Indeed, for these reasons, executives need to be attentive to such visible indicators of quality—whether they reflect true differences in patient care—since these indicators may be used by prospective customers to choose where they go for care. More broadly, licensing, accreditation, tort law, and regulations associated with quality control abound in health care. Even when they use standards based on widely held beliefs rather than on evidence of their import for quality, they have an ability to influence organizational performance regardless of the validity of the claim.

Factors Associated with Effective Performance

Despite the difficulties involved, studies have identified a number of factors generally associated with higher quality of care (Aiken, Sochalski, & Lake, 1997; Flood, 1994; Flood & Fennell, 1995; Flood & Scott, 1987; Kimberly & Minvielle, 2000; Miller & Luft, 1994):

- Quality of professional staff
- High standards
- Experience with other cases of the same type
- More formally organized professional staffs with well-defined coordination and conflict management processes
- Participative organization cultures emphasizing team approaches
- Timely and accurate performance feedback
- Active management of environmental forces
- Type of ownership, competition, staffing continuity, and compensation
- Higher levels of differentiation and coordination of medical staff

Evidence related to peer review through quality assurance and continuous quality improvement is discussed in the following section.

In nursing homes, higher levels of staffing by registered nurses is associated with improved physical functioning, lower mortality, a greater likelihood of being discharged to home, and less unnecessary hospitalizations. In home health care services, it is also associated with greater patient satisfaction. In regard to the quality of professional staff, key factors are recruitment, retention, and having people work within their professional abilities. This involves concentrating the work of professionals in such a fashion that greater experience produces better patient-care outcomes over time. As noted, many studies have found higher volume of patients treated by both institutions and individual physicians to be associated with more positive patient-care outcomes (Birkmeyer & Dimick, 2004; Flood, Scott, & Ewy, 1984; Halm, Lee, & Chassin, 2002; Luft, Granick, Mark, & McPhee, 1990; Taub et al., 2004).

Setting high standards is compatible with professional values. A key factor involves strict admission requirements and exerting strong control in enforcing standards. More tightly organized professional staffs assist in this process by providing regular forums for problem management and conflict resolution (Shortell & LoGerfo, 1981). In nursing homes, greater control over medical staff admitting privileges is associated with less inappropriate drug prescribing; staffing continuity and compensation are associated with greater resident satisfaction and better physical functioning. Coordination also plays an important role in overall effectiveness.

A participative organizational culture emphasizing team approaches is particularly important when the environment is changing rapidly. An ongoing team approach allows ideas to be communicated and discussed quickly by the professionals that will be most affected by the changes involved. A participative culture helps to develop good work habits on the part of all involved and reinforces appropriate peer group pressure. Further, teams generally do a better job of solving complex problems than individuals. For example, work focused on hospital intensive care units found that efficiency of utilization and perceptions of higher quality of care were related to good conflict management—including communication, problem solving, and leadership—combined with a patient orientation (Shortell, Zimmerman, Gillies, et al., 1990). Many studies suggest that structures allowing for greater coordination and communication across disciplines that participate in the care of the elderly contribute to better outcomes. For example, the use of multidisciplinary teams bears favorably on both physical and psychosocial outcomes in nursing homes and patient satisfaction with home health care services.

Timely and accurate feedback raises the visibility of behavior in the organization such that accountability requirements are met, and deviation from performance standards is assessed. Nursing homes and home health agencies are beginning to tie together financial and clinical data in negotiating rates for various levels of services with managed care organizations. A good clinical-financial management information system enables corrective action to be taken more quickly. Finally, more active management of the external environment enables the organization to educate external groups (e.g., licensing and accreditation bodies, regulatory groups, third-party payers) about quality objectives and practices and the associated challenges involved. For example, university teaching hospitals, which have established their own hospital-specific governing boards separate from the university governing boards, have been better able to negotiate with relevant external groups and more clearly communicate their mission and objectives.

As the incentives to form more integrated delivery systems grow, there is great need to assess the performance of such systems from both an efficiency and effectiveness perspective. The existing evidence is largely mixed while the issue of quality of care provided by such systems is largely unexplored (Bazzoli, Chan, Shortell, & D'Aunno, 2000; Bazzoli, Shortell, Dubbs, Chan, & Kralovec, 1999; Dubbs, Bazzoli, Shortell, & Kralovec, 2004; Shortell, Morrison, & Friedman, 1990).

In sum, managers must recognize the limitations of each class of performance indicator as well as understand the interests of the various constituency groups—including their own—that have a stake in the functioning of their organization. Only such awareness will enable them to correct for these bi-

ases and balance the often conflicting interests of the several parties involved.

Managerial Issues in Assessing Performance

The need for managing quality is central to any organization. Health care organizations, coming under increasing pressure to be cost-effective, have been turning away from old models of assuring quality to a new model of quality improvement, which has been effective in helping industries worldwide to improve their products or services. The old model in health care relegated quality to the quality assurance (QA) department; the new model emphasizes quality improvement (QI) teams, which cut horizontally across functions and reach vertically across hierarchical lines to involve the entire management and staff. The old model solved problems and held individuals culpable for mistakes; the new one prevents problems by continuously improving the true source of defects— the process. The old model was based on peer review and focused on upholding minimally acceptable standards of care; the new borrows from principles applicable to any industry and encourages striving for excellence. The form and function of the old model was required by external accreditors and third-party payers for quality of care; the new permeates all processes and requires a strong internal culture to support it. The differences are profound enough to require a major paradigm shift—not necessarily to displace all of the activities of QA but to restructure most of the way quality is managed. In this section, both models are presented and their strengths and weaknesses contrasted. To set the stage, general issues in evaluating professionals and other staff and unintended responses to evaluation are presented.

Evaluating Professional Performance: The Professional Model

In the classic professional model, the foremost means to ensure that professionals produce high-quality

IN PRACTICE

Stakeholder Interests: Corporate Responsibility for Disclosure of Scientific Evidence in Medicine

In a novel claim testing the way that the $400 billion worldwide pharmaceutical industry is regulated, the New York State attorney general, Eliot Spitzer, sued the British-based drug giant GlaxoSmithKline [June 2, 2004], accusing the company of fraud in concealing negative information about its popular antidepressant medicine Paxil.

The civil lawsuit, filed in State Supreme Court in Manhattan, contends that GlaxoSmithKline engaged in persistent fraud by failing to tell doctors that some studies of Paxil showed that the drug did not work in adolescents and might even lead to suicidal thoughts. Far from warning doctors, the suit contends, the company encouraged them to prescribe the drug for youngsters.

A spokeswoman for the FDA would not comment on the lawsuit but noted that the agency required companies to submit all data related to the safety of their drugs. Because so much drug company data submitted is considered proprietary, it is up to the FDA to decide when to disclose possible safety concerns. That is what it did [in 2003], when it warned doctors on the use of Paxil for adolescents and children. [In 2004], it required antidepressant makers to strengthen suicide warnings on labels.

Mr. Spitzer's lawsuit is part of a broad assault by prosecutors on the drug industry's marketing practices. [In May 2004], for example, federal prosecutors in Boston announced a settlement with the world's largest drug maker, Pfizer; the company agreed to pay $430 million and to plead guilty to charges that its Warner-Lambert unit promoted the drug Neurontin to doctors for the treatment of conditions where no benefit had been proved.

At issue in most of these investigations . . . is the marketing of approved drugs for off-label uses—

those not specifically approved by the FDA. While doctors are free to prescribe an approved drug for any use, the manufacturers are supposed to limit their marketing to those uses with FDA clearance.

The new wrinkle in Mr. Spitzer's suit is his argument that a drug maker is committing fraud if it does not tell doctors about trials of a medication that raise safety concerns. "I'm certainly not the person to determine whether Paxil is appropriate or not for any given patient," Mr. Spitzer acknowledged. "But what I can do is ensure the information to doctors is fair and complete so that those equipped to make this determination can do so."

Dr. Barry Perlman, president of the New York State Psychiatric Association, said, "Whenever we don't have the complete picture, we can't prescribe ethically and appropriately, and that's an enormous obstacle to good care."

Pharmaceutical companies sponsor most clinical trials of drugs and, in many cases, they jealously guard the data that results. If a test suggests that a drug is effective in treating a certain condition, the company will push to get its results published in a prestigious journal. If the results reflect poorly on the drug, they often never appear in public.

Experts have long criticized the tendency in the industry to publish only positive clinical trials, arguing that this distorts medical practice and undermines the scientific process. Some have suggested that the results of all clinical trials should be published in a federal registry. But some say that doctors are unlikely to consult such a registry and will continue to be influenced by trial results published in leading journals.

Mr. Spitzer's suit is the first to suggest a way of resolving such matters. If a company's marketing message is at odds with the results of its own suppressed clinical trial, he argues, the company is liable for damages under consumer fraud laws.

In the case of Paxil, GlaxoSmithKline, sponsored five trials of the drug in adolescents suffering from major depression . . . . to qualify for a six-month extension of Paxil's patent granted under a federal law that encourages the testing of drugs in children. But it published only one of the trials, which showed mixed effect. The unpublished trials failed to show any benefit for the drug and suggested that it might increase the risk of suicide.

An internal memo cited in the suit said the company should have "effectively managed the dissemination of these data in order to minimize any potential negative commercial impact." And, according to the suit, the company told its sales representatives that "Paxil demonstrates remarkable efficacy and safety in the treatment of adolescent depression." The suit contends that sales representatives passed this on to doctors.

Source: Excerpted from Harris, G. (2004, June 3). Spitzer sues a drug maker, saying it hid negative data. *New York Times*.

work is to give them the skills, training, and values needed to produce life-long devotion to excellence. However, to weed out any "bad apples" and to inspire them to continue learning, professional workers can be held accountable by making their work visible to others whose opinion counts. In professional work, peer review is needed because only peers can truly judge the quality of one's work. These notions, for physicians in particular and nurses to a more limited extent, are backed up by a potential for malpractice litigation against sub-standard care and by financial fines or professional reprimands for poor performance (Hall, 1988).

Health care organizations have always operated by using both professional and bureaucratic forms of control. Some have argued that there are two independent lines of authority, one for physicians and the other for everyone else. In their exposition of work in hospitals, Geogopoulos and Mann (1962) implied that these two lines of authority acted more like a lobotomized brain rather than an integrated right and left brain in coordinating activities. But others, like Scott (1982), describe three alternative models that can be used to embed professionals ef-

fectively into an organization: *autonomous*, in which professionals retain independent authority to control and evaluate themselves as a group; *heteronomous*, in which professionals are subject to more line-authority control; and *conjoint*, in which professionals and administrators coexist in a mutually interdependent setting in which each group is roughly equal in power and in the importance of their functions. The hospital that Geogopoulos and Mann were describing fit the autonomous model; but the modern health care organization is moving toward the third model, in which mutual understanding and cooperation play key roles for organizational effectiveness.

In health care organizations, because of the high percentage of professionals involved and their diversity, health care executives need to understand and accommodate the varying professional requirements of each group. Physicians, in particular, have high need for achievement and autonomy in clinical decision making. Other groups have less highly developed claims to autonomy but desire organizational settings in which they can practice their full range of professional skills. Job autonomy, for example, is associated with less conflict, increased job satisfaction, and greater client satisfaction (Weisman & Nathanson, 1985).

Almost all professionals have high standards of excellence, and therefore organizations and managers that emphasize high-performance expectations and provide the necessary support for obtaining excellence are likely to be more effective. Achieving such standards is a function of both specification of rules and procedures as well as informal communication and use of ad hoc task forces that involve relevant groups. Rules and procedures help to define and handle many problems, but because of the complexity and uncertainty of much professional work, informal and ad hoc mechanisms must also be used to deal with nonroutine problems. Examples include emergency cases; patients with multiple diagnoses; elderly patients with chronic care needs that cut across many specialties and even organizations; and patients with illnesses involving complicated moral, legal, economic, or ethical issues.

Involving professionals in the development of standards, norms, rules, policies, and practices is essential. Studies indicate that such involvement is associated with greater professional satisfaction and can play an important role in staff retention. Increasingly, professionals want to be involved not only in deciding what will have an immediate impact on their work but also in some of the larger organizational issues that may affect their future practice. Examples include the organization's relationship with third-party payers, regulators, and competitors. Thus there exists growing physician involvement in management and governance issues and new forms of joint venture relationships (also see Chapters 9 and 11) (Alexander, Morrisey, & Shortell, 1986; Barr & Steinberg, 1983; Robinson, 1999; Shortell, Morrisey, & Conrad, 1985).

In sum, existing studies suggest that evaluating and coordinating professional work is facilitated by high standards and clear expectations, specified rules and procedures combined with job autonomy, flexibility in coordinating work, and a high degree of professional involvement in decision making.

These practices place a premium on the manager's conflict management (see Chapter 5), communication and coordination (see Chapter 8), and organization design skills (see Chapters 6, 7, 9, and 10).

Evaluating Nonprofessional Work: The Bureaucratic Model

Comparing observed performance values with established standards is also seldom a simple mechanical process but one requiring experience and judgment. It is to accommodate these skills that the appraisal function is typically assigned to a supervisor—a person selected on the basis of seniority or merit and located close to the work site. Experience and proximity allow these individuals to detect nuances in performers' activities and to take into account special circumstances that affect performance values and their associated outcomes. Many of the complaints and problems associated with supervisor-worker relations may be attributed to disagreements over performance appraisal and may signify both the complexities and the sensitivities associated with this process. In nursing homes, research shows that who does performance evaluation can make a difference. Nurse aide turnover is higher in nursing homes in which the director of nursing, as opposed to the floor charge nurse, writes performance evaluations.

In the modern health care organization, these tasks of evaluating performance—particularly in the context of maximizing organizational performance—are made more difficult by the complexity of occupations and people involved in providing care. More and more, in recognition of the different skills and perspectives necessary to perform such tasks, interdisciplinary teams rather than individuals become the basic accountability unit within the organization, necessitating new means for evaluating work and improving the process. This task becomes even more difficult as stakeholders outside the traditional provider setting expand their roles and responsibilities in providing information about the effectiveness of technologies used in health care (see In Practice, p. 432).

DEBATE TIME 13.1   What Do You Think?

An article in the *Journal of the American Medical Association (JAMA)* described a study of serious medical "missteps" based on anonymous responses from 114 interns and residents regarding their own most significant errors in the previous year. The main categories of serious missteps and examples of each are indicated below.

It is possible that the problems may *not* have been due to individual error but rather to underlying processes and systems involved in patient diagnosis and treatment. For each category of missteps, develop an argument that the error was due to problems in the underlying process rather than from the individual physician's mistake.

Example	Outcome*
ERRORS IN DIAGNOSIS—38 Cases (33%)	
Failed to diagnose bowel obstruction in patient with fluid buildup in abdomen	Death
Failed to examine and diagnose fracture in crack cocaine user	Delayed treatment
EVALUATION AND TREATMENT—24 cases (21%)	
Treated malignant hypertension on the ward instead of in an intensive care unit	Stroke
Incompletely cleaned a diabetic foot ulcer	Amputation
PRESCRIBING AND DOSING—33 Cases (29%)	
Did not read syringe and gave 50 times the correct dose of a thyroid drug	None apparent
Inadvertently stopped asthma medication at time of hospitalization	Respiratory failure
PROCEDURAL COMPLICATIONS—13 Cases (11%)	
Removed pulmonary artery catheter with the balloon inflated	Small amount of bleeding
Placed intravenous line in main vein without a follow-up X-ray	Fatal lung collapse
FAULTY COMMUNICATIONS—6 Cases (5%)	
Failed to put do-not-resuscitate order in chart and failed to inform spouse	Resuscitation performed against patient's wishes
Failed to obtain consent before placing intravenous line in main vein	Fatal complication after procedure

*Cause and effect cannot be determined.

Source: Adapted from Wu, A.W., Folkman S., McPhee S.J., and Lo, B. Do house officers learn from their mistakes? *JAMA*, 265(16):2090. Copyright 1991, American Medical Association.

IN PRACTICE   Applying Root Cause Analysis To Improve Health Care

In the factories of Toyota Motor Corp., any worker who spots a serious problem can pull a cord and stop the assembly line. Richard Shannon, chairman of medicine at Allegheny General Hospital in Pittsburgh, is applying the Toyota technique to an intensive-care unit here.

Just the other day, a nurse brought the medical "production line" to a halt. Candice Bena thought a 76-year-old patient needed a new intravenous line but couldn't get the radiology department to install one immediately. Fearing the patient would develop an infection, the nurse phoned Dr. Shannon.

That was the equivalent of pulling "the 'andon' cord," says Dr. Shannon, using the Japanese word for "lantern." He immediately called the hospital's chairman of radiology, who within two hours installed the new IV line himself. "That's the Toyota production system. No problem should be left unsolved."

Toyota is widely considered an exemplar of what has been popularized as "lean" management. The term spans a wide variety of practices, including "mistake-proofing"—or digging for the root cause of mistakes in real time and taking countermeasures. Another is "value stream mapping," in which frontline workers map the many steps in a production process, then cut out those that customers—or patients—don't value. The auto maker . . . also helped pioneer the now-famous just-in-time approach to obtaining supplies from vendors only as they are needed in the factory.

At Allegheny General, the two intensive-care units had been averaging about 5.5 infections per 1,000 patient days, mostly blood-stream infections from catheters inserted into patients. That infection rate was a bit higher than the Pittsburgh average but a bit lower than the national average, says Dr. Shannon. Over the prior 12 months, 37 patients,

already some of the sickest people in the hospital, had 49 infections. Of those, 51% died.

Dr. Shannon and the staff in the two units—doctors, residents, nurses—applied the Toyota "root-cause analysis" system, investigating each new infection immediately. Their main conclusion: A femoral intravenous line, inserted into an artery near the groin, had a particularly high rate of infections. So the team made an all-out effort to replace these lines with less-risky ones in the arm or near the collarbone. Dr. Shannon, who oversees the two units, gave the directive to keep femoral lines to an absolute minimum.

It's good medicine, he says. . . . The result: a 90% drop in the number of infections after just 90 days of using the new procedures.

It's also good business: By reducing infections, the new procedures have saved almost $500,000 a year in intensive-care-unit costs. "It's not in my interest to be putting in lines all day long," says Paul Kiproff, chairman of radiology. But with infections down, "this is clearly advantageous."

Similar things are happening in at least a dozen hospitals across the country. The Toyota system emphasizes the smoothest possible flow of work—accomplished by, say, mapping out work processes and eliminating unnecessary steps, and using teamwork to identify and fix problems as soon as they crop up. Hospitals are using the tactics to reduce patient waiting times, slash wheelchair inventories, prepare operating rooms faster and move patients through a hospital stay or doctor visit quickly, seamlessly and error free.

Employers are looking at steep increases in health care costs and saying, "Hey, guys, this is broken. You really have to fix it," says John Toussaint, chief executive of ThedaCare Inc., a three-hospital nonprofit group in Appleton, Wisconsin. ThedaCare's board "demands this of me," Mr. Toussaint says. Board members include executives of Kimberly-Clark Corp., Bemis Co. and Banta Corp., companies that pay the tab for employees treated by ThedaCare hospitals. ThedaCare recently hired consultants steeped in the Toyota system after seeing their results at a nearby snowblower maker.

Hospitals aren't factories, though. Doctors, nurses, and other hospital staffers don't think of themselves as assembly-line workers or their patients as anything resembling a Camry under construction. Sarah Klahsen, a hospital manager who helped teach the Toyota techniques at Pella Regional Health Center, says employees were initially skeptical of the experts who soon would arrive from the window company. "I think there's a fear, a sense that, 'We save lives. What do you do?'" says Ms. Klahsen.

To ease the potential culture clash, many hospitals play down the Toyota name. But the conflict between the culture of efficiency and the culture of caring is never far from the surface.

One recent afternoon, eight ThedaCare employees struggled to cut the 14 days it takes to send bills for certain surgeries to insurers. They mapped every step in the process, and saw an obvious bottleneck: A medical technician held onto patient-billing records until making a call to the discharged patient to check on post-surgical health. Skipping that step would save 72 hours.

When Jean Muhowski, the surgery-department manager, met with a group of managers and presented a plan to drop the follow-up call, many protested. "My wife had surgery five times and appreciated those calls," said public-affairs manager John Gillespie. So Ms. Muhowski and her team surveyed 40 patients, and discovered more than half did value the call.

The eventual compromise: Upon discharge, patients are offered the option of a follow-up call. And the staffers who call get summary sheets, not actual patient records, so bills can go to insurers more quickly.

Source: Adapted from Wysocki, Jr., B. (2004, April 9). Industrial strength: To fix health care, hospitals take tips from factory floor; Adopting Toyota techniques can cut costs, wait times; Ferreting out an infection; What Paul O'Neill's been up to. *Wall Street Journal* (Eastern edition).

The Impact of Evaluation on All Types of Performers

All attempts to evaluate a performance may be expected to have effects on that performance. The setting of standards, the selection of indicators, the sampling of performance, and the comparison of performances with standards all affect the performance itself (Dornbusch & Scott, 1975). The primary purpose of any evaluation system is to exert influence on the performance of participants—if not the performance immediately under review, then subsequent ones. But equally important and less obvious are the unintended effects of performance evaluation. People basically prefer to receive a good evaluation; therefore, workers will seek to improve their evaluation irrespective of whether that change actually improves the quality of their performance. Ideally, of course, the evaluations made are accurate and appropriate; but if not, *reactivity* to the performance criteria can result in an appearance of improvement in performance rather than motivating the worker to seek true changes in quality. Or, as W. Richard Scott once paraphrased an old song, "When you're not near the goal that you love, you love the goal that you're near."

These biasing or diverting effects occur because it is often difficult or overly costly to devise evaluation systems and indicators that accurately reflect the complexity of desired outcomes to which the performance is addressed. Thus, although examinations are developed to test learning, their repeated use is likely to influence what is taught or, more importantly, what is learned. And if diagnostic thoroughness is signified by the number of laboratory tests ordered, then the number of tests ordered may far exceed the number required by the patient's medical condition. In particular, hard measures—measures that are specific, capable of being quantified, and easy to observe—tend to drive out soft measures.

Nonetheless, there is some evidence that physicians will respond to evaluations by peers for its own sake. For example, physicians have responded to internally imposed peer review (Wennberg, Blowers, Parker, & Gittelsohn, 1977). Dyck and his colleagues (1977) found that rates of healthy tissue removal associated with appendectomy dropped significantly when criteria about "acceptable" rates were made explicit, absent any need to reprimand physicians. However, physicians knew that peers were going to monitor their rates in the future with undetermined consequences. Physicians have also responded by dropping the rate of prescribing drugs when a computerized system with the capability to monitor prescriptions was introduced, even though the system was intended for another purpose (Cohen, Flood, Himmelberger, Mangini, & Moore, 1980).

Finally, the work by the Maine Medical Foundation (MMF) and the Minnesota Clinical Comparison and Assessment Project and the Center for the Evaluative Clinical Sciences at Dartmouth provides many examples of how a study group of physicians, when given feedback on utilization with evidence that some physicians were unusually high, can result in a reduction of the outlier rates over time (Borbas, Stump, Dedecker, et al., 1990; Keeler, Chapin, & Soule, 1990; Keeler, Soule, Wennberg, & Hanley, 1990; Nelson et al., 2002). However, there is some evidence that suggests that physician profiles showing the relative use rates of services, when divorced of any apparent consequences, appear to have no effect on behavior (Wones, 1987).

Two Models for Changing Performance

Quality Assurance. **Quality assurance (QA)** refers to "the formal and systematic exercise of identifying problems in medical care delivery, designing activities to overcome these problems, and carrying out follow-up steps to ensure that no new problems have been introduced and that corrective actions have been effective" (Brook & Lohr, 1985). In reviewing 25 years of QA activities, Williamson (1988) noted agreement on five principles for assuring quality.

- Successful QA requires individual and organizational commitment to develop the values and incentives of excellence.

- Responsibility for excellence must be decentralized so that the professionals and staff responsible for the care have the power to review and implement necessary changes.

- At the same time, QA requires an approach that is comprehensive of all the groups in the hospital that can affect quality, including education, administration, and support services.

- At the same time, QA is best targeted toward prioritized, specific needs rather than being based on a shotgun approach to identifying problems.

- QA itself should be continuously monitored for its effectiveness and adaptiveness to current organizational needs to ensure that its contributions outweigh its costs.

The evidence that QA has been successful in changing physician's behavior is scant (Jessee, 1984; Luke, Krueger, & Modrow, 1983; Mittman & Siv, 1992). As Luke, Krueger, and Modrow (1983) remarked, "It is clear that quality assurance has until now been both expensive and, in general, marginally effective." The general conclusion is that the primary problem has been a failure to focus on the means to secure changes in organizations or physicians rather than on the techniques to assess quality (Fifer, 1983; Jessee, 1984; Shanahan, 1983; Wyszewianski, 1988). In reviewing the evidence on changing physician's behavior and assuring quality, Eisenberg (1986) discusses the importance of an environment conducive to high quality, including strong professional leadership and diffusion of up-to-date innovations in medicine as well as face-to-face interactions with colleagues—not necessarily found in most QA activities. These arguments have been supported by work based on QA in a primary care setting (Kind, Fowles, & McCoy, 1987; McCoy, Kind, Fowles, & Schned, 1987).

Many are calling for greater integration and coordination of QA activities as well. For example, a study by the U.S. General Accounting Office found several reasons for concern about the systems for monitoring quality in Medicare. There is little evidence of the effectiveness of the review methods being used; there is poor coordination across groups reviewing quality with little or no sharing of information; the data used are of questionable accuracy and generalizability; and there are inadequate strategies for developing the methods and knowledge needed to correct the situation and inadequate resources being allocated to redress these concerns (Medicare, GAO 1988).

While most have called for increased coordination and integration of these activities as well as standardization of the procedures, others have warned of information overload, which overwhelms the system and stymies action and largely symbolic evaluations—going through the motions of QA—which can attend too centralized and extensive of reviews. To solve these problems, many propose to increase coordination and integration of these activities as well as standardize the procedures. Others caution against too much information gathering, which can overload the system and stymy action or create largely symbolic evaluations—going through the motions without impacting the substance (Fifer, 1983; Heatherington, 1982; Rosen & Feigin, 1982; Shanahan, 1983; Vuori, 1980).

Quality Improvement. Quality improvement is the promise put forward to address the problems—real and imagined—in quality assurance in Ameri-can health care delivery. **Quality improvement (QI)** is a management philosophy to improve the level of performance of key processes in the organization. In particular, this approach insists that "quality is an organizational problem" (see Debate Time 13.1, p. 435), that is, that variation in quality is as much due to the way in which care is organized and coordinated as it is to the competence of the individual caregivers (Kimberly & Minvielle, 2003, p. 205). It was developed originally by several industrial quality experts and applied successfully in a variety of industries worldwide (Crosby, 1979; Deming, 1986; Juran, 1988). The principles espoused by these experts differ little but have helped spawn several terms used interchangeably with QI: *total quality management (TQM), industrial quality control,* and *continuous quality improvement (CQI).* Key philosophical concepts include:

- Productive work involves processes. Most work implies a chain of processes whereby each worker receives inputs from suppliers (internal or external to the organization), adds value, and then passes it on to the customers, who are defined to include everyone internal or external who receives the product or service of the worker.

- The customer is central to every process. Processes are improved to meet the customer's needs reliably and efficiently.

- There are two ways to improve quality: eliminate defects in the process and add features that meet customers' needs or preferences better.

- The main source of quality defects is problems in the process. Workers basically want to and succeed in carrying out the process correctly. The problems derive from the process being wrong.

- Quality defects are costly in terms of internal losses by lowered productivity and efficiency, increased requirements for inspection and monitoring, and dissatisfied customers. Preventing defects in the process by careful planning saves resources.

- Focus on the most important processes to improve. Use statistical thinking and tools to identify desired performance levels, measure current performance, interpret it, and take action when necessary.

- Involve every worker in QI. Use new structures such as teams and quality councils to advise and plan QI strategies.

- Set high standards for performance; go for being the best.

Benchmarking is the process of establishing operating targets based on the leading performance standards for the industry or what the Japanese call *dantotsu*, the "best of the best." But it should not simply be a metric—determining a standard against which to measure performance; benchmarking is a philosophy to guide the process of proactive, structured practices needed to achieve excellence. Camp (1989) describes this process in four steps.

1. **Know your operation.** That is, assess your organizational strengths and weaknesses.

2. **Know the industry leaders** or your direct competitors.

3. **Incorporate the best.** Don't hesitate to copy or modify, but be sure you start with the best.

4. **Gain superiority.**

An example of this philosophy applied to a clinical situation in a hospital is illustrated in the case of Allegheny General Hospital (see In Practice, p. 436).

The philosophical approach of QI in some senses is similar to that of such groups as the MMF (Keeler, Kahn, Draper, et al., 1990). Both start with the premise that wide variation in practice indicates that something is amiss—not all rates can be right, even if one doesn't know which rate is right. But the two part company in their philosophical approaches to which rate is right—in the sense of being desirable. The MMF approach targets the outliers (usually high utilization) with the view that outlying providers should alter their performance to look more like the typical performance of their peers. All others are okay as is. The QI approach, in contrast, argues that the outliers on the side of good quality should become the benchmark against which everyone else should strive—to try to be the best, not typical.

The evidence that QI will help improve performance in health care comes mostly from other industries since its application is so new to the health industry. Many groups have turned to QI, and accreditation bodies such as the Joint Commission of Healthcare Organizations has revised its accreditation rules to foster this approach (Roberts, 1992). Berwick, Godfrey, and Roessner (1991) report on demonstrations carrying out QI in 21 health care organizations including hospitals, group practices, and HMOs. While some organizations did not complete their reports and few tackled clinical quality of care issues, most felt that they had made significant progress. The authors (Berwick, Godfrey, & Roessner, 1991, p. 25) conclude:

> The evidence that quality management can help in manufacturing and business processes is overwhelming, and it is a very safe bet that the analogous processes in health care (billing, information transfer, equipment maintenance, and the like) stand to gain as much. . . . The same goes for *service* processes, like making appointments, providing telephone access, and moving patients efficiently from place to place. . . . It requires a little more imagination to see how quality management can help technical medical care . . . yet these areas still await complete exploration.

A study of Pennsylvania nursing homes indicates that quality improvement adopters, when compared with facilities that practice only quality assurance, are more likely to report improvements in the quality of resident care and in employee relationships resulting from their quality monitoring program. In addition, nursing home quality improvement adopters report being more satisfied with their quality control program and are more likely to report reductions in mortality and infection rates, reduction in food delivery times, and reduction in employee absenteeism.

In a study of adoption of quality improvement techniques in hospitals, Westphal, Gulati, and Shortell (1997) found that early adopters reformed programs to suit their own needs, but later adopters took on programs that had become normative. They found that only those who customized programs gained performance efficiencies from their introduction, though later adopters gained legitimacy even if no efficiencies resulted.

In the process of implementing QI, a balance between the basic components—implementing the technique, establishing the culture, and planning appropriate strategy—needs to be maintained to be effective (Berwick, 1991). Sometimes proponents try to implement only one component, such as data gathering and problem solving by the interested parties. But evidence from other industries suggests that the package, to be successful, requires implementation of all features. Based on the experiences with QI at the Henry Ford Health System, Sahney (1992) identified several major barriers to successful implementation and urged preventive or corrective attention be paid by managers.

- Middle management is unsure of its role and lets teams tackle insignificant processes or complex problems with insufficient support.

- The pace of improvement is often glacially slow as people brainstorm and flounder on how to proceed. Feedback and rewards for time invested are insufficient.

- Changing the culture is difficult, and members can lose faith in the process.

- Evangelistic devotion to QI can block free discussion and inventive solutions. Likewise, cynical use of QI can divert resources and energy with no real benefit to the organization as a whole.

- Time availability to carry out QI must be sufficient at all levels, including senior and middle management.

- Results of QI, if not shared broadly internally to the organization, are unknown beyond the few people involved.

A basic premise of QI is that every process has variation in how well it produces a service or product. In order to reduce the variation, the first step involves a careful and information-driven analysis of what can cause a failure of the process, with what frequency such problems occur, and the extent to which problems vary over time. Understanding the process and developing and implementing corrective action by a group process requires being able to communicate the information effectively. Simple and direct statistical tools such as histograms, bar charts, and scattergrams help ensure that anyone throughout the organization can understand and use them. In addition, some tools have been developed specifically to help QI teams, such as flowcharts, Pareto diagrams, and control charts (Batalden & Buchanan, 1989; Ishikawa, 1985; Stewart, 1986; Wheeler & Chambers, 1987). They serve multiple purposes in the process of improving quality: gathering information about processes and probable causes of problems, displaying information and testing theories, and monitoring and controlling a process after a remedy has been applied (Plsek, 1991; Plsek, Onnias, & Early, 1989). One such tool, the cause-and-effect diagram, is used to condense a large array of information about processes in an organized way. The ultimate effect (e.g., an adverse event such as medication errors) is at the end of the arrow. Each major antecedent cause is represented by a branch attached to the arrow. Figure 13.1 is a cause-and-effect diagram portraying the overall process of producing health services. (See Debate Time 13.2. p. 443)

Finally, both advocates and critics of QI note the special challenges presented by involving professionals—particularly physicians—in QI systems to evaluate clinical processes. Combining general lessons about how to implement innovations in organizations with the special requirements of professionals, Kaluzny, McLaughlin, and Kibbe (1992) advise taking several precautions when designing QI strategy in health care organizations.

- Use physicians' time wisely. Use them as consultants or on subteams that focus on clinical issues needing their expertise. Recognize that their involvement will be episodic and related to specific interests and topics.

- Peak physicians' interests. Capitalize on physicians who are most interested in QI, nurture their involvement, and focus on issues that make them curious.

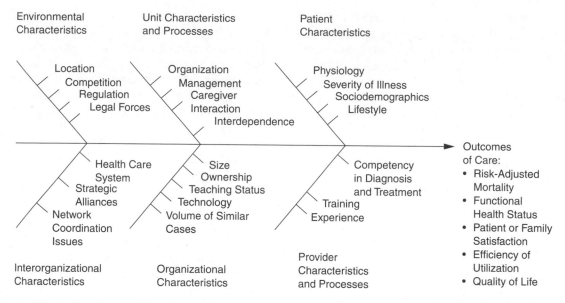

Figure 13.1. Cause-and-Effect Diagram for Continuous Improvement in Health Services Organizations

- Empower physicians' participation. Involve them early on in the process.

- Respect professional values. Avoid statistics and reviews that threaten physicians' competency. Be flexible. Balance the needs for autonomy with the requirements of QI initiatives.

- Diagnose and capitalize on which of the four stages of adoption specific units and groups have reached: recognizing a problem in need of a solution, identifying QI as a valued solution, implementing QI strategies related to the problem, or institutionalizing QI thinking and techniques into everyday clinical practice.

THE MANAGER'S ROLE IN CREATING HIGH-PERFORMANCE HEALTH CARE ORGANIZATIONS

The problems in defining and measuring performance, which occur in all organizations, are partic-ularly challenging for health care organizations. This is because, as noted in Chapter 1, the product of health care organizations is frequently difficult to define and measure. In addition, many of the activities that influence the performance of health care organizations are not directly controllable by managers but rather are under the direction of physicians and other health care professionals. Add to this the environmental forces of inflation, regulation, competition, new technology, and changing consumer preferences, and it is no wonder that some have referred to the health care executive's job as attempting to steer a wayward bus down a hill in which physicians control the brakes, and other groups (trustees, third-party payers, etc.) have their foot on the accelerator. Thus it is tempting to wave the white flag and conclude that there is relatively little that managers can do to define, measure, or influence performance. Nothing could be further from the truth.

It is precisely because the task of defining, measuring, and influencing performance is so difficult that management can play a key role. As discussed in Chapters 2 and 4, defining the organization's core values and reasons for being and translating

---

✤ DEBATE TIME 13.2 What Do You Think?

Figure 13.1 provides a framework for thinking about quality improvement in health services organizations. Some people believe that the greatest improvement opportunities lie with increasing clinicians' competence and skills. Others believe greater improvement results from changes in the organization and management of patient care units. Still others believe that the quality of care is largely a function of the availability of sophisticated technology or the degree of teaching activity going on. What do you think? Where would you place the most emphasis? What factors, conditions, or variables influence your decision?

---

these into operational reality lies at the heart of **transformational leadership**. Transformational leaders think about performance in terms of controllable and noncontrollable factors and constantly work to convert uncontrollable factors into factors that can be controlled. Figure 13.2 provides a continuum of such factors.

As shown, events such as natural disasters, international relations, and national economic policy are relatively uncontrollable by health care executives. In contrast, issues concerning the organization's wage and salary administration, marketing plans, and patient-care policies and practices are, for the most part, directly controllable by executives. In between are factors involving intermediate degrees of control. These include factors largely internal such as the organization's mission and culture, labor mix, and organization design as well as external factors such as system consolidation, growth, and third-party payment trends on the one hand and external regulation, competition, and new technological developments on the other.

A major point of Figure 13.2 is that more effective managers not only focus on variables on the right side of the page that are most directly controllable but also attempt to extend their influence over factors moving to the left, involving health industry trends and external regulatory, competitive, technological, and legal forces. They do this by refusing to accept these forces as givens and viewing them instead as opportunities for expanding their organization's mission and potential effectiveness. For example, many health care companies have developed, on their own or in joint ventures with insurance companies, the ability to provide health insurance services and other third-party financing, which can channel more patients into their delivery system. Many hospitals are changing their size by reducing in-patient bed capacity and converting formerly unused capacity to long-term-care beds or outpatient programs. Nursing homes are rapidly expanding into subacute and rehabilitation services in response to the growth in Medicare managed care.

Other organizations have gained control over new technological developments through linkages with medical schools and research centers and through investment in biomedical and biological product companies. In similar fashion, these organizations are proactive in shaping consumer preferences and tastes through market research and new product-development strategies rather than merely reacting to changes in consumer preferences.

A recent major report from the Institute of Medicine (IOM), a branch of the National Academy of Sciences, exposed the high prevalence and enormous financial and health consequences of clinical errors in health care (IOM, 2001). This problem is illustrated in the opening scenario. In subsequent attempts to prevent and correct such safety problems, health care has borrowed and adapted quality control concepts and techniques from systems engineering and models such as airline safety and

Relatively
Uncontrollable

Relatively
Controllable

Natural Disasters	Health Care System	Consolidation	Organizational Mission	Wage and Salary
International Relations	External Regulation	System Growth	and Culture	Administration
National Economic Policy	and Accreditation	Organization Size	Labor Mix	Capital Investment
(e.g., Inflation	New Technological	Ownership Status	Human Resources	Strategy
Unemployment)	Developments	Third-Party Payment	Development	Financial Goals
Population Demographics	Competition	Trends	New Product or New	Marketing Plans
(e.g., Changing Age	Physician Surplus or	Teaching Affiliation	Market Development	Patient Care Policies
Mix of the Population)	Shortage	Medical Staff	Vertical and Horizontal	and Practices
Stock Market	Nurse Surplus or	Organization and	Integration (e.g.,	Problem Identification
Social Problems	Shortage	Characteristics	Acquisitions, Alternative	and Management
(e.g., Riots)	New Legal	Purchaser Demands	Delivery System	Conflict Management
Immigration Patterns	Developments	for Preferential	Development)	Practices
	Societal Preferences	Conditions	Organization Design	QA Practices and
	and Tastes		(e.g., Coordination,	Policies
			Centralization of	
			Decision Making)	

Figure 13.2. Factors Affecting Health Care Organizational Performance Arranged on a Continuum of the Degree to Which Managers Can Exert Control

controls for pilots (Ferraco & Spath, 2000; Hart & Hart, 2002; Nelson et al., 2002; Thomas & Helmreich, 2002). These techniques emphasize the examination of processes in detail to uncover the sources for error and reduce variation in error rates.

In the context of trying to gain control over processes and eliminate sources of errors, some have cautioned that reducing variation in errors is not the only goal in health care (so is *improving* quality by reducing the overall rate of error) and that not all surprises are dysfunctional and undesirable. McDaniel, Jordan, and Fleeman (2003) propose borrowing principles from "complexity science" so as to also foster creativity and learning in health care organizations. They note that "status quo" is not a realistic nor desirable goal in complex, dynamic settings such as health care and a healthy balance between control and creativity is needed.

These attempts to broaden the influence base involve macropolitical strategies of networking, coalition building, and joint venturing (see Chapters 9–11 for related discussions). They involve actively managing the environment and not merely managing one's own organization. Priorities must be set, and tradeoffs must be made. Nonetheless, all stakeholders

would agree that the organization needs to obtain necessary resources (people, money, legitimacy) for its continued existence; to coordinate, manage, and integrate these resources in providing desired services and products; and to achieve a reasonable degree of goal attainment in those areas that are deemed most important. Thus the discussion and guidelines that follow are organized around the issues of acquiring necessary resources, making wise performance trade-offs, and managing a high-performance health care organization for the twenty-first century.

Resource Acquisition

The way in which health care organizations obtain resources has changed radically in the past few years. Philanthropy has declined to the point where it is no longer a major source of support, and much greater emphasis is given to the debt and, for investor-owned organizations, equity markets. At the same time, mergers, consolidations, affiliations, and opportunities to join multihospital systems have enabled many hospitals to obtain resources otherwise not available (Ermann & Gabel, 1984). As a result, it has become increasingly important for health care organizations to have positive operating margins and strong balance sheets regardless of whether they are investor owned or not-for-profit. Overall, **resource acquisition** needs to be more carefully targeted than in the past to conform with the organization's overall strategic plan (see Chapter 14). New areas for strategic growth include same-day surgery, satellite clinics, home health care, diagnostic imaging, ambulatory alcoholism and psychiatric care, health promotion, sports medicine, and related ventures.

The forces just listed have meant a different role in the resource acquisition process for the organization's board of directors. Previously, effective health care organizations selected board members primarily for their ability to provide and maintain rapport with community groups as a linkage to philanthropic sources; today's boards require greater experience and expertise in marketing, finance, risk taking, and entrepreneurship. Taking hospitals as an example, bridges to the community and other links to the external environment are still important, but the linkage requires board members to possess expertise and experience to help hospitals make the transition from acute care inpatient institutions to more diversified health care organizations emphasizing outpatient and primary care. The emphasis shifts from board members being the stewards of the hospital's assets to becoming active builders of a more diversified resource base. This is a particular challenge for rural, inner-city, public, and some university teaching hospitals. These groups face a variety of resource acquisition issues: low occupancy and financial instability (e.g., many rural hospitals), a high percentage of Medicaid and medically indigent patients (e.g., many inner-city and public hospitals), and diminished revenues from state governments coupled with increased competition from surrounding community hospitals (e.g., many teaching hospitals affiliated with state medical schools).

The issues of resource acquisition is particularly important in competitive environments. A study focused on hospitals found that organizations in competitive environments whose boards are entrepreneurial tend to be more successful in obtaining needed resources (money, patients, and staff) than those with boards not so oriented (Barrett & Windham, 1984). This study also suggests that in any environment, whether competitive or noncompetitive, effectiveness in obtaining resources is increased when there is greater congruence of interests between the CEO and the board chairperson.

Failure of a given organization to attract sufficient resources on its own may result in corporate reorganization, consolidation, merger, affiliation membership, or multihospital system membership. With the exception of internal corporate reorganization, all of these represent to varying degrees a networking strategy designed to attract capital, strengthen political clout, create possible economies of scale, compete for managed care contracts, and perhaps most importantly, achieve integration of clinical services. Failure to successfully negotiate such relationships is likely to result in suboptimal performance and possible closure.

A second important resource acquisition issue involves the ability to recruit and retain physicians, nurses, and related professional staff, which in turn can help attract patients. The existing shortage of primary care physicians represents a major new challenge not only to acquire such staff but potentially to restructure and retrain current staff to meet these needs. To meet this challenge, recruitment efforts need to be carefully targeted. Restructuring efforts may involve nurses playing an even greater role in delivering primary care or some specialists retraining to provide general care. Such restructuring of the professional staff, to be successful, needs to be extra sensitive to issues of control and motivation in professional work (see Chapters 3–5).

Managing Trade-offs

Health care organizations are confronting an increasingly competitive environment in which the public will hold managers accountable not only for the cost of care but for the quality of care provided within their institutions. A natural reaction to this type of demand is to tighten existing controls, define lines of authority, clarify role definitions, and implement a range of performance-evaluation systems. These actions may symbolically fulfill the expectations of those within and outside the organization that somebody is finally taking control. In reality, however, this approach may camouflage serious problems.

What is really needed is a shift in paradigms away from the mechanical model of control based on surveillance, inspection, and discipline to a new model of commitment and a cycle of continuous improvement as previously discussed. Each department in the organization determines who its customers are and what they want. The department then develops systems to meet the needs of its constituent groups and to monitor performance, assuring continuous improvement in the quality of services provided.

Many observers believe that there are inherent trade-offs between efficiency and effectiveness—between containing costs and providing high-quality care. It is felt that attempts to become more efficient and productive will be made at the expense of quality. For example, patients may be discharged too soon, they may receive fewer services, the quality of the services they receive may be reduced, and hospitals may not keep up with the latest technology advances to provide state-of-the-art care. All of these behaviors may indeed erode the quality of care provided as perceived by one group or another.

But a contrasting view may also be taken. Specifically, it is possible that attempts to become more productive and efficient may be associated with improvements in quality. For example, productivity improvements that reduce length of stay may facilitate patient discharge to more appropriate outpatient settings or home environments, which may facilitate the healing process and reduce patients' susceptibility to hospital-acquired infections and illnesses. Fewer tests and procedures reduce the risk of possible side effects and mistakes. It also requires that caregivers be better diagnosticians and provide more focused treatment. Given the lack of evidence supporting strong relationships between process and outcomes of care, it is uncertain how changes in the process of care may affect outcomes, al-

though it is recognized that there are thresholds beyond which outcomes may not improve and may, indeed, even deteriorate. Reductions in the quality of inputs involving patient-care amenities may reduce patient satisfaction but are not likely to affect mortality or functional health status measures. Finally, the fact that not all hospitals will be able to have state-of-the-art technology may actually improve quality by channeling patients to selected high-tech hospitals where more qualified professionals exist to use the technology appropriately and where sufficient volume of cases exist to promote better patient outcomes (Flood et al., 1984; Luft, 1981; Shortell & LoGerfo, 1981).

Which of the scenarios described above is most likely to occur depends on a number of key variables. It would appear that the greatest potential for diminished quality exists in health care organizations that are financially stressed, serve a relatively high percentage of uninsured patients, operate in highly competitive markets, have difficulty recruiting highly qualified staff, and serve a patient population in which there is inadequate home and social support networks.

It is clear that the trade-off issue will not go away. It places health care managers squarely in the center of the tension between those who view health care primarily as an economic good and those who view it primarily as a social good.

It is also important to recognize that improving the performance of individual health care organizations is not the same as improving an individual's performance or the overall ability of health care systems and communities to deliver cost-effective services. Nonetheless, as the delivery of health care becomes more consolidated both horizontally and vertically, improvements in individual organizational performance are likely to have ripple effects. Conversely, failure to improve performance has pervasive negative effects throughout the system. Thus a major challenge for health care managers in the future lies not only in improving individual organizational performance but in improving the performance of networks, coalitions, affiliations, and systems. In the process, it will be important to remember that there is something wrong with every available measure of performance. Thus effective managers will use many indicators to assess individual, group, organizational, and network performance.

Systemic Change

Managers of individual health care organizations can do much to improve the effectiveness of health care but, on their own, they will not be able to achieve the level of quality for which we all aspire. The sobering report on errors in health care from the Institute of Medicine (2001) concludes that:

> Redesign is not aimed only at the health care organizations and professionals that comprise the delivery system. Change is also required in the structures and processes of the environment in which those

organizations and professionals function. Such change includes setting national priorities for improvement, creating better methods for disseminating and applying knowledge to practice, fostering the use of information technology in clinical care, creating payment policies that encourage innovation and reward improvement in performance, and enhancing educational programs to strengthen the health care workforce.

Organizations are bit players in the wider system of health care. Their participants must not only pursue improvements within their own boundaries but also contribute to change efforts underway at regional, state and national levels if progress is to take place and be sustained (Scott, Ruef, Medel, & Caronna, 2000).

MANAGERIAL GUIDELINES

Maintaining and Improving Quality of Care

1. Develop a participative, team-oriented organizational culture that encourages input from professionals and other workers from all levels of the organization.
2. Establish high standards that appeal to professional standards. Link professional values and goals to those of the organization.
3. Develop information systems that provide relevant, timely, and accurate data for purposes of taking corrective action and reaching ever-higher standards. Use statistical thinking and tools to identify desired performance levels, measure current performance, interpret it, and take action when necessary.
4. Look for opportunities to improve quality by detecting and preventing potential

problems in the process. Focus on the most important processes to improve.
5. Design work to make the best use of professionals' experience and expertise.
6. Develop reward systems that reinforce participation and high performance. Don't blame individuals for defects in the process.
7. Develop organizational structures that promote communication, coordination, and conflict management.
8. Actively manage the external environment to recruit the best available talent.

Evaluating Professional Work

1. Professionals working in health care organizations are largely self-motivated. Thus setting high standards consistent with professional norms of excellence promotes effectiveness. *(continues)*

MANAGERIAL GUIDELINES *(continued)*

2. Any organization requires rules and procedures. In health care organizations, the rules and procedures must be based as much on professional needs, values, and aspirations as on the needs, values, and aspirations of the organization.

3. The professional's need for autonomy must be kept paramount in all organization design decisions.

4. The special needs of professional work demand that flexible mechanisms be used to coordinate such activity.

5. Professionals want to participate in decisions that will affect the professional nature of their work.

6. Increasingly, professionals want to participate in larger issues that will affect the nature of their work in years to come.

Acquiring Resources

1. Boards of directors need to adopt more corporate forms of organization with emphasis given to strategic planning, entrepreneurial, and risk-taking activities.

2. Linkages must be formed with new types of stakeholders, including employers, business coalitions, and special-interest consumer groups.

3. Executives need to make more use of macropolitical strategies involving the negotiation of network relationships, which will form larger resource pools.

4. The effective health care organization needs to become more proactive in managing its environment in order to compete more effectively.

5. The organization needs to become adept at developing specialized market niches and initiating products and services for targeted market segments where sufficient resources exist to gain a distinctive long-run competitive advantage.

6. In order to be effective in the long run, organizations need to learn how to continuously differentiate their product or service relative to competitors.

Improving Productivity and Efficiency

1. Develop accurate, timely, and useful management information systems. Remember that all data are not useful.

2. Concentrate productivity improvement programs in large departments where big payoffs will result.

3. Consider streamlining and consolidating departments and functions.

4. Develop scheduling systems consistent with professional values. Focus on areas where quality can be maintained or even enhanced through better scheduling of staff and support resources.

5. Cross-train staff to gain greater flexibility.

6. Develop productivity-based incentives based on work activities under the control of organizational members.

7. Set high standards by establishing "best practices" in one's own organization as well as using comparisons from competitors and industry leaders.

8. Involve organizational members, particularly professionals, in the development, implementation, and monitoring of productivity and efficiency initiatives.

9. Focus energy on working smarter, not necessarily harder.

DISCUSSION QUESTIONS

1. Take the perspective of the CEO of a large group practice, which owns its own managed care health plan. Describe three major ways that you could improve the access, quality, and cost containment of health care in your organization. Critique your solutions regarding the extent to which your solution may cause other problems to surface [what kind?] and the extent to which you as the CEO should have the responsibility and power to implement these changes.

2. Using a health care organization that you know well, provide three examples each of possible structural, process, and outcome measures of effectiveness. Would you expect these measures to be highly associated? Why or why not?

3. Consider a community hospital, a major teaching hospital, and a hospital in a large for-profit system. For each, list the major constituency groups (both internal and external). Indicate what kinds of effectiveness criteria each group would be most likely to promote.

4. Hospital A and Hospital B both have as their major goal for this year the implementation of a QI program. Hospital A hired a consultant firm and sent its top managers to a program to learn how to change the corporate culture and to set up quality teams to investigate problems. They formed teams to plan strategies of meaningful QI in two specific areas: billing and use of the emergency room. Hospital B, lacking funds, tried to have study groups and use self-teaching but involved everyone from the CEO to the janitor. Which hospital do you think will succeed in implementing QI? Why?

5. Clinic Q was a large multispecialty group practice with a major emphasis on specialist care. Because they were worried about not having enough referrals for specialist care,

their major goal for the year was to set up two new branches of primary care providers. To attract primary care providers, they discovered that they had to offer salaries higher than the average salary of other physicians at the clinic. Start-up costs were also high. Using concepts such as strategic planning, effectiveness, productivity, and efficiency, discuss how to evaluate whether this expansion was a "success" for the organization.

REFERENCES

Aaronson, W. E., Zinn, J. S., & Rosko, M. D. (1994). Do for-profit and not-for-profit nursing homes behave differently? *Gerontologist, 34,* 775–786.

Aiken, L. H., Sochalski, J., & Lake, E. T. (1997). Studying outcomes of organizational change in health services. *Medicare Care, 35,* NS6–NS18.

Alexander, J. A., Morrisey, M. A., & Shortell, S. M. (1986, September). The effects of competition regulation and corporatization on hospital-physician relationships. *Journal of Health and Social Behavior, 27,* 220–235.

Alexander, J. A., & Rundall, T. G. (1985, March). Public hospitals under contract management: An assessment of operating performance. *Medical Care, 23,* 209–219.

Ancona, D., Kochan T., Scully, M., Van Maanen, J., & Westney, D. E. (1996). *Managing for the future: Organizational behavior and processes.* Cincinnati, OH: South-Western College Publishing.

Argyris, C. (1982). *Reasoning, learning, and action.* San Francisco: Jossey-Bass.

Barr, J. K., & Steinberg, M. (1983, Spring). Professional participation in organizational decision making: Physicians in HMOs. *Journal of Community Health, 8*(3), 160–173.

Barrett, D., & Windham, S. R. (1984, Fall). Hospital boards and adaptability to competitive environments. *Health Care Management Review,* 11–20.

Batalden, P. B., & Buchanan, E. D. (1989). Industry models of quality improvement. In N. Goldfield, & D. B. Nash (Eds.), *Providing quality care: The challenge to clinicians.* Philadelphia: American College of Surgeons.

Bazzoli, G. J., Chan, B., Shortell S. M., & D'Aunno, T. (2000). The financial performance of hospitals belonging to health networks and systems. *Inquiry, 37*(3), 234–252.

Bazzoli, G. J., Shortell S. M., Dubbs, N., Chan, C., & Kralovec, P. (1999). A taxonomy of health networks and systems: Bringing order of chaos. *Health Services Research, 33*(6),1683–1717.

Berle, A. A., & Means, G. C. (1932). *The modern corporation and private property.* New York: Macmillan.

Berwick, D. M. (1991, Summer). Blazing the trail of quality: The HFHS quality management process. *Frontiers of Health Services Management, 7*(4), 47–50.

Berwick, D. M., Godfrey, A. B., & Roessner, J. (1991). *Curing health care: New strategies for quality improvement.* San Francisco: Jossey-Bass.

Birkmeyer, J. D., & Dimick, J. B. (2004). Potential benefits of the new Leapfrog standards: Effect of process and outcomes measures. *Surgery, 135*(6), 569–575.

Borbas, C., Stump, M. A., Dedecker, K., et al. (1990, February). The Minnesota Clinical Comparison and Assessment Project. *Quality Review Bulletin, 16,* 87–92.

Bradford, D. L., & Cohen, A. R. (1984). *Managing for excellence.* New York: John Wiley & Sons.

Brook, R. H., & Lohr, K. N. (1985). Efficacy, effectiveness, variations and quality: Boundary-crossing research. *Medical Care, 23,* 710–722.

Burnham, J. (1941). *The managerial revolution.* New York: John Day.

Burns, J. M. (1978). *Leadership.* New York: Harper & Row.

Cameron, K., & Whetten, D. A. (1981). Perceptions of organizational effectiveness across organizational life cycles. *Administrative Science Quarterly, 26,* 525–544.

Camp, R. C. (1989). *Benchmarking: The search for industry best practices that lead to superior practices.* Milwaukee, WI: American Society for Quality Control, Quality Press.

Campbell, J. P. (1977). On the nature of organizational effectiveness. In P. S. Goodman & J. M. Pennings (Eds.), *New perspectives on organizational effectiveness.* San Francisco: Jossey-Bass.

Choi, T., Allison, R. F., & Munson, F. (1986). *Governance and management of university hospitals:* *External forces and internal processes.* Ann Arbor, MI: Health Administration Press.

Cleverly, W. O. (1981). Financial ratios: Summary indicators for management decision making. *Hospital and Health Services Administration, 26,* 26–47.

Cohen, S. N., Flood, A. B., Himmelberger, D. U., Mangini, R. J., & Moore, T. N. (1980). *Development, implementation, and evaluation of the monitoring and evaluation of drug interactions by a pharmacy oriented report system (MEDIPHOR) HS00739.* (Final Report to the National Center for Health Services Research). Springfield, VA: National Technical Information Service.

Collins, J. C. (2001). *Good to great: Why some companies make the leap—and others don't.* New York: Harper Business.

Collins, J. C., & Porras, J. I. (2003). *Built to last: Successful habits of visionary companies.* New York: Harper Business.

Connor, R. A., Feldman, R. D., Dowd, B. E., & Radcliff, T. A. (1997). Which types of hospital mergers save consumers money? *Health Affairs, 16*(6), 62–74.

Coyne, J. S. (1982, Winter). Hospital performance in multi-hospital systems: A comparative study of system and independent hospitals. *Health Services Research, 17,* 303–329.

Crosby, P. B. (1979). *Quality is free.* New York: New American Library.

Cyert, R. M., & March, J. G. (1966). *A behavioral theory of the firm.* Englewood Cliffs, NJ: Prentice-Hall.

Davies, H. T., & Rundall, T. G. (2000). Managing patient trust in managed care. *Milbank Quarterly, 78*(4), 609–624.

Deming, W. E. (1986). *Out of the crisis.* Cambridge, MA: Massachusetts Institute of Technology.

Donabedian, A. (1966). Evaluating the quality of medical care. *Milbank Memorial Fund Quarterly, 44*(2), 166–206.

Donabedian, A. (1980). *Explorations in quality assessment and monitoring, vol. 1: The definition of quality and approaches to its assessment.* Chicago: Health Administration Press.

Dornbusch, S. M., Scott, W. R., with Busching, B. C., & Laing, J. D. (1975). *Evaluation and the exercise of authority.* San Francisco: Jossey-Bass.

Dubbs, N. L., Bazzoli, G. J., Shortell, S. M., & Kralovec, P. D. (2004). Reexamining organizational configurations: An update, validation, and expansion of the taxonomy of health networks and systems. *Health Services Research, 39*(1), 207–220.

Dyck, F. J., Murphy, F. A., Murphy, J. K., Road, D. A., Boyd, M. S., et al. (1977). The effect of surveillance on the number of hysterectomies in the province of Saskatchewan. *New England Journal of Medicine, 296,* 1326–1328.

Eisenberg, J. M. (1986). *Doctors' decisions and the cost of medical care: The reasons for doctors' practice and ways to change them.* Ann Arbor, MI: Health Administration Press Perspective.

Ermann, D., & Gabel, J. (1984). "Multihospital systems: Issues and empirical findings." *Health Affairs, 18,* 585–596.

Fennell, M. L., & Alexander, J. A. (1989). Governing boards and profound organizational change in hospitals. *Medical Care Review, 46,* 157–187.

Ferraco, K., & Spath, P. L. (2000). Measuring performance of high-risk processes. In P. L. Spath (Ed.), *Error reduction in health care: A systems approach to improving patient safety.* San Francisco: Jossey-Bass, p. 17–95.

Fifer, W. R. (1983). Integrating quality assurance mechanisms. In R. D. Luke, J. C. Krueger, & R. E. Modrow (Eds.), *Organization and change in health care quality assurance.* Rockville, MD: Aspen System Corporation.

Fleming, G. V. (1981). Hospital structure and consumer satisfaction. *Health Services Research, 16,* 43–64.

Flood, A. B. (1994). The impact of organizational and managerial factors on the quality of care in health care organizations. *Medical Care Review, 51*(4), 381–428.

Flood, A. B., Bott, D. M., & Goodrick, E. (2000). The promise and pitfalls of explicitly rewarding physicians based on patient insurance. *The Journal of Ambulatory Care Management, 23*(1), 55–70.

Flood, A. B., & Fennell, M. L. (1995). Through the lenses of organizational sociology: The role of organizational theory and research in conceptualizing and examining our health care system. *Journal of Health and Social Behavior, 36,* 154–169.

Flood, A. B., Fremont, A. M., Jin, K., et al. (1998). How do HMOs achieve their savings? The effectiveness of one organization's strategies. *Health Services Research, 33*(1), 79–99.

Flood, A. B., & Scott, W. R. (1987). *Hospital structure and performance.* Baltimore: Johns Hopkins Press.

Flood, A. B., Scott, W. R., & Ewy, W. (1984, February). Does practice make perfect? Part I: The relationship between hospital volume and outcomes for select diagnostic categories. *Medical Care, 22,* 98–114.

Georgopoulos, B. S., & Mann, F. C. (1962). *The community general hospital.* New York: Macmillan.

Gillies, R., Shortell, S., & Anderson, D. (1993, Winter). Conceptualization and measuring integration: Findings from the health systems integration study. *Hospital and Health Services Administration, 38*(4), 467–489.

Haberstroh, C. J. (1965). Organization design and systems analysis. In J. G. March (Ed.), *Handbook of organizations* (p. 1182). Chicago: Rand McNally.

Hall, M. A. (1988). Institutional control of physician behavior: Legal barriers to health care cost containment. *University of Pennsylvania Law Review, 137,* 431–536.

Halm E. A., Lee, C. & Chassin, M. R. (2002). Is volume related to outcome in health care? A systematic review and methodologic critique of the literature. *Annals of Internal Medicine, 137*(6), 511–520.

Harrison, J. S., & Freeman, R. E. (1999). Stakeholders, social responsibility and performance: Empirical evidence and theoretical perspectives. *Academy of Management Journal, 42,* 479–485.

Hart, M. K., & Hart, R. F. (2002). *Statistical process control for health care.* Pacific Grove, CA: Duxbury.

Heatherington, R. W. (1982). Quality assurance and organizational effectiveness in hospitals. *Health Services Research, 17,* 185–201.

Institute of Medicine. (2001). *Crossing the quality chasm: A new health system for the 21st century.* Washington: National Academy Press.

Ishikawa, K. (1985). *What is total quality control?* Englewood Cliffs, NJ: Prentice-Hall.

Jessee, W. F. (1984). Quality assurance systems: Why aren't there any? *Quality Review Bulletin, 10,* 408–411.

Juran, J. M. (Ed.). (1988). *Juran's quality control handbook* (4th ed.). New York: McGraw-Hill.

Kaluzny, A. D. (1990, April). The role of management in quality assurance: The case of Smith vs. ACE Management Company. *Quality Review Bulletin,* 134–137.

Kaluzny, A. D., McLaughlin, C. P., & Kibbe, D. C. (1992). Continuous quality improvement in the clinical setting: Enhancing adoption. *Quality Management in Health Care, 1,* 37–44.

Kanter, R. M. (1981). Organizational performance: Recent developments in measurement. *Annual Review of Sociology, 7,* 321.

Keeler, E. B., Kahn, K. L., Draper, D. M., et al. (1990). Changes in sickness at admission following the introduction of the Prospective Payment System. *Journal of American Medical Association, 264,* 1962–1968.

Keeler, R. B., Chapin, A. M., & Soule, D. N. (1990). Informed inquiry into practice variations: The Maine Medical Assessment Foundation. *Quality Assurance in Health Care, 2,* 69–75.

Keeler, R. B., Soule, D. N., Wennberg, J. E., & Hanley, D. F. (1990). Dealing with geographic variations in the use of hospitals: The experience of the Maine Medical Assessment Foundation Orthopedic Study Group. *Journal of Bone and Joint Surgery, 72*(A), 1286–1293.

Kerr, S. (1975). On the folly of rewarding A while hoping for B. *Academy of Management Journal, 18,* 769–783.

Kimberly, J. R., & Miles, R. H. (Eds.). (1980). *The organizational life cycle.* San Francisco: Jossey-Bass.

Kimberly, J. R., & Minvielle, E. (2000). *The quality imperative: Measurement and management of quality in health care.* London: Imperial College Press.

Kimberly, J. R., & Minvielle, E. (2003). Quality as an organizational problem. In S. S. Mick & M. E. Wyttenbach (Eds.), *Advances in health care organization theory.* San Francisco: Jossey-Bass.

Kind, E. A., Fowles, J., & McCoy, C. E. (1987, September). *Effectiveness of the primary profile in changing physician practice styles.* Presented at the American Medical Review Research Center Annual Meetings, Washington, DC.

Komaroff, A. L. (1985). Quality assurance in 1984. *Medical Care, 23,* 723–738.

Landau, M. (1973). On the concept of a self-correcting organization. *Public Administration Review, 33,* 533–542.

Luft, H. S. (1981). *Health maintenance organizations: Dimensions of performance.* New York: John Wiley & Sons.

Luft, H. S., Granick, D. W., Mark, D. H., & McPhee, S. J. (Eds.). (1990). *Hospital volume, physician volume and patient outcomes: Assessing the evidence.* Ann Arbor, MI: Health Administration Press.

Luke, R. D., Krueger, J. C., & Modrow, R. E. (1983). *Organization and change in health care quality assurance.* Rockville, MD: Aspen System Corporation.

Managing Hospital Marketing at AMI. (1984, June). Beverly Hills, CA: American Medical International.

McCoy, C. E., Kind, E. A., Fowles, J., & Schned, E. S. (1987). Measuring quality in an HMO: The primary care practice profile. In *Managing quality health care in a dynamic era* (pp. 112–117). Washington, DC: The Group Health Association of America.

McDaniel, R. R., Jordon, M. E., & Fleeman, B. F. (2003). Surprise, surprise, surprise! A complexity science view of the unexpected. *Health Care Management Review, 28*(3), 266–278.

Mechanic, D. (1998). The functions and limitations of trust in the provision of medical care. *Journal of Health Politics, Policy and Law, 23*(4), 661–686.

Medicare: Improving quality of care assessment and assurance: Report to the Chairman, Subcommittee on Health, Committee on Ways and Means, House of Representatives. (1988). (GAO/PEMD-88-10). Washington, DC: US General Accounting Office.

Menke, T. J. (1997). The effect of chain membership on hospital costs. *Health Services Research, 32*(2), 177–196.

Miller, R. H., & Luft, H. S. (1994). Managed care plan performance since 1980. *Journal of the American Medical Association, 271*(19), 1512–1519.

Mittman, B. S., & Siv, A. L. (1992). Changing provider behavior: Applying research on outcomes and effectiveness in health care. In S. M. Shortell & U. E. Reinhardt (Eds.), *Improving health policy and management.* Baxter Health Policy Review, Ann Arbor, MI: Health Administration Press.

Moss, M., & Adams, C. (1998, April 7). For Medicaid patients, doors slam closed; Langreth R. After seeing profits from the poor, some HMOs abandon them. *The Wall Street Journal* (Eastern Edition) p. B1.

Nauert, R. C. (1996). The quest for value in health care. *Journal of Health Care Finance, 22*(3), 52–61.

Nelson, E. C., Batalden P. B., Huber, T. P., Mohr, J. J., Godfrey, M. M., Headrick, L. A., & Wasson, J. H. (2002). Microsystems in health care: Part 1. Learning from high-performing front-line clinical units. *Journal on Quality Improvement, 28*(9), 472–493.

Nelson, E. C., Mohr, J. J., Batalden, P. B., & Plume, S. K. (1996). Improving health care, Part 1: The clinical value compass. *The Joint Commission Journal on Quality Improvement, 22*(4), 243–258.

Nerenz, D. R., & Zajac, B. M. (1991). *Indicators of performance for vertically integrated health systems: Final report of 1990 Ray Woodham Visiting Fellowship.* Detroit, MI: Center for Health System Studies, Henry Ford Health System.

Ohsfeldt, R. L. (1993). Contractual arrangements, financial incentives, and physician-patient relationships. In J. M. Clair & R. M. Allman (Eds.), *Sociomedical perspectives on patients' care.* Lexington, KY: University of Kentucky Press.

Pauly, M. V., Hillman, A. L., & Kerstein, J. (1990). Managing physician incentives in managed care: The role of for-profit ownership. *Medical Care, 28,* 1013–1024.

Pearson, S. D., & Raeke, L. H. (2000). Patients' trust in physicians: Many theories, few measures, and little data. *Journal of General Internal Medicine, 15*(7), 509–513.

Peters, T. K., & Waterman, R. A., Jr. (1982). *In search of excellence.* New York: Harper & Row.

Plsek, P. E. (1991). Resource B: A primer on quality improvement tools. In D. M. Berwick, A. B. Godfrey, & J. Roessner (Eds.), *Curing health care: New strategies for quality improvement.* San Francisco: Jossey-Bass.

Plsek, P. E., Onnias, A., & Early, J. F. (1989). *Quality improvement tools.* Wilton, CN: Juran Institute.

Proenca, E. J., Rosko, M. D., & Zinn, J. S. (2000). Community orientation in hospitals: An institutional and resource dependence perspective. *Health Services Research, 35*(5), 1011–1035.

Prottas, J. M. (1979). *People-processing* (p. 74). Lexington, MA: Lexington Books.

Roberts, J. S. (1992). Peer review and continuous quality improvement. In *Bridging the gap between theory and practice.* Chicago: Hospital Research and Educational Trust.

Robinson, J. C. (1999). *The corporate practice of medicine: Competition and innovation in health care.* Berkeley, CA: University of California Press.

Rosen, H. M., & Feigin, W. (1982). Medical peer review and information management: The deadend phenomenon. *Health Care Management Review, 7,* 59–66.

Rosko, M. D., Chilingerian, J. A., Zinn, J. S., & Aaronson, W. E. (1995). The effects of ownership, operating environment, and strategic choices on nursing home efficiency. *Medical Care, 33,* 1001–1021.

Sahney, V. K. (1992). Implementation, observed barriers, and management of continuous quality improvement (CQI). In *Bridging the gap between theory and practice: Exploring continuous quality improvement.* Chicago: Hospital Research and Educational Trust.

Scott, W. R. (1977). Effectiveness of organizational effectiveness studies. In P. S. Goodman, & J. M. Pennings (Eds.), *New perspectives on organizational effectiveness.* San Francisco: Jossey-Bass.

Scott, W. R. (1982). Managing professional work: Three models of control for health organizations. *Health Services Research, 17,* 213–240.

Scott, W. R. (1993). The organization of medical care services: Toward an integrated model. *Medical Care Review, 50,* 271–304.

Scott, W. R., Ruef, M., Medel, P. J., & Caronna, C. A. (2000). *Institutional change and healthcare organizations: From professional dominance to managed care.* Chicago: University Press.

Senge, P. (1990). *The fifth discipline: The art and practice of the learning organization.* New York: Free Press.

Shanahan, M. (1983). The quality assurance standard of the JCAH: A rational approach to patient care evaluation. In R. D. Luke, J. C. Krueger, & R. E. Modrow (Eds.), *Organization and change in health care quality assurance.* Rockville, MD: Aspen Systems Corporation.

Shortell, S. M. (1983). Physician involvement in hospital decision-making. In B. Gray (Ed.), *The new health care for profit: Doctors and hospitals in a competitive environment* (pp. 73–102). Washington, DC: National Academy Press, Institute of Medicine.

Shortell, S. M. (1985, July–August). High performing health care organizations. Guidelines for the pursuit of excellence. *Hospital and Health Services Administration, 30,* 7–35.

Shortell, S. M., Gillies, R. R., Anderson, D. A., et al. (1996). *Remaking health care in America: Building organized delivery systems.* San Francisco: Jossey-Bass.

Shortell, S. M., & LoGerfo, J. P. (1981, October). Hospital medical staff organization and quality of care: Results for myocardial infarction and appendectomy. *Medical Care, 19,* 1041–1055.

Shortell, S. M., Morrisey, M. A., & Conrad, D. (1985, December). Economic regulation and hospital behavior: The effects on medical staff organization and hospital-physician relationships. *Health Services Research, 20,* 597–627.

Shortell, S. M., Morrison, E. M., & Friedman, B. (1990). *Strategic choices for America's hospital: Managing change in turbulent times.* San Francisco: Jossey-Bass.

Shortell, S. M., Waters, J. M., Clarke, K. W. P., & Budetti, P. P. (1998). Physicians as double agents: Maintaining trust in an era of multiple accountabilities. *Journal of the American Medical Association, 280*(12), 1102–1108.

Shortell, S. M., Wickizer, T. M., & Wheeler, J. R. C., Jr. (1984). *Hospital-physician joint ventures: Results and lessons from a national demonstration in primary care.* Ann Arbor, MI: Health Administration Press.

Shortell, S. M., Zimmerman, J. E., Gillies, R. R. et al. (1990, May). Continuously improving patient care: Practical lessons and an assessment tool from the National ICU Study. *Quality Review Bulletin, 5,* 150–155.

Steers, R. M. (1975). Problems in the measurement of organizational effectiveness. *Administrative Science Quarterly, 20,* 546.

Stewart, W. A. (1986). *Statistical method from the viewpoint of quality control.* New York: Dover Publications.

SUPPORT: Study to Understand Prognosis, Preferences for Outcomes, Risks, and Treatment project. (1990). *Journal of Clinical Epidemiology,* 43.

Taub, D. A, Miller, D. C., Cowan, J. A., Dimick, J. B., Montie, J. E., & Wei, J. T. (2004). Impact of surgical volume on mortality and length of stay after nephrectomy. *Urology, 63*(5), 862–867.

Their, S. O., & Gelijns, A. C. (1998). Improving health: The reason performance measurement matters. *Health Affairs, 17*(4), 26–28.

Thomas, E. J., & Helmreich, R. L. (2002). Will airline safety models work in medicine? In M. M. Rosenthal & K. M. Sutcliffe, (Eds.), *Medical error: What do we know? What do we do?* San Francisco: Jossey-Bass.

Vuori, H. (1980). Optimal and logical quality: Two neglected aspects of quality of health services. *Medical Care, 18,* 975–985.

Weick, K. E. (1977). Re-punctuating the problem. In P. S. Goodman and J. M. Pennings (Eds.), *New perspectives on organizational effectiveness.* San Francisco: Jossey-Bass.

Weisman, C. S., & Nathanson, C. A. (1985, October). Professional satisfaction and client outcomes: A comparative organizational analysis. *Medical Care, 23,* 1179–1192.

Wennberg, J. E., Blowers, L., Parker, P., & Gittelsohn, A. M. (1977). Changes in tonsillectomy rates associated with feedback and review. *Pediatrics, 59,* 821–826.

Westphal, J. D., Gulati, R., & Shortell, S. M. (1997). Customization or conformity? An institutional and network perspective on the content and consequences of TQM adoption. *Administrative Science Quarterly, 42,* 366–394.

Wheeler, D. J., & Chambers, D. S. (1987). *Understanding statistical process control.* Knoxville, TN: Statistical Process Controls.

Williamson, J. M. (1988). Future policy directions for quality assurance: Lessons from the health accounting experience. *Inquiry, 25,* 67–77.

Wones, R. G. (1987). Failure of low-cost audits with feedback to reduce laboratory test utilization. *Medical Care, 25,* 78–82.

Wu, A. W., Folkman, S., McPhee, S. J., & Lo, B. (1991). Do house officers learn from their mistakes? *Journal of American Medical Association, 265*(16), 2090.

Wyszewianski, L. (1988). The emphasis is on measurement in quality assurance: Reasons and implications. *Inquiry, 25,* 424–436.

Zinn, J. S. (1994). Market competition and the quality of nursing home care. *Journal of Health Politics, Policy & Law, 19,* 555–582.

FIVE

Charting the Future

THE NATURE OF ORGANIZATIONS: FRAMEWORK FOR THE TEXT

Organizations and Managers
- Organization Theory and Health Services Management (Chapter 1)
- The Managerial Role (Chapter 2)

Need to Motivate and Lead People and Groups	Need to Operate the Technical System	Need to Position the Organization	Need to Chart the Future
by	by	by	by

Need to Motivate and Lead People and Groups

by

Satisfying Individual Needs and Values
- Motivating People (Chapter 3)

Providing Direction
- Leadership: A Framework for Thinking and Acting (Chapter 4)

Encouraging Cooperation
- Conflict Management and Negotiation (Chapter 5)

In Response to Problems of Personnel
- Commitment
- Turnover
- Apathy
- Conflict among Professionals

Need to Operate the Technical System

by

Determining Appropriate Work Groups and Design
- Groups and Teams (Chapter 6)
- Work Design (Chapter 7)

Establishing Communication and Coordination Mechanisms
- Coordination and Communication (Chapter 8)

Exertin g Influence
- Power and Politics (Chapter 9)

In Response to Problems of Technical Performance
- Productivity
- Efficiency
- Quality
- Consumer Satisfaction

Need to Position the Organization

by

Determining Appropriate Organization Design
- Organization Design (Chapter 10)

Acquiring Resources and Managing the Environment
- Managing Strategic Alliances (Chapter 11)

Managing Change and Innovation
- Organizational Innovation, Change, and Learning (Chapter 12)

Attaining Goals
- Organizational Performance: Managing for Efficiency and Effectiveness (Chapter 13)

In Response to Problems of The Environment
- Environmental Complexity and Uncertainty
- Technological and Social Change
- Competitive Forces
- Multiple Performance Demands

Need to Chart the Future

by

Managing Strategically
- Strategy Making to Health (Chapter 14)

Anticipating the Future
- Creating and Managing the Future (Chapter 15)

In Response to Problems of Survival and Growth
- Long-Run Survival
- Long-Run Performance and Growth

Organizations are components of a larger environment and are influenced by an unfolding series of events over time. Success of an organization depends upon its ability to chart the future given the events of time. The two chapters in this section highlight a number of future trends that will influence health care and various approaches to manage the organization given these trends.

Chapter 14, "Achieving Competitive Advantage: The Case for Strategy" focuses on the idea of strategic management and how the principles of strategic management can increase the success of the organization in its changing environment. Specifically, the chapter addresses the following questions:

- What is strategic management, and how does it relate to competitive advantage, corporate structure, and market structure?

- What are the major structural features of markets and market structure, and how does this affect the development of a management strategy?

- What strategic models are available, and how might they be used within the health care setting?

The last chapter, "Creating and Managing the Future," identifies the major trends likely to affect the delivery of health care over the next decade. Attention is given to understanding the changing role of health care providers and, specifically, the challenges facing management. Questions include:

- What larger societal forces are shaping the health care system?

- How are the changing roles of physicians, nurses, and other health professionals likely to influence the delivery of health care?

- What are the major future challenges to health care managers?

Upon completing these final two chapters, readers should be able to identify the major trends likely to affect the operations of health services organizations and the strategic approaches required to meet these challenges over the next decade.

CHAPTER 14

Achieving Competitive Advantage: The Case for Strategy

Roice D. Luke, Ph.D. and Stephen L. Walston, Ph.D.

CHAPTER OUTLINE

LEARNING OBJECTIVES

After completing this chapter, the reader should be able to:

1. Define the concepts of strategy, competitive advantage, and market structure.

2. Understand the differences between the market structure and resource-based views.

3. Understand the interrelationships between environment, market structure, and strategy.

4. Understand the major sources of competitive advantage, including some important examples of strategy for each source.

5. Understand the relationship between hospital-system ownership type and patterns of strategy.

6. Identify the major sources of threat in the Porter five forces model and be able to use these in conducting strategy analysis.

7. Gain insight into how strategy and strategy analysis applies to real markets and organizations in the health care industry.

8. Understand the difference between strategy at company versus local market levels.

9. Understand the unique strategic features of hierarchical models as pursued by local hospital clusters.

KEY TERMS

Activities
Analyzer
Company-Level Strategy
Costs of Coordination,
    Compromise, Inflexibility
Defender
Dual Advantages
Environment
First Movers

Generic Strategies
Hierarchical Configuration
Imitation
Learning Curve
Local-Level Strategy
Market Power
Market Structure View
Niching
Positioning Dynamics

Product Differentiation
Prospector
Reactor
Resource-Based View
Spatial Dispersion
Sustainability
SWOT Analysis
Value Chain

✦ IN PRACTICE   Achieving a Competitive Advantage— The Mayo Clinic

Prior to 1986, the Mayo Clinic, an internationally respected physician-based health care system centered in Rochester, Minnesota, made news primarily through its many clinical, research, and educational accomplishments. But in 1986, Mayo took its first expansionary steps toward building a regional and possibly national health care system. In that year, Mayo integrated the Clinic and two Rochester Hospitals—Saint Mary's Hospital and Rochester Methodist Hospital—putting them under a common governance structure. And, in that same year, Mayo opened a clinic in Jacksonville, Florida (located approximately 1,200 miles to the south). A year later, Mayo expanded further in Jacksonville, by acquiring St. Luke's Hospital, and also in that year opened a clinic in Scottsdale, Arizona. Five years later, in 1992, Mayo started up a regional network surrounding its Rochester sites, initiating a process of acquiring and affiliating with a large number of physician practices and hospitals. Mayo

Clinic's primary site remains concentrated around Rochester and accounts for about 70% of their revenues. Mayo through their Mayo Health System has now acquired 15 hospitals and over 60 clinics and other provider facilities in 64 communities in southern Minnesota, northern Iowa, and western Wisconsin, in a radius of 150 miles from their base in Rochester. Then, in 1998, Mayo opened a hospital in Phoenix, Arizona, to support the clinic it had already established in that area. Recently, it announced plans to sell its Jacksonville Hospital to St. Vincent's (an Ascension hospital) and build a new hospital closer to its existing clinic in Jacksonville. In 2004 the Mayo Clinic consisted of a 1,626 physician group practice in Rochester, MN; a 316 physician group practice in Jacksonville, FL; a 332 physician group practice in Scottsdale, AZ; two large hospitals in Rochester, MN, Saint Marys Hospital (1,157 beds) and Rochester Methodist Hospital (794 beds); St. Luke's Hospital in

(continues)

CHAPTER PURPOSE

Like the Mayo Clinic, many health care organizations became appreciably more strategic over the last decade, primarily because they foresaw the consequences of government policy and industry preferences favoring the use of market forces. Significantly, they saw a growing willingness to rely on managed care to bring under control the continuing and staggering increases in health care costs. As a result, health care organizations across the country anticipated that their markets would undergo major structural changes, as existing rivals, new entrants, nichers, buyers, sellers, and many other types of organizations would become increasingly more involved in competitive activities.

The subsequent flood of strategic responses was not limited to one or a few sectors in the health care industry. In the distribution sector, for example, McKesson, the San Francisco-based distributor of pharmaceutical and medical/surgical products, altered rather dramatically its approach to competition. Entering the 1990s, McKesson had emerged as one of the leading distributors of pharmaceuticals in the country. However, as it watched the new emphasis on market consolidation and system integration among provider organizations, McKesson altered its overall approach to the market. In 1997, it diversified its distribution business by acquiring General Medical, the third largest distributor of medical/surgical products. Two years later, McKesson attempted to position itself to better respond to the increased emphasis on system integration among its client organizations, by merging with HBOC, a major health care information company.

Undoubtedly, the hospital sector became the most intensively involved in strategy in the 1990s. Among the more interesting developments were the decisions made by many Catholic-sponsored multi-hospital systems to come together, forming still larger and more powerful "cosponsored" hospital systems (e.g., Catholic Healthcare West, Ascension, Trinity, etc.). The for-profit hospital systems also got into the act, merging and acquiring one another, resulting in a small number of systems, many of which rank among the very largest in the country (e.g., HCA, Tenet, Community Health Systems, etc.).

Not-for-profit hospitals and systems were among the most active strategically in this period, as is dramatically illustrated by the percentages shown in Table 14.1. From 1989 to 2003, the number of hospitals that became members of not-for-profit multi-hospital systems increased by 66%, which compares to a small decline and small increase, respectively, in the numbers of hospitals that entered for-profit and Catholic multi-hospital systems. More strikingly, the number of not-for-profit systems increased by nearly 300% in this period, compared to declines in the numbers of systems in the other two ownership types (of course, the declines

Table 14.1. Percentage Changes from 1989 to 2003 in the Level of Acute Care General Hospital Participation in Multi-Hospital Systems

	# Hospitals Systems*	# Systems	# Hospitals per System
Not-for-Profit	66%	292%	−36%
For-Profit	−8	−31	34
Catholic	10	−69	132
All	27	30	−3

*Note: The number of acute care general hospitals declined by about 9% in this period.

in the number of for-profit and Catholic systems reflects the mergers that occurred between systems within these two ownership categories). The Mayo Health System (see In Practice, p. 459) is an example of a not-for-profit system that grew rapidly over the past decade.

Clearly, health care executives now must be capable of formulating strategies, if they hope to ensure that their organizations remain viable well into the future. This is an especially important development, given the degree to which mission continues to influence the decision making of many health care organizations. But even the most community-oriented of these organizations recognize that no mission can be sustained without their remaining strategically viable. Strategy, in other words, now plays a key role in coloring and shaping how health care organizations view and attempt to enact their futures.

This chapter focuses directly on the concept of strategy as applied to health care organizations. It does so first by defining the concept itself, second by sketching out a framework for the analysis of strategy, and finally by exploring five major sources of advantage that form the bases for most competitive strategies.

THE CONCEPT OF STRATEGY

All organizations create strategies to guide them in their decision making. They form strategies to help them manage the supply channel, invest in information systems and other technologies, restructure their organizations, replace facilities, train staff, and so on. Each of these strategies identifies the means (the strategic ideas) by which organizations hope to accomplish specific ends (the strategic objectives).

Competitive strategies are no different in this regard; they express the ideas that organizational leaders believe will help them achieve certain objectives in the marketplace. In one important respect competitive strategies differ from these other types of strategy—their ends are assessed substantially in relative terms by the degree to which organizations implement their strategic ideas, gaining a degree of advantage over (or relative to) their rivals.

In other words, competitive strategies incorporate ideas not just about what actions organizations might take, but the assumptions and interpretations those organizations make, however implicitly, about the actions, accomplishments, and plans of rivals. A decision by two local hospitals to merge, for example, might reveal as much about the economic conditions facing the two hospitals as their assessments of the strengths and weaknesses, prospective moves, etc., of their rivals. Again, competitive strategies are conceived in a context of competitive combat, with all of its concomitant threats and opportunities. And its primary end is to produce advantage for an organization over what might have been attained by its rivals.

What then is competitive advantage? There are many specific indicators of competitive advantage— a better sales force, deeper financial reserves, superior image among consumers for quality, more efficient management systems, greater negotiating power, improved ability to react rapidly to market changes, and so on. Most organizations seek these and many other advantages as they formulate their competitive strategies. And each of these gives organizations a greater ability, than might otherwise be the case, to influence the decisions and behaviors of competitors and consumers in their markets. Put another way, gains in competitive advantage translate into increased **market power** for one organization relative to another.

Economists generally consider the ability of organizations to charge higher prices than might be possible under more ideal market circumstances to be presumptive evidence of market power (Scherer & Ross, 1990). An organization that attains a dominant market share (a specific strategic objective) increases its ability to charge higher prices or, in other words, increases its market power. Strategists, on the other hand, take a broader view of market power. They consider any advantage that gives organizations an ability to affect the market behaviors— price and non-price—of rivals, customers, and others to be evidence of relative market power (Porter, 1980). A hospital that distinguishes itself as a high-quality provider in its local market, for example, not only gains an ability to charge higher

prices, but also to negotiate forcefully with managed care organizations, attract physicians to admit and do surgery in that hospital, bargain with suppliers, attract patients, and even be more selective about the kinds of local and national organizations with which it might wish to merge or become aligned, or by which it might prefer to be acquired. Competitive advantage is thus attained when an organization experiences some increment in market power, relative to that attained by its competitors.

Defining Strategy

After years of searching for how best to define competitive strategy (see Barney, 1991; Gluck, Kaufman, Walleck, & Steven, 1980; Peteraf,1993; Porter, 1985, 1996), the field now appears to be resolved that its end is to gain competitive advantage. Thus, building on this trend, we offer the following definition (Luke, Walston, & Plummer, 2003):

> Strategies are those key concepts and ideas that organizations use (or have used) to achieve and sustain competitive advantage over their rivals.

This definition incorporates some important components of competitive strategy that need additional explanation. First, it recognizes that strategies are mostly conceptual. They incorporate those ideas upon which organizations rely as they seek advantage in the marketplace. These ideas are sometimes rather grand and overarching, reflecting the vision and resolve of organizational leaders. The formulation of grand strategies often serves to motivate and focus the efforts of employees, boards, and other stakeholders. But, as Mintzberg (1994) has argued, such ideas can be too "grand," in that they easily become enshrined and institutionalized within organizations, preventing them from adapting and learning as new information is gained and markets and organizations change. Regardless of how dramatic they might be, organizations use strategic ideas to guide them as they invest resources and take actions designed to gain competitive advantage.

We would note that not all strategic ideas are new and course changing, nor do they necessarily lead to major commitments of new resources. Often, organizations conclude that they should "stick to the knitting," so to speak; that is, they should continue to focus on existing sources of advantage, emphasizing refinements and implementation, rather than grand (and often highly risky) new strategic initiatives.

Second, the definition of strategy contains two key verbs—achieve and sustain. It is often easy to overlook the fact that strategies, once attained, might not be so easily sustained. Many hospitals learned this lesson in recent years, as they invested heavily in information technologies in hopes that by doing so they would generate considerable competitive advantage, only to discover to their dismay that their rivals imitated their moves, negating any advantage they might have attained in the short term. Competitive advantage is dynamic. It must be weighed and updated, as competitors make counter moves and consumer tastes and behaviors change. Organizations thus must apply the dual tests of advantage and **sustainability** when assessing existing positions and possible new organizational moves in the marketplace.

Third, competitive strategies are much more than the sum of new ideas and arguments for new undertakings. They are also deeply embedded within a series of past decisions and investments that result in distinctive resources, capabilities, business models, acquisitions, and so on, all of which provide the foundations upon which organizations establish competitive advantage. Thus, analysts can learn a great deal about the strategies of organizations by weighing existing strengths and weaknesses as well as possible new moves those organizations might take to expand upon and sustain competitive advantage. For example, the strategies of a locally dominating hospital system might be deduced by examining its past actions—the number, sizes, and types of hospitals it has acquired; whether it has moved into nearby rural areas; what other provider businesses it has established in the market; what integration strategies it has pursued across its

provider units; whether it is invested in physician practices; what investments it has made in IT and other technological resources; and so on. Thus, strategy represents as much the moves organizations have already taken as those highly proprietary decisions they might make during proverbial strategy retreats. In other words, strategy is often reflections of distinctive *business models* or approaches organizations adopt as they seek advantage in the marketplace over time.

STRATEGY ANALYSIS FRAME

Just over two decades ago, the strategy field seemed more focused on the processes organizations use in strategic decision making than on analyzing with any depth the determinants of strategy (Schendel & Hofer, 1979). This is primarily because the field at that time lacked many of the essential concepts and tools (Mintzberg, 1990, 1998) needed for strategy analysis. Since then, however, important progress has been made in filling in some of the voids in strategy analysis. Two intellectual streams of thought are especially important in this regard—the market structure and the resource-based views of strategy. The first is closely linked to the work of Michael Porter (1980, 1985), an economist who translated the concepts and tools of industrial organization economics (which historically had been applied to policy analysis) into terms and frames of reference that could be used in the study of competitor behaviors, competitive advantage, and the market drivers of strategy. The resource-based view focused internally on how organizational capabilities, resources, activities, structures, and other factors produced distinctive and sustainable competitive advantage (Barney, 2001; Collis & Montgomery, 1995; Grant, 1998).

Together, these and other areas of intellectual development have greatly enhanced our ability to conduct thoughtful analyses of strategy for individual organizations. Ironically, much of this work has confirmed the widely recognized and rather simplistic logic of the **SWOT** (strengths, weaknesses, opportunities, and threats) **analysis** framework (Andrews, 1971; Henderson, 1979). The **market structure view** elaborates on external threats and opportunities; the resource-based view elaborates on internal strengths and weaknesses.

Central to the market structure view is a hypothesized relationship between the structures of markets and the conduct of competitors in those markets (Scherer & Ross, 1990). Market structure refers to the organizational features of markets that condition or influence the strategies of competitors; and conduct refers to the actions or strategies organizations take collectively in response to environmental and market stimuli. Three structural features are generally considered to be among the most important (Bain & Qualls, 1987):

1. Degree of concentration

2. Height of entry barriers

3. Level of product differentiation in the market.

Each of these influences strategic decision making directly. Higher levels of market concentration, higher entry barriers, and greater **product differentiation** all increase the market power of established competitors and, in the process, diminish price competition as well. But they also influence many forms of non-price competition, all of which means that market structure is often a major determinant of strategic choice.

Porter's contributions are thus highly important. First, he reinforced the conclusion that market structure can have a powerful impact on strategy. Second, he enriched our understanding of the number and variety of structural drivers one might need to evaluate in a thorough strategy analysis. He is perhaps best recognized for his five forces framework (see Figure 14.1), which frames the primary sources of threat most organizations face in market competition. Threats come most directly from immediate rivals. But they also come from sources just outside

of the markets—from potential entrants, buyers, sellers, and substitutes. We list in the figure some of the structural features identified by Porter that are important for studying health care strategy.

By contrast, the **resource-based view** emphasizes the important role distinctive resources and capabilities play in building competitive advantage. Resources refer to the more tangible elements within organizations—manpower, plant, equipment, location—and capabilities, to the intangibles—talent, skills, management systems, coordinating mechanisms, experience, and organizational knowledge. An important contribution of the resource-based view is its emphasis on sustainability. Advantages could easily be eroded, if rivals are able to imitate or substitute for the distinctive resources and/or capabilities attained by any given competitor. Resource-based scholars have thus focused on such counterbalancing characteristics as rarity, inimitability, durability, and transparency, which are associated with the difficulty rivals sometimes face in duplicating the internal resources and capabilities of competitors (Barney, 2001; Collis & Montgomery, 1995; Grant, 1998).

Interestingly, Porter (1985), who is closely associated with the externally focused market structural view, added to the thinking about how internal organizational factors impact competitive advantage. He argued that to improve their external positions, organizations needed to do a better job managing and coordinating the specific **activities** they perform in producing goods and services. Strategically important activities can be found in a number of areas, including marketing, production, distribution, acquisition, financing, and so forth. Competitors, he suggested, should evaluate all critical activities in what he called their "value chains" to see how the congruence, complementarity, and fit among them might be improved and their contributions to competitive advantage enhanced.

An emphasis on resources and capabilities as well as on activities might be especially important in health care, for two reasons. First, health care organizations focused on both technical and service quality are directly dependent on the quality and

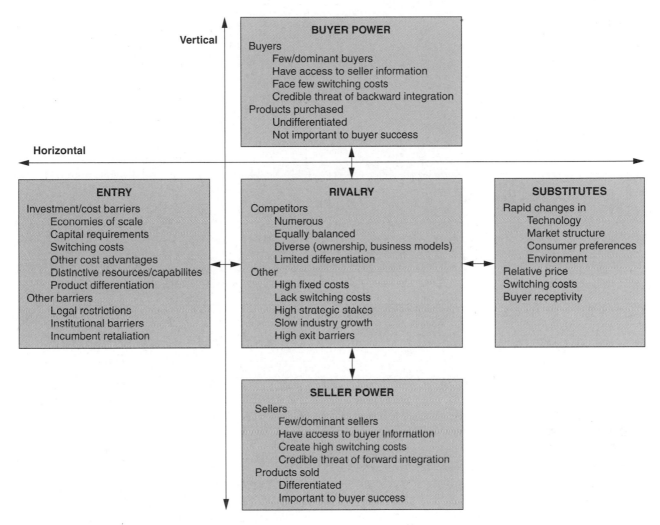

BUYER POWER
Buyers
    Few/dominant buyers
    Have access to seller information
    Face few switching costs
    Credible threat of backward integration
Products purchased
    Undifferentiated
    Not important to buyer success

Vertical

Horizontal

ENTRY
Investment/cost barriers
    Economies of scale
    Capital requirements
    Switching costs
    Other cost advantages
    Distinctive resources/capabilites
    Product differentiation
Other barriers
    Legal restrictions
    Institutional barriers
    Incumbent retaliation

RIVALRY
Competitors
    Numerous
    Equally balanced
    Diverse (ownership, business models)
    Limited differentiation
Other
    High fixed costs
    Lack switching costs
    High strategic stakes
    Slow industry growth
    High exit barriers

SUBSTITUTES
Rapid changes in
    Technology
    Market structure
    Consumer preferences
    Environment
Relative price
Switching costs
Buyer receptivity

SELLER POWER
Sellers
    Few/dominant sellers
    Have access to buyer information
    Create high switching costs
    Credible threat of forward integration
Products sold
    Differentiated
    Important to buyer success

Figure 14.1. Porter's Five Forces Framework

SOURCE: Adapted with the permission of Free Press, a division of Simon & Schuster, Inc. from *Competitive strategy: Techniques for analyzing industries and competitors* by Michael E. Porter. Copyright © 1980 by the Free Press.

management of resources and systems. Second, health care organizations are very complex, especially now that so many providers and facilities are coordinated at the local market level, which makes it essential that they find ways to better integrate internally and interorganizationally. Third, these organizations are increasingly dependent on complex technologies, which place heavy demands on system integration

and control to ensure that they are utilized efficiently and with high quality. Those organizations that discover the formulas for system integration will surely be better able to gain advantage in the ponderous world of health care competition.

Figure 14.2 joins these two perspectives to form a framework for strategy analysis. The market structural view is shown on the right and the

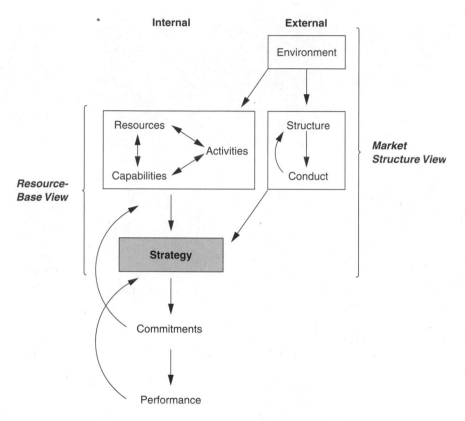

Figure 14.2. Strategy Analysis Frame

SOURCE: Adapted Luke, R. M., Walston, S. L., & Plummer, P. M. (2003). *Healthcare strategy: In pursuit of competitive advantage* (p. 46). Chicago: Health Administration Press.

resource-based view, on the left. Strategic evaluations of both internal and external factors lead to conceptualizations about strategy and this, to commitments of resources needed for strategy implementation.

Some organizations will emphasize internal factors, while others, external factors. A rural hospital that enjoys a near monopoly will likely focus more on internal assessments, while a major urban system that is in competition with another such system might emphasize external factors. Also, the importance of internal versus external factors will vary over time. In the 1990s, for example, most hospitals and hospital systems concentrated on external

factors—threats from managed care companies, opportunities for merger and acquisition, and threats from local and national physician organizations. In today's environment, with somewhat diminished external threats and much of the local merger and acquisition opportunities now gone, hospital systems are tending to concentrate much more on internal refinements as bases for gaining competitive advantage.

In coming years, market conditions could shift the emphasis again to external factors. It is likely, for example, that with increased threats in funding and growth in complex and costly technologies, health care systems might need to be much larger than they are now. This could ignite a new wave of cross-market mergers and acquisitions, not just in the hospital, but in many other sectors within health care.

SOURCES OF COMPETITIVE ADVANTAGE

While in discussing the concept of strategy it can be noted that a growing consensus at that the end of strategy is competitive advantage, there is somewhat less resolution as to what the means for achieving this end might be (e.g., see Barney, 2001; Eisenhardt and Martin, 2000; Foss, 1999; Grant, 1991; Porter, 1996). The primary arguments come from the two perspectives discussed earlier, from the resource-based and market structure views.

The resource-based view takes a longer-term perspective, suggesting that organizations need to develop an ability to compete over time, if they hope to sustain distinctive competencies and adapt to changing circumstances. Such organizations, they argue, will thus be better able to win the competitive war, rather than a few market skirmishes here or there. In other words, organizations that have strong management, excellent products, well-honed systems of decision making and control, etc., should be able to prevent imitation and substitution by rivals and to move with strength and resolution when it is necessary. The counter view, put forward specifically by Porter, is that no market battle can be won if a competitor lacks a strong position in the marketplace. It matters little, he suggested, how competent an organization's administrative team might be or how sophisticated its IT strategy, if that organization lacks products and services that are preferred by consumers (Porter, 1996). Such an organization simply would be unable to win any competitive battles.

Without detailing the pros and cons of each of the arguments, we simply conclude that they are both correct. Advantages, whatever their sources might be, are advantages. A hospital that is able to draw upon the deep pockets of a large parent organization (internal source of advantage) might be better able to adapt to future market and environmental shifts than will one that is at the moment more favorably viewed by the consuming public (an external source), but lacks the capital to respond to unanticipated changes in its markets. The point is, any source of advantage can be important to strategy, so long as it enhances the competitive advantage of an organization relative to its rivals.

Furthermore, it is important to understand that internal and external sources of advantage are highly interdependent. A company that has a high-quality medical staff and established and effective management systems (both of which are internal sources of advantage) should be better able to project an image of quality in the marketplace (an external positioning advantage). A system that has attained, through a series of mergers and acquisitions, an unassailable position of dominance in its local market (an external advantage), might be better able to take the time to refine its resources and capabilities (an internal advantage).

It is also true that which source of advantage might be the most important strategically will depend on the conditions inherent in the markets and broader **environment**. In the 1990s, for example, a time in which there was considerable market change and uncertainty, a number of hospitals took seriously the recommendations coming from some quarters that they refine internal systems of management. They in turn invested heavily in such programs as total quality management and organizational reengineering (Walston & Bogue, 1999; Walston & Kimberly, 1997) and, unwittingly, left the door open to their competitors to win in the acquisitions business (an externally focused strategy). As a result, their competitors gained unassailably dominant positions in their local markets. Timing and sequencing were the key here, not so much which advantage was inherently more important conceptually.

In the end, does it really matter which source of advantage—internal or external—is correct? Any source of advantage can be important, so long as it contributes to competitive advantage and is feasible, ethical, legal, and consistent with an organization's mission. In sum, gaining and sustaining advantage is the end of strategy, and the various sources of advantage—all of them—are its means.

The Major Sources of Competitive Advantage

While there are many sources of competitive advantage, most can be grouped within five major categories. The five are given labels beginning with the letter "P" for ease of remembering them (Luke, Walston, & Plummer, 2003):

- Potential—Access to distinctive and superior capabilities and resources
- Performance—Superior operations and the implementation of strategy
- Position—Projection of distinctive and valued images to consumers
- Power—Accumulation and effective use of organizational mass
- Pace—Measured timing and intensity of strategic action

The first two of these—potential and performance—are internal sources of advantage and the second two—position and power—are external. The last source, pace, is neither. It applies to both internal and external approaches to building competitive advantage.

Each of these sources can be and often is interrelated with the others. The buildup of organizational power through a series of acquisitions and/or mergers (power strategy), for example, could occur because an organization took a strategically more aggressive approach (pace strategy) to strategy. Such a buildup could also produce economies of scale and thus contribute to improved efficiencies (performance strategy) and, as a consequence, enable the organization to charge lower prices in the marketplace (position strategy). And it could enable the organization to acquire more sophisticated IT capabilities and enhance its technology overall (potential strategy).

In the remainder of the chapter, each of the five sources of competitive advantage will be explained. At the end of the chapter, expansion on the one source—power—which has become so important in transforming the hospital and a number of other sectors within the health care industry, will be covered.

PACE

Management consultants have tended to emphasize pace as a primary source of competitive advantage. This is because the timing, level of risk taking, and aggressiveness of strategic actions are somewhat more amenable to leadership and structural and cultural factors within organizations than are many of the other sources of advantage. In their now classic book, for example, Peters and Waterman (1982) identified eight essential attributes of excellence that they concluded contributed to the success of the 75 major corporations they studied. The first of the eight was a "bias for action," which, they argued, if adopted by organizations, would help them become early movers strategically and thus to gain market advantages over time.

A number of pace-related concepts have emerged in the organizational and strategy literatures, including, for example: adaptability (Chakravarthy, 1982), flexibility (Harrigan, 1985), surprise (Rothschild, 1984), initiative (MacMillan, 1984), learning (Mintzburg, 1978), innovation (Young, Charns, & Shortell, 2001), and defense (Porter, 1980). Indeed, **first movers** and the **learning curve**, two pace-related concepts, are well-established ideas in the strategy literature. The idea behind the experience curve (Henderson, 1979) is that organizations learn with time and thus are able to achieve manpower efficiencies, production standardization, specialization, refinements in the use of technology, and many other advantages, simply because they moved early to invest in new businesses and management capabilities. Early moving organizations thus potentially gain distinct advantages over late movers, presumably because the latter would have to enter at the same high-cost positions as did the early movers and would have to pass through the same learning processes to lower their costs and become more competitive over time. Also, early movers, given their established advantages, should be able to capture dominant positions in their markets and to erect market barriers that slow the progress of late moving rivals. A local hospital system, for example, that invests early in ambulatory surgery centers and other service lines and integrates these into its broader hospital-based systems should be able gain strong, even unassailable positions in its markets that later-moving rivals might not easily overcome (Parker, Charns, & Young, 2001).

On the other hand, the evidence supporting early movers is mixed, at best (Lieberman & Montgomery, 1998). Early movers, for example, might not be able to sustain their presumed advantages, if their rivals are able to learn and adapt by studying the early movers, imitating their decisions, and/or recruiting away their skilled clinical staff and leadership teams. There is also the possibility that late movers will learn from the mistakes of early movers by not adopting the information technologies acquired by first movers, if those technologies are no longer the most cost-effective and sophisticated of those currently available. Also, there is the problem that early moving carries with it considerable risk. A number of high-profile health care organizations have moved first and failed strategically—Columbia/HCA, Phycor, MedPartners, and many others illustrated the downsides of early moving in the prior decade.

One of the more widely recognized conceptualizations of pace-related strategies is the typology of strategic orientations developed by Miles and Snow (1978). They suggested that organizations tended to fall within one of four strategic orientations, reflecting their aggressiveness and willingness to take risks in strategic decision making. The four are:

- **Prospector**—Organizations that frequently search for new market opportunities and regularly engage in experimentation and innovation
- **Analyzer**—Organizations that maintain stable operations in some areas but also search for new opportunities, often following the lead of prospector organizations
- **Defender**—Organizations that rely on established approaches to growth and seldom make adjustments to existing, proven strategies
- **Reactor**—Organizations that perceive opportunities and turbulence but are not able to adapt consistently or effectively

Prospector-type organizations obviously would be the most strategically aggressive of the four. With their emphases on innovation and early movement, these are the ones most likely to encounter the wide swings between risk and opportunity often encountered by early movers. By contrast, defender organizations would tend to focus on existing sources of advantage, emphasizing refinements in existing products and improvements in efficiencies. One might expect competitors that dominate their markets (e.g., large hospital clusters in large urban markets and sole-provider competitors in rural markets) to shift from the more aggressive postures that might have helped them attain their dominant positions to more cautious and defensive orientations, designed to prevent upstart competitors from eroding the dominant players' established market positions.

The analyzer orientation falls somewhere in between. As conceptualized by Miles and Snow (1978), analyzers tend to let others make the early moves, while they search for evidence that such will produce advantage. Organizations that assume this orientation will thus tend to emphasize market research and testing over intuition and flair in strategic decision making. The reactor differs from all of these in that they either lack a clear vision and sense of direction or face inalterable constraints on their ability to act strategically when opportunities present themselves. Many public hospitals fall into this category, since so many of them are constrained by institutional rigidities and conflicting missions.

Which of these or other strategic orientations is preferred will depend very much on the specifics of the competitive situation faced by given organizations as well as their overall sources of competitive advantage. Competitors located in markets that are in the throes of change, for example, might need to assume more aggressive strategic postures. Just such a situation existed in the 1990s, a decade in which many health care organizations became much more aggressive strategically to avoid being left in the competitive dust. For those located in more stable environments, which orientation is best often depends on an organization's ability to respond to perceived threats and opportunities.

In their study of the strategic orientations of hospitals in the 1980s, for example, Shortell, Morrison, and Friedman (1990) found that hospital aggressiveness in strategy varied widely, depending significantly on organizational cultures and leadership style. They found that while many hospitals shifted their strategic orientations over time, they tended to move toward orientations that were not too different from the ones they had initially adopted. They thus suggested that hospitals operate within strategic *"comfort zones,"* meaning that their approaches to strategy shifted only marginally over time. This is consistent with Miles's finding (1982) that tobacco firms tended to maintain their strategic orientations over time, which consistency he attributes to the important role culture and management structures play in shaping or constraining the willingness of organizations to take strategic risk. Figure 14.3 shows the comfort zones identified by Shortell and colleagues (1990). As can be seen, if they shift at all, both prospectors and defenders are likely to shift to the analyzer orientation rather than make more dramatic moves to the other end of the strategic spectrum. By contrast, since they are more or less in the middle with respect to their willingness to assume risk, both analyzers and

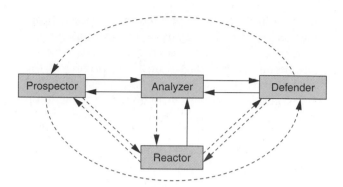

Figure 14.3. Strategic Comfort Zones for Shifting Pace Strategy Orientations

SOURCE: Adapted from Shortell, S. M., Morrison, E. M., & Friedman, B. (1990). *Strategic choices for America's hospitals* (p. 37). San Francisco: Jossey-Bass.

reactors would be expected to shift toward any one of the other strategic orientations.

POTENTIAL AND PERFORMANCE

The resource-based view mentioned earlier ties competitive advantage directly to the distinctive internal competencies available to individual organizations, which we encapsulate using two of the five sources of advantage—potential and performance. Potential refers to the unique resources and capabilities upon which organizations rely as they pursue advantage over their rivals. And performance refers to how well they are able to execute organizational activities, most especially those that impact strategic outcomes. Neither potential nor performance contributes directly to competitive advantage. Rather, as illustrated in Figure 14.4, they produce advantage indirectly if: (1) they enhance other sources of advantage and (2) subsequent gains in advantage can be sustained. A local multihospital cluster that has created a superior IT system might convert this into competitive advantage by hardwiring physicians to

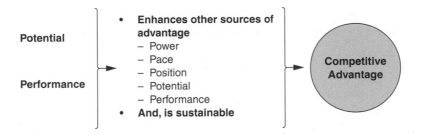

Figure 14.4. Potential and Performance Contribute Indirectly to Competitive Advantage

SOURCE: Adapted Luke, R. M., Walston, S. L., & Plummer, P. M. (2003). *Healthcare strategy: In pursuit of competitive advantage* (p. 163). Chicago: Health Administration Press.

its system, thereby, hopefully, "capturing" physician commitment (by raising the costs of switching to rival hospitals) to admit to their facilities. These two are emerging as highly important sources of advantage in the current decade, especially for hospital systems. Having passed through a rather active period of mergers and acquisitions, many hospital clusters now need to concentrate their energies on consolidating services and management capacities. This is true for two reasons—few opportunities for additional acquisitions and mergers remain within most local markets (on the other hand, cross-market possibilities are still very much available) and many local clusters now have the time (and the need) to consolidate their gains, by taking advantage of scale and scope economies and close spatial proximities. Many hospitals and hospital systems are thus seeking to gain competitive advantage by enhancing internal capabilities and improving performance overall.

Potential

As displayed in Table 14.2, resources and capabilities differ in the degree to which they are tangible—resources being more tangible and capabilities, less so. Internal resources and capabilities are strategically highly important in health care, given the complexity, technical sophistication, and general quality imperatives that distinguish this industry. (From this point on, we will use the term *capabili-*

ties generally when referencing both resources and capabilities).

As argued by the advocates of the resource-based view, sustainability is key to ensuring competitive advantage based on internal capabilities. Rivals counter the advantages of competitors primarily in two ways, by imitation or by substitution (Ghemawat, 2001). **Imitation** occurs when rivals duplicate the internal capabilities of a given competitor. Substitution occurs when rivals find alternative approaches for gaining advantages based on internal capabilities. Sustainability depends directly on how difficult it is for rivals to duplicate or imitate an organization's distinctive capabilities. Table 14.2 lists four general barriers to imitation. While all are important in health care, we emphasize one of these for purposes of illustration—strategic complexity, system interconnectedness.

Hospitals and hospital systems are such multifaceted entities that many internal capabilities derive their advantages as much from multiple, highly interrelated organizational elements as from the specific capabilities themselves. Thus, even if a rival were able to duplicate some critical capability, it would be less likely that it could copy the entire system of interrelationships that account for that capability's distinctiveness.

Sentara, a six-hospital system in the Virginia Beach–Norfolk area, has invested heavily in a capacity to manage the distribution and handling of its medical/surgical supplies. It runs a major warehouse,

Table 14.2. Resources and Capabilities of an Organization

Tangible (resources)

Financial (structure, cash flow, capital base, profitability)

Physical plant, property (condition, age, modernity)

Service capacity/mix

Organization structure (tightness, centralization)

Partnerships, alliances

Systems (information systems, control systems, clinical integration, etc.)

Technology

Clinical and/or administrative manpower

Location

Intangible (capabilities)

Experience

Reputation

Culture

Specialized skills and knowledge (e.g., "system" skills, clinical, management)

Communication, analytic, interactive skills

Distinctive organizational "routines"

Motivation

Innovativeness

orders direct from manufacturers and receives direct shipment from many of them, negotiates many of the prices on products (rather than to rely so much on GPO contracts), redistributes shipped supplies to its facilities and physician offices, etc. By taking on nearly all of its distribution functions, Sentara has been able to save millions of dollars in supply costs per year. The question is, can its competitors imitate this distinctive capability? Although there might be little mystery as to how each element in the supply chain is managed, few local hospital systems have been willing or able to separate themselves from their primary distributors and group purchasing organizations to the degree Sentara has.

A close look at Sentara reveals that its ability to manage the supply channel is tied to many other factors—it has an innovative and competent administrative team, is sufficiently large and geographically concentrated for supply coordination to be financially feasible, and has invested heavily in IT and other technological areas that are crucial for success in this area. In other words, it is not just technical knowledge about the supply channel that is needed for this to be done internally, but a highly intertwined configuration of systems, skills, resources, management systems, and other resources that make it possible for a system like Sentara to pull off and sustain this unique approach to supply channel management.

Another example is the growing use of advanced communications technologies, which are capabilities that might not be accessible to all competitors in given markets. Sutter Health, for instance, has attained a degree of advantage as an advanced caregiver by establishing three eICU centers that support a number of its hospitals regionally. The three have been placed strategically in its three major markets, Sacramento, San Francisco, and the East Bay area (Berkeley and Oakland). The eICUs utilize telecommunication and sophisticated information technologies to enable specially trained nurses and intensivist physicians to manage from remote sites the care provided to seriously ill patients. Sutter is thus taking advantage of its overall size and local concentration to create an integrated multi-organizational system of intensive care. It is also heavily investing in IT, which will enhance the capability offered by the eICU as well as other distinctive clinical capabilities being created by Sutter. Sutter Health is thus creating complex sets of competencies that might be difficult for its rivals to duplicate.

PERFORMANCE

Performance can take one into a wide realm of administrative functioning and organizational structuring, although our focus here is on those areas of performance improvement that affect competitive advantage directly. In particular, the focus is on advantages that are derived from the implementation of strategy.

It is common for strategies to fail solely because of broad management and system failures. (Although strategic outcomes can be tied to small, seemingly inconsequential failures—recall the adage that a war was lost, because of a failure to nail a horseshoe properly onto a horse.) Mintzberg (1994), for example, argued that strategic planning often fails because organizations are unable to implement planning models effectively. He identified the "great divides" that too often lead to failed strategies—failures for objectives and goals to be tied to strategies, strategies and budgets to be coordinated, budgets and strategies to drive programmatic activities, and so on. Individual rigidities and turf protection, unrecognized organizational complexities, and general uncertainty too often diminish the idealized role of corporations to provide management direction, coordination, monitoring, and control (Lorange, 1980). It is possible that such problems are even more challenging in health care than in other industries, given the highly institutionalized and constrained environments within which most health care organizations operate.

An alternative perspective on performance as a strategic concept can be found in Porter's (1985) conceptualization of the **value chain**. He argued that significant competitive advantages can be derived out of a better, more systematic management of identified "activities" within the value chains of organizations. The value chain is a conceptual disaggregation of organizational activities in both the support and actual production of products (Hill & Jones, 1998). An organization that carefully identifies each of the critical activities it performs should be able to identify areas where small improvements in performance generate cumulatively rather substantial improvements in how strategy is implemented. Porter argued:

> Competitive advantage cannot be understood by looking at a firm as a whole. It stems from the many discrete activities a firm performs in designing, producing, marketing, delivering and supporting its product . . . The value chain disaggregates a firm into its strategically relevant activities in order to understand the behavior of costs and the existing and potential sources of differentiation. (1985, p. 33)

Porter drew a distinction between "primary" and "support" activities. The former refer to those administrative tasks and processes that are directly involved in production (acquisition of inputs, production, sale of products) and the latter, to those that would be identified with the infrastructure of an organization. In addition to assessing the activities themselves, Porter suggested that organizations also need to evaluate the interrelationships among activities. He said:

> Value activities are related by linkages within the value chain. Linkages are relationships between the way one value activity is performed and the cost or performance of another. . . . Linkages can lead to competitive advantage in two ways: optimization and coordination. (1985, p. 48)

This is where trade-offs, optimization, and coordination would be made as organizations identify better ways to configure and administer strategically important activities.

The analysis of value chain activities can and should be done within individual facilities as well as between interrelated facilities that are combined within larger systems. The latter need is especially important in health care, given the complex systems of interrelationships that exist between providers and facilities at the local level. The so-called integrated system (IDS), for example, was conceived as an approach by which local provider collectives might coordinate the care for individual patients (AHA, 1990, 1992; CHA, 1992). While the IDSs have yet to attain their much touted potential, many are discovering the power of local proximities, system restructuring, and interorganizational coordination (e.g., see the Sentara example, p. 472) as the bases upon which overall system performance can be improved.

In general, management experts have paid considerable attention to integration and its many related management terms: economies of scale, economies of scope, synergies, dominant logic, complementarities, and corporate coherence (Ansoff, 1965; Milgrom & Roberts, 1995; Prahalad & Bettis, 1986; Teece, Rumelt, Dosi, & Winter, 1994). Each such term refers to somewhat different ways by which complex organizations gain advantage through coordination and integration. Complementarities, for example, are attained when performance and outcomes are improved when different competencies and/or products are joined; economies of scale refer to efficiency gains attributable to expanding the use of fixed assets; and synergies refer to gains that result from joint operation of activities or business units.

The evidence supporting the benefits of integration, it should be mentioned, are mixed, in general (Mahajan & Wind, 1988) and for health care specifically (McCue, Clement, & Luke, 1999). There are many reasons for this, not the least of which are the many costs associated with coordination. Three types of costs are especially important (Porter, 1980):

1. **Costs of coordination**

2. **Costs of compromise**

3. **Costs of inflexibility**

Coordination between two hospitals, for example, even if owned by the same multihospital system can be very challenging. Hospitals have long enjoyed high levels of organizational autonomy. And their medical staffs, boards, and other important stakeholders often resist cooperation when called upon to make major commitments to change. Interestingly, some same-system hospitals have taken the additional step of formally merging in hopes of stripping away some of the barriers that otherwise interfere with compromise, cooperation, and strategic adaptability. Clearly, health care organizations face many formidable challenges in translating performance improvement into competitive advantage. But, for those that succeed in this effort, the opportunities for making major gains in competitive advantage relative to "performance-challenged" rivals can be very great.

POSITION

Porter not only argued that positioning is the essential basis upon which organizations gain competitive advantage, but suggested that most organizations ideally should pursue only one of three **generic strategies**:

1. Low cost

2. High differentiation

3. Focus (pursue customer niches with either low-cost or high-differentiation strategies)

He argued that organizations should not attempt two of these at once, since each of the generic positions required organizations to evolve distinctive cultures, structures, management systems, even leadership capacities to pull them off successfully. A hospital, in other words, might not be able to emphasize high quality/high technology, while at the same time pursue a low-cost strategy in its markets. But is Porter correct in this?

Ghemawat (2001) suggested that significant advantages might be attained if organizations were to pursue **dual advantages**—that is, simultaneously to pursue both differentiation and low-cost positions (p. 56). While organizations might be better able to achieve efficiencies in production and management by pursuing one or the other of the generic strategies, it is certain that an organization that achieves a dual advantage will trump any that attain only one, either low cost or high differentiation.

This, of course, is an argument about feasibility more than of desirability. A form of dual advantage is the middle position—moderate quality and costs—which straddles the two primary generic positions. Significantly, this is the most common position attained by most health care providers. Few seek low-cost (or, more accurately, low-price) positions, although they all will see strategic advantages (better cash flow, ability to generate needed capital for development and growth, etc.) in bringing their costs under control. Low-cost positions simply are too easily associated with low quality, which in health care is a highly undesirable position to be in. It is true that if the managed care model had really taken off, as conceived in the 1990s, low-cost positions might have provided considerable competitive advantage. Low-cost providers would likely have been better positioned to win competitive managed care contracts.

But this model has not developed as expected and thus low cost has become more an internal performance goal than a strategic positioning objective.

Interestingly, most community general hospitals occupy middle positions with regard to quality. They achieve positioning advantages by capturing unique locations, emphasizing service, promoting their medical staffs, advertising high technology investments in selected clinical services, building networks of ambulatory surgery centers, and so on. The highly desirable high-quality positions are not easy to attain by hospitals and other health care providers. In the hospital sector, the high-quality position tends to be dominated by the relatively small number of large academic and nonacademic referral centers. In Memphis, for example, preeminence in quality positioning is fought out by two major medical centers—the 696-bed Methodist University Hospital and the 706-bed Baptist Memorial Hospital–Memphis. To strengthen them in their strategic battles, these two hospitals have evolved strong local hospital clusters—Methodist Healthcare and Baptist Memorial Health Care—that now dominate the Memphis and surrounding areas (added together, their clusters control around 70% of the metropolitan market). The remaining seven acute care general hospitals in the market (out of a total of 16) are forced to compete for positioning advantages in other areas—service niches, quality niches, other health care businesses (e.g., ambulatory surgery), and so forth. Notably, many flagship hospitals are able to extend some of their distinctive positioning status to their local systems members (e.g., see the Partners Health System in Boston, Johns Hopkins in Baltimore, Memorial Hermann in Houston, and Orlando Regional Health System in Orlando).

In a few large markets, a fairly large number of hospitals compete for high-quality positions (e.g., the large number of large medical centers located in New York, Chicago, and Philadelphia). In most small markets, at most only one hospital is sufficiently large and sophisticated to claim a high-quality position (examples include the New Hanover Regional Medical Center in Wilmington,

North Carolina, Sacred Heart General Hospital in Eugene, Oregon, and Greenville Memorial Hospital in Greenville, South Carolina).

A growing trend is for specialty hospitals to compete for selected positions within markets. Often local hospital systems, groups of local physicians, or outside proprietary firms use specialty **niching** in local markets to gain advantage. The jury is still out, however, as to whether the specialty strategy will be successful in capturing focused high-quality positions such that demand is drawn away from the larger, more complex medical centers. These latter hospitals and systems often anticipate entry by specialty hospitals and establish their own specialty entities, often as extensions of their flagship facilities.

A good example of a strictly specialty company is the Cancer Treatment Centers of America (CTCA), a three-facility system located in some fairly competitive markets—Chicago, Seattle, and Tulsa (and with plans to expand into some additional important markets). CTCA positions itself as an alternative to the big, high-prestige (and frequently too impersonal and institutional) cancer centers often associated with major academic medical centers. They emphasize patient empowerment in the choice of treatment options and a more sensitive approach to dealing with the sick individuals and their families as they battle the emotionally draining disease of cancer.

It is also possible that, once systems that happen to be centered around high-quality positioned flagship facilities have had sufficient time to consolidate recent mergers, acquisitions, and new business development, they will use their established positions to enter (by merger, acquisition, and/or new construction) new, more distant markets. The moves by the Cleveland Clinic into two locations in Florida and by the Mayo Clinic into Florida and Arizona hint at a possible major new strategy that could be pursued by well-positioned hospital systems seeking opportunities for growth.

The above and other positioning strategies might also be greatly enhanced by the continued explosion in telecommunications and sophisticated clinical technologies (e.g., eICUs, robotic surgery, telecommunication-based consultations, and other outreach services). It is very possible, for example, that prestigious institutions will be able to provide service support to providers located at considerable distances away—regionally, nationally, even internationally. They would be able to enter such distant markets in this way primarily because they have established reputations for (or positions in) high quality.

The aforementioned and other trends together suggest that positioning could in the future emerge as a major source of competitive advantage within the health care industry. And changes in positions could occur much more rapidly than in the past. This also suggests that positioning needs to be viewed in much more dynamic terms. Rivals might more easily than in the past be able to erode the established **positioning dynamics** of dominant players. All health care organizations thus might need to be increasingly diligent in assessing their positions and adjusting them as necessary over time.

Importantly, position shifting could move in many directions. Figure 14.5 illustrates diagrammatically possible movements in the spectrum of positions. The figure shows three levels each (low, medium, high) for cost and differentiation options, resulting in a total of nine possible positions. The so-called generic positions can be found along the diagonal—the middle position, in this case, is treated as if it were one of the generic positions. Off-diagonal positions represent various dual-advantage options, with high cost/low differentiation being the least desirable and low cost/high differentiation being the ideal. Obviously, all competitors will seek to move in the southeast direction in the matrix in search of improvements over their existing positions in their markets. For example, a hospital located in a low cost/low differentiation position might be expected to move along the diagonal to a middle position or to the right, to capture a low cost/moderate differentiation position. It is also possible, of course, that such a competitor might seek to reinforce and strengthen its low cost/low differentiation position, believing that it has few significant rivals in this area.

Clearly, with rapid changes in technology and growing turbulence in the markets due to an increasingly challenging reimbursement environment,

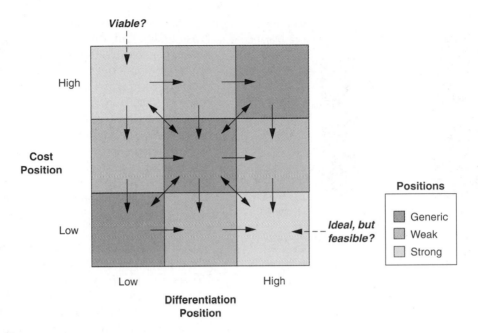

Figure 14.5. Dynamics of Positioning

SOURCE: Adapted Luke, R. M., Walston, S. L., & Plummer, P. M. (2003). *Healthcare strategy: In pursuit of competitive advantage* (p. 46). Chicago: Health Administration Press.

health care organizations will need to engage assertively in position assessments. Positioning threats are likely to come from many directions, from existing (often increasingly powerful) rivals, externally based specialty organizations, and, in the case of hospitals, even from their own medical staffs. Positioning analyses need to focus not just on an organization's image in the market, but on all of the marketing elements that go into positioning—product selection, location, price, and promotion (Kotler & Armstrong, 1996).

POWER

Power strategies constitute some of the most important approaches to achieving competitive advantage in most industries, including in health care. This is

because of the close association that exists between size and the ability of competitors to dominate and sustain advantages over time. Power strategies, however, can be viewed from a number of perspectives, two of which we emphasize here. The first distinguishes them by the degree to which advantages are derived from absolute versus relative organizational size. The second focuses more on the model type, as determined by how organizations combine business units to gain competitive advantage.

Power Strategies—Absolute versus Relative

The essential difference between absolute and relative power is illustrated in Figure 14.6. The overall size of an organization—absolute power—is associated with the depth of resources that an organization is capable of bringing to bear in any given competitive battle. Absolute size is thus correlated

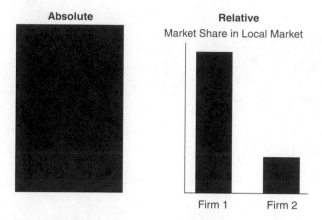

Figure 14.6. Two Ways to Project Market Power

SOURCE: Adapted Luke, R. M., Walston, S. L., & Plummer, P. M. (2003). *Healthcare strategy: In pursuit of competitive advantage* (p. 175). Chicago: Health Administration Press.

with such strategically important factors as financial resources, managerial and support staff, market visibility, purchasing power, advertising power, political clout, economies of scale, ability to enter markets, and so on. Because its overall absolute size, for example, HCA, the largest private hospital chain in this country, is able to penetrate individual markets and make selective investments with greater speed and surprise than are most of its smaller rivals. And it is able to use its size-related strengths to ward off threats from these competitors.

By contrast, relative power derives advantages from the concentration of resources within individual markets. Given its relative power (about a 40% market share), Orlando Regional is able to negotiate from strength for managed care contracts. And it is able to derive a number of other important advantages from its relative power, including system integration, a solidly established high-quality position, physician commitment, patient loyalty, and local supply-chain efficiencies. Orlando Regional's strengths in that market offset many of those attributable to the absolutely larger, but locally smaller HCA (with its two hospitals and roughly 7% share).

Similar advantages accrue to many other smaller (absolutely), but often dominating local systems across the country. As shown earlier in Table 14.1, it was the smaller, mostly not-for-profit systems that proliferated in that critically important period. And many of these now dominate their local markets, in large part because of the advantages attributable to relative size. (We note that the focus of antitrust enforcement on market dominance testifies to the importance of relative power, by contrast to absolute power, as a source of competitive advantage.)

Many systems combine absolute and relative power in various and often innovative ways. In its Denver, Kansas City, Richmond, and a number of other markets, HCA is a lead player that captures the advantages of both absolute and relative power. However, it has only one hospital in the Washington, DC, market, located in the suburb of Reston, and functions as a small, niched (suburban) player in that market. Triad, a large for-profit system, specializes in small sole-provider markets and thus draws upon overall company size as well as local monopoly power to derive competitive advantage. The Mayo Clinic in Rochester (a relatively small urban area) dominates its market as well as the surrounding nonurban markets, having established an extensive network of hospitals, clinics, and other services in that area. Sutter Health (mentioned earlier) and the Intermountain Health Care (headquartered in Salt Lake City) have expanded regionally to become a medium-sized system (in absolute size terms) that dominates their local urban are rural areas (relative power).

Power Strategies—Model Types

Four major power strategy models are commonly considered in the study of strategy:

Same Businesses

1. *Horizontal expansion*—expansion in the scale of existing business activities (e.g., the merger of two or more hospitals)

Different Businesses (also referred to as diversification)

2. *Vertical integration*—the combination and co-ordination of businesses that share input-output relationships (e.g., integrating hospital and managed care companies)

3. *Horizontal integration*—the combination and coordination of different types of businesses that are not vertically related (e.g., jointly managing hotel and hospital companies)

4. *Portfolio*—the combination and financial co-ordination of different types of businesses; the exclusive focus on financial is the primary difference between portfolio and horizontal integration

One should note that the term *horizontal* describes two different power strategies. The first, horizontal expansion, is a model in which integrative learning and scale advantages are captured by expanding within the same business area. The second, horizontal integration, draws on similar sources for advantage, but as a consequence of expanding and integrating across different types of business. Vertical integration, which is commonly identified as a separate business model, is in many respects a subset of horizontal integration since it involves the combination and integration of different types of business. The distinction is that vertical specifically and exclusively refers to the combination of businesses related to each other as buyers and sellers. Similarly, portfolio (or conglomerate-type model) could be seen as a subset of horizontal integration, since it involves the combination of different businesses. It is separately identified because of the lack of emphasis on interorganizational integration. In effect, each combined business within a portfolio model is run independently of one another, with the exception that corporations engaged in this business model approve and monitor the budgets of and move funds across the various owned businesses.

The portfolio model, which is very common outside of health care, is rarely found within the health care industry. Hillenbrand is a notable exception to this. Hillenbrand currently owns two companies—Hill-Rom, the leading supplier of bed and wall systems to the acute care sector, and Batesville Casket, a leading supplier to the funeral services industry. Hillenbrand does not integrate these two businesses, but does engage in corporate approvals, monitoring, and financial control over its operating companies.

Horizontal expansion is by far the most commonly pursued model in most industries, for obvious reasons. Expansion within one's own industry is usually the least risky approach to growth. Competitors understand their own businesses, know their competitors, understand the structures and competitive forces within their markets, and are generally well positioned to identify targets for acquisition and merger. The other three models, by contrast, take organizations into business arenas with which they are less likely to be familiar and, as a result, introduce them to greater risk than might be present if they were to grow through horizontal expansion. It is interesting that the health care industry seemed poised to move aggressively into vertical integration in the 1990s, based on vastly overstated assumptions about the interdependence between managed care payment and delivery (Conrad & Dowling, 1990; Conrad & Shortell, 1996; Enthoven, 1980; Mick, 1990; Mick & Conrad, 1988). Some health care companies did succeed with vertical integration, coming out of the 1990s, but most did not. Sentara and Intermountain Health Care did put together strong vertically integrated systems. Primarily hospital companies, these two and a few others built their own HMOs and invested in physician practices. IHC now even prefers to identify itself more as a vertically integrated than an exclusively service provider company. On its own Web site, for example, IHC emphasizes its integrative structure:

> IHC consistently ranks as the nation's top integrated health system. Integration means that doctors, hospitals, and health plans work together in a coordinated manner for the benefit of the patient.

In the past decade, vertical just seemed to make a lot of sense. From a policy perspective, full integration between managed care and provider systems offered the prospects that strong incentives for cost containment could be introduced. By placing provider services within HMOs, the presumed ideal vertical model, incentives would be created to minimize services since payment would be tied to anticipated rather than actual service provision. From a strategic perspective, vertical also seemed to be a logical business model. Health care providers and payment systems were highly interdependent, which meant that efficiencies would likely be captured if service provision were integrated within payment (managed care) systems. Such reasoning is fully consistent with the logic of exchange theory (Mick, 1990; Ouchi, 1977), which predicts organizational (vertical) integration when exchanges between buyers (in this case, managed care companies) and sellers (hospital, physician, and other provider organizations) become intense, complex, and uncertain. All of these conditions characterized managed care/provider exchanges moving into the 1990s, which contributed to the predictions that vertical models would proliferate in this industry.

However, vertical did not grow to the degree expected, for a variety of reasons. Importantly, consumers did not generally accept the restrictions on access associated with vertical models. Many providers, especially physicians, resisted integration. Vertical integration meant that physicians and hospitals would lose considerable autonomy, as they would become mere cost centers within managed care organizations if they were internalized within vertical systems. And they did not like the idea that many traditional provider/patient relationships would be broken, if patients were forced to select a managed care company that did not "own" the patients' particular doctors or hospitals.

By contrast, horizontal expansion succeeded far beyond expectations in the prior decade. Most significantly, hospitals joined systems as they sought to build unassailable positions of power within local markets in order to ward off the many threats they believed were present. The rush to horizontal

is clearly reflected in the numbers presented in Table 14.1, although buried within those numbers are some strategically very important models that need to be understood. We discuss these briefly in the next section.

Horizontal Expansion Models

It is important to understand some of the key model types that have evolved in the last few years, especially within the hospital sector. First, one should distinguish between horizontal expansion strategies pursued at **company-level strategy** versus **local-level strategy** levels. HCA has a horizontal strategy for its collective of hospitals nationally and individual horizontal strategies that it pursues within each of its local markets. In Denver, for example, HCA built up a seven-hospital system as a strategy for competing (horizontally) against two other strong system clusters in that market, Centura (five local hospitals) and Exempla (three local hospitals). We note that for many systems, these two levels of strategy—company and local market—are virtually the same. The Cleveland Clinic Health System, for example, covers only the Cleveland market and thus its company and its local market strategies are identical. (Note that half of the multihospital systems are single market companies and 90% of these are not-for-profit, the rest are either for-profit or Catholic systems.)

Second, horizontal expansion strategies, whether examined at the company or local levels, differ across systems in some additional important respects. We focus here on two strategically very important dimensions—size and pattern of spatial dispersion.

Clearly, system size is important strategically for many of the reasons already discussed. At the company level, multihospital systems range in size from 2 hospitals (37% of the systems) to nearly 200 (HCA being the largest). The ways in which these systems derive advantage differ significantly by how big they are. The large systems, for instance, are able to use overall mass to build advantage within local markets and to negotiate with suppliers. They also face many more challenges than do smaller systems in coordinating, standardizing, and creating appropriate organizational structures across their hospitals and markets. Small systems, on the other hand, will tend to intermingle company-level and local market strategies. Because of their small size, they are more likely to be influenced in their strategic thinking by local stakeholders, institutional constraints, and conflicts among individual hospitals and other provider entities.

At the local level, system size is best measured in relative terms, by the market shares individual competitors have attained within given markets. Systems that dominate their markets locally will tend to pursue competitive advantage differently than those that have much smaller local shares. Dominant systems, for example, will tend to offer full spectrums of services, ranging from the most complex tertiary care to primary care. And because of their relative mass, they will be relatively more able to negotiate from strength with both buyers and sellers, achieve desirable high-quality positions and attract top-quality health care manpower. More minor players locally will tend to build advantage through niching geographically (e.g., by dominating suburbs) and along selected service lines, partnering with larger competitors, and emphasizing quality.

In addition to size, horizontal strategies for hospital systems also differ greatly by the degree of **spatial dispersion**, at both the company and local levels. At the company level, more geographically clustered systems will tend to focus more on the interdependencies among their facilities. For example, they will tend to pursue market dominance, achieve allocative efficiencies in service distributions/offerings, integrate service delivery, build information networks, and negotiate from strength for local managed care contracts. More widely dispersed companies are less able to capture the advantages attributable to spatial proximities. They will tend to focus more on the traditional corporate concerns of standardization, monitoring, control, and management structures.

Given the importance of dispersion differences between health care companies, it is helpful to compare two systems that are about the same size, but differ dramatically by their relative dispersion. Two

medium-sized systems—Sutter Health and Catholic Health East—operate around 24 hospitals. But, Sutter is tightly clustered within the Northern California region—the average distance between each of Sutter hospitals and its corporate headquarters is about 71 miles—whereas Catholic Health East (CHE) is much more widely dispersed—the average distance for CHE hospitals is around 280 miles. These two very different dispersion patterns mean that these systems will likely pursue competitive advantages in distinct ways. Because of its regional concentration, Sutter will likely seek many of the advantages for tightly clustered models just mentioned—service rationalization and integration, information networking, consolidation, etc. Few of these advantages are available to the more dispersed Catholic Health East. Thus, CHE can be expected to concentrate strategy around individual facilities (e.g., niching, partnering with rivals, standardization, and focusing on organizational structuring) and regions where CHE might have more than one facility.

Dispersion patterns are also highly important at the local level. A pattern that is especially distinctive within the hospital sector is the degree to which the facilities are **hierarchically configured**. Over the last several decades, many large (and mostly not-for-profit) hospitals initiated local system development, resulting in systems that have a number of smaller hospitals, physician practices, ambulatory surgery centers, and other provider entities clustered around large, highly complex and visible referral centers. The result is a form of local horizontal expansion that is highly distinctive to the hospital sector—which might be called hierarchical or hub-spoke models (Fox, 1986). The joining of complex tertiary and quaternary service providers—the "hub" hospitals—with various levels of both general and specialized providers creates a kind of functional interdependency that few other model types are able to attain. Strategically, these distinctive model types not only tend to dominate their markets, they are potentially able, because of close geographic proximities and the logic interdependencies attributable to the hub-spoke design, to create comprehensive, integrated delivery arrangements. This configuration facilitates referral flows from spoke to hub, rationalization of service distributions (centralization of some services, dispersion of others), and most of the other advantages expected of geographically clustered hospital systems. It is very common for one or two examples of such models to be present in most urban markets. The two Memphis companies discussed earlier represent two hub-spoke models that compete head to head in a single market. Baptist Memorial Healthcare has 17 hospitals within the region that center around its 706-bed flagship hospital, Baptist Memorial Hospital–Memphis. Methodist Healthcare runs seven hospitals and other provider entities, all within the Memphis metropolitan area, that center around the flagship, Methodist University Hospital, a 696-bed referral and academic center.

Note that the urban and rural clusters vary considerably in the "steepness" of the hierarchical structure. Some are much flatter than is the case for the examples presented above, with only minor variations in size and complexities among the cluster members. Some combine very small hospitals and some very large hospitals. The New York City Health and Hospitals Corporation, for example, runs 11 acute care general hospitals in the New York area, most of which range well above 300 beds per hospital. And some local clusters are clumped very close together downtown or in a suburb and others are spread throughout a metropolitan area, even into nearby rural areas. Each of these spatial configurations offers different challenges and opportunities for how competitive advantage is gained. And, together, these models, as well as those that can be observed at the company level, illustrate the great diversity in approach to horizontal expansion that exists within the hospital sector.

CONCLUSION

It is important to remember that many of the models and strategic approaches to gaining competitive advantage discussed in this chapter are rather new to the health care field. Accordingly, many health care organizations might not have captured all of the advantages attributed to their particular business models and approaches to strategy. However, with time, it is likely that these organizations will become more and more experienced with system building and strategy and increasingly discover novel ways by which to extract competitive advantage from the particular systems they have created and given the unique features of their markets. They will also learn what they have to do to assure that any gained advantages are sustained over time.

Health care is a unique industry and, as such, competitors within this industry will pursue strategies in both similar and distinctive ways from those one might observe outside of health care. The strategy analyst must not only understand the concepts and approaches to strategy analysis, but be aware of how these might uniquely be applied to this most distinctive of industries. Health care strategists must learn how growing organizational size and complexity translate into advantage, how advantage is attained uniquely at local versus company levels, how company/corporate strategies interact with those at the local market level, how advancing technologies will be utilized to gain advantage, how timing and risk taking contribute to short- and long-term success, and how distinctive positions can offset advantages attributable to unassailable size and resources.

Further, the health care strategist must remember that while health care organizations are now deeply imbedded within competitive and strategically active environments, they have lost none of their obligations to serve community and individual needs. The health care strategist will need to find creative ways to balance mission against vision and assure the participation of diverse stakeholders in strategic decision making. These and many other needs place a high premium on health care leaders who combine knowledge and vision with a special understanding of the idiosyncrasies and expectations of this most important industry.

MANAGERIAL GUIDELINES

1. Develop a clear understanding of the concepts of and interrelationships among environmental forces, market structure, and strategy. The vagaries and indirections of market competition can only be understood if interpreted within the context of valid and workable conceptual frameworks. The strategy analyst must draw a number of conceptual frameworks that together address threats and opportunities in markets and the broader environment as well as strengths and weaknesses within individual organizations, including rivals.

2. Develop a clear understanding of what competitive strategy is and how it is pursued within the health care industry. Strategy is not the mere selection of business opportunities among those that have the best financials. Rather, it is the formulation of those concepts and ideas organizational leaders think will help them gain and sustain competitive advantage over their rivals. While all organizations pursue many kinds of strategies, competitive strategy is unique, given its focus on rivals and the pursuit of advantage. Competitive advantage is a relative concept; it contrasts one organization's gains in market power to gains attained by rivals. The five P's discussed in this chapter— power, pace, performance, potential, and positioning—summarize the means by which organizations gain competitive advantage relative to their rivals.

3. Develop a clear understanding of the important relationships between organizational structure, implementation capabilities, and strategy. While discussed only briefly in this chapter, a strategy analyst will ultimately be confronted with the challenge of creating an organizational structure and implementation strategy that will facilitate and sustain the objectives of intended and emergent strategies. This is especially important for complex organizations in which strategy often leads to the joining of multiple business units, and it may be even more important for a health care field that is becoming ever more integrated and elaborate. With the many interorganizational relationships that will need to be managed in the modern health care company, new structures and approaches to implementation may well become the lynchpin of a successful strategy. It will likely be of little value, for example, to visualize the strategic power of a regionalized health system if there is no way to bring physicians, partnering hospitals, and other health care providers into a unified whole. Structure and implementation skills could be the keys to unlocking the full potential of well-conceived strategies in the health care field.

4. Grasp the close linkage between strategic objectives and the public interest in health care. Strategy may well be the equivalent of an ill-shaped suit when fitted onto health care organizations charged with meeting the public interest. By its very nature, competitive strategy is self-serving and aggressive. Thus, most health care organizations will be confronted by the often-difficult question: "Does this strategy serve the community interest?" For example, while power strategies may prove very effective in assuring survival in highly competitive and

(continues)

MANAGERIAL GUIDELINES (continued)

oligopolistically structured hospital markets, they may not add to an objective of maximizing competition or generating innovation. A low-cost strategy may not prove to be in the best interests of patients whose lives hang in the balance of critical resource-allocation decisions. Or an aggressive expansion in health care business lines could simply add to the duplication of an already too costly health care system.

Strategy need not be in conflict with the public good. The pursuit of a power strategy in a local market could facilitate the integration of care across a fragmented delivery system, much-needed investments in IT, and a more rational distribution of service capacities among otherwise duplicative provider entities. Health care providers therefore operate in a unique environment in which there will inevitably exist a tenuous balance between public and private interests. In the

pursuit of advantage, health care strategists must carefully weigh how their decisions will impact the cost, quality, and accessibility of services provided to local populations and, in some cases, consider engaging in collaborative as opposed to more strictly competitive interactions with rivals.

5. Recognize that strategies considered to be ideal at one point in time might not be appropriate as time passes and markets and the environment change. Once commitments are made to particular strategic courses of action, risks become deeply immersed in strategic implementation and control at the expense of vigilance, learning, and adaptability to changing conditions and rationalities. Thinking while doing and doing while thinking should be the hallmark of effective strategy making, especially in a rapidly changing industry such as health care.

DISCUSSION QUESTIONS

1. Two very unique systems have made some similar, but very unusual moves. They are the Mayo Clinic (see In Practice on p. 459) and the Cleveland Clinic Health System (http://www.cchs.net). Both systems are centered around large, highly specialized, complex, highly prestigious, physician-centered hospitals/clinics. Both are in the Midwest. And, both have acquired facilities in the South (the Cleveland Clinic in Fort Lauderdale and Naples, FL, and Mayo in Jacksonville, FL, and Phoenix, AZ).

Despite their similarities, these two systems face very different market situations in their primary markets. Both dominate their

primary markets—Mayo controls approximately 87% of a small urban market (Rochester, MN, has a metropolitan population of about 170,000) and Cleveland Clinic has about a 40% market share in a very large market (Cleveland has a metropolitan population of about 2.2 million). Not counting its two locations in Florida, all of Cleveland Clinic's nine Ohio hospitals are in the Cleveland metropolitan area. Mayo has two large hospitals in Rochester and operates 15 hospitals and clinics in the surrounding nonurban areas in Iowa, Minnesota, and Wisconsin.

Review the In Practice material about the Mayo Clinic at the beginning of the chapter, review the Mayo and Cleveland Clinic Web sites, and then answer the following questions.

- How are differences in their primary markets likely to affect the strategies these two systems will pursue in and around those markets?
- How important do you think each of the five primary sources of competitive advantage—power, pace, position, performance, and potential—has been to each of these two systems in the recent past? In the future?
- What strategic rationale do you think led them to enter markets far to the south? Will this logic likely lead them to enter other distant markets? If so, into what types of markets might they enter, based on their unique sources of competitive advantage?
- Given their similarities in strategy and system type, is it reasonable to expect that these two systems will merge with one another in the future?

2. Now, look at the following three medium-sized health systems and compare these to one another and to the Mayo and Cleveland Clinic health systems:
   - St. Joseph Health System (*http://www.stjhs.org*) (an Orange County, CA-based Catholic system with facilities in Southern California, Northern California, Texas, and New Mexico).
   - Sutter Health (http://sutterhealth.org) (a Sacramento, CA-based not-for-profit system with facilities only in the Northern California area), and Iasis Healthcare (http://iasishealthcare.com) (a Nashville, TN-based for-profit system with facilities in Arizona, Florida, Nevada, Texas, and Utah).

   Given their differences as companies—in ownership type, system size, geographic dispersion patterns, sizes of hospitals, degree to which they dominate their local markets, sizes of the markets, involvement of physicians in leadership, ownership or not of clients, etc.—what role might the corporate headquarters for each of these five systems play in strategic decision making (i.e., the centralization of deci-

sion making regarding the formulation, funding, and control of competitive strategies for their individual hospitals and local hospital clusters)? What structural models might they use (across their system as a whole) to accomplish their strategic objectives? While all of these systems are in the same size range (11–20 hospitals), they differ in their ownership types. How might such differences affect how they pursue competitive advantage? How does mission factor into your assessments?

Look more closely at the facility locations for these systems and describe how their patterns of dispersion might affect how they each pursue competitive advantage.

How might these systems differ in how they use the five primary sources of competitive advantage—power, pace, position, performance, and potential—as bases for gaining competitive advantage?

3. Review the Web sites of the following four 6-hospital, not-for-profit systems:
   - Orlando Regional Healthcare (http://www.orlandoregional.org) (Orlando; average dispersion: 11 miles)
   - MedStar Health (http://www.medstarhealth.org) (Baltimore, Washington, DC; average dispersion: 27 miles)
   - Shands HealthCare (http://www.shands.org) (Gainesville, Jacksonville; average dispersion: 53 miles)
   - Baptist Healthcare System (http://www.bhsi.com) (Louisville and other markets in Kentucky; average dispersion: 79 miles)

   Compare and contrast the approaches each of these four systems might take in the pursuit of competitive advantage.

   How important is a hierarchical (hub-spoke) configuration to each of these systems?

REFERENCES

American Hospital Association. (1990). *Section for health care systems. Renewing the U.S. health care system.* Washington, DC: The Office of Constituency Sections.

American Hospital Association. (1992). *Overview: AHA's national reform strategy.* Chicago: American Hospital Association.

Andrews, K. R. (1971). *The concept of corporate strategy.* Homewood, IL: Irwin.

Ansoff, H. I. (1965). *Corporate strategy: An analytic approach to business policy for growth and expansion.* New York: McGraw-Hill.

Bain, J. S., & Qualls, D. (1987). *Industrial organization: A treatise,* (6), Part A. Greenwich, CT: JAI Press.

Barney, J. (1991). Firm resources and sustained competitive advantage. *Journal of Management, 17*(1), 99–120.

Barney, J. B. (2001). Resource-based theories of competitive advantage: A ten-year retrospective on the resource-based view. *Journal of Management, 27*(6), 643–650.

Catholic Health Association. (1992). *Setting relationships right: A working proposal for systemic healthcare reform.* St. Louis, MO: Catholic Health Association.

Chakravarthy, B. S. (1982). Adaptation: A promising metaphor for strategic management. *Academy of Management Review, 7*(3), 35–44.

Collis, D., & Montgomery, C. (1995). Competing on resources: strategy in the 1990s. *Harvard Business Review, 73*(4), 118–128.

Conrad, D. A., & Dowling, W. (1990). Vertical integration in health services: Theory and managerial implications. *Health Care Management Review, 15*(Fall), 9–33.

Conrad, D. A., & Shortell, S. M. (1996). Integrated health services: Promises and performance. *Frontiers of Health Services Management, 13*(1), 3–40.

Eisenhardt, K. M., & Martin, J. A. (2000). Dynamic capabilities: What are they? *Strategic Management Journal, 21*(10–11), 1105–1121.

Enthoven, A. C. (1980). *Health plan: The only practical solution to the soaring cost of medical care.* Boston: Addison-Wesley.

Foss, N. J. (1999). Research in the strategic theory of the firm: "Isolationism" and "integrationism." *Journal of Management Studies, 36*(6), 725–755.

Fox, D. M. (1986). *Health policies, health politics: The British and American experience, 1911–1965.* Princeton, NJ: Princeton University Press.

Ghemawat, P. (2001). *Strategy and the business landscape: Core concepts.* Upper Saddle River, NJ: Prentice-Hall.

Gluck, F. W., Kaufman, S. P., Walleck, A. S., & Steven, A. (1980, July/August). Strategic management for competitive advantage. *Harvard Business Review, 58*(5), 154–161.

Grant, R. (1998). The resource-based theory of competitive advantage: Implications for strategy formulation. In S. Segal-Horn (Ed)., *The strategy reader,* (pp. 179–199). Malden, MA: Blackwell.

Grant, R. M. (1991). Resource-based theory of competitive advantage: Implications for strategy formulation. *California Management Review, 33*(3), 114–136.

Harrigan, K. (1985). *Strategic flexibility: A management guide for changing times.* Lexington, MA: Lexington Books.

Henderson, B. D. (1979). *On corporate strategy.* Cambridge, MA: Abt Books.

Hill, C., & Jones, G. (1998). *Strategic management.* Boston: Houghton Mifflin Company.

Kotler, P., & Armstrong, G. (1996). *Principles of marketing* (7th ed.). Englewood Cliffs, NJ: Prentice Hall.

Lieberman, M. B., & Montgomery, D. B. (1998). First-mover (dis)advantages: Retrospective and link with the resource-based view. *Strategic Management Journal* (19) 1111–1125.

Lorange, P. (1980). *Corporate planning: An executive viewpoint.* Englewood Cliffs, NJ: Prentice-Hall.

Luke, R. D., Walston, S. L., & Plummer, P. M. (2003). *Healthcare strategy: In pursuit of competitive advantage.* Chicago: Health Administration Press.

MacMillan, I. C. (1984). Seizing competitive initiative. In R. Lamb (Ed), *Competitive strategic management* (pp. 272–296). Englewood Cliffs, NJ: Prentice-Hall.

Mahajan, V., & Wind, Y. (1988). Business synergy does not always pay off. *Long Range Planning, 21*(1), 59–65.

McCue, M. J., Clement, J. P., & Luke, R. D. (1999). Strategic hospital alliances do the type and market structure matter? *Medical Care, 37,* 1013–1022.

Mick, S. (1990). Explaining vertical integration in health care: An analysis and synthesis of transaction-cost economics and strategic management theory. In S. Mick (Ed), *Innovations in health care delivery: Insights for organization theory* (pp. 207–240). San Francisco: Jossey-Bass.

Mick, S. S., & Conrad, D. A. (1988). The decision to integrate vertically in health care organizations. *Hospital & Health Services Administration, 33*(3), 345–360.

Milgrom, P., & Roberts, J. (1995). Complementarities and fit: Strategy, structure, and organizational changes in manufacturing. *Journal of Accounting and Economics, 19*, 179–208.

Miles R. (1982). *Coffin nails and corporate strategies.* Englewood Cliffs, NJ: Prentice-Hall.

Miles, R. E., & Snow, C. C. (1978). *Organizational strategy, structure, and process.* New York: McGraw-Hill.

Mintzberg, H. (1978). Patterns in strategy formation. *Management Science, 24*(9), 934–948.

Mintzberg, H. (1990). Strategy formation: Schools of thought. In J. W. Fredrickson (Ed.), *Perspectives on strategic management* (Chapter 5). New York: Harper Business.

Mintzberg, H. (1994). *The rise and fall of strategic management: Reconceiving roles for planning, plans, planners.* New York: The Free Press.

Mintzberg, H. (1998). *Strategy safari: A guided tour through the wilds of strategic management.* New York: The Free Press.

Ouchi, W. G. (1977). Review of markets and hierarchies. *Administrative Science Quarterly, 22*, 541–544.

Parker, V., Charns, M., & Young, G. (2001, July). Clinical service lines in integrated delivery systems: An initial framework and exploration. *Journal of Healthcare Management, 46*(4), 261–276.

Peteraf, M. (1993). The cornerstones of competitive advantage: A resource-based view. *Strategic Management Journal, 14*(3), 179–191.

Peters, T., & Waterman, R. (1982). *In search of excellence.* New York: Harper and Row.

Porter, M. (1980). *Competitive strategy.* New York: The Free Press.

Porter, M. E. (1985). *Competitive advantage: Creating and sustaining superior performance.* New York: The Free Press.

Porter, M. E. (1996). What is strategy? *Harvard Business Review, 74*(6), 61–78.

Prahalad, C., & Bettis, R. (1986). The dominant logic: A new linkage between diversity and performance. *Strategic Management Journal, 485–501.*

Rothschild, W. E. (1984). Surprise and the competitive advantage. *The Journal of Business Strategy, 4*(3), 10–18.

Schendel, D., & Hofer, C. (1979). *Strategic management: A new view of business policy and planning.* Boston: Little Brown.

Scherer, F. M., & Ross, D. (1990). *Industrial market structure and economic performance.* Boston: Houghton Mifflin.

Shortell S. M., Morrison, E. M., & Friedman, B. (1990). *Strategic choices for America's hospitals: Managing change in turbulent times.* San Francisco: Jossey-Bass.

Teece, D. J., Rumelt, R. P., Dosi, G., & Winter, S. G. (1994). Understanding corporate coherence: Theory and evidence. *Journal of Economic Behavior and Organization, 23*, 1–30.

Walston, S., and Bogue, R. (1999). The effects of reengineering: Fad or competitive factor? *Journal of Healthcare Management, 44*(6), 456–476.

Walston, S., & Kimberly, J. R. (1997). Reengineering hospitals: Experience and analysis from the field. *Hospitals & Health Services Administration, 42*, 143–163.

Young, G. J., Charns, M. P., & Shortell, S. M. (2001, October). Top manager and network effects on the adoption of innovative management practices: A study of TQM in a public hospital system. *Strategic Management Journal, 22*(10), 935–951.

CHAPTER 15

Creating and Managing the Future

Arnold D. Kaluzny, Ph.D. and Stephen M. Shortell, Ph.D.

CHAPTER OUTLINE

- ⚜ The Organization and the Environment
- ⚜ Individuals and Groups within the Organization
- ⚜ The Managerial Role

LEARNING OBJECTIVES

After completing this chapter, the reader should be able to:

1. Identify the major trends likely to affect the delivery of health care.

2. Understand the changing role of physicians, nurses, and other health care professions.

3. Understand the changing role of management and the competencies required to function in the managerial role.

KEY TERMS

Community Care Networks
Disintermediation
Ethnic Composition
Evidence-Based Management
Evidence-Based Medicine
Future Scenarios
Hospitalist

Horizontal Integration
Just-in-Time Management
  (JIT)
Organizational Learning
Organized Delivery Systems
Pay-for-Performance
Social Experimentation

Social Norms and
  Expectations
Strategic Alliance
Technology Assessment
Value or Supply Chain
  Networks
Vertical Integration

❧ IN PRACTICE   Mrs. Dorothy Peterson

Mrs. Dorothy Peterson was a 72-year-old widow living alone. She had high blood pressure but was not compliant with her medication. On February 1, she was found unconscious in her apartment and was taken to the emergency room of the local hospital. The ER conducted its first assessment, asked her niece to provide Mrs. Peterson's advanced directives and within a few hours, she was transferred to the hospital's medical unit with a diagnosis of stroke. Her niece indicated that the advanced directives were given to the hospital during a prior elective admission.

The medical unit conducted a second assessment and developed the first nursing plan. Mrs. Peterson progressed nicely and soon was transferred to the rehabilitation unit where a third assessment was conducted and a second nursing plan developed. Staff found no cognitive impairment but some neuromuscular weakness, which needed intense therapy.

While in the rehabilitation unit, Mrs. Peterson developed a urinary tract infection, was readmitted to the nursing unit, where still another assessment and nursing plan were developed. Three days later, she was discharged to a home care program, where yet another assessment was conducted. Mrs. Peterson had no children, so she went to live with her niece because she needed assistance between the visits by home health staff. The care plan developed by the staff included instructing her niece on how to care for Mrs. Peterson.

Two weeks later, she was readmitted to the ER with an elevated temperature and dehydration, where she received her sixth assessment and was admitted to the medical unit. In the medical unit, she was again evaluated and received another nursing plan. At this point, staff again asked her niece about Mrs. Peterson's advance directives. Her niece replied that she had already submitted that information during four previous assessments.

Two days later, Mrs. Peterson was discharged to Beacon Nursing Home and received her eighth assessment and sixth nursing care plan. On the fourth day at the nursing facility, she complained of shortness of breath, and was readmitted to the emergency room, where, despite all efforts, personnel were unable to resuscitate her, and Mrs. Peterson was pronounced dead. It was never clear to her niece if Mrs. Peterson's advance directives had been available to ER staff during this last admission.

During these 38 days, Mrs. Peterson experienced a caring staff, state of the art technology, along with eight assessments, six nursing care plans, eight admissions, 14 attending physicians, and 24 separate bills totaling over $200,000, of which only $60,000 were reimbursed.

SOURCE: Adapted from the video "Mrs. Dorothy Peterson, A Care Study." Permission granted by Advocate Healthcare. Available from Terra Nova Films 1-800-779-8491 http://www.terranova.org

DEBATE TIME 15.1   What Do You Think?

Scenario 1: Business as Usual

Health care policy vacillates between marketplace fixes and government intervention. Costs remain on an upwardly sloped roller coaster. Gains in managing chronic disease and decreasing disability at the end of the lifespan (Fries, 2003; Singer & Manton, 1998) are crowded out by growing obesity among children and aging baby boomers (Sturm, Ringel, & Andreyeva, 2004). Consumer information and choice grow but overwhelm many individuals (Stone, 2004). Health care quality improves, but challenges remain (McGlynn, et al, 2003), particularly in long-term care (IOM, 2001). The number of uninsured increases and the disparities in care among racial and ethnic groups persist (Kressin & Petersen, 2001; IOM, 2002).

Scenario 2: Hard Times/Government Pressured

Recurrent hard times and a revolt by the states against their rising burden of health care costs for the poor and uninsured (Hoadley, Cunningham, & McHugh, 2004) threaten the health care system. After programs to provide health care for children and long-term care for the elderly and disabled are frozen by the states, the federal government is forced to provide relief. A more frugal national health system is the result. Some successful innovations emerge during the transition, and a national information infrastructure is implemented at last (Thompson & Brailer, 2004). But, those who can afford to often choose to "buy-up" to affluent, higher tech care. Ethical issues related to access to care, particularly for terminal patients, persist.

Scenario 3: Health Care as an Economic Development Issue

Tying health care coverage to employment becomes recognized as a drag on the development of a flexible, responsive workforce able to compete in a global economy (Clinton, 2004). Employer coalitions push for development of coverage that is more independent of the workplace and predictable in cost (Mercer, 2003). Employees and retirees want an affordable system that allows them to maintain relationships with trusted providers. The resulting reforms resemble a mutual insurance system. But the transition to the system is rocky. How to finance care for those who cannot afford it is a major and continuing political issue as the baby boomers retire (Daniels, 2002). Public health initiatives and biomedical research get sidelined in the ensuing debate over personal coverage.

Scenario 4: Health Care as a Shared Vision

The 15 years before 2015 are a time of vision and design for health care. Health care providers, government, and the individuals and communities they serve join together to develop a powerful, shared vision. A unifying theme for that vision is caregiving across the generations. Goals are set for health care that transcend both organizational allegiances and political cycles (IOM, 2002). Ethical issues, such as end-of-life care for the victims of Alzheimer's disease, are addressed in the context of caring communities (Beauchamp, 1999).

SOURCE: Leak, 2004

CHAPTER PURPOSE

Like so many, Mrs. Peterson is a victim of the system. How might this have been prevented? Better technology? More caring people? Perhaps, but clearly the structure within which care is provided influences the provision of care; this, in turn, is dependent on larger secular trends. Four **future scenarios** are presented in Debate Time 15.1 that may influence whether Mrs. Peterson is an isolated event or a constant reminder of a delivery system with fundamental problems (Leak, 2004). It is likely that elements of each scenario will combine to influence the future provision of health services.

A number of forces will play a key role in the emerging health care system. This chapter begins by considering changes likely to occur in the organization and its environment, discusses the future of individuals and groups within organizations, and ends with consideration of the managerial role. The intent is to be provocative yet realistic, building on issues developed in preceding chapters. A central theme is that health services organizations and their leaders can actively influence their environment and thereby create and actively manage their future, and if past is prologue "nothing is written."

THE ORGANIZATION AND THE ENVIRONMENT

Health services organizations, functioning as corporate actors, are the major repository of power within health services. Health care expenditures represent a significant percentage of the gross national product (GNP), and as federal and state governments and major employers continue to be major purchasers of care, the influence of health services corporate actors will increase. The collective decisions of individual hospitals, multihospital systems, alternative delivery systems, nursing home chains, regulatory groups, suppliers, insurance companies, public health agencies, and other corporate actors within the health services field will significantly affect the basic structure and characteristics of services provided.

Health care organizations have been described as operating in and affected by an increasingly complex and unpredictable environment, an environment characterized by the difficulty of predicting both the occurrence and content of change (Stefl, 1999; Zuckerman, 2002). For example, decisions about health care may in fact be made on factors quite independent of the substantive issues involved with health care. Specifically, as health services consume greater portions of the gross national product, their effects on other sectors of the economy are pervasive. Thus, other criteria, such as local employment or employment in a variety of other support ancillary areas, become important criteria affecting decisions within health services.

Along with increasing complexity and unpredictability of the environment will come a demand for greater organizational responsiveness and accountability from different groups. The organization will face the problem of reconciling incompatible objectives. For example, the federal government often defines accountability in terms of cost control, while local consumer groups may see accountability in terms of added facilities and services and greater consumer participation in decision making. In short, the future involves major issues centering on the organization's ability to adapt to divergent demands. This effort will require innovation, the ability to manage external dependencies, and at the same time the ability to learn and restructure relationships. Yet perhaps much of this uncertainty may be overestimated, and compared to the environments of other industries may be fairly certain and predictable (Begun & Kaissi, 2004). Consider some of the major trends and their implications.

Changing Social Norms and Expectations

The underlining **social norms and expectations** are important guides to behavior within health services, and changing norms and expectations will serve to shape the fundamental questions and issues that will guide the public policy debate regarding the future character of health services. Questions of access, quality, safety, and accountability will continue to play a central role and be shaped by fundamental norms and expectations and can no longer be ignored. Moreover, the added burden of preparedness to deal with community disasters in a post–9/11 environment will have profound implications for the management of health service organizations. As described by the IOM report *Crossing the Quality Chasm,* (Chassen, et al., 1998) "the burden of harm conveyed by the collective impact of all our health care quality problems is staggering." As a society, we have valued equality of access and opportunity as well as placing a great deal of emphasis on individualism. It is unlikely that the future will see a resolution of all of our quality problems or a resolution between the underlying values of universal access to quality health care, preparedness, and individual freedom.

Imposed upon these underlying values is the growing need for accountability and the recognition that accountability must include both clinical and financial criteria. Simply holding down costs without paying attention to the quality of services provided the impact on patient health status and overall preparedness of the organization is unacceptable. The new accountability will emphasize value—the relationship between quality, cost, and preparedness or between benefit, cost, and preparedness that meets the needs, demands, and expectations of the purchaser, the consumer, and the larger community. The new accountability, however, will place a significant burden on provider and regulatory organizations as well as insurance carriers as they try to track prevention, treatment, and outcomes as well as manage and assess risk within a post–9/11 environment. The greater the account-

ability the more likely the choice of provider will be limited since plans or provider organizations will only reimburse providers meeting accountability criteria (Weinstein, 1998). The level and focus of accountability are not clear. Most likely the country will evolve toward a system of shared accountability involving the private and public sector at multiple levels requiring the active participation and dialogue among many parties, many of which have not heretofore been involved.

The particular configuration is likely to be influenced by three emerging trends:

- *Health care as a political issue*—While the intersection of politics and health is not new, the late 1990s signaled the dramatic shift prompting one observer to comment, "something new is happening in Washington—Congress is practicing medicine." Policy is increasingly being shaped by political personnel and special-interest groups rather than objective scientific inquiry. (U.S. House of Representatives Committee on Government Reform, 2003). Issues involving stem cell research, contraceptive technology, health care disparities, and end-of-life decisions are likely to be the primary focus in the years ahead. As health care and medical technology become more important to an aging population, and the population has access to politicians, it is likely that evidence-based decisions are increasingly likely to be influenced by political as well as scientific judgment.

- *Deprofessionalization of the medical care process*—In order to meet the challenges of accountability, competition, preparedness, and health services have increasingly taken on the characteristics of industrial organizations. This is really *part of a larger trend* to redefine health care as a commercial as well as professional activity (Hurley, 1998). Through this redefinition, health care has assumed the characteristics of industrial-type organizations with "product lines," "medical loss ratios," "finder fees" for terminally ill patients requiring hospice care, and "direct to consumer advertising"—to illustrate just a few of the challenges underlying the principles of patient care (Glasser, 1998). It will also require the medical profession to share accountability with numerous other groups including payers, consumers, and the community (Shortell, Waters, Clarke, & Budetti, 1998).

- *System change through litigation*—The commercialization of health services has resulted in the emergence of litigation or threat of litigation as a force in shaping business strategy and market behavior of health care providers (Bloche & Studdert, 2004). While a great deal of attention has been given to "tort reform" within the context of medical malpractice, the potential of class action litigation has been underestimated. Legal conflict and the potential for adverse outcomes are likely to influence business strategies in the future, particularly as they affect the future implementation of aggressive cost management strategies.

Demographic Composition and Epidemiology

Managing the future requires a thorough understanding of the evolving demographics and epidemiological characteristics of the population. For example, it is estimated that 125 million Americans have at least one chronic disease (e.g., heart disease, diabetes, asthma, etc.) and 50% of these have more than one condition. The care and treatment of these individuals represents three-fourths of the total U.S. health care expenditures (Lopez, 1997). Equally significant is the changing character of the population, and specifically, the increase in the percentage of elderly people in the population. The proportion of the total population composed of those 65 and over is expected to increase in all states. Over a 30-year period, California and Florida would continue to rank first and second respectively in having the largest number of elderly. By 2025, Texas will rank number three, passing New York and Pennsylvania, and Florida is expected to be the "oldest" state with more than 26% of its population age 65 or older. In fact, the number of elderly is projected to more than double in the United States between 2000 and

2050 from 35,061,000 to 86,705,000 people (U.S. Census Bureau, 2004).

Equally important for managing the future is the racial and **ethnic composition** of the population. Two groups of particular importance that will affect our ability to manage the future are African Americans and Hispanic Americans. Both groups currently remain outside the mainstream of health services and will greatly challenge the ability of the health system in the future. It is expected that African Americans will grow as a percentage of the population from 12.7% in 2000 to 14.6% in the year 2050. Today, the Hispanic American population is equal to the African American population; by the year 2050 the Hispanic population is projected to surpass the African Americans to reach 24.4% of the population. Both groups will represent the youngest part of the population requiring services that are fundamentally different from those required by the elderly portion of the population (U.S. Census Bureau, 2004).

The demands of the population will be further reflected in the epidemiological trends of the population. Diseases of aging, lifestyle, and behavior will present major challenges to the delivery system. Heart disease and cancer are the top two causes of death and they will remain causes of death in the twenty-first century. However, age-adjusted reductions in mortality occurred for both heart disease and cancer in 2002 (Kochanek & Smith, 2004) and for the first time cancer has surpassed heart disease as the most common cause of death among Americans younger than 85 (Associated Press, 2005). The reduction in heart disease mortality is consistent with a downward trend since 1950; cancer mortality has followed a downward trend only since 1992 and then stabilized in 1995 with a slight increase. African Americans and people of low socioeconomic status have the highest rate of both new cancer and cancer deaths (National Cancer Institute, 2003, American Cancer Society, 2005). It is estimated that in the United States, men have a 1 in 2 lifetime risk of developing cancer, and for women it is 1 in 3. The cancer rate is anticipated to double from 1.3 million people in 2000 to 2.6 million in 2050 (National Cancer Institute, 2002). In 2003 there were 1,334,000 Americans diagnosed with cancer. Based on trends 63% are expected to survive for at least five years after diagnosis (National Cancer Institute, 2003).

Alzheimer's disease (AD) will also present major challenges to the system as the population increases in age. In 2001 and 2002 AD was the eighth leading cause of death. The number of patients in nursing homes with AD was 231,900 in 1999, and they represented 14.2% of the nursing home population. The average length of stay for residents with AD is 620 days (National Center for Health Statistics, 2004a). It is projected that by 2015 there will be 2.9 million Americans who will have some form of the disease (Ernst & Hay, 1994). Medicare expenditures are three times higher for patients with AD. In ten years Medicare costs will increase by 55% to $50 billion (Alzheimer's Association, 2004).

Diseases of lifestyle and behavior will present the most difficult challenges to the health services system. Perhaps most traumatic will be the continued toll taken by acquired immune deficiency syndrome (AIDS). Not even listed as a leading cause of death in 1985, the human immunodeficiency virus (HIV) was the eighth leading cause of death in 1995. As of 2002, HIV was not in the top 15 causes of death (it has dropped to 23) for deaths of people of all ages. However, for people ages 24 to 44, HIV is the fifth significant cause of death (National Center for Health Statistics, 2004b). The cost in human suffering is immeasurable, and the lifetime medical expenses associated with AIDS treatment are estimated to be more than $195,000 per person (Kahn, Pinkerton, & Holtgate, 2002).

In the past twenty years, behavior, environment, and genetic factors have created a major epidemic in obesity in the United States. Indicators suggest that the problem will worsen in the future. According to the Nutrition Examination Survey in 1999–2000, 64% of U.S. adults are either overweight or obese—body mass index (BMI) of 25 or more. Since 1970, the percentage of children and teens that are overweight has doubled and now 15% are overweight. All adults with a BMI of 25 or more are at risk for premature death and disability, and these risks increase with the severity of obesity. The prevalence of obesity in adults climbed from 19.8% to 20.9% between 2000 and 2001 and diagnosis of diabetes increased from 7.3% to 7.9% during that same period. These increases occurred in every population group, regardless of gender, race, age, or educational background. Obesity prevalence in adults among U.S. states is the highest in Mississippi, West Virginia, Michigan, Kentucky, and Indiana (listed in order from first to fifth) (National Center for Chronic Disease Prevention and Health Promotion, 2004).

Technology Development, Assessment, and Outcomes

Technology development in both treatment, prevention, and early-detection activities will continue to have a major impact on health services in the future. Such developments will raise questions involving the very development and use of the technology, who will have access to new technological developments, to what degree the decision to use new technology will be centralized, what effect new technology will have on provider-patient relationships, and what new ethical considerations must be considered (Thompson & Brailer, 2004).

In addition, it is likely that the use of complementary and alternative medical practices will expand and have an impact on health services. For example in 2002, 36% of U.S. adult aged 18 years and older used some form of complementary or alternative medicine including chiropractic, homeopathy, and diet-based therapies. When prayer specifically for health reasons is included the number of U.S. adults using some form of complementary and alternative practices increased to 63%. Interestingly, 28% used complementary and alternative methods because they believed that the conventional methods would not help their particular health problem. This is in contrast to previous findings that users of conventional and alternative methods were not dissatisfied with conventional medicine (Barnes, Powell-Griner, McFanne, & Nahin, 2004).

IN PRACTICE — "Personalized Medicine" Can Help Patients and Drug Firms

Biotech giant Genentech barely had time to rejoice over the promising result of a new cancer drug trial before a Wall Street analyst shot out an alert that would have popped the balloons at many firms. The experimental drug Taceva, the analyst told investors, may actually help as few as a tenth of lung cancer patients. A pending diagnostic study could identify that smaller groups of individual who have an abnormal gene. And that could mean Tarceva might not be a huge seller for Genetech, he said.

A few days later however, when a scientist in Boston did unveil that genetic analysis, there was fresh jubilation at Genentech instead of gloom. "What a great week!" said Dr. Susan Hellmann, Genetech's president of product development.

Hellmann's reaction might mystify executives at other drug companies. The prospect of a possible blockbuster drug being reduced to a modest niche product is exactly what worries some executives about the research approach that is called "personalized medicine," pharmacogenomics or molecular diagnostics. But Genentech is part of a growing movement of drug developers who are betting that the interplay of diagnostic and drug design will yield across-the-board gains for patients, insurance companies, and pharmaceutical firms. As described by Dr. Hellmann "Diagnostics can both reduce the cost of drug development and allow health insurance companies to offer better patient care at a lower cost." While the challenges are great "We're starting to have a menu of therapies that can be aligned with a menu of diagnostics. . . . That's the kind of thing that could change the world."

SOURCE: Bernadette Tansey. (2004). *San Francisco Chronicle.*

New developments will change our paradigm of disease and health. The paradigm of diagnosis and treatment will be replaced by one of prediction and early-stage management of the illness. The availability of genetic testing presents great possibilities for saving lives through prevention, early detection, and treatment. It also raises important questions concerning the psychological consequences this knowledge presents for individuals and their families as well as questions of privacy and confidentiality. Similarly, the evolving ability to measure genes and proteins and thus the potential of developing personalized medicine in which patients' risks and preferences are used to choose diagnostic and therapeutic strategies will have profound implications for the health services delivery system (Califf, 2004).

New developments in prevention, early detection, and health-promotion activities will have similarly important implications, particularly as they are implemented in health care delivery systems involving defined populations. Although not as dramatic or as heroic as the basic technological development described above (see In Practice), significant progress is occurring in the control of hypertension, coronary disease, cancer, and certain disabling forms of mental illness. For example, biomarkers and chemoprevention agents—such as the breast cancer prevention agents, tamoxifen and raloxifene, for women at increased risk of developing breast cancer—are important developments having profound implications on the health services system.

Moreover, increasing attention will be given to the role of social factors in determining health. Despite significant improvements in overall health status and an impressive technology, there exists significant—in fact, embarrassing—variation in health status among social groups (Amick, Levine, Tarlov, & Walsh, 1995). Unequal distribution of social resources and well-being are fundamental determinants of health and disease. Emphasizing the role of social determinants of health provides an opportunity to develop and implement more effective social and public health interventions for population-based health improvement. Many of these initiatives will be outside the traditional health community, involving industry, education, and other nonhealth personnel, and have a significant impact on overall health status.

Developments of both conventional and alternative treatments as well as preventive and health-promotion strategies will be accompanied by greater concern for assessment of costs and efficacy. Increasingly, attention will be given to outcomes and the development of evidence-based disease management—that is, an approach to care that emphasizes coordinated, comprehensive care along the continuum of disease and across health care providers in which the approach to practice integrates patho-physiological rational, caregiver experience, and patient preferences with valid and current clinical research evidence (Ellrodt et al., 1997).

Organizational Arrangements

While evolving social norms and expectations, demography, epidemiology, and technologies will affect organizational arrangements, the very nature of the organizations themselves and their interactions will affect the management challenges of the future. New organizational forms will be developed, and existing forms will change, forging new relationships with other organizations in the environment. In the world of health services, a great deal of attention has been given to the configuration of service-delivery organizations transcending existing organizational entities. While both **vertical** and **horizontal integration** represent interorganizational efforts, to be more responsive to changing environmental conditions, the unrelenting demand of cost containment, improving quality, and assuring technology transfer and accountability, will force managers to increasingly consider other forms of organizational arrangements. These include the development of **organized delivery systems** (Shortell et al., 1996), **community care networks** (Weiner & Alexander, & Shortell, 1998) and employer-sponsored delivery systems, or more loosely coupled **strategic alliances** such as joint ventures, purchasing coalitions (Satinsky, 1997), alliances to facilitate the transfer of state-of-the-art technology to local communities (Kaluzny, Warnecke, et al., 2001; Lamb, Greenlick, & McCarty, 1998), and perhaps in the future **value or supply-chain networks** (Burns & Wharton School Colleagues, 2002). The latter form is a widely accepted configuration among industrial organizations involving a virtual network of organizations involved with the production of a product. While this is a very emergent concept in health services, it is likely to receive increased attention in the years ahead.

The watchword among many of these configurations has been *integration*. While a growing percentage of health care organizations and providers of various types participated in these arrangements throughout the 1990s, there is now evidence suggesting that the particular structure affects financial performance of the participating hospitals. Hospitals in health systems that had a unified ownership generally had better financial performance than hospitals in a contractually based health network. Among network hospitals, highly centralized network had better financial performance than decentralized networks. Hospital networks or systems with little differential or centralization experience the poorest performance (Bazzoli, Chan, et al., 2000).

Particular attention needs to be given to the growth of specialty hospitals. (See Debate Time 15.2). The growth of these niche hospitals has been

⚜ DEBATE TIME 15.2   What Do You Think?

For nearly 20 years, Dr. Bruce E. Murphy, a cardiologist and the son of a Baptist minister, has admitted patients to hospitals operated by Baptist Health, the dominant hospital system in Little Rock, Arkansas. In February, he received a letter from Baptist Health saying it might end his hospital privileges.

Dr. Murphy recalled thinking, "It's not a very Christian thing to do, is it?"

But religion, or health care for that matter, is not really the main issue. Dr. Murphy is one of the doctors with an ownership stake in a nearby competitor, the Arkansas Heart Hospital, where he also serves as medical director and where he sends many of his patients. And after seven years of watching Arkansas Heart vie for patients, Baptist Health, the largest health care organization in the state, is warning Little Rock's cardiologists that to invest in the competing hospital could mean no longer treating patients at a Baptist Health hospital.

Hospitals argue that the doctors are threatening their viability by skimming off the most profitable cases, while leaving the hospitals with too many of the patients least able to pay their bills or those whose complicated conditions run up high expenses. They say the doctor's primary interest is in specialties like cardiac care or orthopedics that make the most money—specialized treatment that community hospitals say they need to provide to subsidize other services, like trauma care, that lose money.

The doctors say, in turn, that as free agents they should be allowed to practice at any hospital they choose. And they warn patients—whose choice of hospital may already be narrowed by the terms of their health care coverage—have the most to lose in any battle over where they should go to get care. The doctors, meanwhile, run the risk of having patients go to another physician if they no longer have privileges at a variety of hospitals in some communities.

The doctors' aggressive pursuit of new sources of profit is largely a result of financial pressure caused by climbing expenses and shrinking payments from insurers. Doing an MRI in the office, rather than sending a patient to the hospital, can shift hundreds of insurance dollars to a doctor. And when doctors have ownership stake in a surgery center or specialty hospital, they share in any profits from facility fees in addition to the professional fees they charge for seeing patients there. A majority of the nation's 4,000 or so ambulatory surgery centers are owned by doctors.

More than money is at stake. As more doctors focus on new ventures—and spend more time in the office to maintain their incomes—many are less willing to volunteer their time in emergency rooms or hospital committee meetings. That kind of involvement has traditionally been expected of doctors who have privileges at a hospital, allowing them to admit and treat patients there.

Many hospitals and doctors say they still need one another. Community hospitals depend on doctors to admit the patients that fill their beds. Doctors want to be able to satisfy a patient's medical needs and preferences—and, sometimes, the patient's insurance requirements—by having ready access to community hospitals.

What do you think? How do you see this development evolving in the future?

SOURCE: Adapted from Abelson (2004, April 13). Barred as rivals, doctors see some hospitals in court. *The New York Times,* Business Section.

driven by physicians who have been dissatisfied with the operations of the more traditional community hospitals. Orthopedic and cardiovascular surgeons have been the leading proponents and have demonstrated considerable success in establishing specialty hospitals in noncertificate of need states (Cain Brothers, 2003). The challenge to existing providers is whether it is to their advantage to oppose the emergence of the specialty hospital or partner with the physicians involved and pursue mutual interests.

While these alliances are not unique to health services, they are clearly different organizational forms from those historically characterizing health services and thus, in profound ways, will change how existing health care organizations operate. Emphasis is given to the interaction process in which there is a constant exchange of products, information, money, and social symbols with the emphasis being on interaction and interdependency on each other in various ways in an effort to "customize" services to meet the demands and expectations of patients and defined population groups (McLaughlin & Kaluzny, 1997). Clearly these are fragile and emerging relationships with the critical challenge being the way management deals with the issues of commitment, control, performance, communication, information, and participation over time.

While health services organizations—particularly hospitals, integrated health networks/systems, and health departments—have prided themselves on their self-sufficiency, the push for efficiency will force attention to new configurations among providers, suppliers, and vendors. Vendors and suppliers are no longer simply providing equipment and supplies. For example, in addition to purchasing GE medical imaging equipment, hospitals are also purchasing GE's widely used industrial productivity enhancing, cost-cutting methodology known as Six Sigma (Gabor, 2004). Six Sigma is a statistical measure that refers to the goal of reducing errors and when applied to a health care setting is a technique for improving patient care and reducing cost. Further experimentation with subcontracting and outsourc-

ing functions to other organizations in the community includes **Just-in-time management (JIT)**, in which organizations can benefit from synchronizing inventory with workflow needs, and outsourcing of functions, which has traditionally been part of normal operations. This and other arrangements are just a few of the opportunities to realize efficiencies once thought impossible.

Equally important will be physician alignment with various forms of delivery organizations and their acceptance of various evidence-based management practices to improve quality and reduce cost. The managerial challenge will be to achieve the appropriate balance between involvement and autonomy among the various participants, particularly the physicians involved (Shortell, Alexander, et al., 2001).

Equally significant are changes taking place in major federal organizations such as the Center for Disease Control and Prevention (CDC) and the National Institutes of Health (NIH). These changes will have important implications for the provision of health services at the local, state, and national level. (See Chapter 8 for a description of the ongoing changes at the CDC.)

Both the CDC and NIH are undergoing change to improve their ability to respond to health care challenges and provide a better link to the provider organizations. The NIH through its Roadmap initiative is an attempt to engage the various institutes in dialogue and develop cross-cutting areas of research transcending the respective institutes. The objective being to achieve integration among the respective institutes such that the whole will be greater than the sum of the parts as well as provide an effective mechanism to be able to translate improved science and technology to improving the health status of the population (Zerhouni, 2003).

The CDC through its Futures Initiative shares a similar objective and has launched a significant reorganization to increase its ability to respond to public health challenges and to improve health impact. The reorganization involves a realignment of various units and functions in a way that will enhance the ability of the CDC to develop partnerships and alliances with other public health agencies, provide a coordinated and integrated set of programs to improve the impact of the services provided, and assure a more effective utilization of available resource (CDC, 2004) (See Chapter 8, In Practice, p. 238).

Financing

The changing demographics and epidemiology and new organizational forms will put added stress on the financing of health services and the manner in which providers are reimbursed. Major segments of the population continue to be without health insurance coverage, and health care expenditures consume a significant portion of the gross national product. For example, throughout the entire 2002 calendar year, an estimated 43.3 million people in the United States (17.3% of the population) were without health insurance—an increase by 2.4 million people from 2001 despite the existence of programs such as Medicaid and Medicare. While most people were covered by private insurance (68% in 2002), the fact that most private insurance is employment-based means that any increase in the unemployment rate would increase the percentage of the population without health insurance, presenting significant stress on provider reimbursement (The Kaiser Commission on Medicaid and the Uninsured, 2003).

Health care expenditures climbed to $1.6 trillion in 2002 accounting for 14.9% of the gross national product (GNP) or $5,440 per person. The increase was twice the rate of growth of the GNP (3.6%). When adjusted for inflation constant dollar growth rose 7.1% per capita in 2002 compared to 4.9% annual growth over the past decade. Hospital spending accounted for nearly a third of the aggregate increase (Levit, Smith, et al., 2004).

Several initiatives are underway that will have important implications for the financing and reimbursement of health services. The increasing visibility that the United States is the only industrialized country (with the exception of South Africa)

that does not guarantee financial access to health care for all of its citizens has resulted in a growing interest, at both national and state levels, in expanding financial access to assure a basic set of benefits for all Americans, or at least segments of the population (e.g., mothers and children, and elderly). Major considerations in developing such a program are what benefits should be considered basic, what the benefits will cost, how they should be financed, and what incentives should be developed for the delivery system to provide cost-effective care in meeting the increased demand.

Moreover, in the unrelenting effort to contain costs, Medicare will allow a wider range of private health care plans to enroll beneficiaries, and states who manage the Medicaid program will continue to move in similar directions. These approaches will offer a wide choice of health care plans to beneficiaries, but, at the same time, provide an opportunity for these programs to operate with a stake in controlling costs. One consequence of this may be cost-shifting and care-shifting responsibilities to other institutions—mainly the families under the rubric of "consumer-driven health care." For example, shorter hospital stays and limited nursing home care benefits require that care be shifted to the responsibility of family units. Families who already share a significant burden in terms of child-rearing responsibilities, as well as both husband and wife working, present a significant challenge. Thus, while the cost may be contained within health services, the cost to other institutions within our society may be significant.

As the percentage of gross national product devoted to health spending grows, and as health premiums increase, continued pressures will be placed on accountability, cost-cutting and cost-shifting initiatives as well as interest in implementing **pay-for-performance** systems to reward providers for delivering high-quality care and motivating quality improvement (Epstein, Lee, & Hamel, 2004).

At present, a number of prototypical models are operational, including the Centers for Medicare and Medicaid Services and Premier Inc. demonstration projects involving a network of not-for-profit hospitals (http://www.cms.hhs.gov.) in which bonuses are provided to hospitals based on performance involving the treatment of heart attack, heart failure, pneumonia, coronary artery bypass surgery, and hip and knee replacement for Medicare recipients. In California the Integrated Health Care Association is working with over 200 medical groups and seven health plans in which the plans pay the groups quality bonuses based on achieving various quality measures including immunization rates, chronic illness quality targets, patient satisfaction, and use of information technology. (http://www.chcf.org) The Bridges to Excellence Program (http://www.bridgestoexcellence.org/), which involves a group of large employers in Boston, Cincinnati/Louisville, and Albany/ Schenectady, provide financial incentives for physicians to improve care and practice. Under the program physicians receive prorated bonuses for meeting target goals involving office practice that reduce error and increase quality and in meeting set criteria in the care of diabetic and cardiac patients. These and a number of other programs are in operation. The emergent interest in pay-for-performance systems (see Chapter 3) is likely to grow in the years ahead (Rosenthal et al., 2004).

Given the movement to redefine health care as a commodity, larger purchasers "want the healthcare industry (under whatever configuration) to cut costs—(yet improve quality), *the way the rest of corporate American has done*" [italics added] (Winslow, 1998). This expectation will force clinicians and health services managers to work together more closely to figure out at what point in the continuum of patient care the greatest value is added. Increasingly, this will be in outpatient settings, in the workplace, and in homes. As noted later, it will involve fundamental transitions in managerial roles.

Social Experimentation, Evaluation, and Learning

Social experimentation, evaluation, and learning will extend beyond **technology assessment** to encompass a wide variety of new approaches, programs, and organizations for delivering more cost-effective health care. The demands for greater accountability under an environment of constrained resources will push the health care system further in the direction of Campbell's classic "experimenting society," in which new demonstration programs are rigorously evaluated. Emphasis will be placed not only on results but also on the process by which the results are obtained and the ability to link this knowledge to improved decision making.

Several contemporary applications of this are in process. For example, in 2002 the Institute of Medicine (Corrigan, Greiner, & Erickson, 2003) in response to a request from the Secretary of Health and Human Services recommended a portfolio of demonstration projects in the areas of primary care, chronic care, information and communications technology infrastructure, state health insurance, and liability. Projects within these areas are to be viewed as experiments with carefully designed evaluations such that the results will provide the basis for health system change.

Focusing on specific management practices the Veterans Administration (VA) has funded a new Health Services Research and Development Center of Excellence, the Center for Organization, Leadership, and Management Research (Charns, Young, & Selim, 2004). Located in Boston, Massachusetts, in collaboration with the VA Boston Healthcare System, the VA New England Healthcare System, and Boston University School of Public Health, the mission of the center is to develop and apply knowledge of innovative management practices to improve the effectiveness and efficiency of health services. Emphasis will be on practices that promote change, improve the quality of care, and develop leadership within the institution. While a number of methodologies will be used the VA health care system is a primary laboratory to implement and evaluate management practices. It provides an opportunity to build on an approach known as Clinical Firm Trials Research, which was initiated in the 1980s at the Cleveland Metro Health Center and, more recently, ongoing in several hospitals throughout the country (Goldberg, 2000). Firm research provides an opportunity to evaluate various changes in programmatic initiatives in the delivery of health care with the rigors of a randomized clinical trial.

An important effect of these initiatives is that health services managers will be increasingly part of a continual organizational learning effort—that is, the capacity or processes within the organization to maintain or improve performance based on experience (Barnsley, Lemieux-Charles, & McKinney, 1998). This activity involves knowledge acquisition, "development of creation of skills, insights, relationships, knowledge sharing, dissemination to others of what has been acquired by some, and knowledge utilization, integration of the learning so that it is assimilated, broadly available, and can be generalized to new institutions" (DiBella, Novis, & Gould, 1996).

As clinicians move toward **evidenced-based medicine**, managers will equally be involved with **evidence-based management**. Under this approach, managers will play an important role in the initiation and facilitation of the evaluation and learning process as well as the mediation of the relationship between the evaluators and organizational personnel and the implementation and use of evaluation results for improved decision making (Veney & Kaluzny, 2004). Managers in collaboration with health service researchers must select management practices for evaluation that are believed to have an impact on the quality, cost, and access to services provided by the organization. The purpose of the evaluation needs to be clearly defined and resources committed. A critical issue and the primary responsibility of the manager is to determine whether and when the organization is ready for the evaluation. Premature evaluation serves no one's ends. The manager will also play an important role in facilitating the implementation of the evaluation. This is particularly true in regard to formulating program objectives, which should be clearly understood by all involved.

The manager can also play an important role in mediating relationships between organizational personnel and evaluators. These relationships are frequently characterized by conflict. Organizational personnel understandably view their activities as beneficial and as contributing to the organization's goals. Evaluators, on the other hand, are charged with maintaining the integrity of the evaluation design and taking an independent view as to whether or not and to what degree the program's objectives have been achieved. Further, the evaluation may consume resources that personnel feel may be better spent on direct services. Managers can help minimize these conflicts by ensuring that sufficient time is allocated for discussion and development of mutual understanding and by engaging in direct problem-solving and conflict-resolution strategies as needed.

Finally, managers play a key role in making use of the evaluation results. Managers who work closely with evaluators can help to ensure that the key questions are being answered in a manner that makes sense to the eventual users. This includes suggesting to the evaluators that the report be written in a language and format understandable to the intended audience.

Past, Present, and Future

Table 15.1 presents each of the major trends involving the organization and the environment. As can be seen, both the organization and the environment are faced with increasing risk and varying levels of uncertainty. Organizations are increasingly being challenged, requiring greater adaptability and creativity. The future obviously will involve activities that have not been done before and will require efforts that have not yet been tried.

INDIVIDUALS AND GROUPS WITHIN THE ORGANIZATION

As an organization functions within a larger environment, individuals and groups function within a larger organizational setting. This interaction is critical to the overall performance of health care institutions in the future role of managers within these

Table 15.1. Environmental Trends

	Past (1960s–1980s)	Present (2006)	Future (2006 and beyond)
Social norms and expectations	Provider dominated	Changing consumer expectations	Deprofessionalization shared accountability and external reporting
Demographics and epidemiology	Aging of population not an issue; infectious diseases	Aging as an emergent issue; chronic diseases	Aging a major focus of activity; diseases of lifestyle and aging; growing ethnic diversity
Technical development, assessment, and outcomes	Rapid development and implementation	Emerging efforts at assessment	Use of randomized trials and metanalysis
Financing and reimbursement	Not an issue; retrospective reimbursement	Emergent concern and shift to prospective reimbursement	Increased financial risk Pay-for-performance initiatives
Organizational arrangement	Cottage industry; large number of individual providers	Systems and emerging organizational forms	Reconfiguration of networks and systems
Social experimentation, evaluation, and learning	Emerging efforts	Pressure on accountability	Collaborative efforts among policy makers, researchers, and managers; evidence-based management

organizations. Several developments likely to affect the interaction of individuals and groups within organizations having profound implications on the managerial role are discussed below.

Changing Role of the Patient

The availability of information through direct marketing or the Internet and the increasing reality of the electronic medical record (EMR) will have a profound effect on the role of the patient and particularly their relationship with the provider community. Direct marketing of drugs and other medical interventions—a process known as **disintermediation**—is pervasive and is receiving mixed reviews by the health care community.

Some doctors say that it improves patient compliance because ads act as a regular reminder to take medication. The ads also bring people into the office to talk about conditions that they rarely asked doctors about before.

"Patients are more educated and empowered to seek solution for sometimes stigmatized conditions" (AMA News, March 19, 2001). Others, however, offer a different opinion.

"Not only do we have to explain to our patients the nature of the medical problems that they have, but we also have to discuss why they don't need the drug that was advertised and what is the best option," said Sandra Adamson Fryhofer, MD, the immediate past president of the American College of Physicians (AMA News, 2001).

Whether disintermediation improves or hinders the health care process remains a question; however, the expenditures involved are remarkable. One estimate is that pharmaceutical companies in 2003 are spending $3.1 billion (25% of their marketing budget) on over-the-counter (OTC) advertising and from all indications is likely to intensify (Raskin, 2003). Moreover, the empowering of the patient coupled with the ascendance of the power of purchaser and large provider organizations is likely to have a profound effect on the physician-patient relationship. As described by Solberg et al. (2006) and their study of primary care physicians:

> The net result of all these changes has been to focus attention and pressure on the clinician, especially those in primary care. They are feeling both stressed and unappreciated as they have to run faster to keep up, while being constantly told that what they do isn't good enough. At the same time, it is becoming clearer that if we are to address the cost and quality conundrums we face, clinicians must not only be involved, they must take the lead in making change happen. (p. 298)

Similarly, the growing recognition that information technology has come of age and the proposal that the electronic health record will be available to most Americans within the next 10 years will greatly affect the provision of care (White House, 2004). While the proposal will have major consequences for the overall delivery system, the presence of electronic health records provides an opportunity to put the needs and values of the patient first and gives patients information they need to make informed clinical and economic decisions in consultation with appropriate health care providers.

Changing Role of the Physician

Changing norms and expectations, demographics and epidemiology, new technologies and their emphasis on assessment and outcomes, and fundamental changes in the configuration of health services resulting in increased scrutiny of health care costs are redefining the role of the physician. These changes are likely to affect the basic role that physicians will play in the emerging health care system, as well as the creation of new roles and specialties. The latter is well illustrated by the expanding role of the **hospitalist** as a specialist in inpatient medicine. A role well established in Canada and Europe, it was initially presented in the United states in the late 1990s and has had important clinical, financial, and policy implications (Wachter & Lee,1996). While many questions remain including the discontinuity of inpatient and outpatient care, its impact on cost and quality, etc., the number has grown from a few hundred to approximately 8,000 with a projected growth to 20,000 (Wachter, 2004). The implications of all these changes are expected to be reflected in greater attention to prevention, the incorporation of consumer preferences into medical decision making, and greater involvement in managerial activities, either as a knowledgeable clinician or a physician executive and the expanding importance of evidence-based medicine/management in the provision of care.

The shifting patterns of morbidity and mortality as well as changes in the demographic composition of the population are increasingly forcing medical practice to focus on the treatment of diseases associated with specific lifestyles or behaviors and chronic degenerative diseases of aging. Cardiovascular and pulmonary diseases, trauma, substance abuse, AIDS and other sexually transmitted diseases, cancer, chronic cognitive impairment, and diabetes are among the major health problems facing the population. Today and into the future, prevention will be the primary focus, and the physician will increasingly be at the vanguard of this movement.

Changes in the organization and delivery of health services and the results of health services research efforts are reflected in outcomes research and evidence-based medicine as the basis of clinical decisions. Outcomes research will produce more knowledge about the consequences of alternative treatments for specific conditions and provide recognition of the importance of consumer participation in the choice of treatment options available. The empirical documentation that all treatment is not equal and the explicit recognition that there are trade-offs will give increasing focus to shared decisions. Moreover, the expansion of direct-to-consumer advertising of drugs and other medical interventions will significantly modify the physician-patient relationship. On the one hand, it empowers consumers to be more proactive in maintaining their own health. It also represents rampant commercialization of health services and a further deprofessionalization of the physician's role.

Finally, the emerging trends within the larger environment will force physicians to explore new models of practice (e.g., Future of Family Medicine Project Leadership Committee, 2004) and become increasingly knowledgeable about and involved with the organizational and managerial environment within which they function. Physicians will become active participants in the decision-making process and will join the growing ranks of physician executives forced to confront and reconcile market-oriented economic self-interest with the values of medical professionalism, emphasizing service to patients. This confrontation will impact medical education, challenging the traditional autonomy of professional education, and require new partnerships with emerging delivery systems and the development of a "new professionalism" sustained by a larger institutional framework (Frankford & Konrad, 1998) and a new "moral fabric" (Shortell, Waters, Clarke, & Budetti, 1998). The latter is based on practicing population-based medicine, new models of managing and governing physician groups, aligning physician incentives, new care-management practices, and outcomes reporting systems. The challenge for the health services executive is to develop a working partnership with the physician community—one that fully recognizes the role of physicians in the managerial process.

The emerging trends and particularly the changing role of the patient and their access to information will greatly affect the future role of the physician. The information explosion will make it impractical for the physician to master, let alone control the information that must be accessed on be-

half of one's patient. The physician's role must be realigned to respect the patient's role in this changing environment. The primary loss will be the monopoly on knowing the science. However, the role of integrating and interpreting information, configuring care routines adapted to the needs and preferences of the patient, and orchestrating its delivery presents new challenges and opportunities within a changing health care system (McLaughlin & Kaluzny, 2006).

Changing Role of the Nurse

Nursing is the largest single profession in health care and facing significant challenges given the larger transformation in the financing and delivery of health services. As a profession, nursing has joined the coalition of managers and physicians who can make a difference in the major challenges involved in providing efficient and high-quality health care. This is particularly true in enhancing the clinical integration of care across the continuum.

The challenges facing nursing center on two issues. First is the growing recognition that health services are facing and will continue to face for the foreseeable future a shortage of registered nurses and other nursing assistant personnel. In the years ahead the demand for nursing services will increase with the increasing population in the age groups most likely to use health services (those over 65 and older) at the same time that the supply is likely to decrease as the nursing population providing care is aging and moving out of full-time employment.

Second, the issue of nursing demand and supply will be addressed within the context of a changing health system having a profound effect on the role of nursing within the system. The commercialization and deprofessionalization of health services will be particularly painful for a group that has historically been grounded in "hands-on, human-to-human, intimate work" (Pierce, 2004). Moreover, the increased demand for and use of unlicensed assistant personnel will require supervision by registered nursing personnel, placing nurses in a critical role in the overall management structures of the delivery organization.

The nurse is the primary resource coordinator and, given the greater emphasis on information management, the linking of financial and clinical information will become a critical component in the managerial decision process. Historically involved with case management and active participants in the development of critical paths, the future role requires that the profession produce quality graduates who:

- Are prepared for clinical leadership in all health care settings.

- Are prepared to implement outcomes-based practice and quality improvement strategies.

- Will remain in and contribute to the profession, practicing at their full scope of education and ability.

- Will create and manage systems of care that will be responsive to the health care needs of society.

To meet this challenge, the American Association of Colleges of Nursing propose that the profession needs to prepare clinical nurse leaders. As described by the Association (2003, p. 4):

> The clinical nurse leader (CNL) is a leader in the health care delivery system across all settings in which health care is delivered, not just the acute care setting. The implementation of the CNL role, however, will vary across settings. The CNL role is not one of administration or management. The CNL assumes accountability for client care outcomes through the assimilation and application of research based information to design, implement and evaluate client plans of care. The CNL is a provider and a manager of care at the point of care to individuals and cohorts or populations. The CNL designs, implements and evaluates client care by coordinating, delegating and supervising the care provided by the health care team, including licensed nurses, technicians and other health professionals.

Many of the trends affecting physicians will affect the changing role of nurses in the future. The emphasis on cost-effective care, changes in the demographics and epidemiology of the population, and the various organizational arrangements within the larger system will continually challenge the role of nursing within the health care system. To meet the challenge, nursing will demand a larger voice in management and governance. The challenge for management is to join in partnership with nursing and implement appropriate roles for nurses, clearly recognizing their professional heritage as well as their importance to emerging health care issues.

Perhaps this is best illustrated by the Magnet Recognition Program administered by the American Nurses Credentialing Center, a subsidiary of the American Nurses Association (http://www.nursingworld.org). This program in operation since 1994 bestows national recognition on health care organizations that demonstrate sustained nursing care excellence. Presently, more than 100 health care organizations have been designated for their excellence in:

- The management, philosophy, and practices of nursing services

- Adherence to national standards for improving the quality of patient care services

- Leadership of the nurse administrator in supporting professional practice and continued competence of nurses

- Understanding and respecting the cultural and ethnic diversity of patients, their significant other and health care providers

Expanding Role of Allied Health Professionals

Comprising more than 60% of the entire health care workforce and including over 200 distinct disciplinary groups, allied health is the largest, most complex, and fastest growing occupational group in the United States. Allied health professionals are involved with the delivery of health and related services pertaining to the identification, evaluation, and prevention of diseases and disorders including nutrition, rehabilitation, and dental services. As a diverse group of health professions, they include dental hygienists, diagnostic medical sonographers, dietitians, medical technologists, occupational therapists, physical therapists, radiographers, respiratory therapists, and speech language pathologists (ASAHP, 2004). This group includes approximately 6 million health professionals providing services in a range of settings including hospitals, clinics, physicians' offices, hospices, extended care facilities, HMOs, community programs, and schools—and over the past decade have experienced severe workforce shortages, particularly in physical and occupational therapy (Jones, Johnson, Beasley, & Johnson, 1996). A recent American Hospital Association workforce survey indicated that these shortages remain in hospitals throughout the country. Hospitals report vacancy rates ranging from 12% to 15% among imaging technicians, pharmacists, and many other allied health care positions (Pollack, 2004).

As with nursing and medicine, the realities of financing, reimbursement, demography, epidemiology, technology, and organizational arrangements will have profound implications on this group of health care providers with subsequent implications for health services management. Perhaps its distinguishing feature is its heterogeneity, size, and overspecialization, and thus the emerging forces within the larger system will greatly affect the role of this particular group of providers.

The challenge is to ensure an integrated and well-trained workforce dedicated to meeting patient needs. As described by the IOM (2003) and its efforts to reform health professions education and thus assure commitment to meeting patient needs:

> All health professionals should be educated to deliver patient-centered care as members of an interdisciplinary team, emphasizing evidence-based practice, quality improvement approaches and informatics.

Dynamic Nature of Individual and Group Configurations

Effective management recognizes the dynamic nature of disciplinary and interdisciplinary work groups and individuals interacting within the organization. Clearly, the emerging and dynamic roles of nurses, physicians, and the range of other health professionals within the context of the larger trends affecting health services delivery involving "micro-units" concerned with the provision of primary care (Mohr, Batalden & Barach, 2006) and long-term care (Christianson, Taylor, & Knutson, 1998, Donaldson & Mohr, 2000) will place a premium on the ability to understand and manage these individual and group configurations.

The implications are substantial. First, the recognition that health services organizations are composed not only of work groups, but also a range of interest groups and coalitions that are constantly shifting in order to compete for resources, provides an opportunity for managers to develop leverage between and among these interest groups and coalitions to enhance the overall operations of the organization. The recognition of these dynamics provides an opportunity to structure situations so that individuals and groups can more effectively monitor and control their own activities.

Second, the increasing role of interdisciplinary groups and work units in the provision of health services raises the issue of work group effectiveness and the education of health care providers to function in truly interdisciplinary teams (Baker et al., 1998; Mohr, Randolph, et al., 2003; Schmitt, 2001). While the business of providing health services is usually done within the context of some group setting, the ability of these groups to function effectively is limited by the individual's own disciplinary perspective and lack of appreciation for the dynamics involved as well as other disciplinary perspectives. The overall effectiveness of the group is constantly threatened by the tendency of one disciplinary perspective to dominate and by a fundamental lack of group dynamics.

Finally, given the importance of interdisciplinary activity and the increasing emphasis given to total quality management, which attempts to focus on the horizontal flow of activities within the organizations, individuals will increasingly occupy boundary spanning roles involving various work groups, interest groups, or coalitions. Boundary spanning involves considerable conflict, and increased attention will be given to the development of skills required for communication, negotiation, and conflict management.

Health Services Policy and Management Research

Health services research and its impact on evidence-based medicine and management has come of age and clearly has made major contributions to the policy issues facing the health services system. Moreover, it is likely that the synthesis and dissemination of health services research will play a continuing role in the process of formulating policy, albeit within an environment characterized by political controversy. Future considerations, however, need to be given to the interdisciplinary nature of health services research and the utilization of research by managers (Walshe & Rundall, 2001).

While clearly the substantive issues facing health services at this point focus on cost containment, increasing attention needs to be paid to the configuration and organizational aspects affecting managerial decision making. The interdisciplinary nature of health services delivery and the critical issues of understanding the process of health services delivery will increasingly place a premium on analytical questions that go beyond simply those of cost and reimbursement. The management of groups, the motivation of personnel, and the integration and coordination of services at various delivery levels and across various organizational forms and the emerging ethical issues facing managers within a complex and dynamic delivery system require the attention of a wide variety of social science disciplines within the health services research community.

A second challenge is the utilization of health services research in the decision-making process. More than anything else, the health services manager of the future must be an innovator, at times a visionary, and always a teacher and mentor applying new learning to improved decision making. A partnership is needed between managers and researchers, whereby the health services research community will be acutely aware, responsive, and have ready access to the substantive issues facing managers, and managers will facilitate such access, and in turn be a beneficiary of greater insight and strategies derived from the learning process. In a sense, this partnership represents an alliance in which both managers and researchers work collaboratively to provide an opportunity to assess performance of ongoing activities, develop predictors of performance, and specify the conditions under which various approaches to health services delivery are most effective. Perhaps most importantly, the development of the partnership provides an opportunity to truly develop meaningful and relevant guidelines for evidence-based management.

Information Management

While emerging trends at the larger environmental level such as outcomes management, community networks, and the development of guidelines are occurring, it has been recognized that existing data systems within organizations are embarrassingly inadequate to meet the information needs and strategies inherent in many of these important developments (Institute of Medicine, 2003). Information systems within health services organizations often have a programmatic or categorical character and thus are greatly hindered in their attempt to integrate clinical outcomes, process of care, and financial information. Existing systems either:

- Do not collect and store the right information
- Are not automated or computerized
- Are not integrated

- Lack sufficiently sophisticated computer hardware, software, and data-entry support to permit retrieval and analysis of information

As compiled by the Markle Foundation (2003) and their effort to develop a public-private collaborative designed to address the barriers to developing an interconnected health information infrastructure, information technology is not being widely used in health care.

- Over 90% of the annual 30 billion health transactions are conducted by phone, fax, or mail.
- Only a third of hospitals nationwide have computerized physician order entry (CPOE) systems completely or partially available. Of these, only 4.9% require their use.
- Only 5% of clinician and 19% of health care provider organizations use fully operational computerized medical records.
- Although illegible handwriting is known to cause a substantial number of medication errors, fewer than 5% of U.S. physicians prescribe medication electronically.
- Forty percent of health care organizations planned to spend 1.5% or less of their total operating budgets on information technology and 36% set spending at 2% to 4%. This is compared with an average of 8.5% in other industries.

To address these problems several initiatives have been launched that are likely to have a significant impact on meeting the information needs of the health care system. This is occurring at both the federal, state, and local level and involving both federal and private monies. At the federal level steps have been taken to coordinate public- and private-sector efforts that will accelerate broad adoption of health information technology including the adoption of health information standards, the allocation of monies for demonstration projects on health care information technology, the creation of a new sub-cabinet-level position to coordinate health information technology (The White House, 2004).

At the local level several communities are experimenting with data-sharing initiatives within a geographic area (Lorenzi, 2003). For example, the Indianapolis Network for Patient Care includes all five major medical systems in the Indianapolis area, all four homeless care organizations in Marion county, all county and state public health departments, 85 primary care providers at 20 sites, 3000 sub-specialists, and 30 pubic school clinics. Together, the network covers over 95% of acute inpatient and non-office-based outpatient clinical care including more that 300,000 emergency room visits and 100,000 inpatient visits per year.

Information management and the health care information technology market in 2003 was estimated to have grown at a rate of 9.3% to $23.6 billion from $21.6 billion in 2002. While historically lagging when compared to other industries, it is estimated that the information technology market will expand with spending expected to grow to $30.5 billion by the end of 2006 (Dorenfest, et al. 2004). A good share of this growth is driven by the need to assure patient safety and it is estimated that a good health information system could save the economy $140 billion a year, or 10% of the U.S. total health care spending (Thompson, 2004).

Past, Present, and Future

Table 15.2 summarizes the trends dealing with individuals and groups within the organizations. As with the environment and larger organizations, individuals and groups within organizations are confronting increasing complexity and varying levels of uncertainty. The future will require the active participation of physicians, nurses, and allied health professionals, with the major challenge being to motivate and preserve human resources available to the organization. These resources will be increasingly involved in interdisciplinary groups and will be informed by a developing research base that will permit new designs and managerial strategies.

Table 15.2. Individual and Group Trends

	Past (1960s–1980s)	Present (2006)	Future (2006 and beyond)
Patient	Passive	Emergent—Interactive	Proactive
Physicians	Solo practice	Group practice	Corporate practice (expanding hospitalist movement) Active involvement in managerial activity; interpreting/integrating clinical information
Nurses	Clinical practice	Emerging as a political force	Active participation in managerial structure and policy; clinical leadership
Allied health	Not an issue	Emerging issue	Key participants in teams that manage care across episodes of illness and pathways of wellness
Management research and assessment	Not an issue	Increased recognition	Integral part of managerial and organizational effectiveness
Dynamic nature of groups	Individual and disciplinary groups dominate	Emergence of interdisciplinary groups	Dominance of interdisciplinary groups
Information management	Not an issue	Emerging efforts	Clinical and financial networking; national information infrastructure

THE MANAGERIAL ROLE

Developments at the environment-organizational level, and the individual-group level of the organization provide a clue to future demands on managers. These demands involve three assumptions and three fundamental implications. The first assumption is that health care will continue to have features of both an economic and social good. Since it is financially impossible to provide unlimited care, there must be a mechanism for allocating resources, and it is likely that this will continue to include some marketplace features. At the same time, health care is an intensely personal, human service, which most Americans believe ought to be available to people in need, who are without the ability to pay for the service. A major responsibility and challenge of health services executives and managers in the years ahead will be to manage the inherent tension between health care as both an economic and a social good.

The second assumption is that the world will not become simpler but, if anything, more complex, ambiguous, and uncertain. If past is prologue, managers of health services organizations will encounter continued, if not increasing, stress; this stress will be reflected in the turnover rates among chief executive officers (CEOs).

Since setting a record high turnover rate among CEOs in nonfederal, short-term, general hospitals in the late 1990s of 17% to 18%, the rate has steadily declined to 14% in 2003, a rate comparable to what was recorded in the early 1980s. However, the overall 2003 rate is quite variable among states ranging from a high of 30% in the District of Columbia to a low of 2% in Maine and Nebraska (Weil, 2004). It is expected that the rate will continue to show a great deal of regional variability and the overall rate will probably increase in the future as the CEO ranks are filled with individuals of diverse background and training.

The third assumption is that health services executives and managers working together and with other health care providers can create the future for themselves and their organization. It is precisely because health care delivery will become even more complex, ambiguous, and uncertain that it is possible for managers to shape their destiny. The external environment not only influences managerial and organizational decision making, but the decisions made by managers on behalf of their organizations will also help to shape and influence the environment.

From the three assumptions come four fundamental implications, each involving a major transition in the managerial role.

- The first involves a transition from managing an organization to managing a market or network of services and joint ventures. Health services executives of the future will increasingly be called upon to manage across boundaries. This will require increased skills in coalition building, negotiation, and the ability to put together strategic alliances and partnerships to serve defined populations. It will require executives who see any given organization as part of a broader whole.

- For middle managers, it involves a transition from managing a department to managing a continuum of care. In brief, the job of the pharmacy department head, laboratory department head, radiology department head, or any other hospital department head is no longer that of a department head but rather a manager of pharmaceutical, laboratory, or radiology services across the continuum of care—most of which will be provided outside hospital settings. This will require these individuals to discard the hospital mindset and develop a broader community-based approach to delivering services. It will place a premium on interpersonal skills and the ability to develop collaborative relationships.

- The third transition involves moving from a mentality of coordinating services to a new mindset of actively managing and improving quality across the continuum of care. This involves adopting a broader view of one's responsibilities. For example, the main focus is no longer on whether intensive care services are coordinated with those of step-down units but rather on coordinating care along the entire episode of illness or pathway of wellness leading from the patient's home, to the physician's office, to the relatively short stay in the intensive care unit, and back out again to the after-care units and into the home. It does little good to coordinate only part of this continuum of care if it has no resulting lasting value or impact on the overall episode of illness or ultimately the patient's health status. Actively managing quality will require health services managers at all levels to move beyond suboptimization and consider the overall interdependent processes involved in patient care—again, most of which will occur outside the hospital.

- The fourth transition involves moving from a relatively simple environment to a more complex setting in which health care executives must balance the needs and interests of individuals, the organization, and the larger community. Balancing these needs and interests places the manager in a position of addressing a variety of ethical issues including the allocation of limited resources to different institutional activities, for example, the purchase of new MRI versus setting up a

IN PRACTICE   Ethical Challenges

- Scenario I: You have withdrawn an offer at the last minute (due to poor references) to an ICU nurse manager candidate who has moved across the country to accept the job. The only way you will avoid a lawsuit is if she is hired somewhere else soon. A close colleague calls to ask you frankly why you withdrew the offer. What do you say?
- Scenario II: You are in the final stages of buying land for a new project. Your CEO has been advocating for a purchase on Grand and Broad

Street. You have just learned that the CEO, two key physicians and a board member are partners in the land at Grand and Broad. What do you do?
- Scenario III: Your CEO asks that you fire your CNO, who you have just given a good performance appraisal. After much debate, the CEO finally reports that the medical staff wants him fired because he is gay. What do you do?

(Janet Porter, personal communication, 2005).

"storefront" primary care clinic; responding to changes in institutional governance and ownership and the implication of that change to various organizational stakeholders; conflict of interest in purchasing decisions; and a range of decisions involving personnel evaluations and recommendations (Harris, 2003).

Consider some of the ethical challenges facing managers. What would you do? (See In Practice above.)

Role Performance and Emerging Challenges

The managerial role within health services is perhaps one of the most complex administrative assignments. As described by Walter McNerney (1985):

> There is more to management than crisp efficiency. In the health field, perhaps more than any other, management involves moral issues and ethical choices. It involves a deep commitment and personal courage. It involves a resolve to be just and right, not only a resolve to win.

Role performance will become even more challenging as managers attempt to deal with emerging public-private partnerships, aligning incentives, resource constraints, and increasing emphasis on health and preventive services that are customer focused, information driven, and outcome based. Particular attention needs to be given to balancing the personal needs of patients and assuring the efficiency and quality of care provided within the organization. Consider the challenges presented to the administration as they attempted to meet the needs of Ms. Livingston (see Debate Time 15.3). To meet these emerging trends, the managerial role requires:

- New knowledge and skill competencies based in practice servicing needs at three levels—individual development, organizational improvement, and health system performance (Baker, 2003).

- A recognition that the rapidly changing environment and the scope and depth of competencies needed by health services managers cannot be provided only at career entry level and requires a lifelong commitment.

- A recognition that managerial competencies must be shared with clinical colleagues to form a partnership to meet the changing demands of

DEBATE TIME 15.3   What Do You Think?

Ms. Connie Livingston is a 31-year old-woman living with breast cancer. Her cancer was diagnosed several years ago and, following a lumpectomy and adjuvant therapy, she is doing well—well enough to plan a future involving marriage.

The wedding was planned and the date was set. A license was obtained, guests were invited, and endless details, usually associated with such events, were slowly coming into place. Unfortunately, while visiting Chapel Hill shortly before the wedding, Ms. Livingston developed a pulmonary embolism and was rushed to the emergency room, the attending oncologist was called, and arrangements were made to transfer her to the oncology unit. Her condition was critical and was deteriorating rapidly. Fearing the worst, Connie and her fiancé Jim Smith requested that the marriage be conducted in the university hospital chapel. They insisted that this be a "legal marriage," not just a ceremony.

The legal marriage required a marriage license (issued in the county where the marriage took place) and new blood tests and certification. It also required the scheduling and coordinating of a

group of people, both within and outside the hospital, who just minutes earlier had no idea who Connie Livingston or Jim Smith were, and time was running out. The administrator-in-charge contacted the county registrar to obtain a marriage license and the state laboratory for certification of the required blood test. What typically is done in weeks was now occurring in minutes. Physicians, nurses, and other hospital managers also played key roles in coordinating and expediting the wedding. Timing was critical; any one of these individuals could have created a delay ending the effort. Instead, "things did happen." The wedding occurred—a wish fulfilled—and three hours later Mrs. Livingston-Smith died.

A tragedy? Yes! A lost life? Yes! But this is the reality of health care—a reality that every day provides an opportunity to demonstrate what people can accomplish given the challenge.

SOURCE: From Graber, D. & Kaluzny, A. (2000). Developing high-involvement organizations for the future. In A. Kilpatrick & J. Johnson (Eds.), *Handbook of health administration and policy*. New York: Marcel Dekker, Inc.

the future (Pew Health Professions Commission, 1995).

Adequate role performance requires a new managerial image of the organization—not one of a "hierarchy of roles," but a "portfolio of dynamic processes" (Ghoshal & Bartlett, 1995). Cutting across departmental and organizational boundaries, the managers of these processes require new skills and competencies in leadership, coalition building, quality improvement and assurance, sensitivity to cost-quality relationships, research utilization, innovation, and problem solving.

Specifically, managers must reaffirm their commitment to leadership as a set of processes that creates organizations in the first place or adopts them to significantly changing circumstances. As described by Kotter (1996), leadership defines what the future should look like, aligns people with that vision, and inspires them to make it happen despite obstacles.

Equally critical will be new skills and competencies in coalition building and a perspective that facilitates networking and partnerships among both public and private organizations. Given the emergence of various alliance-type arrangements involving various specialty and primary care providers along with expanding outsourcing arrangements, managers of the future will need skill and vision to integrate the clinical professions and institutions into organizations that provide predictable, cost-effective care. The managerial role here will require group leadership skills, coalition building, negotiation, and conflict management, as well as an overarching systems perspective.

A third competency is in the area of policy and political acuity. While currently managers know how to make improvements, they often lack access to the levers to change the system. Often they are not rewarded for doing the right thing and are punished for thinking globally. Managers of the future will require political skills including interagency analysis, coalition building, and understanding the realities of partisan politics.

Similarly, the entire area of quality improvement and assurance will be fundamental to role performance in the future. Purchasers—whether individual consumers, third-party payers, or governmental units—increasingly demand accountability of health services providers for an appropriate return on investment and increasingly expressed in terms of improved health status and outcome. To function within this set of expectations, managers will require skills in the area of quantitative, statistical, and epidemiological reasoning; outcome interpretation; and application.

Future role performance also requires that managers have a sensitivity to the cost-quality relationship. Individual consumers, third-party payers, and governmental units increasingly demand the provision of health services within the constraints of budgetary limits in all their diversity. Increasingly managers will be called upon to demonstrate their abilities in budget-based resource management, resources creation and allocation, and management within limits and constraints.

New dimensions of role performance are also required in **organizational learning** and innovation. Future role performance will require practitioners to have skills in the area of health services research, management assessment, and application. Many health services managers fail to recognize problems

that are, in fact, researchable and fail to apply knowledge from existing research to enhance organizational performance. There is a serious and growing need for managers to become informed consumers of health services management research to improve organizational performance and services outcomes. Finally, future role performance requires that managers apply knowledge to assure benefit. In an area where the demand for greater productivity and improved outcomes with finite resource limitations predominate, the health services administrator must create workable solutions to operational and system problems.

Another challenge facing the future of role performance of the administrator is the recognition that, given the rapidly changing environment, the scope and depth of competencies needed by health service administrators cannot be provided only at career entry level. The acquisition of new competencies will be needed throughout their entire careers. Health services managers will increasingly come from a variety of educational backgrounds, and thus enhanced lifelong learning is required to equip the manager to address the issues in a rapidly changing environment.

A major breakthrough in management education and leadership development is occurring with the systematic development of leadership competencies for the field (Baker, 2003; NCHL, 2004). These are based on wide input from practitioners and academics alike and behavioral event interviews that identify characteristics that distinguish outstanding leaders from those less successful (NCHL, 2004). These major competency domains have been described as transformational, executional, and people-orientation. *Transformational* competencies involve visioning, energizing, and stimulating a change process that coalesces communities, patients, and professionals around new models of health care and wellness. *Executional* competences involve translating vision and strategy into optimal organization performance. *People-orientation* involves creating an organizational climate that values employees from all backgrounds and provides an energizing environment for them. It also includes leaders' responsibility to understand their impact on others and to improve their capabilities as well as the capabilities of others (NCHL, 2004). These competencies or some variation of them are being incorporated into management education and leadership development programs and accreditation and certification processes.

Finally, role performance in the future will increasingly require the support and participation of clinical professions. Clinicians have increasing impact on the management of the health service system. Thus, if the managerial role is to meet its expectations, it must join in a partnership with the clinicians exposing them to the basic core of the organization and policy knowledge to support role performance in the future. At a minimum, clinical colleagues require a basic understanding of the health services system and the impact of clinical practice and decision making on organization, delivery, and cost (Nolan, 1998).

Preparing Future Managers

Health services managers are playing an increasing role in all segments of the health services delivery system. Initially developed to improve the management of large acute care hospitals, the demand for professional administrators has expanded greatly to include all the private and public organizations that are involved in financing, regulating, assessing, supplying, assisting, and generating policies for health services. While limited training is provided at the undergraduate and doctoral levels, major effort in health services education is at the master's degree. Although commonly referred to as the MHA, the degrees conferred include health management specialization within the MBA, MPH, MPA, MS, MA, MSHA, and others. The degrees reflect a variety of settings in which the programs are based, including schools of medicine, public health, business, public affairs, and allied health. Moreover, the commercialization of health services has been accompanied by the increase in the number of individuals with generic business training as measured by the number of new associates joining the American College of Healthcare Executives (ACHE). For example, in 1970, only 6.57% of the new associates had generic business degrees (no formal training in health ser-

vices management). This number has increased to 27.2% in 2003 with 46.2% of the new ACHE associates having degrees in health care management (Weil, 2004). In the public health sector it is estimated that only 15% have the MPH degree although formal training in public health is included in the various professional and administrative public health manpower categories (Gebbie, 2004).

To meet the changing challenges and opportunities, several strategies need to be considered (Pew Health Professions Commission, 1995; NCHL National Invitational Symposium, 2003; Leatt, Grady & Prybill et al., 2004):

- *Core Curriculum Reform:* Develop an integrated core curriculum that embraces the new competencies, including leadership, coalition building, a community perspective, quality improvement, and the principles of organizational learning. These must be presented in an integrated manner—not as freestanding courses, but as modules that can be "mixed and matched" to meet the learning needs of the student. Moreover, these content areas must be linked to personal assessment such that the role of the manager becomes part of a larger socialization process that begins with the very initiation of the educational experience (Mintzberg 2004).

The development of educational materials and methods must emphasize adaptability and the development of skills to manage the characteristics of the health care system of the future. Given the demographic changes in the community and the workforce composition of health service organizations, it is imperative that students and academic faculty reflect this diversity.

- *Quality Partnerships between University and Practice Professionals:* Expand the university-practice interface to assure the relevance of health services administration curricula to broader health care fields and return the research and educational products that yield improved administrator and organizational performance. The practitioner-academic interface requires a major expansion of the range or provider organizations involved and a redefinition of the mutual benefits accruing to each party. Special emphasis needs to be given to identifying and establishing a broad range of relationships with operating health services organizations, particularly those exhibiting the characteristics of the system of the future, and using these as teaching and research models and focal points for training administrators (Prybill, 2003). Idealized relationships with the future include:

- experiential learning opportunities such as mentoring, internships, residencies, postgraduate fellowships, and administrator training programs in a variety of health service settings including, finance, pharmaceutical, and equipment and supply organizations.

- joint degree opportunities such as MHA-MPH, JD-MHA, MD-MHA, MBA-MHA, and MBA-MPH.

- development of a national recruitment program/strategy to attract talented and committed individuals to health care management as a first career choice (Loebs, 2004).

- middle-management congresses by academic programs for provider organizations participating in experiential learning programs.

- executive-in-residence or visiting-health-care-executive programs bringing operational managers to the classroom.

- leadership forums for multidisciplinary management teams from health care organizations, providing them with training in areas of self-identified skill and competency deficiencies.

- collaborative research efforts between faculty and health care systems that focus on operational problems.

- *Stage Career Competency and Professional Development:* Management education for health services management must be tied to critical career transitions and linked to specific competencies (Warden & Sinioris, 2004). Given the dynamics of the health care system, managers will be in constant need to update and expand their ability to function within the system. Relevant content areas include epidemiology, biostatistics, negotiation skills, health behavior, the organization and management sciences, preparation in community development, and training in ethics and principles of social justice.

The temptation is to "add" new courses in an attempt to meet the knowledge needs of practicing executives. Perhaps a more efficient approach is to introduce such content into existing learning situations familiar to the student (Batalden, 1998). For example, rather than requiring a separate course on ethics, ethical content would be built into many existing courses throughout the curriculum.

- *Management for Clinical Professions:* Health services management programs need to serve as key managerial-policy education resources by supporting and teaching health care organization and management to the clinical professions. This obviously is a collaborative endeavor, taking a variety of forms including joint appointments, collaborative teaching, research, and service activities, but also serving as a resource to prepare clinical faculty to teach their students health services management and policy issues. As our industrial colleagues have learned so long ago, the world is too complex to go it alone.

- *Distance Learning Opportunities:* Whether the student is a clinician interested in management or a manager who is interested in further preparation, all are extremely busy, and many are inaccessible to conventional teaching modalities and traditional residential educational programs. Through teleconferencing, the information highway complemented with two-way television, it is possible to provide state-of-the-art education to thousands of students throughout the country and the world (Umble, Shay & Sollecito, 2003).

Past, Present, and Future

Table 15.3 presents the summary of trends dealing with the managerial role. As can be seen, the role has made a number of major transitions, and more will be required to meet the challenges of the new millennium and beyond. The field is rich

Table 15.3. Managerial Trends

	Past (1960s–1970s)	Present (2006)	Future (2006 and beyond)
Role performance and changing values	Coordinating role subordinate to professional providers	Ascendance of managerial ability; financial and strategic expertise	Continued prominence of managers and recognition of role in managing human resources and interorganization relationships vs. simply financial resources
Preparing future managers	Relatively isolated from mainstream management and organizational theory	Emerging integration yet differentiated from industrial management	Competency-based learning: fully integrated into management training/ lifelong learning/ distance learning

with challenges and opportunities, and as never before, the manager is truly a significant player in determining the future provision of health services.

Returning to Mrs. Peterson and whether hers was an isolated event or chronic system problem, health care managers are likely to face elements of all four future scenarios as they deal with the organization and the environment, individuals and groups within the organization, and their own roles. The challenge will be to identify tractable elements within each option and their inevitable combinations and to direct limited resources and energy to those elements that make a difference in the provision of health services. Issues of quality and efficiency will remain paramount, confounded by fundamental moral and ethical choices heretofore considered only in the abstract. Our ability and contribution to determining the future provision of health services will depend on a critical mix of abilities, insight, and courage. Failure to meet the challenge will sideline managers to simply observing rather than influencing the future and ensure that others will repeat the events experienced by Mrs. Peterson in the years ahead.

DISCUSSION QUESTIONS

1. Recalling the four alternative futures presented at the beginning of the chapter, speculate on the implications of each scenario as it affects efforts at cost containment, changing the organization's culture, and the role of management.

2. Design an idealized educational program for incumbent managers to enhance their overall effectiveness. Be specific about the types of problems you anticipate and how the training program will resolve or mitigate these problems.

3. Compare and contrast how an organized delivery system would be most likely to respond to the challenges outlined in this chapter. Compare the most likely responses of the organized delivery system with those of an individual hospital/health department or group practice. Specifically address issues related to cost containment, changing social norms and demographic composition, technology development and social experimentation, changing roles of physicians and nurses, organizational culture, and the incorporation of women and minorities into management positions.

4. Return to the opening case regarding Mrs. Peterson, what mechanism and/or strategies might one use to prevent or minimize the problem encountered? What are the

advantages and disadvantages of each, and how feasible are these under the various scenarios?

REFERENCES

Alzheimer's Association. (2004). *Medicare.* Retrieved June 2004, from http://www.alzorg/advocacy/priorities/medicare.

AMA News (March 19, 2001) Patient orders: When patients ask for specific drugs, http:ama-assn.org.

American Association of Colleges of Nursing. (2003, May). *Working paper on the role of the clinical nurse leader.*

American Cancer Society. (1998). *Facts & figures.* Atlanta: American Cancer Society, 1999.

American Cancer Society. (2005). *Cancer facts and figures 2005 graphs and figures.* Retrieved January 2005, from http:// www.cancer.org/docroot/MED

American Nurses Credentialing Center. (2003). *Magnet recognition program—Certifying excellence in nursing services.* Silver Spring, MD.

Amick, B., Levine, S., Tarlov, A., & Walsh, D. (1995). *Society and health.* Oxford: Oxford University Press.

Associated Press. (2005, January 20). Cancer passes heart disease as top killer. *New York Times Magazine.*

Association of Schools of Allied Health Professionals. (2004). *Definition: Allied health professionals.* Retrieved June 2004, from http://www.asahp.org

Baker, G. R. (2003). Identifying and assessing competencies: A strategy to improve healthcare leadership. *Healthcare Papers, 4*(1), 49–58.

Baker, R., Gelmon, S., Headrick, L., Knapp, M., Norman, L., Quinn, D., & Neuhauser, D. (1998, Winter). Collaborating for improvement in health professional education. *Quality Management in Health Care, 6*(2), 1–11.

Barnes, P., Powell-Griner, E., McFanne, K., & Nahin, R. (2004, May 27). Complementary and alternative medicine use among adults: United States 2002. *CDC Advance Data Report, 343.*

Barnsley, J., Lemieux-Charles, L., & McKinney, M. M. (1998). Integrating learning into integrated delivery systems. *Health Care Management Review, 23*(1), 18–28.

Batalden, P. B. (1998). If improvement of the quality and value of health and health care is the goal, why focus on health professional development? *Quality Management in Health Care, 6*(2), 52–61.

Bazzoli, G. J., Chan, B., et al. (2000, Fall). The financial performance of hospitals belonging to health networks and systems. *Inquiry, 37*(3), 234–252.

Beauchamp, D. (1999). Community: The neglected tradition of public health. In D. Beauchamp & B. Steinbeck (Eds.), *New ethics for the public's health.* New York: Oxford University Press.

Begun, J. W., & Kaissi, A. A. (2004, January). Uncertainty in health care environments: Myth or reality? *Health Care Management Review, 29*(1), 31–39.

Bloche, M. G., & Studdert, D. M. (2004, March). A quiet revolution: Law as an agent of health system change. *Health Affairs, 23*(2), 29–53.

Burns, L. R., & Wharton School Colleagues. (2002). *The health care value chain: Producers, purchasers and providers.* San Francisco: Jossey-Bass.

Cain Brothers. (2003, March). If you're niched, it might be your fault: Physician-driven specialty hospitals and ambulatory surgery centers. *Strategies in Capital Finance, 39,* 1–14.

Califf, R. M. (2004, Jan.). Defining the balance of risk and benefit in the era of genomics and protcomics. *Health Affairs, 23*(1), 77.

Campbell, D. T. (1969). Reforms as experiments. *American Psychologist, 24,* 409–429.

Campbell, P. (1997, May). Population projections: States, 1995–2025. *Current population reports, Census Bureau, Issues, 25–1131.*

Cassileth, B. (1998). *The alternative medicine handbook.* New York: W. W. Norton.

Centers for Disease Control & Prevention. (2004, June). *Reorganization of CDC units: Office of Communication, Epidemiology Program Office, Public Health Practice Program Office.* Retrieved June 2004, from http://intranet.cdc.gov/od/futures

Charns, M., Young, G., & Selim, A. (2004, January). *The Center for Organizational, Leadership, and Management Research. A research and development program proposal submitted and funded by the Department of Veterans Affairs.* Boston: VA Boston Healthcare System.

Chassen, M., et al. (1998). *Crossing the quality of chasm: The IOM health care quality initiative.* Washington, DC: The National Academic Press.

Christianson, J., Taylor, R., & Knutson, D. (1998). *Restructuring chronic illness management.* San Francisco: Jossey-Bass.

Clinton, H. (2004, April 18). Now can we talk about health care? *New York Times Magazine.*

Corrigan, J. M., Greiner, A., & Erickson, S. M. (Eds.). (2003). *Fostering rapid advances in health care: Learning from system demonstrations.* Washington, DC: The National Academies Press.

Daniels, N. (2002). Justice, health and health care. In R. Rhodes, M. Batlin, & A. Silvers, (Eds.), *Medicine and social justice.* New York: Oxford University Press.

DiBella, A. J., Novis, E. C., & Gould, J. M. (1996). Understanding organizational learning capability. *Journal of Management Studies, 33*(3), 361–379.

Donaldson, M. S., & Mohr, J. J. (2000). *Improvement and innovation in health care microsystems* (a technical report for the Institute of Medicine Committee on the Quality of Health Care in America). Princeton: Robert Wood Johnson Foundation.

Dorenfest, S., et al. (2001, April 23). Healthcare information technology spending is growing rapidly. News release. Sheldon I. Dorenfest & Associates, Ltd.

Ellrodt, G., Cook, D., Lee, J., Cho, M., Hunt, D., & Weingarton, S. (1997, November 26). Evidence-based disease management. *Journal of the American Medical Association, 208*(20), 1687–1692.

Epstein, A. M., Lee, T., & Hamel, M. (2004). Paying physicians for high-quality care. *New England Journal of Medicine, 305*(4), 406–410.

Ernst, R. L., & Hay, J. W. (1994, August). The U.S. economic and social costs of Alzheimer's disease revisited. *American Journal of Public Health, 84*(8), 1261–1264.

Fries, J. (2003). Measuring and monitoring success in compressing morbidity. *Annals of Internal Medicine, 139*(5 Pt 2), 455–459.

Frankford, D. M., & Konrad, T. R. (1998, February). Responsive medical professionalism: Integrating education, practice, and community in a market-driven era. *Academic Medicine, 73*(2).

Future of Family Medicine Project Leadership Committee. (2004). The future of family medicine: A collaborative project of the Family Medicine Committee. *Annals of Family Medicine, 2,* Supplement, 3–99.

Gabor, A. (2004, February 22). Running a hospital like a factory, in a good way. *New York Times.*

Gebbie, K. (2004, June). Center for Health Policy and Doctoral Studies, Columbia University School of Nursing. Personal communication.

Gebbie, K., Rosenstock, L., & Hernandez, L. M. (Eds.). (2003). *Who will keep the public healthy? Educating public health professionals for the 21st century.* Institute of Medicine. Washington, DC: The National Academies Press.

Ghoshal, S., & Bartlett, C. A. (1995, January-February). Changing the role of top management: Beyond structure to processes. *Harvard Business Review, 73*(1).

Glasser, R. J. (1998, March). The doctor is not in. *Harpers Magazine,* 35–41.

Goldberg, H., et al. (2000, March). A controlled time-series trail of clinic reminders: Using computerized firm systems to make quality improvement research a routine part of mainstream practice. *Health Sciences Research, 34*(7), 1519–1534.

Graber, D., & Kaluzny, A. (2000). Developing high-involvement organizations for the Future. *Handbook of Health Administration and Policy.* New York: Marcel Dekker, Inc.

Greene, B., & Kelsey, D. (1998). From case management to medical care management. In E. O'Neil & J. Coffman (Eds.), *Strategies for the future of nursing.* San Francisco: Jossey-Bass.

Greiner, A. C., & Knebel, E. (Eds.). (2003). *Health professions education: A bridge to quality.* IOM Committee on the Health Professions Education Summit. Washington, DC: The National Academies Press.

Halverson, P. K., Mays, G., Kaluzny, A. D., & House, R. M. (1997, Spring). Developing leaders in public health: The role of executive training programs. *The Journal of Health Administration Education, 15*(2).

Harris, D. M. (2003). *Contemporary issues in healthcare law and ethics.* Chicago: Health Administration Press.

Herzlinger, R. (1997). *Market driven health care, who wins, who loses in the transformation of America's largest service industry.* Reading, MA: Addison-Wesley Publishing.

Hoadley, R., Cunningham, P., & McHugh, M. (2004). Popular Medicaid programs do battle with state budget pressures. *Health Affairs, 23,* 143–154.

Hurley, R. (1998). Approaching the slippery slope: Managed care as industrialization of medical practice. In P. Boyle (Ed.), *Rationing sanity: The ethos of mental health.* Washington, DC: Georgetown University.

Ibrahim, M. A., House, R. M., & Levine, R. H. (1995). Educating the public health work force for the 21st century. *Family Community Health, 18*(3), Aspen Publishers, Inc., pp. 17–25.

Institute of Medicine. (2001). *Improving the quality of long-term care.* Washington, DC: National Academy Press.

Institute of Medicine. (2002). *Executive summary of unequal treatment: Confronting racial and ethnic disparities in health care.* Washington, DC: National Academies Press.

Institute of Medicine Committee on Data Standards for Patient Safety, Board on Health Care Services. (2003, July 1). Key capabilities of an electronic health record system. Washington, DC: Institute of Medicine of the National Academies, The National Academies Press.

Jones, W., Johnson, J., Beasley, L., & Johnson, J. (1996, Summer). Allied health workforce shortages: The systemic barriers to response. *Journal of Allied Health, 25*(3), 219–232.

Kahn, J. G., Pinkerton, S. D., & Holtgate, D. R. (2002, January). Can cost-effectiveness analysis help in HIV prevention? Center for AIDS Prevention Studies. Retrieved June 2004, from http://www.caps.ucsf.edu/costeffetiverev

The Kaiser Commission on Medicaid and the Uninsured. (2003). Health insurance coverage in America, 2002 update. Washington, DC: Kaiser Family Foundation.

Kaluzny, A. & Warnecke, R., (eds) (2001). *Managing a health care alliance: Improving community cancer care.* San Francisco, CA: Josee-Bass Publishers.

Kaluzny, A. D., Zuckerman, H., & Rabiner, D. (1998, June). Interorganizational factors affecting the delivery of primary care to older Americans. *Health Services Research, 33*(2), Part II, 381–401.

Kochanek, K. D. & Smith, B. L. (2004, February). Deaths: Preliminary data for 2002. *National Vital Statistics Report, 51*(13). Centers for Disease Control & Prevention.

Kotter, J. P. (1996). *Leading change* (pp. 25–30). Boston: Harvard Business School Press.

Kressin, N., & Petersen, L. (2001). Racial differences in the use of invasive cardiovascular procedures: Review of the literature and prescription for future research. *Annals of Internal Medicine, 135,* 352–366.

Lamb, S., Greenlick, M., & McCarty, D. (Eds.). (1998). *Bridging the gap between practice and research: Forging partnerships with community-based drug and alcohol treatment programs.* Washington, DC: National Academy Press.

Leak, S. C. (2004, June). Associate in Residence, University of North Carolina at Chapel Hill, Institute on Aging. Personal communication.

Leatt, P., R. Grady, L. Prybill, et al. (2004). The Final Report of the Blue Ribbon Task Force on Accreditation. *Journal of Health Administration Education 21.*2, 121–166.

Levit, K., Smith, C., et al. (2004, Jan.). Health spending rebound continues in 2002. *Health Affairs, 23*(1), 147.

Loebs, S., (2004). A Study of Decision Factors for Careers in Health Administration. *The Journal of Health Administration Education, 21.4,* 485–528.

Lopez, L. (1997). Providing care, not cure, with chronic conditions. In *The Robert Wood Johnson Foundation Anthology,* volume 2. Robert Wood Johnson Foundation. Retrieved July 2004, from http://www.rwjf.org/publicationsPdfs/anthology1999/chapter_08.html

Lorenzi, N. (2003, December). *Strategies for creating successful local health information.* Report. Nashville, TN: Vanderbilt University Department of Biomedical Informatics.

Markle Foundation. (2003). *Connecting for health: Facts and stats.* Retrieved June 2004, from http://www.connecting forhealth.org/

McGlynn, E., et al. (2003). The quality of health care delivered to adults in the United States. *The New England Journal of Medicine, 348,* 2635–2645.

McLaughlin, C. P., & Kaluzny, A. D. (1997). Total quality management issues in managed care. *Journal of Health Care Finance, 24*(1), Aspen Publishers, Inc., pp. 10–16.

McLaughlin, C. P., & Kaluzny, A. D., (2006). Quality: From professional responsibility to public policy. In C. P. McLaughlin & A. D. Kaluzny (Eds.), *Continuous quality improvement in health care* (3rd ed.) Sunbury, MA: Jones and Bartlett Publishing Inc.

McNerney, W. J. (1985). Managing ethical dilemmas. *The Journal of Health Administration Education, 3*(3), 331–340.

Mercer Human Resource Consulting. (2003, December 8). Surprise slow-down in U.S. health benefit increase. Press release.

Meyer, H. (1998). Focused factories. *Hospitals and Health Networks, 72*(7).

Mintzberg, H. Managers Not MBAs, Berrett-Koehler, San Francisco, 2004.

Mohr, J. G., Randolph, et al. (2003). Integrating improvement competencies into residency education: A pilot project from a pediatric continuity clinic. *Ambulatory Pediatrics, 3*(3).

Mohr, J. J., Batalden, P. and Barach, P. (2006). Inquiring Into the Quality and Safety of Care in the Academic Clinical Microsystem. McLaughlin, C. P. and Kaluzny, A. D. (eds). Continuous Quality Improvement in Health Care. Jones and Bartlett Publishers, Boston, MA.

National Cancer Institute. (2002). *Annual report shows overall decline in U.S. cancer death rates. Cancer expected to rise with an aging population.* Retrieved June 2004, from http://www.cancer.gov/newsletter

National Cancer Institute. (2003). *Cancer progress report: 2003 update.* Retrieved June 2004, from http://progressreport.cancer.gov

National Center for Chronic Disease Prevention and Health Promotion. (2004). *Nutrition and physical activity.* Retrieved June 2004, from http://www.cdc.gov/nccdphp/dnpa/obesity

National Center for Healthcare Leadership. (2004, June). *Health leadership competency model.* Version 2. Chicago, Illinois.

National Center for Health Statistics. (2004a). *Fast stats: Alzheimer's disease.* Retrieved June 2004, from http://www.cdc.gov/nchs/fastats/alzheimer

National Center for Health Statistics. (2004b, February). *U.S. life expectancy at all time high, but infant mortality increases.* Retrieved June 2004, from http://www.cdc.gov/nchs/pressroom/04news/infantmort.htm

NCHL 2003 National Invitational Symposium proceeding published in Journal of Health Administration Education, Volume: Future of Education and Practice in Health. Management and Policy: Proceeding from the National Summit.

Nelson, E., Batalden, P., Mohr, J., & Plume, S. (1998). Building a quality future. *Frontiers of Health Services Management, 15*(1), 3–32.

Nolan, T. (1998, February 15). Understanding medical systems. *Annals of Internal Medicine, 128*(4), 293–298.

Parsi, K. (2001, July 7). Is it covered of not? Health plans and experimental procedures. *American Medical Association News,* 16.

Pew Health Professions Commission. (1995, November). *Critical challenges: Revitalizing the health profession for the twenty first century.* The Third Report of the Pew Health Professions Commission. San Francisco, CA.

Pierce, S. (2004, March/April). Why is nursing important? *North Carolina Medical Journal, 65*(2), 78–79.

Pollack, R. (2004, June 30). Personal communication to the Honorable Maria Cantwell, U.S. Senate in support of S.2491, the Allied Health Reinvestment Act.

Porter, Janet. (2005). University of North Carolina at Chapel Hill, School of Public Health. Personal communication.

Prybill, L. D. (2003, July). Challenges and opportunities facing health administration practice and education. *Journal of Healthcare Management, 48*(4), 223–232.

Raskin, A. (2003, May). Physician sell thyself. *Business, 2,* 109–113.

Resident population, by age and sex: 1990 to 1996. (1997). *Statistical abstract of the United States, 1997* (117th ed.). (No. 14, p.21). Washington, DC: Government Printing Office.

Rosenthal, M. B., Fernandopulle, R., Ryu Song, H., & Landon, B. (2004). Paying for quality: Providers' incentives for quality improvement. *Health Affairs, 23*(2), 127–141.

Satinsky, M. (1997). *The foundation of integrated care: Facing the challenges of change.* Chicago: American Hospital Publishing.

Schmitt, M. H. (2001). Collaboration improves the quality of care: Methological challenges and evidence from U.S. health care research. *Journal of Interprofessional Care, 15*(1), 47–66.

Shortell, S. M., Alexander, J. A., et al. (2001, July). Physician-system alignment: Introductory overview. *Medical Care, 39*(7), 1–8.

Shortell, S. M., Gillies, R. R., Anderson, D. A., Morgan-Erickson, K., & Mitchell, J. B. (2000). *Remaking health care in America: Building organized delivery systems.* San Francisco: Jossey-Bass.

Shortell, S. M., Waters, T. M., Clarke, K. B. W., & Budetti, P. P. (1998). Physicians as double agents:

Maintaining trust in an era of multiple accountabilities. *Journal of the American Medical Association, 280*(12), 1102–1108.

Singer, B., & Manton, K. (1998). The effects of health changes on projections of health service needs for the elderly population of the United States. *Proceedings of the National Academy of Sciences, 95,* 15618–15622.

Solberg, L. I., Kottke, T. E. and Brekke, M. (2006). Quality Improvement in Primary Care: The Role of Organization, Collaboratives, and Managerial care. In McLaughlin, C. P. and Kaluzny, A. D. (eds.) Continuous Quality Improvement in Health Care. Jones and Bartlett Publishers, Boston, MA. 297–317.

Stefl, M. E. (1999). Editorial. *Frontiers of Health Care Management, 16*(1), 1–2.

Stone, D. (2004). Shopping for long-term care: A daughter questions market theories after watching her parents make decisions about long-term care. *Health Affairs, 23,* 191–196.

Sturm, R., Ringel, J., & Andreyeva, T. (2004). Increasing obesity rates and disability trends. *Health Affairs, 23,* 199–205.

Tansey, B. Genentech a big believer in diagnostics: "Personalized medicine" can help patients and drug firms. *The Chronicle.* May 17, 2004.

Thompson, T. (2004, May 6). *Health information technology summit.* Retrieved June 2004, from http://www.hhs.gov/news/speech/2004/040506.html

Thompson, T., & Brailer, D. (2004, July). *The decade of health information technology: Delivering consumer-centric and information-rich health care.* Report issued by the Office of the Secretary, National Coordinator for Health Information Technology. Department of Health and Human Services, Washington, DC. Retrieved July 2004, from http://www.hhs.gov/onchit/framework/hitframework.pdf

Umble, K. E., Shay, S., & Sollecito, W. (2003). An interdisciplinary MPH via distance learning: Meeting the educational needs of practitioners. *Journal Public Health Management Practice, 9*(2), 123–135.

U.S. Bureau of the Census. (2004, March). *U.S. interim projections by age, sex, race, and hispanic origin.* Retrieved June 2004, from http://www.census.gov/ipc/www/usinterimproj/

U.S. House of Representatives Committee on Government Reform. (2003, August). *Politics and science in the Bush administration.* Minority staff special investigations division, prepared for Rep. Henry A. Waxman. Washington, DC.

Veney, J., & Kaluzny, A. (2004). *Evaluation and decision-making for health service programs* (3rd ed.). Chicago: Health Administration Press.

Wachter, R. M. (2004). Hospitalists in the United States— Mission accomplished or work in progress? *New England Journal of Medicine, 350*(19), 1935–1936.

Wachter, R. M., & Goldman, L. (1996). The emerging role of hospitalists in the American health care system. *New England Journal of Medicine, 335*(7), 514–517.

Walshe, K., & Rundall, T. (2001). Evidence-based management: From theory to practice in health care. *The Milbank Quarterly, 79*(3).

Warden, G. & M. Sinioris, NCHL 2003 Annual Report, National Center for Health Care Leadership, Chicago, IL., July 1, 2004.

Weil, P. A. (2004, June). American College of Healthcare Executives. Personal communication.

Weiner, B., & Alexander, J. (1998). The challenges of governing public-private community health partnerships. *Health Care Management Review, 23*(2), 39–55.

Weiner, B. J., Alexander, J. A., & Shortell, S. M. (2002). Management and governance processes in community health coalitions: A procedural justice perspective. *Health Education & Behavior.*

Weinstein, M. M. (1998, May 31). Whiplash: In health care, be careful what you wish for. *The New York Times,* Late Edition, p. 4.1.

The White House. (2004, April). *The White House, A new generation of American innovation.* Washington, DC: The White House.

Winslow, R. (1998, May 19). Health-care inflation revives in Minneapolis despite cost-cutting. *The Wall Street Journal,* section 1A.

Zerhouni, E. (2003, October 2). The NIH Roadmap. *Science, 302,* 63–72.

Zuckerman, H. S. (2002). Foreword. In: A. Ross, F. J. Wenzel, & J. W. Miltyng, (Eds.), *Leadership for the future: Core competencies in health care.* Chicago: Health Administration Press.

GLOSSARY

Absolute Power A source of competitive advantage grounded in the overall size and/or resources of an organization.

Accommodation Giving the other party in a conflict what they want without resistance; capitulation.

Accountability The responsibility for actions or decisions.

Acquisition The purchase of one company by another; the assets and liabilities of the seller are combined with those of the purchaser.

Activities Specific, identified, and interrelated business functions that organizations refine and share across business units in pursuit of competitive advantage. Organizations identify such activities within two major components of their value chains—primary value chain activities (inbound logistics, operations, outbound logistics, marketing and sales, and service) and support activities (procurement, technology development, human resource management, and firm infrastructure).

Adaptation An organization's adjustment to changes in its environment.

Adaptation Function Within the open system view, this is one of the key management functions. The adaptation function helps the organization to anticipate and adjust to needed changes.

Adaptive Learning A form of learning that occurs when problem solvers adjust their behavior and work processes in response to changing events or trends. Adaptive learning does not change the underlying structure of the system. Single-loop learning promotes adaptive learning.

Administrative Conflict Awareness by the involved parties that there are controversies about how task accomplishment will proceed.

Adoption The decision to make use of an innovation.

Agenda Setting The ongoing process within organizations through which organizational members identify important problems and search for innovations to address these problems.

Alliance Problems vs. Symptoms This distinction highlights that there is often disagreement as to why alliances fail, and that this disagreement is often rooted in mistaking a root cause for a mere symptom.

Alliance Process This refers to the flow of activities in the life cycle of a strategic alliance.

Alliance Risk The risk that the alliance will fail. Must be balanced against the expected rewards.

Alliances Informal, voluntary agreements among individuals or groups of similar or complimentary interests for purposes of achieving objectives.

Analyzer One of four business orientations identified in the Miles and Snow typology. Typically, an analyzer seeks to maintain stable operations in some areas of business activity while searching for new opportunities, often following the lead of prospector organizations.

Analyzing Work Breaking work into distinct tasks in the horizontal and vertical division of labor.

Approaches to Work Design The two primary approaches to work design are psychological and technical.

Arbitrator Manager who intervenes in a dispute as a third party by taking control over the outcome but not the process of the dispute.

Aspiration Level A challenging but attainable outcome a negotiator would ideally like to achieve in the negotiation; target; goal.

Assessment for Design Important stage in preparing to redesign an organization to identify strengths and weaknesses in relation to the mission. It includes consideration of the mission, external environment, internal organization, culture, human resources, and political processes.

Attributes Characteristics of a person or thing.

Attribution Theory A theory that holds that a manager's selection of a leadership style depends upon the way in which follower behavior is perceived and interpreted. Managers notice some things and are unaware of others; what is perceived is always filtered through a manager's distinctive cognitive frame and reshaped by it.

Authority A source of power in organizations that is formally sanctioned, often expressed by the role or position of an individual within the organizational hierarchy.

Avoidance A response to conflict that consists of ignoring it and taking no action to resolve it.

Awareness The initial stage of the organizational change process in which individuals recognize that there is a discrepancy or gap between what the organization or work unit is currently doing and what it should or could be doing.

Balancing Feedback Loops Create dynamic complexity by counteracting or opposing whatever is happening in a system. A thermostat regulates room temperature through a balancing feedback loop.

Bargaining Zone In a negotiation, the set of agreements both parties prefer over impasse, found by determining the range of outcomes across which negotiators' reservation prices overlap; if there is no overlap, the bargaining zone is negative.

Behavior and Performance Norms Behavior norms are rules that standardize how people act at work on a day-to-day basis, while performance norms are rules that standardize employee output by governing the amount and quality of work.

Behavior Modification A technique for applying the concepts of reinforcement theory to modify employee behavior in organizations by providing rewards for desired behavior and sanctions for undesired behavior.

Behavioral Masking Behavioral masking, known as "free riding" or "social loafing," occurs when individuals in large teams are able to maintain a sense of anonymity and gain from the work of the group without making a suitable contribution. When behavioral masking occurs, a member of the team obtains the benefits of group membership but does not accept a proportional share of the costs of membership.

Behavioral Perspective A theoretical school of leadership focused on describing the behaviors of leaders (style) and their differential effectiveness.

Benchmarking The process of establishing operating targets based on the leading performance standards for the industry.

Best Alternative to a Negotiated Agreement (BATNA) What a negotiator will do if a negotiation ends in an impasse.

Biological Organisms One of the metaphors of health care organizations. This metaphor identifies health care organizations as biological organizations that must adapt to their environments in the process of birth, growth, decline, and eventual death.

Boundary Spanning The management role that facilitates adaptation and change of the organization in response to changes in the external environment.

Boundary Spanning Function Another key function of the health care organization as a system. (See *Adaptation Function* previous page.) The boundary spanning function focuses on the interface between the organization and its external environment.

Brains The metaphor of organizations as brains places emphasis on the importance of learning, intelligence, and information processing.

Building and Maintenance Roles Building and maintenance roles are social-emotional behaviors aimed at helping the interpersonal functioning of the team. These behaviors are necessary to keep group members feeling good about the team and interacting effectively with one another.

Bureaucratic Organization An organization structured on bureaucratic principles with clear roles, lines of authority and accountability, procedures, rules, and policies for how work is performed and several levels in the hierarchy.

Bureaucratic Theory Classical bureaucratic theory is consistent with the closed system approach to organizations. Building on five key characteristics, the bureaucratic organizational form can achieve technical superiority under certain stable conditions.

Buyer Threats Threats from buyers, which depend on the market structure, environmental changes, and the relative competitive advantages of buyers and rivals.

Centralization and Decentralization Centralization occurs when decision making is concentrated at the top of the organization. Decentralization occurs when decision making is delegated or decentralized to lower levels in the organization.

Change Any modification in organizational composition, structure, or behavior—new or not new to the organization. Change is a broad concept. Innovation implies change, but not all change involves innovation.

Charismatic Leadership A social relationship between a leader and followers in which the leader presents a revolutionary idea or transcendent image. The follower accepts this course of action not because of its rational likelihood of success, but because of an emotional attachment to the extraordinary qualities of the leader.

Clinical Care System(s)/Management Role(s) Business processes within the health care organization designed to assure appropriate, safe, effective, and efficient patient care to clinically similar patient populations. Management roles involve managing clinical care system-oriented business processes.

Clinical Guidelines or Protocols Whereas critical pathways standardize the treatment approach for a given clinical condition, clinical guidelines standardize the decision process for adopting a treatment approach. Clinical guidelines address the appropriateness of care by specifying the indications for either tests or treatments. Various government agencies and professional associations are involved in the development of guidelines.

Clinical Mentality The cognitive frame of clinicians (e.g., physician or nurse) developed through professional education and experience. Clinicians are thought to have a "mentality" that differs from managers.

Clinical Microsystem A group of clinicians and staff working together with a shared clinical purpose to provide care for a population of patients.

Closed System The closed system view assumes that at least parts of an organization can be sealed off from the external environment. The need for predictability, order, and efficiency is consistent with a closed system view of an organization. Contrast with *open systems view*.

Coalitions See *alliances*.

Code of Ethics A formal set of principles and guidelines that are used in an organization as the basis for defining the boundaries between good and unethical (not always illegal) business practice. These principles and guidelines are visible and made known to all within the organization, as well as external stakeholders.

Collective Innovations Innovations that require the active, coordinated use of multiple members of the organization or social network in order to return benefits (e.g., electronic medical records or computerized physician order entry systems).

Collectivist-Democratic Organization Authority lies with the collective. There is no identifiable manager or hierarchy, and decision making is by consensus.

Combinatorial Complexity Also known as "detail" complexity, combinatorial complexity arises from the number of constituent elements of a system or the number of interrelationships that might exist among them.

Communication The creation or exchange of understanding between sender(s) and receiver(s). Effective communication plays a vital role in both programming and feedback coordination mechanisms.

Communication Channels The channels or methods of communication are the means by which messages are transmitted. Channels include face-to-face or telephone conversations involving individual and/or groups of senders and receivers, e-mail, facsimile messages, letters, memos, policy statements, operating room schedules, reports, electronic message boards, web pages, video teleconferences, newspapers, television and radio commercial spots, and newsletters for internal or external distribution.

Communication Networks Patterns of downward, upward, horizontal, and diagonal communication flows within organizations combined into patterns called *communication networks,* which are communicators interconnected by communication channels. The five common networks are chain, Y, wheel, circle, and all-channel.

Communication Structure The communication structure is the network that develops in teams that allows members to exchange information. The speed and accuracy of the team communication are determined by this structure.

Community Care Networks An integrated system of medical care, public health, and human service organizations that is formed to: (1) serve a common population defined at the community level; (2) provide consistent and coordinated access to services across care settings and along the continuum of care; (3) implement mechanisms for ensuring accountability to patients and to the general public; (4) manage the delivery of services within the context of fixed financial resources, such as through risk-adjusted capitation payments or global budgets; and (5) pursue the objective of improving community health status as well as the health status of enrolled populations.

Company-Level Strategy This term is used to differentiate the overall strategy of an organization from that pursued within local markets or for distinct business units. See *corporate strategy.*

Compatibility An attribute of innovations that refers to the degree to which the innovation is consistent with the values, beliefs, history, and current practices of the potential users.

Compatible Issues Issues for which negotiating parties have the same preferences.

Competition Parallel striving by multiple parties toward a goal that all parties cannot reach simultaneously.

Competitive Advantage The characteristics of a firm that enable it to outperform its rivals; could be called "key success factors" as well.

Complexity An attribute of innovations that refers to the degree to which organizational members perceive the innovation as difficult to understand or use.

Complex Adaptive Systems Are comprised of people and activities that mutually influence each other in complex ways with often-unpredictable outcomes. Elements of the system coevolve as they move forward together and interact over time.

Concentration An expression that characterizes the degree to which a small number of competitors control a market (by capturing market shares).

Conceptual/Mental/System Models Schematic depiction of the working (or operation) of more complicated systems. Used as a heuristic to assist managers in problem formulation/resolution and in developing and executing plans and actions.

Conceptual Skills The ability to form ideas, schemes, or methods in the managerial mind from experiences and/or creative thought.

Conflict Occurs when a concern of one party is frustrated, or is perceived to be frustrated, by another party.

Confrontation Meeting Brings together a large segment of the organization for problem identification and action planning in the event of an immediate threat or a need for rapid action in order to provide direction in a short time period.

Consideration The extent a manager exhibits concern for the welfare of its group, stresses the importance of job satisfaction, expresses appreciation, and seeks input from subordinates on major decisions.

Consolidation The pattern of competitors combining, usually through merger and acquisition, into larger and larger organizational arrangements.

Contingency Perspective A theoretical school that holds that the most effective leadership style is dependent upon a series of contingencies, the most important being: characteristics of the leader (e.g., his or her preferences and competencies), characteristics of followers (e.g., their level of maturity and motivation), and the nature of the situation in which leader and follower interact (e.g., time).

Contingency Theory Posits that the selection of the most appropriate form of organization is dependent upon the particular circumstances of the environment in which the organization operates. Contingency theorists do not advocate an either/or approach but rather view the process as a continuum from more or less bureaucratic (i.e., mechanistic) to more or less organic forms.

Contingency View of Coordination Recognizes that organizations typically use some combination of various coordination mechanisms, but that a particular mechanism or combination of mechanisms will achieve different levels of success depending upon characteristics of specific situations. A contingency approach to intraorganizational coordination requires that managers match the most appropriate coordinating mechanism or mechanisms to a given situation.

Continuing Education Provides health services personnel with the knowledge required to keep themselves and their organizations aware of new technology and service delivery programs.

Continuous Improvement Commitment to quality is a hallmark of successful organization. Recognizing the centrality of quality not only internally but also in terms of the perceptions and expectations of key external constituencies and stakeholders is leading health care organizations toward the principles of continuous quality improvement (CQI) and total quality management (TQM).

Continuous Quality Improvement (CQI) A participative, systematic approach to planning and implementing a continuous organizational improvement process.

Control of Information A situation in which an individual or group within the organization has sole authority over or access to key business information (e.g., financial, marketing, quality), thus providing that individual or group with a degree of power.

Cooptation Attempts to gain the support of a political faction by appointing influential members of such factions to legitimate roles (e.g., special committees, task forces, board of trustees) in a context supportive of the organization.

Coordinating Mechanisms Mechanisms for managing the interconnectedness of work.

Coordination A means of dealing with interdependencies by effectively linking together the various parts of an organization or by linking together two or more organizations pursuing a common goal. This conscious activity is aimed at achieving unity and harmony of effort in pursuit of shared objectives within an organization or among organizations participating in a multiorganizational arrangement of some kind.

Cope with Uncertainties A source of power for individuals and groups by virtue of their ability to handle nonroutine and unpredictable factors that influence the day-to-day operations and strategies of an organization (see *uncertainty*).

Corporate Strategy Those key concepts and ideas that relate to the selection, financing, and integration of business units and/or markets for the purpose of gaining and sustaining competitive advantage for the organization as a whole.

Cost-Effectiveness Is a composite measure that takes into account the degree of goal attainment and the costs to achieve them. To compare the overall cost-effectiveness of a set of alternative strategies, a common unit of measurement, such as cost per life saved, is used to summarize the likelihood and benefits and costs of achieving all possible outcomes under each strategy.

Costs of Coordination, Compromise, and Inflexibility These are costs commonly incurred when organizations engage collaboratively in strategic activities with other businesses. They include the costs of having to coordinate with partners (communicating, boundary spanning, operating complex committee structures, etc.), compromise with partners (give and take to resolve disagreements), and inflexibility (constraints to strategic action because of established commitments to business partners).

Cost Reduction vs. Revenue Enhancement This distinction highlights that the strategic intent behind alliances may differ on fundamental dimensions, such as cost versus value, and that such differences imply different bases for evaluating the success of an alliance.

Countervailing Power A strategy whereby buyers (or sellers) seek to increase their competitive advantage relative to sellers (or buyers), usually by use of power strategies to counteract the power of the other.

Critical Pathways Also known as *clinical pathways, care maps*, and *critical paths*, critical pathways are plans for managing patient care that display goals for patients and provide the corresponding ideal sequence and timing of staff actions to achieve those goals with optimal efficiency. Thus, for a given diagnosis or condition, a critical pathway specifies the work activities in advance.

Cultural Assessment The assessment of an organization's culture through questions such as, "What is it like to work here?" Indications of culture can be derived from employees' favorite stories about heroes, traditions, and language used. Organizations may be multicultural and have strong or weak cultures.

Decision Making Decision making is a process by which teams attempt to apply all available information to the problem at hand so as to make correct decisions. Some of the problems that prevent good decision making are free riders, polarization, and groupthink.

Declining Market A market in which there is an absolute decline in growth over a sustained period of time.

Defender One of four business orientations identified in the Miles and Snow typology. Typically, a defender is an organization that relies on established approaches towards growth and seldom makes adjustments to existing, proven strategies.

Delphi Technique The Delphi technique is a structured group decision-making method that elicits group members' opinions prior to judgments about those opinions. Through this technique, alternative ideas get to the table and are objectively debated by the team members, thereby decreasing the chance of groupthink.

Dependency Relationships Relationships in which an individual or group of individuals depends upon another individual or group of individuals within an organization. This situation describes an unequal relationship where one party to the relationship has political, economic, or social authority and resources, which the other party lacks and needs to function in their everyday work and job.

Design Outcome Design outcome is the organization chart produced at the end of the design process that represents who has authority to make which decisions. It is usually transitory because of changes in the external and internal environments.

Design Preparation The activities preceding organizational design including assessment for design.

Design Process The process of rethinking how authority, responsibility, and accountability should be distributed in an organization.

Designing Individual Jobs Individual jobs can be designed with an eye to motivation, skill requirements, or information flow.

Designing Work Groups to Address Coordination Needs Coordination is simplified when interconnected tasks are assigned to members of a single work group.

Differentiation Refers to the ability of an organization to create products and services that are different from its competitors.

Diffusion A passive process in which a growing body of information about an intervention, product, or technology is initially absorbed and acted upon by a small body of highly motivated recipients.

Disintermediation A process in which individuals have direct public access to the relevant information previously the province of a limited few professionals.

Direct Supervision A way of coordinating work that occurs when someone takes responsibility for the work of others, including issuing them instructions and monitoring their actions. Direct supervision entails some form of hierarchy within the organization.

Direct Work Effort that directly contributes to the accomplishment of an organization's goals.

Dissemination An active process where special efforts are made to ensure that intended users become aware of, receive, accept, and use an innovation.

Distributive Dimension of Negotiation The dimension along which any gain to one party necessarily corresponds to an equivalent loss for another party; the negotiated outcome stated in terms of the relative distribution among the individual parties of the resources being negotiated.

Diversity Training Provides individuals with new experiences and data to disconfirm old belief structures and replace them with fairer judgments regarding gender, ethnicity, race, or sexual orientation.

Divisional Design The organization is divided into several operating units, and decision making is decentralized to these units.

Double-Loop Learning A complex form of learning whereby problem solvers attempt to close the gap between desired and actual states of affairs by questioning and modifying those organization's policies, plans, values, and rules that frame organizational problems and guide organizational action. Double-loop learning promotes generative learning.

Dual-Advantages Strategy The simultaneous pursuit of both high differentiation and low-cost positions, which, while not easy to attain, would produce for highly sustainable levels of competitive advantage. This is a hybrid position, as compared to the so-called "generic" positions of low cost or high differentiation.

Dynamic Complexity A form of complexity that arises from the operation of feedback loops.

Effectiveness In organizations is the degree to which organizational goals and objectives are successfully met.

Efficiency Is defined as the cost per unit of output.

Emerging Market A newly formed or reformed market in which there remains a high degree of uncertainty as to the essential characteristics of the market or the strategic behaviors of the competitors.

Emotional Conflict Awareness of interpersonal incompatibilities among those working together on a task; characterized by negative emotions and dislike of the other person.

Empowerment Empowerment is a strategy in which employees are given information, knowledge, and power to make decisions when the traditional hierarchical management structure and command and control-management techniques are no longer viable. Teams, when used as an extension of the general employee empowerment strategy, occur along four dimensions: potency, meaningfulness, autonomy, and consequences.

Enterprise System(s)/Management Role(s) Business processes within the overall health care business enterprise designed to assure access to strategically critical resources (i.e., capital, human resources, physician manpower, organizational legitimacy, community support, etc.) required for investment and support of the enterprise's clinical care systems. Enterprise management roles involve managing enterprise-level business processes.

Entrant Threats Threats that new competitors will enter the market, where entry is dependent on the height of entry barriers.

Entry Barriers Technological, economic, regulatory, institutional, and other factors that inhibit firms from engaging in new businesses or entering new markets.

Environment As applied to strategy, this term refers to all drivers of strategy (e.g., technological change, demographic change, change in the economy, etc.) that are external to the focal organizations and their specific markets. Environmental factors influence the structures of markets, conduct of rivals, and individual firm strategies.

Environmental Assessment Assessment of the main factors in the external environment that influence how the organization can operate.

Environmental Barriers to Communication Characteristics of an organization and its environmental context that block, filter, or distort communications. Such barriers can be nothing more than the fact that people have too little time to communicate carefully. Other environmental barriers include the organization's managerial philosophy, multiplicity of its hierarchical levels, and power/status relationships between senders and receivers.

Environmental Context The environmental context of a team refers to the external factors that may affect team performance. Examples of these factors are other teams along with the intergroup relationships and conflict that exist, organizational resources, top management support, and the reward and incentive systems.

Equality Fairness Norm A guiding rule stating that every negotiating party should get the same absolute amount of resources in a negotiation.

Equity Fairness in relationships among individuals and groups. In equity theory, employees compare their perceived inputs and outcomes with their perceptions of other's inputs and outcomes.

Equity Fairness Norm A guiding rule stating that negotiating parties should be allocated an amount of resources proportional to their inputs along some relevant dimension.

Ethnic Composition The relative size and distribution of defined ethnic groups within a given population or community. A broad range of constructs may be used in defining ethnic groups, including origin, culture, and race—but most definitions are constructed from self-reported indicators of group membership.

Evidence-Based Management The continual identification and application of available scientific knowledge to improve administrative decision making in health care or other industries. Scientific knowledge may include information about optimal clinical staffing levels, compensation and incentive structures, organization and team design, health care financing arrangements, health care demand and supply projections, consumer preferences, cost-effectiveness information regarding health technologies and services, and information regarding the adoption and diffusion of clinical practices and technologies.

Evidence-Based Medicine The systematic identification and application of available scientific information for clinical decision making by health care professionals. Scientific information includes findings related to process and outcome-based measures of quality, as well as findings related to cost and cost-effectiveness. This process is supported by various mechanisms including clinical practice guidelines, clinical information systems, computer-based medical records, practice profiling and provider feedback mechanisms, health care report cards, and performance measurement systems.

Executive Leadership Role Executive management role(s) responsible for formulating and guiding the organization's strategic processes and for initiating and managing organizational adaptation processes required to achieve its strategic goals.

Execution Skills Performance skills required to achieve organizational accountability expectations, including strategic goals and objectives.

Expectancy The perceived link between effort and performance (e.g., the relationship between how hard an employee tries and how well he or she does in terms of job performance).

External Environment The complex of social, policy, competitive, technological, financial, and community conditions and expectations within which the health care enterprise operates and to which it must relate for access to critical resources and legitimacy.

Feedback Feedback approaches to coordination entail the exchange of information among staff usually while work is being carried out. Feedback approaches permit staff to change or modify work activities in response to unexpected requirements. Feedback also refers to the part of the communication process through which sender and receiver engage in a two-way process of communication. It reverses the sender and receiver roles so that information can be shared, recycled, and fine-tuned to achieve an unambiguous and mutual understanding in the communication process.

Feedback Approaches to Coordination Managing interconnections among tasks through interaction and communication among those who perform those tasks.

First Mover Advantage The advantage an organization attains by being the first competitor to pursue a particular source of competitive advantage. By moving early, first movers often, but not always, gain advantages of scale and learning (reducing costs with learning before second and later movers are able to pursue this source of advantage).

Five Forces Framework A framework, developed by Michael Porter, designed for use in analyzing market structure and competition. The focus is on five primary sources of competitive threat: from rivals, buyers, sellers, entrants, and substitutes.

Follower A person who carries out the directions from a leader.

Formal and Informal Leadership Leadership refers to the ability of individuals to influence other members toward the achievement of the team's goals. Teams may have multiple leaders. Formal leaders have legitimate authority over the team, and since their power has been granted by the organization, these leaders have the ability to use formal rewards and sanctions to support their authority. Informal leaders, on the other hand, are not recognized by the organization and therefore have no legitimate authority; however, they are able to influence the group members and should be considered a powerful force.

Formal Authority System Rights and obligations that create a field of influence within which an individual or department can legitimately operate with the formal support of those with whom they work.

Formal Groups Formal groups are formally organized work teams that operate within an organizational context and interact with a larger organization or organizational subunit. These groups are intact social systems with boundaries, interdependence among members, and differentiated member roles.

Four-Firm Ratio The sum of shares of the top four firms in a market, defined by their relative market shares; this is an indicator of market concentration.

Fragmented Market A market in which no firm has sufficient market share to have a strong influence on the strategic behaviors of competitors.

Functional Design The organization is divided into departments according to the function to be performed (e.g., finance, nursing, pharmacy, purchasing, and so on).

Future Scenarios A set of descriptive profiles that forecasts the performance of a given product, organization, market, or industry over an established period of time. Profiles are based on (1) the extrapolation of current and past performance trends, (2) expectations of future market developments, and (3) assumptions about key managerial decisions that are made during the period. Alternative performance profiles are generated by varying key assumptions, expectations, and managerial decisions across all plausible values. Scenarios are used to facilitate organizational strategic planning under uncertainty by identifying the range of possible outcomes associated with each potential action.

Gain Sharing A process of rewarding employees for increased productivity and/or cost containment by sharing a portion of the realized savings with employees.

Gender Gap The way in which one gender perceives themselves along a set of dimensions (e.g., aspects of the managerial role, leadership style) versus how they are perceived by the other gender.

Generative Learning A form of learning that occurs when problem solvers attempt to eliminate problems by changing the underlying structure of the system. This underlying structure includes the "operating policies" of the decision makers and actors in the system (e.g., their values and assumptions). Double-loop learning promotes generative learning.

Generic Strategies The label Michael Porter gave to two prominent position strategies—low cost and high differentiation. He had argued that most firms naturally gravitate to one or the other and thus called these "generic" positions. In health care and many other retail businesses, the highly common "middle" positions are also, in effect, generic.

Goal Accomplishment The primary objective of leadership; exercising leadership in order to accomplish goals that are so large and/or complex that they cannot be achieved by individuals working alone.

Governance Function When viewed from the systems approach, this is one of six key functions. This area is being given increasing attention because of the important public trust and social accountability responsibilities of health services organizations.

Groupthink Groupthink is a phenomenon that occurs in groups when the desire for harmony and consensus overrides members' efforts to appraise group judgments and decisions realistically. In other words, groupthink occurs when maintaining the pleasant atmosphere of the team becomes more important to members than coming up with good decisions. Self-censorship, collective rationalization, stereotyping others, and pressures to conform are some of the signs that groupthink may be present.

Growth/Share Matrix A graphical representation of and tool for analyzing the businesses/divisions within a multibusiness company; businesses/divisions are arrayed by market share and market growth rate; the matrix was first developed by the Boston Consulting Group.

Health Networks Strategic alliances that are contractual arrangements among hospitals, physicians, and other health services organizations.

Health Systems Arrangements among hospitals, physicians, and other provider organizations that involve direct ownership of assets on the part of the parent system.

Herfindahl-Hirschman Index The sum of the squared shares of competitors within a market (often multiplied by 10,000); this is an indicator of market concentration.

Hierarchical Model A local strategic configuration in which a hospital-based cluster is composed of a large referral center surrounded by one or more nearby smaller community hospitals, physician practices, and other provider entities. Synonym: hub/spoke model.

Hierarchy of Needs Five psychological need levels that must be satisfied sequentially in order to motivate an employee. In terms of rank from lower to higher, these include physiological needs, security needs, belongingness needs, esteem needs, and self-actualization needs.

Holograms Another metaphor for health care organizations. This is an object in which each of the parts contains the entire essence of the overall object or image. Designing health services organizations as holograms emphasizes the need for flexibility, creativity, change, and innovation.

Horizontal Division of Labor Dividing work into tasks to be completed by different people at the same level of the organization.

Horizontal Expansion A power strategy in which similar types of businesses are combined to achieve competitive advantage through the expansion in the scale of existing business activities (e.g., the merger of two or more hospitals).

Horizontal Integration A power strategy in which different types of businesses that are not vertically related are combined to achieve competitive advantage (e.g., jointly managing hotel and hospital companies).

Hospitalist A specialist in internal medicine responsible for managing the care of hospitalized patients.

Human Relations School The focus of the human relations school is on the individual. This is one of the classical perspectives on organizations and has been applied in the health care sector to emphasize the usefulness of participatory decision making.

Human Relations Skills The complex of skills required to develop, maintain, and manage relationships between and among personnel within the organization and the community served, to motivate performance aimed at achieving strategic goals and objectives, and to establish priorities while resolving conflict effectively.

Human Resources Assessment An assessment of the availability of individuals with appropriate knowledge and skills to carry out the mission of the organization.

Human Resources Change Strategies Concerned with changing the attitudes, values, skills, and behaviors of personnel within the organization.

Hybrid Organization An organization that combines two or more firms to achieve coordination or control, but without the use of ownership arrangements (the mingling of assets and liabilities).

Hygiene Factors Factors related to the work environment (i.e., extrinsic factors) whose presence prevents dissatisfaction but does not lead to satisfaction or motivation.

Identification The second stage of the change process that involves an attempt to address the discrepancies or performance gap identified in the awareness stage.

Imitation Proponents of the resource-based view coined this term to refer to threats to the sustainability of competitive advantage, where rivals copy or duplicate a competitor's advantages that are attributable to superior resources and/or capabilities.

Implementation The transition period during which targeted organizational members ideally become increasingly skillful, consistent, and committed in their use of an innovation.

Implementation Effectiveness The overall consistency and quality of targeted organizational members' use of an innovation. Implementation effectiveness is a necessary, but not sufficient condition for innovation effectiveness.

Implementation Policies and Practices A shorthand phrase for the formal strategies that an organization employs in order to put the innovation into use, and the actions that follow from those strategies.

Industrial Organization A field of economics that involves the study of how market structures and processes affect the behaviors and strategies of competitors as they seek to meet consumer demands.

Influence Actions that, either directly or indirectly, cause a change in the behavior and/or attitudes of another individual or group. The primary effect of leadership.

Influence Systems Political activity and informal systems of power that often arise in attempts to influence decisions and activities outside the formal system of authority.

Informal Communication Coexisting with formal communication flows and networks within organizations are informal communication flows, which have their own networks. Like informal organization structures, informal communication flows and networks result from the interpersonal relationships in organizations.

Informal Groups Informal groups are not recognized by the organization but are found in all organizations. They may have a positive effect on the organization, but they can also be powerful enough to undermine the formal authority structure of the organization.

Initiating Structure The degree a manager defines and organizes the work that is to be done and the extent attention is focused on accomplishing objectives established by a manager.

Innovation The process by which an organization puts a technology or practice to use for the first time, regardless of whether other organizations have previously used the technology or practice.

Innovation Effectiveness The benefits the organization realizes from innovation use. Innovation effectiveness depends in part on implementation effectiveness.

Inquisitor Manager who intervenes in a dispute as a third party by taking control over both the process and outcome of the dispute.

Institutional Theory Institutional theorists emphasize that organizations face environments characterized by external norms, rules, and requirements that the organization must conform to in order to receive legitimacy and support.

Institutionalization Stage of the change process in which change is integrated into the ongoing activities of the organization.

Instrumentality The perceived link between performance and outcomes based on the extent to which employees believe that attaining a particular job outcome depends on or is conditional to their performance.

Integrating Skills Skills required to integrate competing concepts, views, and priorities within a competitive environment in order to develop distinctive competencies and effective strategies, and to achieve strategic goals and objectives.

Integration Structures and processes that tie the various units of an organization together so as to increase coordination and collaboration.

Integrative Dimension of Negotiation The dimension along which one party can gain without another party necessarily incurring an equivalent loss; allows mutually beneficial outcomes to be discovered.

Integrators Individuals who, because of specialized knowledge and because they represent a central source of information, are able to facilitate coordination. Examples of effective integrators are found among all health professionals. In most health care organizations, individual nurses, regardless of formal position, often function as integrators linking physicians to the organization's formal administrative structure.

Interconnectedness of Work Interdependencies among tasks, where the completion of one task depends upon the completion of another.

Interdependence The condition of mutual dependence between or among people and organizational units (including entire organizations) that exists whenever work activities are interconnected in some manner—physically or intellectually.

Interdependency Whenever one actor does not entirely control all the conditions necessary for the achievement of an action or for obtaining the outcomes desired from the action.

Interests Aims and objectives of individuals or groups that can differ from and compete with larger organizational goals and objectives or from the aims and objectives of other individuals or groups.

Intergroup Conflict Intergroup conflict occurs when different teams interact, and disagreements occur between the groups. Most intergroup conflict is due to factors related to interdependence among work groups. For example, when two groups are dependent upon each other to do their work, conflicts can easily result when information-transfer procedures are ineffective or lacking.

Internal Environment The conditions within an organization including culture, stakeholder relationships, structures, and processes.

Interorganization Relations An organization's formal and informal relationships with other firms and regulatory agencies.

Interorganizational Relationships As the health services environment grows in complexity and accelerates its rate of change, a key component of many organizations' strategies is to form relationships with other organizations.

Interpersonal Conflict Conflict between two or more individuals.

Intragroup Conflict Conflict among members of the same group.

Intrapersonal Conflict Conflict within one person who is attempting to choose among multiple options in making a decision.

Job Skill and Knowledge Requirements The skills and knowledge required for the successful completion of a particular job.

Job Redesign Altering certain aspects of a job to better satisfy an employee's psychological needs. Examples include task identity, skill variety, task significance, knowledge of results, and feedback.

Just-in-Time Management (JIT) A managerial strategy designed to achieve operational efficiencies by reducing the need for excess or "slack" human, capital, and intellectual resources. Reductions in slack are achieved by implementing processes to secure resources rapidly on an "as-needed" basis rather than maintaining large resource inventories for future use. Similarly, operational processes within the organization are engineered to produce both internally consumed products and externally consumed products at the time of demand.

LEAD Model A model suggesting that leadership style can be described along two dimensions: the amount of attention accorded to developing/ sustaining relationships, and the amount of attention accorded to accomplishing tasks. The most appropriate style is a function of individual/group maturity.

Leadership Providing direction in group activities and influencing others to achieve common goals.

Leadership Match Model The first comprehensive model of leadership style. The underlying theory holds that leaders are unable to alter their style to any appreciable degree. Hence, leadership effectiveness depends not on fitting one's style to the situation (as most contingency theories hold), but rather selecting situations that are conducive to one's style.

Leadership Role One of the roles of a manager: intentionally influencing individuals and groups in order to accomplish a goal.

Leadership Styles (S1, S2, S3, and S4) S1 is a leadership style characterized by a large amount of attention accorded to task accomplishment, and little accorded to building/sustaining relationships with followers. S2 is a leadership style characterized by a large amount of attention accorded to both relationships and task. S3 is a leadership style characterized by a large amount of attention accorded to building/sustaining relationships and little accorded to accomplishing tasks. S4 is a leadership style that accords little attention to either relationships or task. (See *LEAD Model.*)

Learning Curve Sometimes called the experience curve, this term expresses the inverse relationship that is generally assumed to exist between learning (and/or experience) and production costs.

Learning Organization A place where people continually expand their capacity to create the results they truly desire, where new and expansive patterns of thinking are nurtured, where collective aspiration is set free, and where people are continually learning together. Alternatively, an organization that is skilled at creating, acquiring, and transferring knowledge, and at modifying its behavior to reflect new knowledge and insights.

Levels of Organization Design Organization design may be considered at different levels including for a position, work group, cluster or work groups, total organization, network of organization, and a system.

Linking Pins People who serve formally as links between various units in the organization—similar to integrators. Horizontally, in such situations, there are certain organizational participants who are members of two separate groups and serve as coordinating agents between them. On the vertical axis, individuals serve as linking pins between their level and those above and below.

Local-Market Strategy This term is used to distinguish between strategies pursued within specific markets by multimarket firms (which contrasts with broader corporate or company-level strategies).

Machines Another metaphor for health services organizations that emphasizes bureaucratic traits.

Macro Approach When selecting the "unit of analysis" in research and observations on organizations, the macro approach leads us to emphasize the organization as a social system in the context of other organizations.

Maintenance Function The maintenance function is concerned with both the physical and human infrastructure of the organization. As the rate of change accelerates and as the external environment becomes more threatening, greater demands are placed on the maintenance functions of health services organizations.

Management Function Management is a distinct function that cuts across all the other functions and subsystems. In a sense, it is the "head" that organizes, directs, and oversees all of the other functions.

Management Teams Management teams coordinate and provide direction to the subunits under their jurisdiction. They may exist at the board, senior management, or departmental level.

Management Work Decision making about the organizational context within which work is performed.

Managerial Accountability Responsibility for achieving organizational/strategic goals and objectives.

Managerial Competencies Specific skills or abilities such as financial, marketing, change management, and performance assessment.

Managerial Mentality Managers owe their alliance to the organization, accountability is shared, the power they exercise is determined by the office they hold, their time frames are long, feedback is typically delayed or vague, and their tolerance for ambiguity high.

Managerial Office A hierarchically superordinate office, occupied by a manager, in an organization or organizational component.

Managerial Roles A collection of expectations attached to an office. Role expectations are defined by the office's charter (job description) in addition to the expectations of superiors, peers, and subordinates. The aspects of managerial roles can be conceptualized in a variety of ways.

Managing Across Boundaries In the changing health care system where continuity of care is becoming more and more essential, the ability to manage across boundaries between and among organizations is becoming increasingly crucial.

Market An arena in which one or more sellers of given products/services and their close substitutes exchange with and compete for the patronage of a group of buyers. Health care markets are typically delimited in geographic (e.g., metropolitan areas) and/or product terms (e.g., general acute medical/surgical care).

Market Concentration A market is concentrated when a small number of competitors exist. As a result, they exercise collectively or individually high levels of market power.

Market Conduct The collective actions that organizations take within markets in pursuit of competitive advantage. Both conduct and strategy refer to the strategic behaviors of competitors. The difference is that conduct refers to the collective and strategy to individual competitors.

Market Power A competitor enjoys market power when it is able to affect the decisions of competitors (e.g., decisions relating to pricing, offering new products, and engaging in a merger) and/or customers in a market context. In terms of strategy, competitors that gain competitive advantage, by definition, gain market power.

Market Share The percentage of the market controlled by a given competitor. For hospitals and hospital clusters, this can be calculated using a variety of measures, including the percentages of beds, patient days, and revenues controlled by given competitors. This is an important indicator of local market (or relative) power.

Market Structure The organizational features of a market (e.g., seller concentration, entry barriers, degree of product differentiation) that condition or influence the conduct and strategies of competitors.

Market Structure View The perspective on strategy that emphasizes the role of market structure in driving competitive behaviors and advantage.

Matrix Design A matrix design is characterized by a dual-authority system. Each worker is accountable to two bosses, each able to exercise authority over the worker.

Maturity A follower's motivation, responsibility, and competence to complete a task. Maturity is

situational and task-specific; a follower may be very mature in one situation and immature in another.

Mature Market A market in which there is sustained moderate, flat, or even slightly declining growth.

Mediator A third party to a dispute who intervenes by taking high control over the process but not the outcome of the dispute.

Mental Models The discipline of constantly surfacing, testing, and improving our assumptions about how the world works.

Merger The combination of companies whereby the assets and liabilities of each are intermingled.

Micro Approach In the micro approach, the emphasis is on organizational behavior to understand organizations. The unit of analysis is the individual, the group, or the department units.

Mission and Values The encompassing ideas of the organization that define its purpose and its principles.

Mission/Goals The organization's mission and associated goals largely dictate the major tasks to be carried out and the kinds of technologies and human resources to be employed.

Monopolistic Market A market in which one firm has a significant (perhaps total) share of the market; many monopoly markets, however, are also "contestable" in that entry barriers are sufficiently low to cause a monopolistic to act as if the market were competitive.

Motivating Potential of Jobs A job's motivating potential score (MPS) is affected by the skill variety, task identity, task significance, and autonomy and feedback experienced by performing a particular job, which depends in turn on the design of that job.

Motivation A state of feeling or thinking in which one is engaged or aroused to perform a task or engage in a particular behavior.

Motivators Factors related to the work content (i.e., intrinsic factors) whose presence increases job satisfaction and motivation but whose absence does not lead to job dissatisfaction. Motivators include achievements, recognition, work, responsibility, and advancement.

Moving The second stage of Kurt Lewin's three-stage change model; moving involves putting into place new strategies, structures, or practices.

Multiskilled Employees Employees whose jobs are designed to encompass multiple tasks in the horizontal division of labor, with the goal of either making the work more meaningful, simplifying coordination, or both.

Mutual Adjustment A way of coordinating work that occurs through informal communications among individuals who are not in a hierarchical relationship to one another; for example, two physicians sharing information about a patient's clinical condition.

Need Fairness Norm A guiding rule stating that negotiating parties should receive an amount of resources proportional to their need for them.

Negotiation The process whereby two or more parties decide what each will give and take in an exchange between them.

Network Centrality Defines the relative position of individuals and groups in the organization vis-à-vis key communication and information dissemination channels. The more central an individual or group is to communication and information flows in an organization, the more power gained by that individual or group.

Network Externalities Characteristics of situations that make the utility or value of an innovation for one person dependent largely or entirely on others also using the innovation (e.g., e-mail). Innovations subject to network externalities are also referred to as collective innovations.

Niche Strategy A strategy in which a competitor seeks advantage by focusing on a single or small number of product lines or population segments.

Nominal Group Technique Nominal group technique is a group decision-making and problem-solving technique that elicits group members' opinions prior to judgments about those opinions. The technique is particularly effective for setting goals and priorities, and gaining a better understanding of complex issues.

Nonsubstitutability Defines a situation in which a resource, skill, or piece of knowledge cannot be replaced easily within the organization, thus providing the individual or group possessing the resource, skill, or piece of knowledge with a degree of power.

Observability An attribute of innovations that refers to the degree to which the results of an innovation are visible to others.

Office An office is point in organizational space to which a role is attached (collection of expectations).

Oligopolistic Market A market in which there are a small number of firms, and the competitors believe that their rivals have sufficient market power to influence their long-term survival; they therefore consciously adapt their strategies in response to their assessments of rival competitive advantages and expected strategic maneuvers.

Open System This view emphasizes that organizations are parts of the external environment and, as such, must continually change and adapt to meet the challenges posed by the environment. The need for openness, adaptability, and innovation is consistent with an open system view.

Opinion Leaders Individuals who serve as hubs in social and professional networks and strongly influence how innovations are perceived in their organizations and others.

Organization Behavior See *Micro Approach*.

Organization Design In contrast with work design, organization design focuses on the overall allocation of power and authority, information processing, and decision-making rules within the organization and how individual work groups, departments, or divisions are themselves linked together.

Organization Learning A method by which organizations continuously improve performance by ensuring that each member continuously develops knowledge, skills, and motivations that are linked with the organization's central mission and objectives.

Organization Structure The apportionment of responsibility and authority among members of an organization; the architecture of an organization.

Organization Theory Organization theory involves the systematic examination of the ways that organizations function. Over time a number of major perspectives of how organizations work have evolved including: classical bureaucratic theory, the scientific management school, etc. These perspectives can be used to gain insight into the structure and functioning of health services organizations.

Organizational Adaptation Change in organizational structure and/or structure required by environmental changes to achieve strategic goals and objectives.

Organizational Decision-Making Processes Processes within organizations that typify how decisions get made, and may fall under aggregate headings such as strategy, hierarchy, participative approaches, etc. Gaining control over one or more decision-making processes provides increased power to the individual or group exercising the control.

Organizational Effectiveness The extent to which an organization accomplishes its basic objectives and maintains its viability.

Organizational Framework A set of assumptions, concepts, values, and practices providing a way of viewing organizational goals, processes, and performance.

Organizational Transformation Assuring the organization's ability to conform to new (and possibly threatening) circumstances or to take advantage of newly identified opportunities.

Organized Integrated Delivery System An integrated network of health care providers, supported by a health care financing and administrative entity, that competes to assume clinical and financial responsibility for the health of defined populations of health care consumers. A continuum of health care services is available through the network of affiliated providers.

Outcome Measures of Quality In health care delivery assess changes that occur in the health outcomes of the person receiving the service that can be attributed to the quality of the services performed.

Outcomes Assessments A way of systematically collecting, monitoring, and reporting performance results. Through such assessments, managers from different organizations or units can detect and attend to undesirable variation in outputs (by changing or modifying work activities as needed over time or relative to competitors).

Ownership vs. Control This distinction refers to the fact that greater ownership stakes do not necessarily result in greater control of an alliance. Control indicates influence, and an influence can come from many sources, of which ownership is only one.

Pace Strategy A strategy whereby a competitor seeks competitive advantage through the use of timing, aggressiveness, and risk-taking behaviors.

Parallel Design The parallel design retains a functional structure that has responsibility for routine activities but also has a parallel structure responsible for solving complex problems that transcend functional units.

Partner Orientation A summary characterization of the degree to which an alliance partner is interested in working cooperatively with his/her partner.

Path-Goal Model A theory of leadership based on the expectancy theory of motivation. Followers' motivation (which the leader attempts to influence) is seen to be a function of expectancies, instrumentalities, and valences.

Patient-Centered Care A multidisciplinary approach to patient care that centers the design of work around patients' needs.

Pay for Performance A program of financial incentives given to providers (hospitals and physicians) to improve quality and reduce cost based on measured performance on selected indicators.

Performance Achievement of a desired result.

Performance Gaps Perceived discrepancies between expected and actual organizational performance. Performance gaps often trigger the innovation processes as organizational members look for new ideas or technologies to bridge the gap.

Performance Norms Rules that standardize employee output and govern the amount and quality of work required of individuals, as well as the amount of time they are expected to work.

Performance Strategy A strategy whereby a competitor seeks competitive advantage through superior operational and/or strategic performance.

Personal Barriers to Communication Barriers that arise from the nature of people, especially in their interaction with others that apply equally to communication within organizations and between them and their external stakeholders. Examples include people distorting the encoding or decoding of their messages according to their frames of reference or their beliefs and values. People may also consciously or unconsciously engage in selective perception, or permit their emotions—such as fear or jealousy—to influence their communications.

Personal Mastery The discipline of individual learning that involves continuously clarifying our individual sense of purpose and vision, and continuously learning how to see the world as it is without distortion.

Personal Roles Personal roles refer to those roles that individuals assume in groups that mainly satisfy individual needs and are thus unrelated to the group's goals. It is important for team leaders to understand personal roles because they may detract from team performance.

Playing Fields Another analogy for health care (and other) organizations. Health services organizations require the inputs of a variety of highly trained professions who each bring his or her own "culture" to the organization. The challenge is to create a larger overall sense of organizational identity and culture that can embrace the individual cultures of the different health professionals.

Policy Resistance The tendency for interventions to be delayed, diluted, or defeated by the response of the system to the intervention itself.

Political Games The exercise of power in the form of political influence expressed as a set of "games," each with its own structure and rules that are played outside the legitimate system of authority.

Political Model of Organizations Model of organizational behavior that emphasizes the existence of power and influence other than that vested in the formal authority system.

Political Process Assessment Assessing the nature of the informal organization including who are the key leaders and how communication flows.

Political Systems Organizations can also be viewed as political systems in which various groups and actors vie for control of important resources. See *Playing Fields* above.

Politics Domain of activity in which participants attempt to influence organizational decisions and activities in ways that are not sanctioned by either the formal authority system of the organization, its accepted ideology, or certified expertise.

Pooled Interdependence Occurs when individuals and units are related but do not bear a close connection; they simply contribute separately in some way to the larger whole.

Pooling vs. Trading Alliances Pooling alliances reflect two or more organizations contributing similar resources for mutual gain, whereas trading alliances are based on the notion of combining dissimilar—but complementary—resources.

Population Ecology Theory Population ecologists argue that the environment "selects out" certain organizations for survival. Organizational success is more dependent upon environmental selection than managerial decision making and implementation.

Population-Based Management In the managed care environment, health care organizations are increasingly being called upon to work to improve the health status of whole populations or some subset of the public.

Porter Model A framework developed by Michael Porter of Harvard University to analyze the five main forces that affect competition in a market.

Portfolio A power strategy in which different types of businesses are combined to achieve competitive advantage through financial coordination and risk sharing (differs from horizontal and vertical integration in that the synergies, other than financial, in business activities are not pursued as a basis for achieving advantage).

Portfolio Strategy A power strategy whereby firms (either under the same ownership or within a strategic alliance) are managed financially by a parent company in order to achieve synergies and greater competitive advantage.

Position Strategy A strategy whereby a competitor seeks competitive advantage by projecting value to consumers; they do this by pursuing a: (1) low-cost position, (2) differentiated position, and/or (3) market niche.

Positioning Dynamics This term refers to the ongoing attempts by rivals to move within the spectrum of market positions, first moving toward the generic positions (low cost, high differentiation, or middle) and, ultimately, toward the more desirable, but more difficult to attain and sustain dual-advantage positions.

Potential Strategy A strategy that emphasizes the pursuit of advantage through the acquisition and sustaining of superior resources (locations, staff, equipment, etc.) and capabilities (IT systems, management capabilities, supply-chain coordination, vertical integration experience, etc.).

Power Ability (or potential) to exert actions that either directly or indirectly cause a change in the behavior and/or attitudes of another individual or group. The potential to exercise influence. As power increases, so does the probability of getting others to think or act in a certain way.

Power Strategy A strategy whereby a competitor seeks competitive advantage by building/acquiring greater size and/or resources.

Pressing Using relatively contentious tactics in a conflict situation to achieve one's goals without regard for the other party's outcome.

Process Consultation Involves an outside consultant helping a client to perceive, understand, and act upon process events that are occurring within the organization. Focus is put on communications, role and function of group members, group problem-solving and decision-making group norms, and the use of leadership and authority.

Process Measures of Quality Focus on evidence relating to the quality of the performer's activities in carrying out the work.

Product Differentiation An approach to positioning that emphasizes the projection of distinctive values to actual and potential consumers. If successful in differentiating itself, a firm, business, or product can enjoy an increase in market power or competitive advantage.

Production Function The production function provides the product or the service and is at the center of most organizational activity.

Productivity Is defined as the ratio of outputs to inputs.

Product-Line or Program Design Product-line management is defined as the placement of a person in charge of all aspects of a given product or group of products (e.g., all health care for a segment of the population such as women, children, or the elderly).

Professional Engaged in one of the learned professions.

Programming Programming approaches to coordination seek to clarify work responsibilities and activities in advance of the performance of work, as well as specify the outputs of the work process and the skills required to perform the work. Programming approaches essentially standardize work activities for all expected requirements.

Programming Approaches to Coordination Managing interconnections among tasks by prespecifying the nature and sequence of tasks, and who is to perform them.

Project-Management Design A structural means for coordinating a large amount of talent and resources for a given period on a specific project. For example, a health care organization may wish to organize services into a comprehensive home health care program for the chronically ill by forming a team organized around the focus of the program— home services for the chronically ill. Team members would be drawn from nursing, social services, respiratory therapy, occupational therapy, pharmacy, and physicians specializing in chronic disease. To market the program and to handle finance and reimbursement issues, expertise would be provided by team members drawn from the organization's administration. A project manager would be responsible for coordinating the activities of team members.

Prospector One of four business orientations identified in the Miles and Snow typology. Typically, prospectors are willing to assume risk or take aggressive action in the pursuit of competitive advantage, by searching for new market opportunities and regularly engaging in experimentation and innovation.

Psychic Prison Organizations can also be viewed as places where people are trapped by their own perceptions, ideas, and beliefs whether consciously or unconsciously. Often this is reflected in the tendency to avoid conflict, to avoid anxiety-provoking situations, or to strive to maintain one's sense of identity and self-esteem.

Psychological Approach to Work Design Designing work with a focus on worker motivation.

Psychological Safety From a team perspective, psychological safety refers to a shared belief that the team is safe for interpersonal risk taking.

Public Good Any resource or information that is made available for use by the public at-large. In the case of an organization, that public may be defined as anyone and everyone from frontline and lower-level employees to the chief executive officer and board of directors.

Quality Assurance Refers to the formal and systematic exercise of identifying, monitoring, and overcoming problems in health care delivery.

Quality Improvement Is a management philosophy to improve the level of performance of key processes in the organization by focusing on the most important processes to improve, understanding the process, setting high standards for performance outcomes, and using statistical and behavioral methods and tools to measure current performance, interpret it, and take corrective action when necessary.

Rational Model of Organizations Model of organizational behavior that emphasizes that managers orchestrate the activities of a team whose members all subscribe to a common set of goals and objectives.

Reactivity To performance criteria refers to the tendency for evaluated persons to react in ways to maximize achieving positive evaluations of their performance rather than to achieve the best performance.

Reactor One of four business orientations identified in the Miles and Snow typology. Typically, a reactor perceives opportunities and turbulence, but is not able to adapt consistently or effectively to change.

Reciprocal Interdependence Occurs when individuals and units bear a close relationship, such that they mutually depend on each other to achieve given tastes.

Refreezing The third stage of Kurt Lewin's three-stage change model, refreezing involves stabilizing the change by integrating the newly adopted strategies, structures, and practices into existing operating procedures and work routines and by reinforcing changes in the attitudes and behaviors of organizational members.

Reinforcement Operant conditioning in which a stimulus elicits a response that has a consequence. A consequence is an outcome following a response that changes the likelihood a response will occur again following that stimulus. Consequences include rewards and punishments.

Reinforcing Feedback Loops Create dynamic complexity by amplifying or intensifying whatever is happening in a system. In everyday language, we refer to reinforcing feedback loops as self-fulfilling prophecies or the "Pygmalion effect."

Relational Coordination The quality of communication and relationship ties between coworkers that help improve the outcome of a task.

Relationship-Oriented Leader Behavior Actions a leader takes to meet the emotional needs of a follower. A leader can have high or low relationship-orientated behavior with a follower. The relationship between the leader and follower changes based on the maturity of the follower.

Relative Advantage An attribute of innovations that refers to the degree to which the innovation is perceived as superior to current practice.

Relative Power A source of competitive advantage that is grounded in a competitor's local market power (based on market share) relative to that of its local rivals.

Reservation Price The point at which a negotiator is indifferent between an impasse and an agreement, stated in terms of whatever units are being negotiated (e.g., dollars).

Resource Acquisition Refers to the ability of an organization to successfully obtain capital and other types of resources needed.

Resource Dependence Theory The resource dependence theory emphasizes the importance of the organization's abilities to secure needed resources from its environment in order to survive.

Resource-Based View The theoretical perspective that emphasizes the need to acquire/develop/sustain unique, inimitable, and strategically valuable resources and/or capabilities to sustain competitive advantage.

Responsibility Charting Technique that identifies decision-making patterns among a set of actors—individuals, units, departments, or divisions within the organization. It provides an opportunity to compare responses of a specific participant about that person's role in a decision with the response of one or more participants about the same participant role, to compare responses across all actors on a specific decision, to examine responses of each actor across a set of decisions, and to compare actual decision patterns with desired activity.

Risk Taking Characterizes proactive and far-reaching actions of health care organizations to step out of the traditional modes of action and develop new programs and services or modify their ways of carrying out their mission and the delivery of care.

Rival Threats Threats from competitors in the market, which depend on the market structure, environmental changes, and the relative competitive advantages of rivals.

Role Differentiation Role differentiation refers to the specialization of work activities in an organization.

Scientific Management A technical approach to work design that attempts to divide jobs narrowly, and to separate management work from direct work.

Scientific Management School Closely related to the classical bureaucratic approach with an emphasis on span of control, unity of command, appropriate delegation of authority, departmentalization, and the use of work methods to improve efficiency.

Self-Actualization Realizing one's potential for continued growth and individual development. The top level of the hierarchy of needs.

Seller Threats Threats from sellers, which depend on the market structure, environmental changes, and the relative competitive advantages of sellers and rivals.

Sequential Interdependence Occurs when one person or unit depends on another for resources or information to accomplish a task.

Shared Vision The discipline of generating a common or shared aspiration that connects people and derives its motivational power by tapping people's personal visions.

Single-Loop Learning A relatively simple error-and-correction process whereby problem solvers look for solutions within an organization's policies, plans, values, and rules. Single-loop learning promotes adaptive learning.

Six Aims Refer to the Institute of Medicine's Quality Chasm report that identified the following six aims to assess health system performance: safety, effectiveness, efficiency, patient-centeredness, elimination of waste, and equity.

Skills Perspective Suggests that effective leadership is based upon three core skills: technical, conceptual, and human.

Social Capital Refers to the networks, together with shared norms, values, and understandings that facilitate cooperation within or among groups. In a team context, social capital refers to the web of cooperative relationships between providers in a service system that involve interpersonal trust, norms of reciprocity, and mutual aid.

Social Experimentation A collection of methods used for evaluating the performance of programs, services, or other interventions at the population level.

Social Loafing Also known as "free-riding" and "shirking," refers to a situation in which individuals exert less effort when they work in a group than when they work alone.

Social Networks Perspective Emphasizes the role of social relationships among individuals and groups in explaining organizational behavior.

Social Norms and Expectations A common set of knowledge, values, and beliefs that is shared by a group of individuals and that shapes the decision making and behavior of group members.

Sources of Power Notion that power can be derived from personal attributes such as sensitivity, articulateness, self-confidence, and aggressiveness, or from structural sources such as where individuals stand in the division of labor and the communications system of the organization.

Spatial Dispersion Refers to the degree to which a health care system's facilities are concentrated within a local or regional area, which contrasts with those that are dispersed widely across the country.

Stages of Change or Innovation This process involves awareness, identification, implementation, and institutionalization.

Stages of Team Development Stages of team development refer to predictable developmental milestones through which teams proceed. The pace at which teams progress through these stages is dependent upon a number of internal and external factors, and the teams may become stymied within a stage or regress to earlier stages of development. Each stage is characterized by different member behaviors and attitudes and requires specific management emphases.

Stakeholder Mapping Provides a systematic assessment of the variance among personnel as stakeholders using stakeholder identification, stakeholder ranking based on attitudes toward change, and assortment of each stakeholder's power within the organization to shape and affect its ultimate utilization.

Standardization of Outputs A way of coordinating work that specifies the product or expected performance, with the process of how to perform the work left to the worker.

Standardization of Work Processes A way of coordinating work that programs or specifies the content of work. Health care organizations standardize work processes when possible, such as standard admission and discharge procedures or standard methods of performing laboratory tests.

Standardization of Worker Skills A way of coordinating work that occurs when neither work processes nor output can be standardized by standardizing the training of workers.

Status Differences Status is the measure of worth conferred on an individual by a group. Status differences refer to variations in the worth of individuals and groups in organizations, and are seen throughout organizations.

Strategic Alliance Any formal agreement between two or more organizations for purposes of ongoing cooperation and mutual gain.

Strategic Management Those aspects of management within a firm that link strategy analysis and planning to operational management.

Strategic Management Orientation A mental view or outlook focusing on achievement of strategic goals and objectives.

Strategic Management Perspective The strategic management perspective emphasizes the importance of positioning the organization relative to its environment and competitors in order to achieve its objectives and assure its survival.

Strategy Those key concepts and ideas that organizations use, or have used, to achieve and sustain competitive advantage over their rivals.

Stretching Refers to a style of management and organizational culture in which very high performance standards are set with the deliberate intent to "stretch" people to their fullest capability.

Structural Change Strategies Concerned with the fundamental design and structure of health services organizations. This involves approaches that change organizational structure, reporting relationships, use of integrating mechanisms within the institution, management and clinical information systems, and financial systems.

Structural Measures of Quality Assess those organizational features or participants' characteristics that are presumed to have a positive impact on organizational performance.

Substitution Threats Threats from firms that produce products and services that differ from, but perform the same function as, those of extant competitors in the market; the threats depend on the market structure, environmental changes, and the relative competitive advantages of rivals and of those firms that produce substitute products and services.

Support Work Work that does not directly result in achievement of an organization goal, but which is needed for effective accomplishment of other work.

Survey Feedback Provides a mechanism for systematically gathering data on the ongoing social-psychological conditions of the organization and confronting work groups with the findings.

Sustainability The characteristic of a source of advantage that rivals are unable (e.g., because it is rare, is integrated within other complex sources of advantage, etc.) to imitate it, capture it (e.g., through acquisition or purchase), or substitute other sources for it.

SWOT Analysis A simple analytical framework that includes assessments of strategically important factors both internal (strengths and weaknesses) and external (opportunities and threats) to organizations.

Symbiotic vs. Competitive Interdependence This distinction highlights that alliances often have mixed motives, whereby parties can create joint value, but often will compete in the claiming of that value.

Synergies The result of two or more competitors (either under the same ownership or within a strategic alliance) combining activities in order to achieve greater competitive advantage than is possible were they to operate separately.

Systems Thinking The discipline of seeing wholes, perceiving the structures that underlie dynamically complex systems, and identifying high-leverage change opportunities.

Tangible vs. Intangible Resources Terms that distinguish between two types of strategically important resources: those that are more visible (commonly referred to as *resources,* namely, manpower, plant, equipment, location, etc.) and those that represent an organization's *capabilities* and, as such, are less tangible/visible (i.e., talent, skills, management systems, coordinating mechanisms, experience, organizational knowledge, etc.).

Task Analysis Method used for facilitating technical change and improving performance that focuses on the redesign of tasks within the organization.

Task Content Conflict Disagreements about the content of a task being performed by organizational members.

Task Design Task design refers to the content and organization of a task or group of tasks for an individual or group. It may also refer to the work processes and technologies necessary to accomplish tasks.

Task Interdependence Task interdependence refers to the interconnections between tasks, or more specifically, the degree to which team members must rely on one another to perform work effectively.

Task Inventory Approach to Work Design A technical approach to work design that inventories the tasks and skills needed for particular jobs.

Task-Oriented Leader Behavior Actions taken by a leader to emphasize getting a task done. A leader can have high or low task-orientated behavior with a follower; if the maturity of the follower is high, then the leader needs to be low-task oriented.

Task-Oriented Roles Task-oriented roles are roles and functions assumed by team members that help to accomplish team goals and reinforce team norms.

Team Cohesiveness Team cohesiveness is the extent to which team members are committed to the group task, attracted to each other, or motivated to stay in the group.

Team Composition Team composition refers to the membership of a team, particularly in relation to variations in gender, age, professional status, and other factors that may affect team performance.

Team Development Strategies that attempt to remove barriers to group effectiveness, develop self-sufficiency in managing group process, and facilitate the change process.

Team Learning The discipline of creating alignment such that team members think insightfully about complex problems, synergize their knowledge and skills, and produce coordinated action.

Team Productivity Team productivity is the quantifiable measurement of a team's effectiveness in terms of output and efficiency.

Team Size Refers simply to the number of members on a team. It is important because of its impact on many aspects of team process and effectiveness.

Technical Approach to Work Design Designing work with a focus on skill requirements and information flow.

Technology Assessment A class of evaluative methods used to examine the technical, economic, health, and social consequences of technological applications. In the health setting, these methods are used to evaluate health technologies in terms of safety, efficacy, effectiveness, cost, cost-effectiveness, legality, and ethics—both in absolute terms and in comparison with competing technologies.

Total Quality Management (TQM) A participative, systematic approach to planning and implementing continuous improvement in quality.

Trait Perspective A theoretical school of leadership holding that personal traits (attributes/characteristics) have a significant effect on leadership effectiveness and success.

Transactional Leadership Clarification of the roles followers must execute in order to reach their personal goals while fulfilling the goals of the organization. The objective of this type of leadership is to get followers to comply by the rules of the game as presently played.

Transformational Leadership Leadership behavior directed toward upsetting the status quo, seeking to alter both the goal and nature of manager-follower interactions. The objective of this type of leadership is to work with followers to alter the rules of the game.

Transformational Leadership Role Executive leadership role focusing on and accountable for achieving organizational transformation.

Trialability An attribute of innovations that refers to the degree to which organizational members can experiment with the innovation on a limited basis.

Turbulent Environment This refers to the situation whereby an organization is facing rapidly changing external circumstances and greater interconnectedness and interdependence between itself and other organizations.

Tyrants Organizations can behave as tyrants or as instruments of domination that exploit their employees and others either unconsciously or by intent.

Uncertainty Inability of organizations or managers to accurately predict the consequences of an action or the future state of an organization and its environment.

Uncertainty Inherent in Work The degree of uncertainty inherent in work affects task and coordination requirements.

Uncertainty Reduction An important benefit of strategic alliances, when compared to alternative approaches to growth, given the exit options typically found in alliance agreements.

Unfreezing The first stage of Kurt Lewin's three-stage change model, unfreezing involves creating an awareness of the need for change and removing any resistance to change.

Valence Employee feelings about job outcomes that can vary in strength and direction ranging from positive to neutral to negative.

Value Chain Analysis An approach to assessing an organization's "activities" (see definition of activities)—which collectively comprise an organization's value chain—that if better performed and integrated should contribute to gains in competitive advantage.

Value Chain Networks The steps or links involved in production of some product from the input of raw material to the output of the final product consumed by the end user. Each input in the process adds value to the preceding input.

Value-Oriented Leadership Committed to clarifying organizational values (i.e., principles, expectations, or qualities considered worthwhile or important to the organization) and using these values to guide all aspects of organizational culture and behavior.

Vertical Division of Labor Dividing work into tasks—management, direct, and support work—to be completed by people at different levels of the organization.

Vertical Integration A power strategy in which businesses that share input-output relationships are combined to achieve competitive advantage (e.g., integrating hospital and managed care companies).

Work Group/Work Design Health care organizations vary in the way that work is organized. How people are grouped together to accomplish the organization's mission is usually a function of the organization's technology and environment.

Work Requirements Personal attributes and skills required for the successful completion of an identifiable element of work.

AUTHOR INDEX

SUBJECT INDEX

Organizational learning. *See* Learning organizations
Organizational performance, 417–447
    assessment of, 420–442
    challenge of performance, 418–420
    classes of measures, 427–430
    definitional issues, 421–424
    different levels of analysis, 422
    domain of activity, 422–423
    factors associated with effective performance,
        430–431
    impact of evaluation on all types of performers,
        437–438
    managerial issues, 431–434
    manager's role in, 442–447
    models for changing performance, 438
    nonprofessional work, 434–443
    preferences for classes of performance measures,
        429–430
    professional performance, 431–434
    stakeholders, 423–424
Organizational structure, systemic, 50–51
Organizational transformation, 56–57
Outcome measures or organizational performance, 427
Outcomes assessments, standardization of direct patient
    care and, 246
Ownership, alliances and, 361

P

Pace strategies, 468–470
Parallel design, 333
Partners in alliances, types of, 377–378
Path-goal model of leadership, 135–136
Patients, changing role of, 502–503
Pay-for-performance plans, 112–113, 499–500
Performance evaluation, 431–442
    future trends in, 500–501
    impact of, 437–438
Performance gaps, 393
Performance norms, 194–195
Performance strategies, 473–474
Performing stage of team development, 189
Personal mastery, learning organizations and, 389
Personnel, motivation of, 108–109
Physician-hospital organizations (PHOs), 336–338
Physician-hospital trading alliances, 366–368
Physicians
    changing role of, 503–504
    motivation of, 105–108

Physiological needs, 86
Plan-do-study-act (PDSA) improvement methods, 31
Playing fields, organizations as, 34
Policy resistance, 384
Political games, 294–297
Political model of organizations, 281–282
Political process assessment, systematic assessment
    before design and, 322, 325
Political systems, organizations as, 34
Politics. *See also* Power
    defined, 280
    developing and using power and, 290–294
    in health services organizations, 278–282
    organization design and, 325, 327, 328
    organizational performance and, 301, 303
    systems of, reasons for emergence of, 280–281
Pooled interdependence, 239
Pooling alliances, 363–364
Population ecology theory, 27–28
Porter's five "Ps" model, 465
Position strategies, 474–477
Positions (jobs), designing, 318–319
Potential strategies, 470–473
Power. *See also* Politics
    absolute versus relative, 477–478
    abuse of, 298–301
    conditions for use of, 290–294
    defined, 280
    developing and using, 290–294
    employee responses to, 297–298
    increasing, strategies for, 288, 289
    in health services organizations, 278–282
    need for, 92
    organizational performance and, 301–303
    sources of, 282–290
    strategies and tactics for using, 294–297
    systems of, reasons for emergence of, 280–281
Power enhancement alliances, 365–366
Power strategies, 477–480
Pressing, as conflict-management strategy, 156
Process measures of organizational performance, 427
Process theories of motivation. *See* Motivation
Product differentiation, 464
Production function, 21
Productivity, defined, 419
Product-line design, 333–336
Program design, 333–336
Programming approaches to coordination, 242